KU-451-513

METABOLIC BONE DISEASE

Volume II

List of Contributors

LOUIS V. AVIOLI

LEONARD J. DEFTOS

JOEL F. HABENER

STEPHEN M. KRANE

CHARLES NAGANT DE DEUXCHAISNES

JOHN T. POTTS, JR.

ELEANOR B. PYLE

JOHN S. RODMAN

ALAN L. SCHILLER

LOUIS M. SHERWOOD

FREDERICK R. SINGER

ROBERT STEENDIJK

METABOLIC BONE DISEASE

Volume II

Edited by

LOUIS V. AVIOLI, M.D.

Department of Medicine
Bone and Mineral Metabolism
Washington University School of Medicine
and The Jewish Hospital of St. Louis
St. Louis, Missouri

STEPHEN M. KRANE, M.D.

Department of Medicine
Harvard Medical School
and Medical Services (Arthritis Unit)
Massachusetts General Hospital
Boston, Massachusetts

THE BRITISH SCHOOL OF OSTEOPATHY
1-4 SUFFOLK STREET, LONDON SW1Y 4H
TEL: 01-930 9254-8

ACADEMIC PRESS   New York   San Francisco   London   1978

A Subsidiary of Harcourt Brace Jovanovich, Publishers

LOM J [LSP K]

COPYRIGHT © 1978, BY ACADEMIC PRESS, INC.
ALL RIGHTS RESERVED.
NO PART OF THIS PUBLICATION MAY BE REPRODUCED OR
TRANSMITTED IN ANY FORM OR BY ANY MEANS, ELECTRONIC
OR MECHANICAL, INCLUDING PHOTOCOPY, RECORDING, OR ANY
INFORMATION STORAGE AND RETRIEVAL SYSTEM, WITHOUT
PERMISSION IN WRITING FROM THE PUBLISHER.

ACADEMIC PRESS, INC.
111 Fifth Avenue, New York, New York 10003

United Kingdom Edition published by
ACADEMIC PRESS, INC. (LONDON) LTD.
24/28 Oval Road, London NW1   7DX

Library of Congress Cataloging in Publication Data

Main entry under title:

Metabolic bone disease.

    Includes bibliographies and index.
    1.   Bones--Diseases.   2.   Calcium metabolism disorders.
3.   Phosphorus metabolism disorders.   I.   Avioli, Louis V.
II.   Krane, Stephen M.   [DNLM: 1.   Bone diseases.
2.   Metabolic diseases.   3.   Bone and bones--Metabolism.
WE200 M587]
RC930.M46   616.7'1   76−27431
ISBN 0−12−068702−X (v. 2)

PRINTED IN THE UNITED STATES OF AMERICA

Contents

List of Contributors   ix

Preface   xi

Contents of Other Volumes   xiii

1   Parathyroid Physiology and Primary Hyperparathyroidism

    JOEL F. HABENER AND JOHN T. POTTS, JR.

    I. Introduction   1
    II. Fundamental Considerations of the Physiology and Biochemistry
        of Parathyroid Hormone   4
    III. Primary Hyperparathyroidism   48
    References   132

2   Renal Osteodystrophy

    LOUIS V. AVIOLI

    I. Introduction   149
    II. Pathogenesis of Renal Osteodystrophy   151
    III. Clinical and Radiological Correlates   166
    IV. Soft Tissue Calcification   177
    V. Dialysis Bone Disease   183
    VI. The Nature of the Bone Lesions   187
    VII. Therapeutic Management   195
    References   205

3   Hypoparathyroidism

    CHARLES NAGANT DE DEUXCHAISNES AND
    STEPHEN M. KRANE

    I. Postoperative Hypoparathyroidism   218
    II. Nonsurgical Damage to the Parathyroid Glands   245
    III. Functional Hypoparathyroidism of Diverse Etiology in the Newborn   251

    IV. Secondary Hypoparathyroidism Due to Hypercalcemia,
        with Special Reference to the Newborn Infant
        of a Hyperparathyroid Mother   257
     V. Secondary Hypoparathyroidism Due to Hypermagnesemia   258
    VI. Acquired Metabolic Resistance to Parathyroid Hormone   259
   VII. Hypoparathyroidism Due to the Secretion of Ineffective
        Parathyroid Hormone   268
  VIII. Idiopathic Hypoparathyroidism   269
    IX. Pseudohypoparathyroidism and Related Disorders   296
     X. Signs and Symptoms of Hypocalcemia   395
    XI. Biological Findings   402
   XII. Treatment   405
  XIII. Concluding Remarks   415
        References   415

4   The Thyroid Gland in Skeletal and Calcium Metabolism

LEONARD J. DEFTOS

     I. Introduction   447
    II. The Thyroid Hormones: T_3 and T_4 448
   III. Calcitonin   458
    IV. Recent Developments   479
        References   481

5   Paget's Disease of Bone

FREDERICK R. SINGER, ALAN L. SCHILLER,
ELEANOR B. PYLE, AND STEPHEN M. KRANE

     I. Introduction   490
    II. Historical Aspects   490
   III. Incidence and Epidemiology   490
    IV. Histopathology   494
     V. Focal Manifestations   505
    VI. Complications   518
   VII. Metabolic Aspects of Paget's Disease   530
  VIII. Systemic Complications and Associated Diseases   545
    IX. Drug Treatment   551
     X. Etiology   564
        References   567

6   Disorders of Mineral Metabolism in Malignancy

JOHN S. RODMAN AND LOUIS M. SHERWOOD

     I. Introduction   578
    II. Effects of Hypercalcemia   578
   III. Clinical Occurrence   585
    IV. Pathogenesis of Tumor-Associated Hypercalcemia   590
     V. Treatment of Hypercalemia   610
        References   622

7 Metabolic Bone Disease in Children

ROBERT STEENDIJK

I. Growth and Development of Skeleton	634
II. Differential Diagnosis of Hypercalcemia	643
III. Differential Diagnosis of Hypocalcemia	658
IV. Normocalcemic Disorders of Mineral Metabolism	672
V. Bone Disease in Disorders of Renal Function	689
References	696

Index 703

List of Contributors

Numbers in parentheses indicate the pages on which the authors' contributions begin.

Louis V. Avioli, M.D. (149), Department of Medicine, Division of Bone and Mineral Metabolism, Washington University School of Medicine, and the Jewish Hospital of St. Louis, St. Louis, Missouri 63178

Leonard J. Deftos, M.D. (447), Department of Medicine, San Diego School of Medicine, University of California, and Endocrine Section, Veterans Administration Hospital, La Jolla, California 92161

Joel F. Habener, M.D. (1), Department of Medicine, Harvard Medical School, and Endocrine Unit, Massachusetts General Hospital, Boston, Massachusetts 02114

Stephen M. Krane, M.D. (217, 489), Department of Medicine, Harvard Medical School, and Medical Services (Arthritis Unit), Massachusetts General Hospital, Boston, Massachusetts 02114

Charles Nagant de Deuxchaisnes, M.D. (217), Rheumatology Unit, Department of Medicine, St. Pierre University Hospital, B-3000 Louvain, Belgium

John T. Potts, Jr., M.D. (1), Department of Medicine, Harvard Medical School, and Endocrine Unit, Massachusetts General Hospital, Boston, Massachusetts 02114

Eleanor B. Pyle, B.A. (489), Medical Services (Arthritis Unit), Massachusetts General Hospital, Boston, Massachusetts 02114

John S. Rodman, M.D. (577), Department of Medicine, Michael Reese Hospital and Medical Center, and The Pritzker School of Medicine, The University of Chicago, Chicago, Illinois 60616

Alan L. Schiller, M.D. (489), Departments of Pathology, Harvard Medical School, and the Massachusetts General Hospital, Boston, Massachusetts 02114

Louis M. Sherwood, M.D. (577), Department of Medicine, Michael Reese Hospital and Medical Center, and The Pritzker School of Medicine, The University of Chicago, Chicago, Illinois 60616

Frederick R. Singer, M.D. (489), Section of Endocrinology, Department of Medicine, University of Southern California, School of Medicine, Los Angeles, California 90033

Robert Steendijk, M.D. (633), Department of Pediatrics, University of Amsterdam, Amsterdam, The Netherlands

Preface

In this volume of "Metabolic Bone Disease," disorders attended by either acquired or inherited alterations in parathyroid hormone production, metabolic and biological action are considered in detail. Although clinical disorders of bone and mineral metabolism characterized by elevated levels of circulating parathyroid hormone were presented in Volume I, it was considered more appropriate that emphasis be given to skeletal and renal function in Volume I rather than to the associated derangements in hormonal secretion and metabolism. The material in this volume is more specific with regard to disorders of parathyroid gland activity. The relationship between hormonal synthesis, biological activity, and documented abnormalities in specific clinical syndromes is emphasized. Studies of the metabolism and structure –function relationships of parathyroid hormone and others revealing interactions with specific receptors in target organs have also provided a basis for some understanding of parathyroid hormone and vitamin D-"resistant" states. This skeletal resistance to hormone action is classically observed in patients with end-stage renal disease and progressive derangements in skeletal metabolism, a syndrome which is reviewed in this volume.

Although it has been well established that thyroxine and tri-iodothyronine are essential for both modeling and growth of the human skeleton, the function of calcitonin in this regard is still uncertain. In fact, the role of calcitonin in human physiology is conjectural at best. The significance and metabolic consequences of high levels of this hormone in medullary carcinoma of the thyroid are also unknown. These concepts as well as those documenting derangements in skeletal metabolism which attend thyroid-excess syndromes are explored in depth.

The mechanisms whereby a variety of disorders, especially malignancies, produce hypercalcemia have yet to be fully elucidated. However, it is possible to interpret the pathophysiology of these disorders with respect to hormone function and homeostatic controls which maintain the concentration of extracellular fluid calcium content. Some would argue that Paget's disease does not officially warrant a place in a book on metabolic bone disease since it is probably a focal skeletal disorder, yet there is historical precedent for its consideration in the book, "The Parathyroid Glands and Metabolic Bone Disease, Selected Studies" by Fuller Albright and Edward C. Reifenstein. It is likely, however, that when one really understands the pathogenesis of Paget's disease of bone, those factors which normally initiate and modulate skeletal remodeling and bone turnover will be defined. The chapter by Dr. Robert Steendijk should provide those concerned with disorders of bone metabolism in children additional and more detailed information with regard to certain pediatric forms of bone disease which are not adequately reviewed in other chapters of Volumes I and II.

As detailed earlier in the Preface to Volume I, we must again note the difference in the approach of the contributors to this volume. In some of the chapters, references are detailed to substantiate each point, whereas in others the authors indicate reviews which can provide access to pertinent data. We thought it best to permit each author latitude in this regard, recognizing that this approach might detract from a uniformity of style. Furthermore, we have not included every skeletal disorder that some might consider appropriate to what is intended as a textbook on metabolic bone disease. Chapters on subjects such as the bone dysplasias and heritable disorders of the skeleton are planned for future volumes.

We continue to be grateful to all our students, house officers, fellows, and staff who have continued to prod us with questions and criticism of both volumes of "Metabolic Bone Disease." We again acknowledge Ms. Linda Graf for her untiring efforts in preparing this volume and Ms. Eleanor Pyle for her editorial assistance. Our gratitude is extended to the Armour Pharmaceutical Company for the donations which helped defray the cost of reproducing illustrations. The staff of Academic Press has continued to be particularly patient and understanding.

Louis V. Avioli, M.D.
Stephen M. Krane, M.D.

Contents of Other Volumes

Volume I

Bone Metabolism and Calcium Regulation
Lawrence G. Raisz

Kidney Function in Calcium and Phosphate Metabolism
Olav L. M. Bijvoet

Alkaline Phosphatase and Metabolic Bone Disorders
Solomon Posen, Coralie Cornish, and
Michael Kleerekoper

The Diagnostic Value of Bone Biopsies
Paul D. Byers

Vitamin D, Rickets, and Osteomalacia
C.E. Dent and T. C. B. Stamp

Osteoporosis: Pathogenesis and Therapy
Louis V. Avioli

Nephrolithiasis
Hibbard E. Williams and Edwin L. Prien, Jr.

1

Parathyroid Physiology and Primary Hyperparathyroidism

JOEL F. HABENER AND JOHN T. POTTS, JR.

I. Introduction 1
II. Fundamental Considerations of the Physiology and Biochemistry of Parathyroid Hormone 4
    A. Expression of Action 4
    B. Chemistry of Parathyroid Hormone 17
    C. Metabolism of Parathyroid Hormone 24
    D. Secretion of Parathyroid Hormone 34
    E. Biosynthesis of Parathyroid Hormone: Precursors of Parathyroid Hormone, Proparathyroid Hormone, and Pre-Proparathyroid Hormone 38
    F. Control of the Biosynthesis and Secretion of Parathyroid Hormone 42
    G. Summary 46
III. Primary Hyperparathyroidism 48
    A. Incidence 49
    B. Etiology and Pathology 50
    C. Clinical Manifestations 65
    D. Diagnosis 93
    E. Differential Diagnosis 107
    F. Treatment 119
    References 132

I. INTRODUCTION

Primary hyperparathyroidism is being recognized with increasing frequency largely because of a growing awareness of many of the fundamental biochemical and physiological processes characteristic of this disorder

1

Copyright © 1978 by Academic Press, Inc.
All rights of reproduction in any form reserved
ISBN 0-12-068702-X

and the more frequent use of routine measurements of serum calcium. The clinical presentation of the disorder is often subtle, and controversies have arisen about optimal approaches in surgical and medical management. At the same time, there is increased interest both in the fundamental role of parathyroid hormone in normal calcium and phosphate homeostasis and in the effects of the hormone in certain disorders of bone metabolism, such as the osteodystrophy that accompanies the secondary hyperparathyroidism of chronic renal failure (Chapter 1). Some investigators have even speculated that certain bone disorders (e.g., osteoporosis) may be caused by disturbances in parathyroid hormone secretion or action, whereas others have recently suggested a therapeutic role for parathyroid hormone (see Chapter 6, Volume I).

It must be emphasized, however, that there is no definite evidence that any disorder of the skeleton is attributable to a disturbance in parathyroid hormone production per se other than that associated with true primary or secondary hyperparathyroidism. On the other hand, a wider knowledge of the physiology, chemistry, biosynthesis, secretion, mode of action, and metabolism of parathyroid hormone is important not only for improved recognition and management of primary hyperparathyroidism, but also for progress in understanding the broader role, if any, of other disturbances in parathyroid hormone function that have been proposed as contributing to the pathophysiology of certain skeletal disorders, as well as for evaluation of any potential therapeutic role of the hormone.

The advances made in multiple areas of research on the chemistry and physiology of parathyroid hormone have been of practical value to clinicians concerned with the management of parathyroid disorders, as well as to physiologists concerned with calcium homeostasis and the effects of calcium in neurological and metabolic function. At the same time, somewhat paradoxically, investigations concerned with the regulation of parathyroid hormone production and turnover have uncovered unsuspected complexities with regard to the biosynthesis, secretion, and metabolism of parathyroid hormone. These findings have led to uncertainties concerning the nature of the active molecular species of circulating parathyroid hormone, despite the advances made in analysis of the chemical features of human and other mammalian parathyroid hormones.

Similarly, although sensitive radioimmunoassays for parathyroid hormone have been developed, aided by progress in the purification, structural analysis, and synthesis of parathyroid hormone, measurements of the concentration of immunoreactive parathyroid hormone in blood do not necessarily reflect the concentration of biologically active hormone. The immunoassays, although highly useful in the differential diagnosis of hypercalcemic states, have not, in the experience of most laboratories, readily discriminated the normal from the abnormal states of parathyroid secretion seen in certain difficult clinical situations, such as that of patients with equivocal hypercalcemia but recurrent calcium-containing kidney stones.

Until its ultimate disappearance from body fluids, parathyroid hormone undergoes several highly specific cleavages during its formation and transport within the parathyroid cell. The hormone is synthesized via two intermediate precursors that are successively converted by proteolytic cleavages within the gland to the storage form of the hormone, the classically recognized parathyroid hormone extracted from the tissues. It is not known whether the precursor molecules, as with proinsulin, are at times secreted into the circulation in addition to the hormone. If they are, the prohormones might be detected as parathyroid hormone by the radioimmunoassay and yet have biological effects quite different from those of the hormone itself. Also puzzling is the metabolic fate of the hormone after secretion. The organ or organs in which the hormone is cleaved are not yet identified. The cleavage products, at least one of which is biologically inactive, re-enter the circulation. It is possible that the gland may release the fragments also. These fragments are present in the circulation at concentrations considerably higher than those of the originally secreted, biologically active, intact hormone. A problem arises in the accurate assessment of the concentration, inasmuch as the fragment or fragments are measured, with varying degrees of sensitivity in different laboratories, by the antisera to intact hormone used in the immunoassays. In patients with certain diseases, such as chronic renal failure (Chapter 2), the metabolism of the hormone may be different from that in normal states, and the discrepancies would be reflected in concentrations of inactive hormonal metabolites that are much higher.

Attempts to refine the application of the parathyroid hormone immunoassay to clinical problems, plus certain unique features of the immunochemistry of parathyroid hormone, have uncovered what may ultimately prove to be a general pathway for the metabolism of many peptide hormones. In any event, the problems involved in measurement of active circulating parathyroid hormone must be resolved to permit full utilization of the radioimmunoassay as a clinically useful diagnostic tool.

It is the purpose of this chapter to review certain aspects of the physiology, mode of action, chemistry, biosynthesis, secretion, and metabolism of parathyroid hormone, and, as well, to present and discuss the present body of clinical information about the etiology, clinical features, diagnosis, and clinical management of hyperparathyroidism.

II. FUNDAMENTAL CONSIDERATIONS OF THE PHYSIOLOGY AND BIOCHEMISTRY OF PARATHYROID HORMONE

A. Expression of Action

Parathyroid hormone exerts its principal action in man on three major organs: bone, kidney, and small intestine. The net result of the action of the hormone on each of these organs is to raise the concentration of calcium in the extracellular fluid. It is logical to discuss the mode of action of parathyroid hormone on its target organs from the standpoint of (1) the overall physiological effects of the hormone on calcium homeostasis and (2) the biochemical mechanisms by which the hormone exerts its effects on the cells of the specific target tissue.

1. Physiological Effects of Parathyroid Hormone

The action of parathyroid hormone on bone, kidney, and intestine increases the concentration of serum calcium (Fig. 1) (Parsons and Potts, 1972; Potts and Deftos, 1974; Rasmussen and Bordier, 1974). In turn, the production of parathyroid hormone is inhibited by an increase, and stimulated by a decrease, in serum calcium through direct effects of calcium on the rate of parathyroid secretion (Habener and Potts, 1976b; Mayer et al., 1976). This feedback system of regulation involving the parathyroid glands is one of the most important homeostatic mechanisms for the close control of the concentration of calcium in extracellular fluid. Any ten-

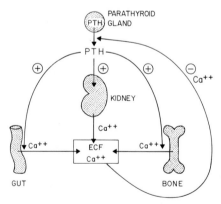

Fig. 1. Physiological actions of parathyroid hormone. The hormone acts directly on receptors in bone, kidney, and, probably indirectly, on gut to raise the concentration of calcium in the extracellular fluid conpartment (ECF). Calcium in the ECF in turn exerts a negative feedback inhibition on the parathyroid gland to reduce the rate of PTH secretion. (Courtesy of Springer-Verlag.)

dency toward hypocalcemia, which might be brought about by intestinal malabsorption or by the phosphate retention that occurs in renal failure (Slatopolsky *et al.*, 1971), is counteracted by an increased rate of secretion of parathyroid hormone. The increased amount of parathyroid hormone in blood then (1) acts to increase the rate of dissolution of bone mineral (and bone matrix), thereby providing an increased flow of calcium from bone into blood, (2) reduces the clearance of calcium by the kidney, returning more of the filtered calcium back into the extracellular fluid, and (3) increases the transport of calcium across the intestinal mucosa, resulting in an increased absorption of dietary calcium. The relative physiological importance of these actions of parathyroid hormone on these three organs is not completely resolved (Nordin *et al.*, 1975; see Chapter 2, Volume I). It is likely that the physiological effects of parathyroid hormone on the gut are mediated through vitamin D metabolites (Tanaka *et al.*, 1973; M. R. Hughes *et al.*, 1975). It has not been definitively established, however, whether there are effects of parathyroid hormone on the intestine that are direct, rather than merely indirect, through mediation of the formation of the active, hydroxylated metabolite of vitamin D (see Chapter 5, Volume I and Chapter 2).

  a. Effect on Bone. The effect of parathyroid hormone on bone has been considered by many workers to be the single most important factor in maintaining calcium homeostasis in the extracellular fluid.

  The potential importance of the effects of parathyroid hormone on bone can be appreciated when it is realized that 99% of the total body calcium resides in the skeleton (Krane, 1970). The skeleton represents one of the largest masses of target tissue directly affected by any hormone and contains approximately 1.5 kg of elemental calcium in the average adult man (Krane, 1970). Despite the enormous reservoirs of calcium in the skeleton, very little (less than 1%) is freely miscible with the extracellular fluid (Walser, 1961; Neer *et al.*, 1967; Krane, 1970). Evidence from calcium kinetic studies indicates a transfer between extracellular fluid and bone of approximately 0.5 gm per day. Active resorption of bone mineral is required to mobilize significant amounts of calcium.

  Metabolic destruction of bone induced by parathyroid hormone was first demonstrated by Barnicot (1948) and by Chang (1951), who showed that grafts of parathyroid tissue adjacent to bone produced osseous erosions. Later, Gaillard (1955) and Raisz *et al.* (1968) showed that extracts of parathyroid glands directly caused resorption of bone in tissue culture. Talmage and Elliot (1956) demonstrated that extracts of parathyroid glands cause hypercalcemia when administered to nephrectomized, dialyzed rats in the fasting state, thereby implicating bone as the source of newly mobilized calcium.

Present evidence derived from *in vivo* studies indicates that there are three temporally related responses of bone to parathyroid hormone (see Chapter 1, Volume I). The initial effects, reflected in blood and urine within minutes after i.v. administration of the hormone, is a fall in plasma calcium (Robinson *et al.*, 1972). Within 1–2 hours, the plasma calcium rises (Robinson *et al.*, 1972; Rasmussen and Bordier, 1973, 1974). A later effect on the skeleton, slower in onset by several hours or even days, is the appearance of increased numbers of osteoclasts and osteoblasts and a general increase in the remodeling of bone, primarily in the direction of dissolution of bone mineral and matrix (see Chapter 1, Volume I).

Recent experimental studies have confirmed the long-standing observation that the very earliest response of an animal to the administration of parathyroid hormone is a transient hypocalcemia rather than hypercalcemia, the latter occurring only later (Fig. 2) (Parsons *et al.*, 1971; Robinson *et al.*, 1972). Kinetic analysis of the distribution of radiocalcium showed that the initial hypocalcemic response is due to a sudden shift of calcium from extracellular fluid into the skeleton. Parsons *et al.* (1971) showed recently that the administration of a small dose of calcium given along with a dose of parathyroid hormone to an animal greatly enhances the mobilization of calcium from the skeleton an hour or two later. To obtain the enhancement in the hypocalcemic response, however, the calcium must be given within several minutes after the hormone is given. The influx of calcium into bone is presumably due to a transient increase

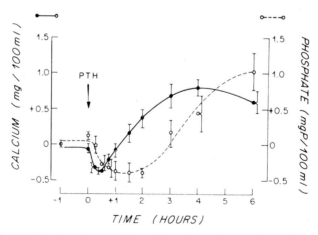

Fig. 2. Mean changes in plasma calcium (●) and inorganic phosphate (○) at selected time intervals after parathyroid hormone injection in a dog. Vertical bars show standard errors of the means. (From Parsons *et al.*, 1971.)

in the permeability of the bone cell membrane to calcium and may serve to activate cellular responses important in net mobilization of bone calcium. The response probably involves increases in intracellular concentrations of both calcium and (cyclic) adenosine $3':5'$-monophosphate (see below) (Chase *et al.*, 1969; Rasmussen and Tenenhouse, 1970).

The time course of the hypercalcemia induced by the action of parathyroid hormone on bone consists of identifiable fast and slow components (second and third temporal responses of bone) (Parsons and Potts, 1972). The earliest hypercalcemic response, following the immediate hypocalcemic response just described, occurs in 1 or 2 hours and represents an outflow of calcium from bone that does not require active protein synthesis and is probably due to activation of preexisting transport systems involved in the mobilization of readily available bone mineral (Parsons and Robinson, 1968; Candlish and Taylor, 1970).

Based on the histological examination of bone after administration of PTH, Rasmussen and Bordier (1973, 1974) concluded that the earliest hypercalcemic effect is manifested by an increase in the resorptive activity of osteocytes (osteocytic osteolysis) manifested by increased size of osteocytes and osteocytic lacunae and increased metachromatic staining of adjacent bone. In addition, there occurred an increase in activity of osteoclasts already present, leading to an increased flow of calcium ion from deep bone to bone surface. This initial series of cellular events is highly sensitive to PTH, requires the constant presence of the hormone, and results in a relatively small flow of calcium out of bone.

It appears that osteocytic responses are of much greater importance than are osteoclastic responses during the early phase of bone resorption. Because of the relatively enormous surface area of bone represented by the osteocytic lacunae and their associated canaliculi (1300 m^2) compared with the surface area covered by active osteoclasts (0.2 m^2), Rasmussen and Bordier (1973, 1974) proposed that osteocytic osteolysis (lacunar–canalicular bone surface) plays a much greater role, albeit immediate and limited, in the maintenance of calcium homeostasis than does the osteoclastic resorption (endosteal and periosteal bone surface). This conclusion takes into account the estimation that only 1% of the bone surface covered by osteocytes is engaged in active bone resorption.

The later, slower component of the hypercalcemic response (third temporal response) occurs in hours to days after the administration of parathyroid hormone and can be distinguished from the earlier response because it is completely abolished by pretreatment of test animals with actinomycin D, an inhibitor of RNA synthesis (Rasmussen *et al.*, 1964) and by inhibition of protein synthesis (Kunin and Krane, 1965).

This third temporal effect of PTH is seen principally as an increase in the numbers of osteoclasts, presumably due to an increased conversion of mesenchymal cells (preosteoclasts) to osteoclasts (Rasmussen and Bordier, 1973, 1974). The magnitude of this later response is potentially great but is inhibited in states of vitamin D deficiency. (The earlier response is not as sensitive to vitamin D.)

In addition to effects on bone resorptive processes, there is evidence that parathyroid hormone modulates bone formation. Rasmussen and Bordier (1973, 1974) have described the effects of the hormone on both function and numbers of osteoblasts. The administration of PTH to parathyroidectomized animals or the sustained excessive secretion of the hormone characteristic of hyperparathyroidism leads to significant changes in bone formation.

The changes that occur in osteoblast function and numbers, as with the changes in osteoclasts, can be divided into two phases. The first and the earliest phase is characterized by an inhibition of activity of individual osteoblasts on bone matrix synthesis (Gaillard, 1961; Heersche and de Voogd van der Straaten, 1965; Nichols et al., 1965; Goldhaber et al., 1968; Heersche, 1969; Milhaud et al., 1971). The later phase is characterized by a greatly increased number of osteoblasts. The osteoblasts, although less active individually than normal because of their greatly increased numbers, thus bring about an increased total rate of bone collagen synthesis (Nichols et al., 1965; Laitinen, 1967).

Parathyroid hormone also exerts important catabolic actions on bone matrix in addition to increased release of bone mineral; release of mineral and matrix elements is coordinated. Parathyroid hormone action leads to destruction of the collagen and ground substance that make up the bone matrix. Matrix destruction accompanies mineral dissolution from bone. Changes in plasma calcium serve as an indicator of destruction of bone mineral, whereas changes in the concentration of hydroxyproline in plasma and its excretion in urine reflect matrix dissolution (Bates et al., 1962; Keiser et al., 1964; Harris and Sjoerdsma, 1966).

It is not clear whether the three effects of parathyroid hormone action on bone (early hypocalcemia, hypercalcemia independent of protein synthesis, and hypercalcemia dependent on protein synthesis) represent completely separate processes differing in biochemical mediation or are a continuous spectrum with a common initiating biochemical event. The earlier of the two hypercalcemic phases is thought to be important in the minute-to-minute regulation of mineral ion flow in and out of bone, whereas the later phase is concerned with remodeling of bone and gross changes in amount of bone mineral and matrix. It is the more chronic actions of parathyroid hormone on bone that result in remodeling of the bone architecture and seem to correlate with the roentgenological and histological picture of the bone disease osteitis fibrosa cystica, which results from long-standing excessive action of parathyroid hormone.

The effect of the hormone on osteocytic osteolysis may be important in the diffuse osteopenia seen in some patients with hyperparathyroidism (Section III, C, 2). Effects of parathyroid hormone on citrate metabolism are considered elsewhere in this volume (Chapter 5).

b. Effect on Kidney. Parathyroid hormone exerts two separate actions on mineral ion transport in the kidney: an increase in phosphate and a decrease in calcium clearance. The nature of the transtubular transport of these ions, the physiological significance of the kidney in calcium and phosphate homeostasis, and effects of excessive or deficient parathyroid action on renal transport processes are reviewed in Chapter 2, Volume I and will be summarized here only briefly to emphasize special features of the renal action of the hormone. The first effect, the earliest to be discovered, is to promote the excretion of phosphate (Greenwald, 1911) by decreasing the resorption of phosphate from the glomerular filtrate.

The marked increase in phosphate clearance induced by parathyroid hormone may be of particular importance in mineral ion balance in view of the abundance of phosphate and relative scarcity of calcium (except in dairy products) in terrestrial existence. When mineral is released from bone, calcium can be conserved, whereas the excess phosphate must be excreted.

For many years, a phosphaturic response was thought to be the sole effect of parathyroid hormone on the kidney (Albright and Reifenstein, 1948). Talmage *et al.* (1955), however, demonstrated that the hormone also acts on the kidney to decrease the clearance of calcium and thereby to conserve extracellular calcium. These workers observed that parathyroidectomy in rats resulted in both hypocalcemia and increased excretion of urinary calcium and that these effects could be prevented by the administration of parathyroid extract.

The effects of parathyroid hormone on reducing renal clearance of calcium in man were demonstrated by Kleeman *et al.* (1958, 1961) and examined further by Nordin and Peacock. Plots relating urine calcium to plasma calcium (an indicator of the filtered load of calcium) show a relative hypoexcretion (despite hypercalcemia) in primary hyperparathyroidism and hyperexcretion (relative to hypocalcemia) in hypoparathyroidism (Fig. 3). Several studies (Nordin and Peacock, 1969; Peacock *et al.*, 1969; Nordin *et al.*, 1972, 1975) have led these authors to draw several conclusions. They have calculated a T_m for calcium in man of 8 mg/100 ml of GFR. Since the exact amount of calcium in the glomerular filtrate is not known, and the reabsorption by different calcium complexes could markedly influence the results, this value cannot be verified experimentally but

Joel F. Habener and John T. Potts, Jr.

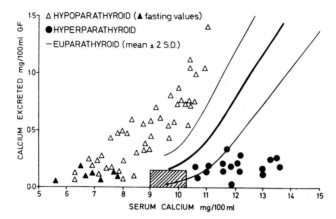

Fig. 3. Relation between urinary calcium excretion (as mg/100 ml of glomerular filtrate) and serum calcium during calcium loading in clinical hypoparathyroidism and hyperparathyroidism. The lines show the mean values ($\pm$2 S.D.) obtained in normal subjects, and the shaded area represents the normal basal range. (Modified from Nordin and Peacock, 1969.)

is deduced from a number of experiments. Nordin, Peacock, and associates emphasize the critical and, to them, predominant role of the kidney in the maintenance blood calcium homeostasis and in preventing hypocalcemia and/or hypercalcemia via either retention or rapid excretion of calcium, respectively. (See Chapter 2 for a critical review of this thesis).

In addition to the studies of Talmage *et al.* (1955) in rats, Biddulph and colleagues (Biddulph, 1972; Biddulph and Gallimore, 1974) have shown similar findings in studies of hamsters, confirming the generality in mammals of a significant calcium-conserving action of parathyroid hormone in the kidney.

It is important to note that, although the renal clearance of calcium is reduced in hyperparathyroid patients, hypercalciuria (defined here as urinary calcium excretion greater than 400 mg per 24 hours) may still be seen in many patients, owing to the predominant influence of hypercalcemia and the consequently greatly increased filtered load of calcium. Some have stressed the value, in differential diagnosis, of tests based on these effects of parathyroid hormone on the renal handling of calcium, in view of the fact that the degree of hypercalciuria in patients with hypercalcemia due to hyperparathyroidism is often much less than that seen in patients with hypercalcemia due to other causes.

The precise nature, anatomic location within the nephron, and controlling influences on overall renal transport and clearance of mineral ions (calcium, phosphate, and magnesium) comprise an active area of investigation by nephrologists and endocrinologists. With regard to overall phosphate excretion and phosphate clearance, it has been widely believed that the bulk of renal phosphate reabsorption occurs in the proximal tubule and that this is the site at which parathyroid hormone exerts its phosphaturic action by inhibition of phosphate reabsorption. Recent data of Knox and Lechene (1975) have suggested, however, a role for the distal tubule in overall phosphate clearance and as a site of action of parathyroid hormone in promoting phosphaturia. Agus *et al.* (1973) had also provided evidence for inhibition of phosphate reabsorption in the distal nephron segments under the influence of parathyroid hormone.

Agus *et al.* (1973), in their studies in dogs, advanced the thesis that phosphate as well as calcium reabsorption in the proximal tubule is closely related to sodium transport. Earlier studies had suggested the importance of sodium ion in phosphate transport *in vitro* in intestine (H. E. Harrison and Harrison, 1963) and kidney (Moroz and Krane, 1963). Studies on the kidney were interpreted to show proportionate inhibition of sodium (and calcium) reabsorption with an even greater inhibition of reabsorption of phosphate induced by parathyroid hormone. Sodium rejected at the proximal tubule is reabsorbed distally but phosphate is not, leading to brisk phosphaturia. The role of the hormone in blocking distal reabsorption of phosphate was not emphasized by Agus *et al.* (1973), but distal action has been stressed more recently by Knox and Lechene (1975).

The studies of Goldberg and associates (Agus *et al.,* 1973), as well as those of Knox and Lechene (1975) and Knox *et al.* (1975), have clarified several aspects of interaction between volume expansion, sodium diuresis, and parathyroid hormone action at both the proximal and distal tubules with regard to phosphate reabsorption. Evidence has been accumulated suggesting that the action of parathyroid hormone on the proximal tubule in which inhibition of phosphate reabsorption occurs can be simulated by volume expansion or saline infusion; the overall phosphaturia caused by parathyroid hormone, however, is much greater than that seen with saline infusion alone. Knox and Lechene (1975) presented evidence that the action of parathyroid hormone on phosphate reabsorption in the proximal tubule involves the inhibition of carbonic anhydrase.

Knox and Lechene (1975) interpreted their findings to indicate that the greatest effect on blockade of phosphate reabsorption occurs in the distal tubule and is uninfluenced by saline infusion, volume expansion, or inhibition of carbonic anhydrase; they believed that the distal tubular locus of action is the most important in bringing about overall phosphaturia. Such effects were first suggested by Nicholson and Shepherd (1959) as a result of their studies in dogs, but continued interest in such an idea was dropped because of results from the stop–flow studies of Samiy et al. (1960, 1965).

The overall handling of calcium by different portions of the nephron and, in particular, the anatomic site in which net calcium reabsorption—identified in physiological studies by Nordin et al. (1975) and Biddulph and Gallimore (1974)—actually occurs, has been the subject of recent investigations. Several studies had established that the renal reabsorption of calcium paralleled that of sodium (Lassiter et al., 1963; Duarte and Bland, 1965). These workers also suggested that the bulk of the calcium reabsorption occurred in the convoluted portion of the proximal tubule and that specific inhibition of sodium transport in the proximal tubule was accompanied by a smaller but significant inhibition of calcium reabsorption. The findings of Agus et al. (1973) using microprobe analysis and micropuncture, referred to above, in which there was a detailed analysis of proximal and distal tubular sodium and phosphate reabsorption in response to parathyroid hormone, also dealt with the tubular handling of calcium in detail. Parathyroid hormone causes not only an inhibition of reabsorption of sodium and phosphate in the proximal tubule, but also of calcium. The blockade in calcium reabsorption was proportionate to that of sodium.

Reabsorption of calcium, on the other hand, in the distal tubule accounted for the overall reduction in calcium clearance noted. The effects of PTH on tubular calcium, phosphate, and sodium reabsorption were simulated by administration of dibutyryl cyclic AMP. The studies were consistent with a view that cyclic AMP might be involved in the distal tubular stimulation of calcium reabsorption, the critical step in overall reduction in calcium clearance. Wesson and Lauler (1959) had suggested, in clearance studies in dogs, a close relationship between the reabsorption of calcium and that of magnesium; none of the more recent detailed analyses of the function of different portions of the nephron have included a localization of magnesium reabsorption, but it is reasonable to assume that the site of magnesium reabsorption may be the same distal tubular site involved in calcium reabsorption.

Parathyroid hormone in large doses, in addition to effects on renal tubular transport of sodium, calcium, phosphate, and magnesium, decreases renal tubular bicarbonate reabsorption, resulting in excretion of an inappropriately alkaline urine and a tendency toward systemic acidosis (Hellman et al., 1965; Morris et al., 1971, 1972).

Although many aspects of the physiological effects of parathyroid hormone on the kidney remain to be clarified, present information can be summarized best by stressing that effects of the hormone occur in two principal sites, the proximal and distal tubule. Proximal tubular effects involve inhibition of bicarbonate reabsorption as well as inhibition of reabsorption of calcium, sodium, and phosphate. At the distal tubular sites there may be an additional and, even more physiologically important, inhibition of phosphate reabsorption; at the same time, there is clearly an opposing effect on calcium, namely, a stimulation of calcium reabsorption. Very little overall increase in sodium clearance occurs from parathyroid hormone action, inasmuch as distal tubular mechanisms that function independently of parathyroid hormone are involved in the reabsorption of sodium presented in excess quantities because of blockade of proximal tubular sodium reabsorption. On the other hand, present evidence suggests that the increased phosphate in tubular fluid resulting from inhibition of proximal reabsorption is not only not reabsorbed distally but may in fact be further actively blocked below normal rates of distal tubular reabsorption of phosphate by the action of parathyroid hormone.

c. Effect on Intestine. The effect of parathyroid hormone on the intestine was the last major action of the hormone to be widely recognized and remains the least understood. It has been appreciated for many years that fecal excretion of calcium is diminished in patients with hyperparathyroidism (Albright and Reifenstein, 1948). Numerous experimental studies in man and in animals have established that parathyroid hormone produces an increase in intestinal absorption of calcium by increasing transport of the ion from the lumen of the upper small intestine (Talmage and Elliot, 1958; Rasmussen, 1959). Efforts to demonstrate direct effects of the hormone on intestinal calcium transport *in vitro* have been generally unsuccessful. There has been one report that stimulation of intestinal calcium transport by parathyroid hormone can be shown to occur when the peptide is added to fluid perfusing an isolated intestinal loop (Olson *et al.*, 1972). (Extensions of this particular study or other examinations of possible direct effects of the hormone on intestinal transport have not been reported or apparently pursued recently. Rather, attention has centered on indirect effects of the hormone on intestinal absorption through effects on vitamin D.)

Parathyroid hormone influences the renal production of $1,25\text{-}(OH)_2D_3$ (Garabedian *et al.*, 1972; Tanaka *et al.*, 1973; M. R. Hughes *et al.*, 1975), the probable metabolically active form of the vitamin in the intestine (Omdahl *et al.*, 1971; Lawson *et al.*, 1971; Holick *et al.*, 1971; Haussler *et al.*, 1971), through stimulation of renal 1-hydroxylase activity. As noted in Chapter 3, it has been possible to treat successfully patients with hypoparathyroidism and pseudohypoparathyroidism using extremely small amounts of $1,25\text{-}(OH)_2D_3$ (Kooh *et al.*, 1975; Neer *et al.*, 1975). The hypocalcemia and impaired intestinal absorption of calcium have been corrected by administration of as little as 0.004 μg of vitamin per kilogram of body weight per day. Doses of vitamin D that were at least one-hundred times higher than those of the dihydroxylated metabolite were required to maintain normocalcemia in these two conditions. These findings suggest that there is impaired conversion of 25-OHD$_2$ to 1,25-(OH)$_2$-D$_3$ in hypoparathyroidism and pseudohypoparathyroidism. Thyroparathyroidectomy of rats on a diet low in calcium had been shown earlier to reduce the production of 1,25-(OH)$_2$-D$_3$ from 25-OHD$_3$ to negligible levels (Garabedian *et al.*, 1972). The administration of parathyroid extract restores the levels of 1,25-(OH)$_2$-D$_3$ to control levels.

This trophic effect of parathyroid hormone on the production of 1,25-(OH)$_2$-D$_3$ may be mediated through a decrease in serum and/or intracellular concentrations of phosphate in the kidney produced by the action of parathyroid hormone on the renal tubule cells (Tanaka *et al.*, 1973; M. R. Hughes *et al.*, 1975). It was observed that rats fed a diet low in phosphorus supplemented with 25-OHD$_2$ show a high intestinal transport of calcium as compared to rats similarly treated but fed a diet containing adequate phosphorus (Tanaka *et al.*, 1973). The increased intestinal calcium transport correlated well with the synthesis of 1,25-(OH)$_2$-D$_3$. Studies employing a radioreceptor assay for 1,25-(OH)$_2$-D$_3$ have provided further evidence that low serum phosphorus concentration or some factor associated with phosphate depletion stimulates the renal synthesis of 1,25-(OH)$_2$-D$_3$ (M. R. Hughes *et al.*, 1975). Direct assay of blood of phosphate-depleted rats has shown a marked increase in the circulating concentration of the dihydroxyvitamin independent of the presence of the parathyroid (and thyroid) glands. Rasmussen *et al.* (1972) found that the 1α-hydroxylase of isolated renal tubules can be activated by parathyroid hormone or its proposed intracellular mediator, cyclic AMP. Since one of the known effects of parathyroid hormone on renal cells is to lower intracellular phosphate, it is possible that both parathyroid hormone and phosphate depletion enhance 1α-hydroxylase through a common intracellular mechanism (M. R. Hughes *et al.*, 1975).

Thus, the principal conclusion that can be drawn at present about the action of parathyroid hormone on the intestine is that the stimulation of calcium absorption seen in states of excessive parathyroid secretion and the deficient absorption seen in hypoparathyroid states reflects an indirect, although physiologically important, effect of the hormone, namely, control of the synthesis of 1,25-(OH)$_2$-D, perhaps mediated by parathyroid hormone directly or by changes in the content of phosphate in the renal cell. Direct actions of the hormone, if any, remain to be confirmed.

d. Effect on Other Organs. Parathyroid hormone exerts an effect on a number of organs other than bone, kidney, and intestine. Parathyroidectomy has been found to increase the calcium content of milk in lactating rats (Toverud and Munson, 1956) and the content of calcium in the salivary gland (Kraintz et al., 1965). A transient hypotension is frequently observed in animals after an injection of parathyroid hormone. Charbon (1968) presented evidence that this hypotensive effect is due to an increase in blood flow to the liver and the kidney. The overall physiological significance of the observations that the vascular system is affected by parathyroid hormone has not been determined, but perhaps alterations in blood flow induced by the hormone in some way influence the metabolism of the hormone. There is also evidence that parathyroid hormone may be important in normal tooth development. (Abnormalities in dentition in hypoparathyroidism are considered in Chapter 3.)

In addition to regulation of calcium and phosphate flux into blood from bone and kidney, parathyroid hormone also has been shown to influence the transport of magnesium in a manner that is qualitatively similar to that found for calcium (MacIntyre et al., 1963; MacIntyre and Robinson, 1969).

2. Biochemical Mode of Action

Over the past several years, evidence has accumulated indicating that parathyroid hormone acts at the biochemical level through the activation of the enzyme adenylyl cyclase and the formation of (cyclic) adenosine 3':5'-monophosphate (cyclic AMP) in the cells of the target tissues. The initial effect of parathyroid hormone on kidney in vitro (Marcus and Aurbach, 1969) and in vivo (Chase and Aurbach, 1967) and on bone in vitro (Chase et al., 1969; Peck et al., 1973; Rodan and Rodan, 1974; Wong and Cohn, 1975) is a stimulation of adenylyl cyclase (Fig. 4). An increase in the activity of adenylyl cyclase results from a specific interaction of hormone with the target-cell membrane in bone and kidney, and leads to an increase in intracellular cyclic AMP.

It seems likely that this rapid increase in intracellular cyclic AMP, which is probably augmented by an influx of calcium into the cell, is the initial biochemical manifestation of the physiological effects of parathyroid hormone. Within minutes after the administration of parathyroid hormone, there is a rise in urinary cyclic AMP that precedes the phosphaturic response of the kidney (Fig. 5) (Chase and Aurbach, 1967). Likewise, the effects on adenylyl cyclase of bone cells can be detected within 1 minute after the addition of parathyroid hormone. In addition, dibutyryl-cyclic AMP, an analogue of cyclic 3':5'-AMP that enters cells more readily, simulates the actions of parathyroid hormone on bone (Vaes, 1968; Raisz et al., 1969; Herrmann-Erlee and van der Meer,

TARGET   CELL

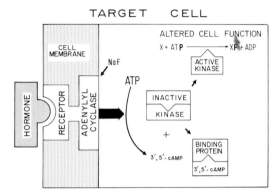

Fig. 4. Proposed cellular model for mechanism of action of parathyroid hormone on target cell (e.g., bone or kidney). Hormone binds to receptor in cytoplasmic membrane leading to activation of the enzyme adenylyl cyclase. The enzyme catalyzes the formation of cyclic 3',5'-AMP from ATP. Cyclic 3',5'-AMP binds to a receptor protein causing its dissociation from kinase and consequent activation of kinase enzyme. Active kinase is believed to be involved in phosphorylation of substrate proteins (X) leading to altered cell function. It is possible that the substrate protein may be part of a transport system for calcium (? microtubules).

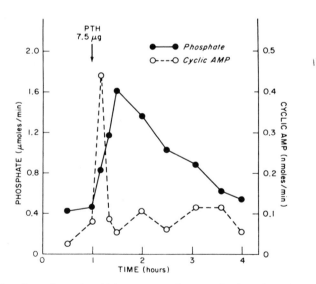

Fig. 5. The effect of parathyroid hormone on the excretion into the urine of phosphate and cyclic AMP by a parathyroidectomized rat. Parathyroid hormone (7.5 μg) was injected intravenously over a 2-minute period at the time shown by the arrow. (From Chase and Aurbach, 1967.)

1974). Dibutyryl-cyclic AMP produces a rise in serum calcium, a lowering of serum phosphate, and an increased excretion of calcium, phosphate, and hydroxyproline in urine (Rasmussen *et al.,* 1968; Russell *et al.,* 1968).

Our understanding of the subsequent intracellular mechanisms through which the effects of increased cyclic AMP are mediated is incomplete. Present evidence indicates that activation by cyclic AMP of protein kinases may be the next step in the chain of events leading to the physiological effects of the hormone (Fig. 4) (Aurbach *et al.,* 1972; Walsh and Ashby, 1973). Specific cyclic AMP-dependent protein kinases have been identified in kidney tissue. Cyclic AMP was shown to bind to a specific binding protein, causing it to dissociate from and thereby to activate the protein kinase (Kuo and Greengard, 1969; Winickoff and Aurbach, 1970). The kinases appear to be responsible for catalyzing the phosphorylations of a number of proteins, such as histones, ribosomal proteins, and microtubular proteins (Goodman *et al.,* 1970; Walsh and Ashby, 1973). Microtubular proteins are thought to be involved in the intracellular processes leading to the transport of calcium across cells and membranes from bone and renal tubular fluid to the extracellular fluid (Aurbach *et al.,* 1972). Microtubules were identified histologically in bone cells (Holtrop and Weinger, 1972), and colchicine, an inhibitor of microtubular function, was shown to produce hypocalcemia in rats (Aurbach *et al.,* 1972; Heath *et al.,* 1972) and to inhibit bone resorption *in vitro* (Raisz *et al.,* 1973).

Whatever may be the cellular sites that are affected by the increased concentration of intracellular cyclic AMP, its role in hormone action seems firmly established. The initial effect of the increased cyclic AMP, which occurs within minutes of the administration of parathyroid hormone, is a hypocalcemia due to a flow of calcium out of blood into, apparently, skeletal cells. Thus, both cyclic AMP and calcium may serve as "second messengers" for mediating the final effects of parathyroid hormone on receptor cells.

A scheme representing the proposed cellular model for mechanism of action of parathyroid hormone on target cells (e.g., bone or kidney) is presented in Fig. 4 (Aurbach *et al.,* 1972).

B. Chemistry of Parathyroid Hormone

1. Chemical Properties of the Natural Products

The first biologically active extracts of parathyroid hormone from bovine glands were made by Collip (1925) using hot 5% hydrochloric acid.

Further purification of the hormone was not achieved until many years later, however, when Aurbach (1959) and Rasmussen *et al.* (1964) developed improved extraction procedures that eventually provided large quantities of relatively pure parathyroid hormone that could be used for the development of a radioimmunoassay (Berson *et al.*, 1963) and studies on the physiological action of the hormone. Further improvements in purification techniques led to the isolation of homogeneous preparations of parathyroid hormone (Keutmann *et al.*, 1971).

The complete amino acid sequences of bovine and porcine parathyroid hormones have been determined using a combination of enzymatic and chemical cleavages of the hormone followed by automated sequential degradation of the resulting peptides (Fig. 6) (Brewer and Ronan. 1970; Niall *et al.*, 1970; Potts *et al.*, 1971; Woodhead *et al.*, 1971; Sauer *et al.*, (1974). Two closely related but distinct isohormonal forms of the bovine hormone have been identified, but analyses of their sequences have not yet been accomplished, owing to lack of sufficient amounts of these minor hormone variants (Keutmann *et al.*, 1971).

Studies of the chemistry of human parathyroid hormone are less complete than those of the bovine and porcine hormone. Keutmann *et al.* (1974) described the isolation, chemical composition, and biological assay of the human parathyroid hormone. Sequence analysis of the first amino-terminal 34 or 37 residues of the human hormone was reported independently by Brewer *et al.* (1972) and Niall *et al.* (1974), and approximately 90% of the sequence of the remainder of the polypeptide is known (Keutmann *et al.*, 1975a). The structure found for this segment of the human hormone closely resembles that of the bovine and porcine hormones (Fig. 6). At present, however, disagreement exists concerning the exact structure of the human parathyroid hormone. One group found that the human differs from the bovine hormone at positions 1, 7, and 16 (Niall *et al.*, 1974), whereas the other found additional differences at positions 28 and 30, and found position 22 to be glutamine in both bovine and human hormone, at variance with the findings of the other group (Brewer *et al.*, 1972; Niall *et al.*, 1970, 1974). Ultimate resolution of these discrepancies in structural analysis will require further chemical and immunochemical studies; these are continuing (Brewer *et al.*, 1975; Keutmann *et al.*, 1975a; Segre and Potts, 1976). Eventual resolution of the disagreements in sequence is important since synthetic human PTH, in which there is interest for physiological and clinical studies, should be based on the correct sequence of the human hormone.

Soon after the establishment of the existence of proparathyroid hormone, a biosynthetic precursor parathyroid hormone (see Section II, E), Hamilton *et al.* (1974) undertook a large-scale purification of the prohor-

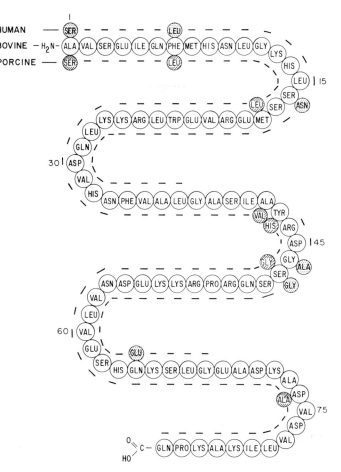

Fig. 6. Amino acid sequences of bovine, porcine, and human parathyroid hormones. The continuous structure shown in open circles is that of bovine PTH. The appended amino acids indicate differences in the sequences of human (stippled circles) and porcine (shaded circles) hormones. Dashed lines indicate that, at specified positions, amino acids are identical to those in bovine hormone sequence. Note that sequence of human PTH is not yet completed. (From Keutmann *et al.*, 1975a.)

mone and isolated a sufficient quantity (approximately 1 mg) to permit a partial determination of its primary amino acid sequence. The prohormone contains an additional hexapeptide sequence at the amino terminus of the hormone (Fig. 7) (Hamilton *et al.*, 1974). Subsequently, with the use of highly sensitive microsequencing techniques applied to the polypeptides labeled with radioactive amino acids, the structures of the human (Jacobs *et al.*, 1974; Huang *et al.*, 1975) and porcine (Chu *et al.*,

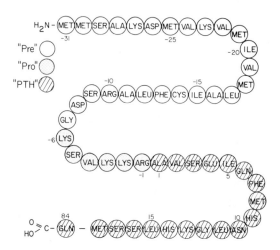

Fig. 7. Amino acid sequence of bovine pre-proparathyroid hormone (Pre-ProPTH) as determined by microsequencing techniques. The radiolabeled pre-prohormone was synthesized *in vitro* in a cell-free extract of wheat germ by addition of parathyroid messenger RNA and radioactive amino acids. The amino acid sequence was determined by sequential Edman degradation. The N-terminal methionine (residue −31) is the initiator amino acid not removed in the wheat-germ system. Note sequence of PTH is interrupted between positions 18 and 84.

1975) proparathyroid hormone-specific sequences were determined and were found to be identical with (human) or similar (porcine) to the structure of the bovine prohormone. The additional prohormone-specific peptide is very basic; four of the six additional amino acids are positively charged (three lysine and one arginine). The high positive charge of the prohormone peptide accounts for its rapid electrophoretic mobility on polyacrylamide gels. The arginine residue adjacent to the amino-terminal alanine of PTH renders the bond between the prohormone hexapeptide and the hormone itself highly susceptible to cleavage by trypsin.

The amino acid sequence of bovine pre-proparathyroid hormone (Pre-ProPTH), the major product obtained from the translation of parathyroid messenger RNA in cell-free systems, has also been determined (Fig. 7). Pre-proparathyroid hormone is thought to be the initial and earliest biosynthetic precursor of parathyroid hormone (Section II.E). It consists of ProPTH with the addition of an additional peptide sequence of 25 amino acids at the NH_2 terminus (Habener *et al.*, 1975b; Kemper *et al.*, 1976b). The sequence in regions specific for the pre-proparathyroid hormone, insofar as it has been determined, appears to be hydrophobic, a property that may be important in relation to its proposed function of facilitating attachment to and transport across the membrane of the endoplasmic reticulum. It has been determined that the NH_2-terminal methionine of pre-proparathyroid hormone is the initiator amino acid that begins the synthesis of the polypeptide in response to recognition of the specific initiator AUG codon of the mRNA (Kemper *et al.*, 1976b).

2. Synthesis of Fragments and Analogues of Parathyroid Hormone and Proparathyroid Hormone: Structure–Activity Relationships

Early work indicated that the full 84-amino-acid sequence for bovine parathyroid hormone was not required for biological activity. It was established, using dilute acid hydrolysis, that the amino-terminal 29 amino acid fragment was biologically active (Keutmann *et al.*, 1972). As sequence data on the amino-terminal region of bovine PTH became available, it became possible to undertake chemical synthesis of amino-terminal fragments of the molecule (Potts *et al.*, 1971; Tregear *et al.*, 1973).

The synthesis of a biologically active amino-terminal 1–34 fragment of the bovine PTH sequence confirmed the earlier observation that the amino-terminal fragments of the molecule were biologically active. The synthetic tetratriacontapeptide was found to possess all the specific physiological and biochemical properties associated with native PTH (Potts *et al.*, 1971). In addition to stimulating adenylyl cyclase in both bone and kidney cells, the synthetic peptide elevated blood calcium in rats and dogs and caused an increase in renal excretion of both cyclic AMP and phosphate in the rat.

In the *in vivo* chick assay, in which the peptide is administered intravenously, the activity of the 1–34 fragment is 7700 U/mg, which is slightly greater on a molar basis than that of the native hormone.

Several fragments representing progressively shorter segments of the amino-terminal region of bovine parathyroid hormone were prepared by solid-phase peptide synthesis and bioassayed in the *in vitro* rat kidney adenylyl cyclase assay and the *in vivo* chick hypercalcemia assay (Tregear *et al.*, 1973). These studies defined the minimum chain length required for activity (Tregear *et al.*, 1973; Potts *et al.*, 1973; Parsons *et al.*, 1975). A list of the peptide fragments synthesized, together with the results of bioassay in the rat adenylyl cyclase and chick hypercalcemia systems, is shown in Table I.

A dramatic loss of biological activity results from deletion of the amino-terminal alanine residue (2–34). Removal of the second residue, valine (3–34), results in a complete loss of activity of bovine PTH in both assay systems. Hence, little deletion is tolerated at the amino terminus. Shortening at the carboxyl terminus of the 1–34 peptide is less critical.

TABLE I

Comparative Biological Activities of Parathyroid Hormone and Fragments of Parathyroid Hormone in Two Different Bioassays[a]

	Rat adenyl cyclase in vitro		Chick hypercalcemia in vivo	
	Potency MRCU/mg[b]	Potency Mole %	Potency MRCU/mg	Potency Mole %
1–84 (native)	3000	100	2500	100
1–34	5400	77	7700	132
2–34	200[c]	3	3800	64
3–34	<10	<0.3	<5	<0.2
1–26	<10	<0.3	—	—
1–27	200[c]	2	—	—
1–28	440	5	<10	<0.3
1–31	740	10	4000	62
1–12 + 13–34	<10	<0.3	<5	<0.2

[a] From Habener and Potts (1976b, based on data of Marcus and Aurbach, 1969, and Parsons et al., 1973).

[b] USP units based on standard provided by the Medical Research Council (MRCU), Mill Hill, England.

[c] Nonlinear response in the assay.

Seven residues may be deleted before the resulting peptide, 1–27, is reduced in potency in the cyclase assay to the stage of a weak nonparallel response. From the overall bioassay results obtained with the synthetic fragments of bovine parathyroid hormone that are shorter than the 1–34 peptide, the minimum length for activity can be defined as a continuous sequence involving residues 2 through 27, with the possibility of further deletion at the carboxyl terminus not yet fully resolved (Table I).

In recent studies it has been shown that the region critical for binding to receptors associated with stimulation of adenylyl cyclase activation in renal cortical membranes is present in the fragment 3–34 and analogues of this sequence (Rosenblatt et al., 1977). These studies have made possible investigation of competitive inhibitors of hormone action useful in investigation of initial steps of hormone/receptor binding and ultimately, possibly, in physiological applications (Rosenblatt et al., 1977). Basic features of structure–activity relations in bovine hormone have been confirmed in human synthetic studies of peptide fragments based on the amino-terminal sequence of the hormone.

These observations of the biological activities of small fragments of the hormone allow one to conclude that any circulating biologically active fragment of endogenous parathyroid hormone must include a continuous polypeptide sequence from the amino-terminal portion of the hormone no shorter than approximately 27 residues, beginning with residue number 2.

The chemical synthesis of a 40 amino acid peptide fragment of the prohormone, consisting of the amino-terminal 34 residues of the hormone plus the prohormone-specific hexapeptide sequence, was accomplished and has led to more extensive biological and immunological testing (Goltzman *et al.*, 1974; Habener *et al.*, 1974a; Peytremann *et al.*, 1975; Habener and Potts, 1976b). Information obtained from such studies with the synthetic peptide confirmed and extended the information obtained previously with tests employing the native prohormone available only in limited amounts.

The results of assays of the biological activity of native proparathyroid hormone and the synthetic fragment of the prohormone in several different assay systems provided the following information: (1) the prohormone is biologically active in *in vivo* hypercalcemia assays in rat (Hamilton *et al.*, 1971a) and chick (Habener *et al.*, 1976b; Herrmann-Erlee *et al.*, 1976), in *in vitro* assays of bone resorption in tissue culture, activation of renal adenylyl cyclase (Goltzman *et al.*, 1974), and conversion of ^{14}C-citrate to CO_2 (Hamilton *et al.*, 1971a); (2) the activity of the prohormone in all systems is considerably less than that of PTH; (3) the relative activity of the prohormone compared to hormone varies among the assay systems used (Habener and Potts, 1976b).

It is likely that the observed activity of the prohormone is not due to inherent activity of the prohormone molecule itself but rather to the activity of the hormone that is formed by enzymatic conversion of the prohormone precursor within the test system. It was possible to assess simultaneously the relative activity of the prohormone and the degree of conversion of prohormone to native hormone and of prohormone fragment to hormone fragment during incubation in the renal adenylyl cyclase assay. Goltzman *et al.* (1975) and Peytremann *et al.* (1975) showed that the addition of the trypsin inhibitor benzamidine to the assay system lowers the activity of the prohormone from 3–4% to less than 0.1% of that of the hormone. The deleterious effects of extension of the peptide chain at the amino terminus on the structure–activity relationships of analogues of parathyroid hormone had been shown earlier; chemical addition of the amino acid tryosine or the tripeptide glycylglycyltyrosine to the amino-terminal alanine of the fully active synthetic peptide 1–34 resulted in a drastic lowering of the biological activity of the hormone (Parsons and Potts, 1972). These studies suggest that the prohormone itself, even if it enters the circulation, is inherently inactive, although it might be rendered active by cleavage by the ubiquitous trypsin-like enzymes present in plasma.

C. Metabolism of Parathyroid Hormone

1. Heterogeneity of the Circulating Hormone

Immunoreactive parathyroid hormone in the circulation consists not only of intact hormone but also of one or more hormonal peptide fragments thought to arise as a result of the peripheral metabolism of the hormone or secretion of fragments from the gland. This information led to new insights into the nature of secretion and metabolism of the hormone, as well as to refinements in the techniques and interpretations of the radioimmunoassay, particularly with regard to the use of antisera that are known to recognize specific antigenic sites of the hormone.

Berson and Yalow (1968) supplied the first data showing that parathyroid hormone in plasma differs in immunochemical properties from hormone extracted from parathyroid tissue. These workers demonstrated that hormone in plasma samples from patients with hyperparathyroidism had a reaction in the radioimmunoassay that was different from that of standard hormone (extracted from parathyroid adenomas), and that the degree of difference in reactivity varied with the particular antiserum used in the assay. Moreover, they observed that the rate of disappearance of hormone after parathyroidectomy was more rapid when measured with one antiserum than with another (Fig. 8).

Although the studies of Berson and Yalow demonstrated immunochemical heterogeneity of hormone in the circulation, the basis for this heterogeneity was not then known. Subsequently, the heterogeneity of immunoreactive PTH was found to be due to the presence of hormonal fragments. Sherwood et al. (1970) and Arnaud et al. (1971a), using in vitro methods, showed that fragments of immunoreactive parathyroid hormone accumulated in the culture media during incubation of parathyroid tissue and that the hormonal fragments were associated with a nonparallel slope of response in the immunoassay. The observations led to the suggestion that only fragments of parathyroid hormone are secreted into the circulation in vivo, and that such fragments, in turn, account for the immunochemical heterogeneity of plasma hormone detected earlier by Berson and Yalow. It was found subsequently, however, by analysis of hormone secreted directly from the parathyroids in vivo, that the hormonal fragments found in the circulation probably arise, at least in part, after the hormone is secreted into the circulation.

The results of gel filtration and radioimmunoassay of hormone secreted in vivo in parathyroid venous effluent blood (Habener et al., 1971b) indicated a predominance of intact hormone with immunochemical properties and apparent molecular weight indistinguishable from those of hormone that can be extracted from the parathyroid tissue (Fig. 9a,b). Fur-

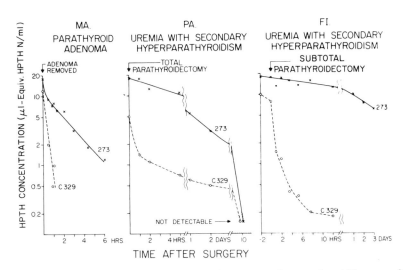

Fig. 8. Differences in the disappearance of immunoreactive parathyroid hormone from plasma after parathyroidectomy in patients with primary or secondary hyperparathyroidism when hormone is measured by different antisera. Plasma samples were assayed with antiserum C329 and antiserum 273 using an extract of a normal human parathyroid gland as standard (HPTH N) and ^{125}I-BPTH as tracer. Plasma concentrations of hormone are given as μl equivalents of the plasma standard of HPTH (see text). (From Berson and Yalow, 1968).

thermore, monolayer cultures of cells derived from human parathyroid adenomas (Martin *et al.*, 1972) and slices of parathyroid glands during short peroids of incubation (less than 6 hours) (Habener *et al.*, 1975a) produced only intact hormone. Secretion of fragments of the hormone by organ cultures of parathyroid glands becomes evident only at long incubation times; it is difficult at present to relate these later tissue-culture events to events *in vivo*.

Immunoreactive parathyroid hormone in the peripheral circulation consists of one or more hormonal fragments that are responsible for the altered immunochemical reactions given by plasma hormone in the immunoassay (Habener *et al.*, 1971a, 1972b; Canterbury and Reiss, 1972; Segre *et al.*, 1972, 1974; Goldsmith *et al.*, 1973; Silverman and Yalow, 1973; Fischer *et al.*, 1974). A large hormonal fragment with an estimated molecular weight of 6000 to 7000 appears to be the predominant form of the hormone in the circulation (Fig. 9a,b), although intact hormone and smaller hormonal fragments have also been detected (Canterbury *et al.*, 1973; Silverman and Yalow, 1973).

Since the parathyroid gland venous effluent contains predominantly hormone that is identical in size to hormone extracted from glands, it was

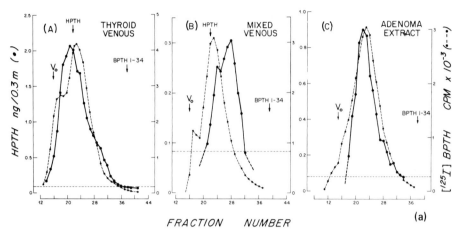

Fig. 9(a). BioGel P-10 filtration patterns of radioimmunoassayable parathyroid hormone (PTH) in samples obtained simultaneously by venous catheterization of (A) inferior thyroid vein (thyroid venous) and (B) superior vena cava (mixed venous) in a patient with a parathyroid adenoma. These patterns are compared to (C) filtration of a partially purified standard hormone extract prepared from human parathyroid adenomas (adenoma extract). Parathyroid hormone concentration in thyroid venous plasma was 150 ng/ml. Indicated hormone concentration in mixed venous samples is only approximate because of nonparallel response in the assay. ^{125}I-Labeled bovine parathyroid hormone (BPTH) was cochromatographed in each filtration as a marker (dotted lines). Arrow marks elution positions of void volume of column (V_o), human parathyroid hormone (HPTH), and the synthetic bovine 1–34 amino-terminal peptide (BPTH) 1–34. The dashed horizontal line indicates the sensitivity limit of the radioimmunoassay (antiserum GP-1; dilution 1 : 250,000). Note that the thyroid venous sample resembles the adenoma extract in eluting at or before the markers of HPTH and ^{125}I]BPTH. In contrast, activity in the mixed venous sample elutes later than the markers. From Habener *et al.*, 1971a.)

concluded that the fragments found in peripheral blood must be derived, largely, from cleavage of the intact hormone after secretion into the circulation. It is apparent that the fate of parathyroid hormone after release from the gland is a more complex process than that of uptake by receptors and simple clearance from the circulation. Further understanding of the process of peripheral clearance and metabolism of the hormone required development of techniques to assess the nature of the cleavage, the site or sites of cleavage, and the biological and chemical properties of the circulating fragments.

The chemical nature and biological significance of the forms of the hormone in the circulation have been evaluated more precisely through characterization and modification of the antisera used for the analysis of plasma samples and of fractions of plasma samples obtained by gel filtra-

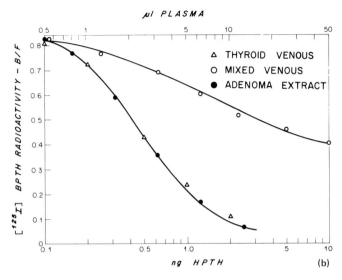

Fig. 9b. Demonstration of immunochemical dissimilarity of parathyroid hormone in peripherally obtained plasma, as compared with plasma from parathyroid gland effluent and to hormone extracted from parathyroid adenomas. The fall in the bound/free ratio of ^{125}I-labeled bovine hormone is shown for different amounts of plasma or the human parathyroid hormone solution used in the gel filtration study of Fig. 1. $\bigcirc$, superior vena cava; $\triangle$, inferior thyroid vein; $\bullet$, standard, human hormone (PTH-1–84), adenoma extract.

tion studies. The results of immunoassay using specific fragments of the bovine hormone, prepared both by chemical synthesis and by enzymatic or chemical cleavage of natural hormone, have indicated that limited regions of the parathyroid hormone appear to satisfy the binding requirements of the various antisera (Segre *et al.*, 1972). The antiserum can then be modified to recognize limited, specific regions of the hormonal molecule by selective absorption of the appropriate fragments of the hormone. Antisera have thus been prepared for exclusive recognition of a limited region of the sequence either at the amino- or carboxyl-terminal end of the hormone.

Although the antisera used were raised against bovine PTH, the amino-terminal-specific components of the antisera react very similarly with both the bovine and human hormones (Segre *et al.*, 1974), a reflection of the fact that the amino acid sequences of the two hormones are closely similar in the sequence region recognized by the antisera (Fig. 6). Studies with radioimmunoassays using the adsorbed antisera indicate that hormone released directly from the gland into the parathyroid effluent blood coelutes from the gel column with the marker of intact hormone and is detected equivalently by both the amino sequence- and carboxyl sequence-specific antisera. In contrast, the large hormonal fragment of 6000–7000 daltons that predominates in the peripheral circulation is recognized by an antiserum that reacts with antigenic determinants in the carboxyl sequence 53–84 but not by an antiserum that recognized antigenic determinants that are amino terminal to residue 30 (Fig. 10). Since this large fragment lacks the critical amino-terminal sequence required for biological activity and the fragment is present in much higher concentrations than native, uncleaved hormone, it is likely that much of the immunoreactive hormone detected in the circulation is biologically inactive.

If the fragment of MW 7000 arises as a result of cleavage by an endopeptidase, one would expect to find a second fragment of MW 2000–4000. Canterbury *et al.* (1973), working with concentrates of human plasma from patients with hyperparathyroidism, detected in addition to the large fragment, a smaller fragment of MW of approximately 4000. Silverman and Yalow (1973). Goldsmith *et al.* (1973), and Fischer *et*

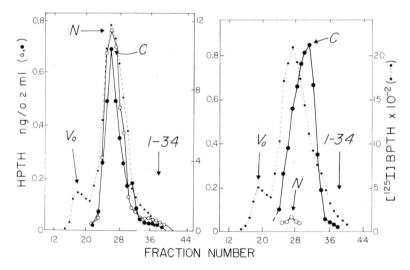

Fig. 10. Gel filtration pattern (BioGel P-10) of immunoreactive parathyroid hormone obtained from the thyroid vein by venous catheterization (left) and from the general circulation by venipuncture (right). Plasma (0.5–0.8 ml) and 50 pg (20,000 cpm) of ^{125}I-labeled bovine parathyroid hormone (^{125}I-bPTH) consisting of native hormone purified from gland extracts were cochromatographed. Immunoreactive parathyroid hormone was measured in aliquots of each gel fraction against a human parathyroid hormone standard using radioimmunoassays that specifically measure an amino-terminal sequence between residues 14–30 (N assay) (○) and a carboxyl-terminal sequence between residues 53–84 (C assay) (●). Arrows indicate void volume of column (V°) and elution position of synthetic bovine peptides 1–34 (1–34). (From Habener *et al.*, 1972b.)

al. (1974) also detected smaller fragments of PTH in plasma. The smaller fragment described by Canterbury *et al.* (1973) was found to be biologically active in an *in vitro* renal adenylyl cyclase assay (the larger fragment was inactive), which indicates that the fragment probably consists of the amino-terminal sequence of the hormone, and that cleavage of the hormone may not necessarily be a process of hormone inactivation.

The reason for the discrepancies in the findings of different groups concerning the presence of an amino-terminal fragment in the circulation is not known. Peripheral cleavage of parathyroid hormone might occur in the vicinity of receptors; thus, in one sense, whether the fragment circulates is less significant than whether it is cleaved in a fashion that preserves biological activity. As illustrated in Fig. 11, if the cleavage occurs amino terminal to position 27, both fragments produced by cleavage would be biologically inactive, based on considerations of structure and activity. If cleavage occurs carboxyl terminal to position 27, the amino-terminal fragment produced might still be active.

Recent investigations involving several different approaches have helped to identify more precisely the site of cleavage. Segre *et al.* (1974) presented chemical evidence that peripheral cleavage of the hormone could result in the production of an active fragment. ^{125}I-Labeled bovine PTH, with radioactive iodine linked to the tyrosine residue at position 43, was infused into dogs. After injection of labeled peptide, there was progressive accumulation of a product corresponding to the large C-terminal fragment (Fig. 12). It was possible to separate the C-terminal fragment from other peaks of radioactivity and then analyze the fragment by sequential degradation using the Edman procedure. Radioactive tyrosine appeared after 7 and 10 steps of degradation, indicating that the fragment of MW 6000 isolated from the circulation of the dog probably consists of at least two fragments closely related in size. One fragment presumably consists of sequence 34 through 84, and the other, 38 to 84. Each of these

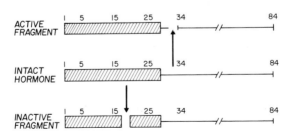

Fig. 11. Model of the two theoretical alternate sites of metabolic cleavage of parathyroid hormone (sequence 1–84). The hatched area indicates the minimal sequence required for biological activity. (From Potts *et al.*, 1973.)

Joel F. Habener and John T. Potts, Jr.

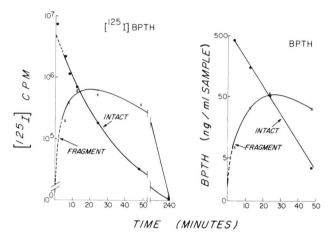

TIME   (MINUTES)

Fig. 12. Disappearance of intact PTH and appearance and disappearance of the C-terminal fragment of PTH after the intravenous injection of bovine ^{125}I-labeled (left) and unlabeled (biologically active) (right) PTH into dogs. (Modified from Segre *et al.*, 1974.)

fragments must be biologically inactive because each lacks the amino-terminal amino acids required for activity. In addition, use of region- or sequence-specific antisera to analyze for the fragment after injection of unlabeled biologically active hormone gives results in close agreement with those obtained with radioactive peptide.

These studies suggested that the C-terminal fragment is indeed a true cleavage product generated peripherally after intact hormone enters the circulation rather than merely intact hormone with altered conformation and immunological properties. If the fragment is generated by a single site-specific cleavage, which might occur by action of an endopeptidase, the smaller coproduct from the amino terminus could be biologically active because it would represent region 1–33, known to be biologically active.

Thus, there could be two active molecular species, the intact hormone and a smaller amino-terminal fragment. Peripheral cleavage could even involve an activation process, rather than degradation and inactivation, i.e., the native hormone might not be active at all before cleavage. Recent studies *in vitro*, however, do suggest that the native hormone is active on renal receptors without cleavage (Goltzman *et al.*, 1976). Alternatively, the spectrum or duration of biological activity of a smaller fragment might differ from that of the intact molecule, and thereby peripheral cleavage might produce two different types of active molecular forms of the hormone.

A schematic depiction of the current concepts describing the peripheral metabolism of parathyroid hormone is shown in Fig. 13. At present, the

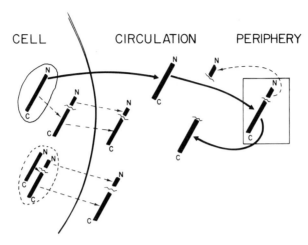

Fig. 13. Schematic model summarizing present information and concepts concerning the secretion and metabolism of parathyroid hormone and the origins of the heterogeneity of immunoreactive parathyroid hormone in the circulation. In addition to release of intact hormone from the parathyroid cell (pathway denoted by heavy arrows), during prolonged incubations of parathyroid tissues *in vitro* there may be release of fragments of PTH formed by proteolytic breakdown of PTH in the cell (interrupted arrow). Fragmentation of the hormone is shown occurring alternatively in the same or different secretory granules that release intact hormone. Uptake of hormone after secretion occurs in peripheral organs (perhaps target organs, e.g., kidney), followed by a second cleavage; the larger and biologically inactive C fragment reenters the circulation, but the fate of the smaller N fragment, which may be biologically active (and be released adjacent to the receptors), is at present uncertain (interrupted arrow). It is likewise uncertain to what extent peripheral metabolism versus glandular release contributes to the hormonal fragments detected in the general circulation.

heterogeneity of circulating parathyroid hormone precludes valid measurements of absolute concentrations of the hormonal species in plasma by radioimmunoassay. Additional studies of the peripheral metabolism of the hormone may ultimately help to clarify disagreement in reports about the diagnostic significance of hormone levels measured in plasma (see Section III, D, 3). It is likely that the antisera used in radioimmunoassays by different workers are sensitive to different limited regions of the hormonal molecule.

Recently, further analyses of the heterogeneity of circulating immunoreactive hormone uncovered findings consistent with secretion of fragments from the parathyroids (Silverman and Yalow, 1973) (see below). Such fragments, however, need not be identical with fragments produced peripherally. At present, it is difficult to assess quantitatively the relative contributions of peripheral metabolism and glandular secretion of fragments to the fragments detected in the peripheral circulation.

Such quantitative analyses would require immunoassay measurements employing standard solutions of immunologically defined fragments that are not yet available.

Despite the complex nature of circulating immunoreactive hormone, experience has demonstrated that the total concentration of immunoreactive parathyroid hormone in blood does correlate with chronic changes in the secretory activity of the parathyroid gland and is, therefore, even at present, helpful in establishing the clinical diagnosis of hyperparathyroidism.

2. Distribution, Disappearance, and Organ Specificity

The rate of disappearance of parathyroid hormone from the circulation has been determined by immunoassay in man and in animals after either exogenous injection of hormone (Sherwood et al., 1968; O'Riordan et al., 1970; Singer et al., 1975) or acute suppression of endogenously secreted hormone by parathyroidectomy or by calcium infusion (Berson and Yalow, 1968; Fang and Tashjian, 1972). Most of the data indicate that the hormone is cleared rapidly from the circulation with a half-time of disappearance of from 5 to 20 minutes. In certain instances, however, such as secondary hyperparathyroidism due to severe, chronic renal failure, the clearance of immunoreactive hormone from the circulation is prolonged. Berson and Yalow (1968) and, more recently, Silverman and Yalow (1973) found immunoreactive hormone in the circulation for as long as several days after total parathyroidectomy in patients with chronic renal failure (Chapter 2). On the basis of these findings, Silverman and Yalow proposed that circulating hormonal fragments may arise exclusively by secretion from the gland. Because it has been established that much, at least, of the hormone secreted by the parathyroid glands consists of intact hormone, this proposal requires that the rate of disappearance of fragments of hormone from the circulation be considerably slower than the disappearance of intact hormone to account for the predominance of fragments in the peripheral circulation.

The heterogeneity of circulating immunoreactive hormone presents problems in the meaningful interpretation of the apparent disappearance times of plasma hormone shown by immunoassay. The actual disappearance rate of biologically active hormone from the circulation is not known. Intact hormone could, in theory, disappear by being cleaved into fragments, and by such alteration escape detection unless a given antiserum could detect the cleavage products as readily as it detects the intact hormone. On the basis of studies in animals with normal renal function, the clearance or metabolism of intact hormone is of the order of minutes, not hours or days (Segre et al., 1974; Habener et al., 1976a).

Uncertainty persists, however, about whether fragments or hormone, secreted from the gland as a small fraction of the secreted hormone, might persist with very long half-time in blood, especially in chronic renal failure.

The volume of distribution of injected parathyroid hormone in the body was determined by extrapolation of the initial disappearance curve back to time zero. The distribution volume corresponds to approximately 30% of the body weight, roughly equivalent to the extracellular fluid volume (Sherwood *et al.*, 1968). Although it is difficult to relate any apparent volume of distribution to any well-defined physiological compartment, such as extracellular fluid, these results suggest widespread distribution of hormone and indicate that the specificity of hormone interaction with target organs is probably dependent on receptor binding rather than on restricted distribution.

There is evidence that the liver and kidney are the organs primarily involved in either the metabolism or clearance of intact hormone or hormone fragments (Fang and Tashjian, 1972; Singer *et al.*, 1975). Simultaneous sampling of arterial and venous blood across various organs in the dog was carried out in experiments with bovine parathyroid hormone infused until a steady state of hormone concentration was achieved (Singer *et al.*, 1975). Under these conditions, radioimmunoassay showed a 20–30% fall in concentration of hormone across kidney and liver; no fall was detected across lung or hind limb. Renal excretion of hormone or, at least, simple glomerular filtration without modification, does not appear to play a role in hormone disappearance, inasmuch as less than 1% of the administered dose of hormone could be detected as immunoassayable hormone in the urine.

In other types of studies, the rate of disappearance, from blood, of immunoreactive parathyroid hormone (without distinction between intact hormone and fragments) has been determined by radioimmunoassay in intact, nephrectomized, and partially hepatectomized rats (Fang and Tashjian, 1972). Bilateral nephrectomy and partial hepatectomy, but not adrenalectomy or splenectomy, each resulted in a significant decrease in the rate of disappearance of hormone, indicating that the kidney and liver contribute importantly to hormone metabolism. Direct perfusion of isolated rat liver *in situ* with parathyroid hormone revealed hormonal fragments in the perfusate (Canterbury *et al.*, 1975). These studies strongly implicate the liver as an important organ for the metabolism of parathyroid hormone.

Zull and Repke (1972) reported a novel approach to the study of PTH metabolism. They prepared a tritiated derivative of PTH through chemical coupling of [*methyl*-³H]acetimidate to the free amino groups of the hormone. After injection of the tritiated hormone in rats, radioactivity rapidly localized to the kidney in the form of low-molecular-weight material, soluble in trichloroacetic acid. If it can be shown that the radioactive hormone itself retains biological activity and that the [*methyl*-^{3}H]-acetimidate group remains covalently attached to the hormone, these studies may eventually lead to useful information about the relationship of receptor binding and metabolism of the hormone by the kidney.

D. Secretion of Parathyroid Hormone

1. Early Physiological Studies in Animals

Early experiments *in vivo* showed that the secretion of parathyroid hormone is inversely proportional to the concentration of ionized calcium perfusing the parathyroid glands (Patt and Luckhardt, 1942; Copp and Davidson, 1961; Care *et al.*, 1966). The studies demonstrated that perfusion of the parathyroids with calcium-deficient fluids resulted in systemic hypercalcemia, presumably due to increased secretion of parathyroid hormone into the circulation. Later studies with specific radioimmunoassay provided confirmation that circulating hormone is increased with hypocalcemia and decreased with hypercalcemia (Sherwood *et al.*, 1966; Mayer *et al.*, 1969).

The immunological techniques permitted assessment of the normal patterns of secretion and the factors that control the production of parathyroid hormone (Care *et al.*, 1966; Sherwood *et al.*, 1966). The studies showed that the hormone is constantly detectable in the plasma of normal animals, suggesting that the secretion of the hormone is continuous; blood calcium was shown to be the primary determinant of parathyroid hormone secretion. Analysis by radioimmunoassay showed that infusions of calcium or EDTA that raise or lower blood calcium induce a fall or a rise, respectively, in concentration of hormone in plasma (Sherwood *et al.*, 1966). With prolonged infusions of EDTA, a five- to sixfold increase in hormone concentration was sustained for many hours. Direct perfusion of goat parathyroid gland *in situ* with calcium (Care *et al.*, 1966) showed that the initial response of the gland to perturbations in calcium concentration occurs within minutes, that the calcium receptor for regulation of hormone secretion is within the gland itself, and that the changes observed in peripheral hormone concentration reflect actual changes in secretory rate.

Detailed analyses of the changes in parathyroid hormone and calcium concentrations in the peripheral plasma showed a linear and inverse relationship between concentrations of hormone and calcium in the blood perfusate (Sherwood *et al.*, 1968; Mayer *et al.*, 1969; Mayer, 1973). The conclusion was that calcium regulates hormone secretion predominantly through a mechanism of proportional control; a suggestion of derivative control was seen, however, under conditions of rapid change in calcium concentration. The syndrome of parturient paresis in cows has been studied as a model of secondary hyperparathyroidism. These animals develop parathyroid gland hyperplasia as an adaptation to the mild, chronic hypocalcemia that occurs during pregnancy (Buckle *et al.*, 1969; Mayer *et al.*, 1969; Mayer, 1970; Blum *et al.*, 1974). The changes in hormone concentration in peripheral blood that occur during spontaneous or artificially induced hypocalcemia in these parturient cows vastly exceed the responses seen in nonparturient cows (Mayer, 1970). The greatest increase in plasma hormone detected after maximal hypocalcemic challenge in nonparturient cows is two- to threefold. In contrast, hormone concentrations may rise as much as 20-fold in blood of parturient cows with parathyroid hyperplasia and secondary hyperparathyroidism.

Even in states of exaggerated hormone secretion (such as seen in parturient cows with secondary hyperparathyroidism), the inverse relationship between hormone and calcium concentrations remained, although the slope of the line relating hormone secretion rate to blood calcium was much steeper in parturient cows with secondary hyperparathyroidism than in the nonparturient cows (Mayer, 1970).

At the time these studies were performed, the heterogeneity of circulating hormone and the variable rate of metabolic clearance of different fragments were not known. Subsequent, direct measurements of secretion rate (see below) have led to better definition of specific details of control of hormone secretion by blood calcium.

2. Determination of Secretion Rate and Reserve of the Parathyroid Gland

The results of studies of hormone levels in peripheral blood in response to changes in blood calcium are not a true reflection of hormone secretion rate, owing to distortion introduced by the heterogeneity of immunoreactive hormone. The true values for concentration of biologically active hormone and for rates of secretion and disappearance cannot be established by studies solely dependent on measurements of peripheral immunoreactive hormone. The observed patterns of secretion and metabolism of hormone are distorted in most immunodetection systems by the presence of multiple forms of hormone that differ in biological activity and metabolic rate.

Mayer (1973) avoided the difficulties introduced by peripheral metabolism of hormone by directly assessing hormone secretion rate in calves by analysis of hormone concentration in parathyroid effluent blood. Parathyroid hormone secretion rate was measured directly in anesthetized calves by determination of the arteriovenous difference in hormone concentration across a superior parathyroid gland. Blood flow was determined by collection of parathyroid venous effluent. Under basal resting conditions, the average rate of secretion was 1 ng/kg/min in three normocalcemic calves. In a 500-kg cow, this would extrapolate to ~ 0.5 μg/min. When calcium concentration of arterial blood perfusing the gland was altered by infusion of either calcium chloride or disodium EDTA into a jugular vein, secretion rate was inversely related to arterial calcium concentration in a graded manner over a relatively narrow range of calcium concentration (Fig. 14). Above 10.5 mg/100 ml, a basal secretion rate (secretion rates were calculated for all glands by extrapolation of the results obtained from a single gland) of approximately 0.3 ng/kg per min was maintained despite induction of hypercalcemia. Below 10.5 mg/100 ml, a slowly induced decline of calcium concentration in three calves elicited a progressive increase in secretory rate, which rose to 1 ng/kg per

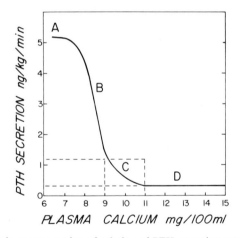

Fig. 14. Schematic representation of relation of PTH secretion rate to plasma calcium based on data obtained from studies on calves. Parathyroid venous effluent was collected from anesthetized calves during periods of induced changes in blood calcium. PTH was measured by radioimmunoassay. Four separate regions are represented on the curve by the letters A–D. Region C lies within the range of physiological regulation; region B reflects the rapid increase in secretion rate that occurs in response to hypocalcemia, reaching a maximum at a plasma calcium of approximately 7 mg per 100 ml. A low but substantial secretion of PTH persists, despite increasing hypercalcemia (region D). Dashed lines indicate range of normal basal plasma calcium and PTH concentrations. (G. P. Mayer, 1973 studies; cited in Habener and Potts, 1976c.)

min at 9 mg/100 ml and approached a maximum of about 5 ng/kg per min near 8 mg/100 ml. Further decreases in calcium concentration induced little or no change in secretory rate.

The steep response in rate of secretion of hormone in the mildly hypocalcemic range suggests a secretory control mechanism more appropriate for calcium homeostasis than a proportional secretory response operating over a wide range of calcium concentration—the latter mechanism having been deduced in the earlier studies (Sherwood et al., 1966). The finding by Mayer et al. (1976) of a persistent rate of secretion under basal conditions independent of blood calcium concentration was an unexpected finding. Hormone secretion continued even when the calcium concentration of the blood was maintained at 16–18 mg/dl for 48 hours (Mayer et al., 1976). It is not known whether the molecular composition of the hormone secreted under these conditions of unusually high calcium concentration is identical to that of intact hormone or whether, for example, the hormone consists of either biologically active or inactive fragments. On the other hand, if the hormone secreted during suppression of the gland by high calcium is biologically active, this situation provides an explanation of the defect in secretory control that is characteristically seen in patients with primary hyperparathyroidism due to adenomas of the parathyroid glands (see below).

Although it is not known whether synthesis of new hormone, which must ultimately replenish that which is secreted, is directly related to increased secretion or is controlled independently by calcium, it appears, from detailed analyses of cows, that hormone secretion in the parathyroid gland is closely coupled to synthesis of new hormone.

Inasmuch as the parathyroid mass in an adult cow is approximately 1 gm (Mayer et al., 1968), and the content of glandular hormone determined by radioimmunoassay is approximately 200 μg/gm wet gland weight (Hamilton et al., 1971b; Habener et al., 1976c), it becomes apparent that the gland contains sufficient stored hormone to provide basal secretory needs for approximately 400 minutes at 0.5 μg/min. When hormone secretion was stimulated, however, either in vivo by induced hypocalcemia via administration of an infusion of EDTA, or in vitro by lowering the calcium concentration in the incubation medium, the rate of secretion of hormone was shown to increase maximally approximately fivefold. These estimates indicate that biosynthesis of new hormone by the parathyroid gland is required within 7 hours under conditions of normal secretion and within $1\frac{1}{2}$ hours under conditions of sustained maximum stimulation.

The secretory reserve of the parathyroid glands is, therefore, somewhat limited compared with other endocrine glands, such as the pituitary (Finkelstein et al., 1972) and pancreatic islet cells (Humbel et al., 1972), where stores are sufficient to meet normal physiological secretory demands for days. The relatively low content of the stored hormone in the parathyroid is consistent with microscopic studies of the parathyroid gland that demonstrated sparse numbers of secretory granules (Roth and Schiller, 1976).

E. Biosynthesis of Parathyroid Hormone: Precursors of Parathyroid Hormone, Proparathyroid Hormone, and Pre-Proparathyroid Hormone

During the past several years, considerable advance has been made in our knowledge of the pathways involved in the biosynthesis of parathyroid hormone. The establishment of suitable *in vitro* systems, which allow for the control of certain nonspecific influences on cellular secretion that may becloud results from studies done in *in vivo* systems, has made it possible to investigate the pathways and specific regulation of intracellular processes in the parathyroid gland.

It is now known that parathyroid hormone is biosynthesized in the cell in the form of two larger precursors termed preproparathyroid hormone and proparathyroid hormone. Hamilton *et al.* (1971b) first suggested the existence of a proparathyroid hormone, an immediate cellular precursor of parathyroid hormone. Subsequently, formal kinetic proof was shown for a precursor-to-product relationship between the prohormone peptide and parathyroid hormone (Kemper *et al.*, 1972; Cohn *et al.*, 1972). Working with both human (Habener *et al.*, 1972a; Chu *et al.*, 1973b) and bovine (Kemper *et al.*, 1972; Cohn *et al.*, 1972; Habener *et al.*, 1973a) parathyroid tissue *in vitro*, it was shown by chromatographic or electrophoretic analysis of parathyroid extracts that proparathyroid hormone is labeled before parathyroid hormone during short incubations of tissue with radioactive amino acids and that the prohormone is progressively converted to the hormone after a delay of approximately 30 minutes (Fig. 15). When further incorporation of labeled amino acids was inhibited after a short initial incubation by addition of an excess of unlabeled amino acids, the radioactivity in the proparathyroid hormone decreased, whereas that in parathyroid hormone continued to increase. Similar results were obtained when protein synthesis was inhibited with puromycin, indicating that the continued synthesis of protein was not required for the transformation of the prohormone to the hormone.

It is important to distinguish conceptually between these studies describing the identification of a prohormone and those of Sherwood *et al.* (1970) and Arnaud *et al.* (1971a) in which the intact hormone itself was incorrectly termed a prohormone. At that time it was believed that the

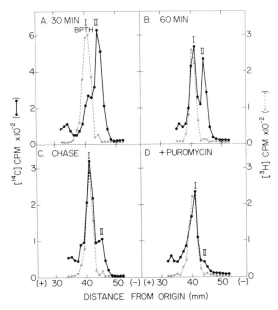

Fig. 15. Electrophoretic analysis of extracts from parathyroid adenoma tissue to illustrate precursor–product relation between PTH (I) and ProPTH (II). Acid–urea extracts of tissue were analyzed after incubation of parathyroid tissue at 37°C under the following conditions: (A) 30-minute and (B) 60-minute incubation in ^{14}C-labeled amino acids: (C) after replacement with a medium containing unlabeled amino acids to block further incorporation of radioactive amino acids; (D) after addition of an inhibitor of amino acid incorporation after 90 minutes. Although incorporation of labeled amino acids was completely inhibited by the addition of unlabeled amino acids and puromycin, peak I continued to rise in concentration, that is, in content of radioactive amino acids, indicating conversion by proteolytic enzymes. The ^{3}H-labeled bovine PTH, previously purified by gel electrophoresis, was added to the extracts before electrophoresis to mark the mobility of PTH. (From Habener *et al.,* 1972a.)

intact hormone was not the form in which hormone was secreted, but rather that hormonal fragments were the principal secretory product (see section II, C; Fig. 13). Thus, intact hormone was described as a prohormone in the sense that it was the predecessor of the secreted form of the hormone. The confusion arose because it was not recognized at that time that under conditions of long-term incubations *in vitro* (greater than 6 hours), proteolytic cleavage of PTH occurs in organ cultures of parathyroid tissue (such cleavage is not seen with shorter periods of incubation) and results in the secretion of fragments of the hormone into the media.

Proparathyroid hormone (see Section II, B; Fig. 7) differs chemically from parathyroid hormone in that it has an additional hexapeptide sequence at the N-terminus of the hormone.

In addition to studies with bovine parathyroid glands, investigations were carried out subsequently using parathyroid tissue of the human (Habener et al., 1972b; Chu et al., 1973b), rat (Chu et al., 1973a), and chicken (MacGregor et al., 1973). Proparathyroid hormones have been identified in all three species, and evidence obtained thus far indicates that their properties are similar to those of the bovine prohormone. A sequence identical to that found in the bovine was found for the human prohormone hexapeptide (Jacobs et al., 1974; Huang et al., 1975).

Recently, however, evidence was obtained showing the existence of a precursor even earlier than proparathyroid hormone. Direct translation of parathyroid messenger RNA in heterologous cell-free systems (wheat germ and Krebs II ascites tumor) resulted in the synthesis of a protein that is larger than ProPTH (Kemper et al., 1974a; Habener et al., 1975c). The additional 25 amino acid sequence of this protein, designated pre-proparathyroid hormone, is at the amino terminus of proparathyroid hormone (Fig. 7) (Kemper et al., 1976a). Pre-proparathyroid hormone has now been identified in intact parathyroid cells by pulse-labeling parathyroid slices for 2 minutes with [^{35}S]methionine (Habener et al., 1976b). Initially, there was the possibility of artifactual production of pre-proparathyroid hormone in the cell-free system, attributable to errors in translation of the messenger RNA (Kemper et al., 1974a); the cumulative evidence strongly indicates, however, that pre-proparathyroid hormone is indeed a short-lived precursor that is converted rapidly to proparathyroid hormone. If the observations indicating the existence of a pre-proparathyroid hormone are valid, similar short-lived prehormones should exist for polypeptide hormones other than parathyroid hormone. In fact, the recent demonstration of other such prehormones of proinsulin, ACTH, growth hormone, and prolactin has substantiated the findings obtained with the parathyroid hormone. Inasmuch as the pool size of pre-proparathyroid hormone in the tissue is extremely low in relation to parathyroid or even proparathyroid hormone, the possibility exists that a significant fraction of pre-proparathyroid hormone may be converted to proparathyroid hormone even before completion of synthesis of the nascent polypeptide chain.

The functions that the biosynthetic precursors for parathyroid hormone fulfill in the cell are unknown. They may serve to facilitate the intracellular transport of the hormonal polypeptide from its site of synthesis on the ribosome to the point of cleavage of ProPTH in the Golgi apparatus (Fig. 16).

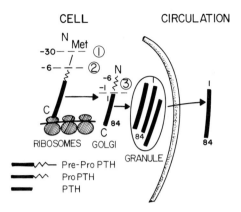

Fig. 16. Schema depicting intracellular pathway of the biosynthesis of parathyroid hormone. Pre-proparathyroid hormone (Pre-ProPTH), the initial product of synthesis on the ribosomes, is converted to proparathyroid hormone (ProPTH) by removal of N-terminal methionine (1) and N-terminal sequence of 24 additional amino acids (2) within seconds after synthesis. By 20 minutes after synthesis, ProPTH is transported to the Golgi region and is converted to PTH by removal of the N-terminal hexapeptide (3). PTH is stored in the secretory granule until released into the circulation in response to a fall in the blood calcium level. (From Habener and Potts, 1977.)

Under unusual circumstances, pre-proparathyroid hormone or pro-parathyroid hormone may not be cleaved and may accumulate in the cell or even be secreted. For example, Wong and Lindall (1973) reported the existence of several proteins from hyperplastic parathyroid tissue that are larger than proparathyroid hormone and that react with antisera to PTH. Benson *et al.* (1974) reported finding immunoreactive material of high molecular weight in blood of patients with ectopic hyperparathyroidism (secretion of parathyroid hormone-like material by tumors not of parathyroid origin). There is no direct evidence as yet, however, to substantiate this thesis.

One aspect of the chemistry of the precursor molecules remains unsettled. Analysis of the amino acid composition of the prohormone preparation that was used for sequence analysis has shown approximately 25 amino acids in addition to those of PTH (Cohn *et al.*, 1972), raising the possibility that these amino acids not accounted for at the amino terminus might represent sequence at the carboxyl terminus of ProPTH. The work of Habener *et al.* (1973a) and Kemper *et al.* (1976a) has not led to any evidence for a carboxyl-terminal extension of the hormone. Hamilton *et al.* (1975) continue to analyze this problem, which remains unsettled.

Radioimmunoassays that are specific for the detection of the bovine (Habener *et al.*, 1974a) and human (Habener *et al.*, 1976c) prohormone have been developed; these assays may prove useful in physiological studies of the prohormone as well as for detection of the peptide in tissue extracts and fluids and in blood. The recognition site of the antiserum used in the assay involves the sequence region at the site of attachment of the prohormone sequence to the hormone. The assay readily detects intact prohormone and synthetic peptides incorporating the prohormone sequence but not the hormone or hormonal fragments such as the pro-hormone hexapeptide sequence alone or the amino-terminal peptides of the hormone itself. Radioimmunoassays that are specific for the detection of pre-proparathyroid hormone have not yet been developed.

F. Control of the Biosynthesis and Secretion of Parathyroid Hormone

Very little information is available at present concerning the biochemical mechanisms through which calcium regulates the synthesis and secretion of parathyroid hormone. Compared with other endocrine glands, important differences are apparent in the effects of calcium on the secretion of parathyroid hormone. In endocrine tissue other than the parathyroids, additional tropic stimulation is necessary to demonstrate effects of calcium in the secretory process, e.g., in pancreatic islets and in the pituitary and adrenal cortex (Rubin, 1970), whereas the parathyroid glands respond to changes in the calcium concentration without the requirement of additional stimulatory agents. In addition, secretion of PTH varies inversely with the calcium concentration, whereas in most other endocrine systems, calcium stimulates secretion. These findings suggest that the response to calcium by the parathyroid cells must differ from that characteristic of other endocrine organs. Figure 17 schematically depicts

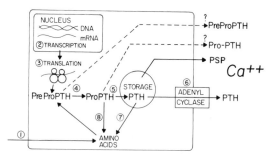

Fig. 17. Model of a parathyroid cell depicting steps in hormone synthesis and transport where calcium may be proposed to exert regulatory effects (circled numbers 1–8). Dotted arrows indicate possible release of precursors; PSP, a protein of MW 150,000, distinct from parathyroid hormone, is known to be released along with PTH in response to changes in calcium content. (From Habener, 1976.)

several proposed points in the functioning of the parathyroid cell where calcium may exert a regulatory influence on the cellular pathways involved in the synthesis and the secretion of parathyroid hormone.

Earlier evidence suggested that calcium may regulate the flow of amino acids into the parathyroid cell (Raisz and O'Brien, 1963), but the observations have not been investigated further by newer techniques. Nothing is known directly about the possible effects of calcium on regulation of messenger RNA synthesis or possible action of calcium on translational events, i.e., peptide initiation, elongation, or termination. It is not even known whether calcium exerts any direct effects on hormone biosynthesis or whether changes in rates of hormone biosynthesis occur only in response to calcium-mediated changes in glandular secretion.

Calcium has been shown to alter biosynthesis of parathyroid hormone *in vitro*. The results of studies by Hamilton *et al.* (1971a) and Habener *et al.* (1975a), however, differed with respect to the amounts of radioactive hormone appearing in bovine parathyroid slices during *in vitro* incubations. The earlier studies of Hamilton indicated that the amount of hormone was inversely related to the calcium concentrations in the media, whereas Habener found a direct relationship. The latter observation indicates that increased storage of hormone occurs as a result of suppression of normal secretion induced by elevated concentrations of calcium and, conversely, that hormone stores are depleted during hypocalcemic stimulation of secretion. The amounts of prohormone, however, were noted to decrease with increasing calcium in the media by approximately 15% over a 4-hour period of incubation of the gland slices (Habener *et al.,* 1975a). The relatively small changes in prohormone synthesis in response to changes in calcium concentration are most consistent with transcriptional rather than translational regulation of hormone synthesis. In these studies, synthesis of nonhormonal proteins was found to be independent of the calcium concentration.

The conversion of proparathyroid hormone to PTH seems to be a likely point in the schema of regulation by calcium. Studies thus far, however, have indicated that calcium probably has no direct immediate effects on the activity of the enzyme(s) involved in proteolytic cleavage of ProPTH to PTH (Habener *et al.,* 1974b). The results of these studies indicate that calcium probably does not serve as an essential cofactor for the activity of the cleavage enzyme. Parathyroid glands that have been chronically suppressed by hypercalcemia, however, appear to convert ProPTH to PTH at a lesser efficiency than do nonsuppressed glands (Chu *et al.,* 1973a). The observations in chronically stimulated glands probably reflect an overall adaptive alteration in the cellular biosynthetic machinery, including the amount of the proparathyroid hormone-cleaving enzyme.

Many studies describe the effects of calcium on parathyroid hormone secretion. Patt and Luckhardt (1942) established that the secretion of parathyroid hormone *in vivo* is inversely related to the concentration of calcium in the blood perfusing the gland. These observations were confirmed by Copp and Davidson (1961) and by Sherwood *et al.* (1966) in studies in which radioimmunoassay was used to measure secretion from isolated perfused glands *in vivo*. In addition to these studies *in vivo*, numerous analyses of hormone secretion *in vitro* (Sherwood *et al.*, 1970; Hamilton *et al.*, 1971b; Oldham *et al.*, 1971; Kemper *et al.*, 1974b; Habener *et al.*, 1975a) supported the observations made *in vivo*. Despite the recognition that calcium controls hormonal secretion, there is little information regarding biochemical mechanisms through which the secretory activity of the parathyroid gland responds to changes in the concentration of extracellular calcium.

Furthermore, although calcium appears to be the principal factor that regulates secretion of PTH, other substances may also affect secretion. Some studies showed that magnesium ion is equivalent to calcium ion in blocking (hypermagnesemia) or stimulating (hypomagnesemia) the release of hormone (Targovnik *et al.*, 1971), whereas others indicate that calcium is 2 to 3 times more potent than magnesium (Mayer, 1974; Habener and Potts, 1976a). It seems unlikely, therefore, that magnesium plays an important physiological role in control of hormone secretion (since magnesium is less potent and yet is present in blood at much lower concentrations than calcium). Recent evidence indicates that severe hypomagnesemia (and/or the accompanying intracellular magnesium deficit), rather than stimulating hormone production, leads to a blockade in hormone release (Anast *et al.*, 1972; Suh *et al.*, 1973; Levi *et al.*, 1974; Rude *et al.*, 1976). Studies in man suggested that infusion of strontium may also suppress hormone secretion.

The divalent cations may not be the sole determinants regulating parathyroid hormone secretion. The hormones glucagon (Cushard *et al.*, 1971), calcitonin (Fischer *et al.*, 1971), and even epinephrine (Fischer *et al.*, 1973; Blum *et al.*, 1975) may stimulate secretion of parathyroid hormone, but the physiological significance of these hormones as secretagogues is still unknown. From studies in cows, Reitz *et al.* (1971) concluded that calcitonin does not have a direct effect but only influences secretory rate secondarily through effects on plasma calcium concentration. On the other hand, at high concentrations (100 ng/ml or greater), calcitonin was reported to release PTH from glandular tissue incubated *in vitro* (Fischer *et al.*, 1971; Sherwood and Abe, 1972). Deftos and co-workers (1971) observed an abrupt increase in the circulating levels of PTH during calcium infusion in several patients with medullary carcinoma of the thyroid (Chapter 4). The hypercalcemia caused not only a release of calcitonin from the tumor, but a paradoxical increase in circulating PTH; the normal response to hypercalcemia would be a decrease in circulating parathyroid hormone due to suppression of secretion. Again the very high levels of calcitonin released in this disease state *in vivo* raised the question that very high levels of calcitonin may release parathyroid hormone; the physiological significance of calcitonin as a secretagogue for PTH, however, has not been shown. Phosphate was shown to have no direct effect on hormone secretion, but stimulates the parathyroid gland through a lowering of the concentration of calcium (Sherwood *et al.*, 1968). There is no evidence for a critical involvement of a specific nerve or blood supply in the regulation of parathyroid glandular activity (Potts and Deftos, 1974).

Adenosine 3':5'-monophosphate (cyclic AMP) has been implicated as an intermediate in the action of calcium on parathyroid hormone secretion. Perfusion of parathyroid glands *in vivo* (Abe and Sherwood, 1972) with solutions containing dibutyryl cyclic AMP, an analogue of cyclic AMP that can freely enter cells, stimulates secretion of bioassayable and immunoassayable parathyroid hormone even in the presence of high concentrations of calcium that ordinarily suppress hormone secretion. In addition, studies on the activity of adenylyl cyclase in canine parathyroid homogenates have shown an unusual sensitivity to calcium (Dufresne *et al.*, 1971). Concentrations of ionic calcium as low as 1×10^{-7} M inhibit activity of the enzyme. These ionic calcium concentrations are less than 1% of those required to produce significant inhibition of adenylyl cyclase in other tissues. The data suggest that adenylyl cyclase may play a specific role in mediating the known effects of calcium on parathyroid function. Studies *in vivo* (Fischer *et al.*, 1973; Blum *et al.*, 1975) and *in vitro* (Sherwood and Abe, 1972) suggest that the stimulation of parathyroid hormone release might involve β-adrenergic receptors. Epinephrine and isoproterenol, but not norepinephrine (all at concentrations of 0.1 mM), release PTH into the media during the incubation of parathyroid tissue *in vitro* (Sherwood and Abe, 1972), and infusion of epinephrine (0.08 μmole/min) into cows *in vivo* results in an increase in the PTH concentration in peripheral plasma (Fischer *et al.*, 1973) and in venous effluent from the parathyroid gland (Blum *et al.*, 1975). The stimulatory effect of the catecholamine was prevented by administration of the β-adrenergic blocking agent propranolol. These observations, which suggest that stimulation of β-adrenergic receptors in parathyroid tissue causes increased hormone secretion, are consistent with the general concept that the action of β-adrenergic agents is mediated by increases in cyclic AMP in target tissues (Ball *et al.*, 1972).

Although many studies have been carried out with parathyroid tissue incubated with labeled amino acids, a systematic analysis of the products of secretion was undertaken only recently. Electrophoresis of the radiolabeled protein secreted into the media during *in vitro* incubation of bovine parathyroid slices with [³H]leucine has shown, in addition to secretion of PTH, another major protein of MW 150,000 (distinct from the ProPTH fraction) secreted by gland tissue (Kemper *et al.*, 1974b). The amount of this protein secreted into the medium is dependent on the extracellular concentrations of calcium, as is PTH. This high-molecular-weight protein, the role of which is still unknown, may have a function in the intracellular transport and secretion of PTH, similar to that of neurophysin (Fawcett *et al.*, 1968). Neurophysin is known to transport oxytocin and vasopressin in the cell and to be secreted from the cells of origin along with these hormones.

It is important to recognize another mechanism of potential importance in the regulation of parathyroid hormone production. Evidence was reported supporting the existence of calcium-dependent degradative pathways for parathyroid hormone (Habener *et al.*, 1975a) and also for pro-parathyroid hormone (Chu *et al.*, 1973a). These conclusions were derived from the experimental observations *in vitro* that the intracellular accumulation and depletion of hormone stores in response to changes in extracellular concentrations of calcium could not be entirely accounted for by formation and secretion of hormone. Additional studies will be required to determine whether this process is important in the overall regulation of hormone biosynthesis and secretion *in vivo*.

G. Summary

Parathyroid hormone undergoes multiple, specific cleavages from the point of initial cellular biosynthesis to ultimate disappearance from the circulation (Fig. 18). The first of these cleavages occurs in the cell when pre-proparathyroid hormone is converted to proparathyroid hormone. Then ProPTH is converted to PTH, the predominant species of the hormone, which is stored in the gland and is secreted into the circulation. After secretion, the hormone then undergoes a third cleavage in the peripheral circulation into at least one biologically inactive fragment of a molecular weight of approximately 7000. A second fragment, which may be biologically active, may also be formed; whether it is present in the general circulation is still not certain. These specific cleavage steps could serve as points of metabolic control regulating both the amount of biologically active hormone available for secretion (intraglandular cleavage) and the concentration of hormonally active peptides circulating and interacting

CELL CIRCULATION PERIPHERAL ORGAN

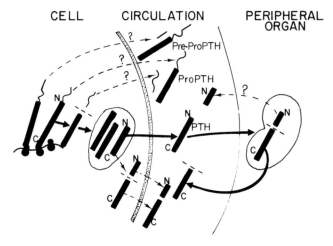

Fig. 18. Schematic model summarizing present information and concepts of biosynthesis, secretion, and metabolism of parathyroid hormone and the origins of the heterogeneity of immunoreactive parathyroid hormone in the circulation. In addition to release of intact hormone from the parathyroid cell (pathway denoted by heavy arrows), there may be release of prohormone or the prohormone-specific hexapeptide after cleavage from the precursor, pre-proparathyroid hormone (the ribosomal precursor of ProPTH), or possibly of fragments of PTH formed by proteolytic breakdown of PTH in the cell (?). Uptake of hormone after secretion occurs in peripheral organs (perhaps target organs, e.g., kidney), followed by a second cleavage; the larger biologically inactive C fragment reenters the circulation, but the fate of the smaller N fragment, which may be biologically active (and may be released adjacent to the receptors), is at present uncertain (?). The N fragment may not reenter the circulation. Fragments of hormone may also arise from peripheral metabolism, as well as be released from the gland. (From Habener and Potts, 1977.)

with receptors in bone and kidney (peripheral cleavage). In addition, the biosynthetic precursors, pre-proparathyroid hormone and proparathyroid hormone, may be secreted into the circulation. Presumably, the prohormones also would undergo specific cleavages, resulting in the formation of hormonal fragments.

Although present evidence indicates that cleavage occurs peripherally after secretion of the hormone in the circulation, other evidence indicates that fragments of the intact hormone are secreted from the gland. The amount of any such secreted fragments, even if small relative to intact hormone, could contribute to the forms of hormone found in the circulation, if the rate of disappearance of the fragments from the circulation was considerably slower than the disappearance of intact hormone, which Silverman and Yalow (1973) suggested may occur in renal failure. Present evidence, however, based on the studies of Habener *et al.* (1971b, 1972b), Segre *et al.* (1974), and Habener *et al.* (1976a), favors the view that peripheral cleavage is the principal source of the circulating fragments of hormone detected.

Many issues remain to be resolved about the biosynthesis, control of secretion, and metabolism of PTH. The nature and specificity of the enzymatic cleavages have not yet been determined. It is also unknown whether the pattern of cleavage and subsequent clearance are the same in any one individual under different physiological circumstances or from one individual to another within the human or other species. The similarity observed in the size and immunochemical characteristics of the large hormonal fragment detected on gel filtration of plasma samples from different patients, as well as the closely similar profiles seen for man, cows, and dogs, suggests that considerable similarities exist in the overall metabolism of parathyroid hormone in the mammalian species. At the center of these issues is the still unclear physiological significance of the peripheral metabolism of parathyroid hormone. Recent studies (Goltzman *et al.*, 1976) have indicated that the intact hormone is active without cleavage in *in vitro* assays employing renal cortical tissue. It still remains possible, however, that peripheral metabolism of parathyroid hormone, at least in part, represents an activation process analogous to conversion of angiotensin I to II. Active fragments produced may have a spectrum or duration of action different from that of the native molecule. Alternatively, the principal role of peripheral metabolism may be merely a catabolic function, namely, the elimination of hormone from extracellular fluid, once it is secreted. An efficient mechanism for hormonal clearance or destruction may be equally as important as careful modulation of secretion in controlling the concentration of hormone in blood and tissue fluids for homeostatic function. In disease states such as chronic renal failure or in altered physiological states, alterations in metabolism may contribute to changes in concentration of circulating hormone.

Systematic studies to assess these fundamental issues in terms of their physiological significance have not yet been reported; when available, the information concerning details of biosynthesis, secretion, and metabolism may considerably refine understanding of the pathophysiology of many diseases involving disorders of parathyroid function.

III. PRIMARY HYPERPARATHYROIDISM

Primary hyperparathyroidism is a disorder due to an excessive secretion of parathyroid hormone (Albright and Reifenstein, 1948). The abnormal concentration of circulating hormone usually leads to hypercalcemia and hypophosphatemia. Associated with these disturbances in mineral ion metabolism may be recurrent nephrolithiasis, peptic ulcers, mental changes, excessive bone resorption, and other more-subtle complications.

This disorder was first recognized as a clinical entity over 50 years ago when it was discovered that surgical removal of parathyroid adenomas led to cure of the malady (Mandl, 1926; Gold, 1928; Barr *et al.*, 1929; Wilder, 1929). Albright and associates contributed considerably toward the understanding of the pathophysiology of this disease and described many of its protean manifestations (Albright *et al.*, 1934; Albright and Reifenstein, 1948). An account of one of the first patients studied in depth was reported by Bauer and Federman (1962).

A number of reviews describing large series of patients with primary hyperparathyroidism have appeared (Norris, 1946; Howard *et al.*, 1953; Cope, 1969, 1966; Deating, 1961; Hellström and Ivemark, 1962; Riddick and Reiss, 1962; Dent, 1964, cited by Pyrah *et al.*, 1966; Riddick, 1967; Lloyd, 1968; Wang, 1971, 1976; Aurbach *et al.*, 1973; Watson, 1974).

A. Incidence

Primary hyperparathyroidism most commonly occurs in adults, with peak incidence between the third and fifth decades, and is 2 to 3 times more common in women than in men (Hellström and Ivemark, 1962; Watson, 1974). The disease has been detected in young children (Chaves-Carballo and Hayles, 1966), and the initial diagnosis has been made also in the elderly (Hellström and Ivemark, 1962; Riddick, 1967).

Patients may go for years with undetected hyperparathyroidism because of minimal symptoms (Randall and Keating, 1958; Riddick, 1967). On the other hand, manifestations of the disease may appear abruptly in a few instances, and some patients may exhibit severe complications, such as marked dehydration and coma associated with severe hypercalcemic "parathyroid crisis" (Wilson *et al.*, 1964).

The disease formerly had been regarded as rare. Recently, however, with improved recognition and wider use of routine screening techniques, the diagnosis has been made much more often than in earlier decades (Cope, 1960; Boonstra and Jackson, 1965, 1971; Purnell *et al.*, 1971).

The increased recognition of asymptomatic hyperparathyroidism is ascribable to the increased frequency of detection of hypercalcemia through routine estimation of serum calcium in annual physical examinations, a practice encouraged by the availability and economy of multiphase automated clinical chemistry procedures.

The discovery of asymptomatic hyperparathyroidism in so many individuals has led to considerable uncertainty about both the absolute incidence and natural history of the disease. If the large number of patients with elevated blood calcium levels but without detectable clinical aberrations are simply in the early stages of their disease (which might be associated with complications in subsequent years), then hyperparathyroidism as a disease entity is considerably more common than earlier estimates would have indicated. Two decades ago the incidence was estimated to be approximately 1 case per 10,000 persons per year—based on detection rates in patients with kidney stones (Melick and Henneman, 1958). Purnell et al. (1974) and Boonstra and Jackson (1965), by contrast, have more recently estimated the incidence to be as high as 1 case per 1000 persons per year based on an index of detection of hypercalcemia in routine examinations of healthy subjects.

If, on the other hand, these apparently healthy patients, more numerous than those with symptomatic disease, have had their hyperparathyroidism for years and continue to be asymptomatic after initial recognition, then the natural history in these individuals must differ greatly from the more severe form of hyperparathyroidism that has been classically recognized. It may be that certain compensatory mechanisms, hormonal or metabolic, block the effects of excessive parathyroid secretion in the asymptomatic, healthy patients. The implications for management of the mild or asymptomatic form of the disease may be different than in symptomatic patients; in the latter group surgical correction is clearly indicated, but it is unclear whether surgery is needed in the asymptomatic patients. Studies in several centers are presently underway in an effort to determine the natural history of apparently asymptomatic hyperparathyroidism (Riggs et al., 1971; Purnell et al., 1974; R. M. Neer, unpublished observations).

B. Etiology and Pathology

Normally four parathyroid glands are present in the neck in tissue adjacent to the thyroid and/or thymus (Fig. 19). In a study of the distribution of normal glands in 160 autopsies of patients dying from causes unrelated to parathyroid disease, 156 subjects had four glands, 3 had five glands, and 1 had six glands (Wang, 1976). The usual position occupied by the upper glands was posteriorly at the cricothyroid junction (77%) or behind the upper pole of the thyroid (22%). Of 312 parathyroid glands examined, only 3 upper glands were found behind the upper esophagus (Wang, 1976). The position of the normal lower glands varied more widely, from within the thymus to regions adjacent to the lower pole of the thyroid (Wang, 1976). The lower glands were ectopically located more frequently than the upper glands. Several were at the carotid bifurcation,

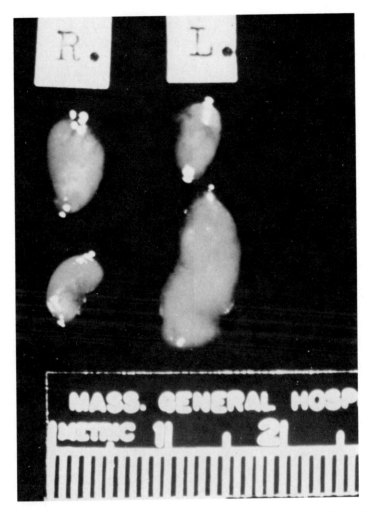

Fig. 19. Gross appearance of four normal parathyroid glands removed at autopsy to illustrate relatively small size and variation in appearance. (Courtesy of the Department of Pathology, Massachusetts General Hospital.)

and the remainder were with thymic remnants near the carotid sheath at the thoracic inlet or within the mediastinum.

Enlargement of only a single gland is sufficient to cause excessive hormone secretion. This is the most common cause of primary hyperparathyroidism (Table II). The enlarged gland is usually classified as a benign adenoma (Fig. 20); only rarely is it a malignant carcinoma (Fig. 21). In 10–15% of cases of primary hyperparathyroidism, enlargement or

TABLE II

Frequency of Causes of Primary Hyperparathyroidism at the Massachusetts General Hospital

	1930–1951	1952–1961	1962–1971	1972–1976	1930–1976
Adenoma	107 (83%)	88 (77%)	185 (81%)	219 (86%)	599 (83%)
Single	104 (81%)	86 (75%)	184 (81%)	219 (86%)	593 (82%)
"Double"[b]	3 (2%)	2 (2%)	1 (0.4%)	0 (0%)	6 (1%)
Hyperplasia	17 (13%)	21 (18%)	32 (14.1%)	35 (13.7%)	105 (15%)
Clear cell	11 (9%)	4 (4%)	1 (0.4%)	3 (1.2%)	19 (3%)
Chief cell	6 (5%)	17 (15%)	31 (13.6%)	32 (12.5%)	86 (12%)
Carcinoma	5 (4%)	5 (4%)	10 (4.4%)	2 (0.8%)	22 (3%)
Total	129	114	227	256	726

[a] Courtesy of Drs. C. A. Wang, O. Cope, B. Castleman and S. I. Roth. Cases include postmortem findings.

[b] Provisional diagnosis only; primary hyperplasia has not been excluded.

hyperplasia of all four glands occurs (Fig. 22). The abnormal gland is often found to develop in the inferior parathyroids and may be found in an unusual location in 6–10% of all patients examined. Such ectopic parathyroid adenomas may be located in the thymus, the thyroid, or even the pericardium as a consequence of incomplete or abnormal migration from their origin in the 3rd and 4th branchial pouches during embryological development (Wang, 1976). Retroesophageal adenomas have also been reported. Adenomas usually vary in size from 0.5 to 5 gm, although tumors as large as 10 to 20 gm are occasionally found. Histological examination most commonly reveals that the adenoma is composed primarily of chief cells (Fig. 23). Rarely, adenomas are composed of oxyphil cells or a mixed population of cells.

Adenoma of a single gland with atrophy in the others was regarded, in the past, as the most common cause of primary hyperparathyroidism (Roth, 1962, 1971). More recently, however, several pathologists and surgeons have subscribed to the view that hyperplasia in multiple glands is the most frequent cause of primary hyperparathyroidism (Paloyan et al., 1973).

Hyperplasia of all four parathyroids occurring in renal failure or other states of chronic hypercalcemia, presumably as a secondary or compensatory mechanism, has been known for many years (Pappenheimer and Wilens, 1935). Hyperplasia as the cause of primary hyperparathyroidism, that is, when the hyperplasia is the cause of a metabolic disorder rather than a compensatory response, has also been recognized. The nature of the stimulus that leads to the hyperplasia is unknown. Hyperplasia involv-

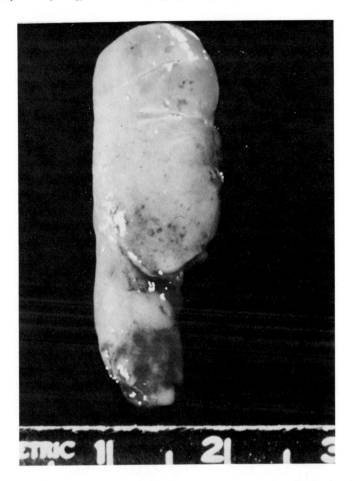

Fig. 20. A 0.2-gm parathyroid adenoma arising from a parathyroid gland to illustrate greater size than normal glands (Fig. 19). Adenoma is at top and is compressing remaining normal parathyroid tissue below. (Courtesy of the Department of Pathology, Massachusetts General Hospital.)

ing clear cells was described many years ago (Albright *et al.*, 1934) (Fig. 24). Later, appropriate emphasis was directed to the frequency of chief-cell hyperplasia as a cause of primary hyperparathyroidism (Cope *et al.*, 1961) (Fig. 23).

Paloyan *et al.* (1973) reviewed some of the concepts regarding the multiple-gland etiology of hyperparathyroidism, considered by some authors (Black and Utley, 1968; Golden and Canary, 1968) to reflect a more accurate picture than the traditional view that disease in a single gland is

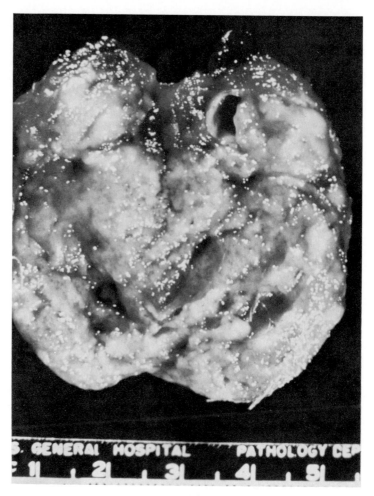

Fig. 21. Cut section of a parathyroid carcinoma showing highly irregular, gritty surface due to extensive fibrosis. (Courtesy of the Department of Pathology, Massachusetts General Hospital.)

usually responsible for primary hyperparathyroidism. Paloyan and associates reported that in approximately 50% of the patients with primary hyperparathyroidism, abnormalities may be found in most of the parathyroid glands if each of the glands is identified surgically, biopsied, and carefully examined. The changes involve either diffuse hyperplasia and/or a nodular hyperplasia. They stressed that most of all four parathyroid glands should be removed to effect true cure of hyperparathyroidism.

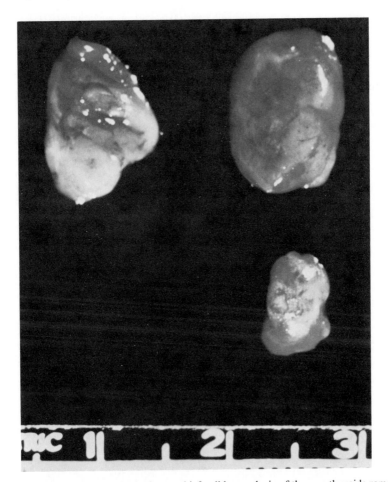

Fig. 22. Gross appearance of primary chief-cell hyperplasia of the parathyroids removed at surgery. Glands are irregular in outline and enlargement is variable. The fourth, a smaller gland, was left in the neck. (Courtesy of the Department of Pathology, Massachusetts General Hospital.)

In contrast, Roth (1971), Wang (1971), and Wang *et al.* (1975) have continued to maintain that, in over 80% of patients with primary hyperparathyroidism, a single abnormal gland or adenoma is the only abnormality (Table II). Wang *et al.* (1975) reported that in only 15% of the cases is multiple-gland disease present—an incidence that has remained relatively constant in the period between 1930 and 1976 (Table II, based on data kindly supplied by Drs. Wang, Cope, Roth, and Castleman).

It is generally agreed by all that it may be difficult by either gross or

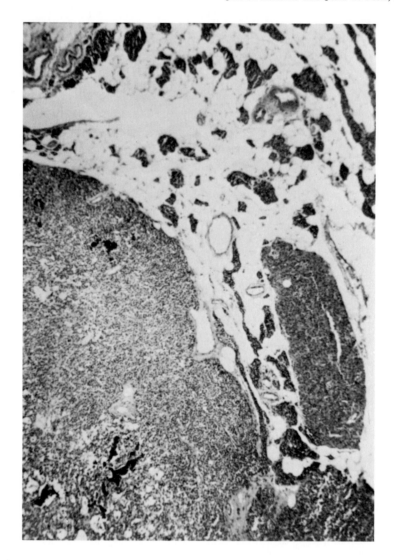

Fig. 23. Microscopic appearance of a chief-cell adenoma of the parathyroid gland. Adenoma is in lower-left half of the field. Normal parathyroid tissue with characteristic fatty stroma and islands of chief cells and oxyphil cells is seen in lower-left field. (Courtesy of the Department of Pathology, Massachusetts General Hospital.)

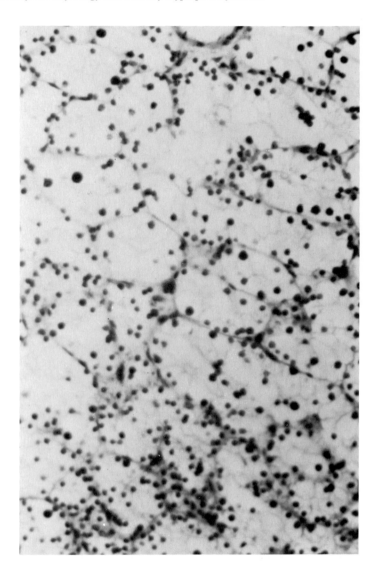

Fig. 24. Microscopic appearance of clear-cell hyperplasia of the parathyroid gland. Large clear cytoplasmic vacuoles and small nuclei are characteristic. (Courtesy of the Department of Pathology, Massachusetts General Hospital.)

histological examination to distinguish between adenoma and hyperplasia or to decide whether abnormalities are present in only one or all four parathyroid glands. Roth (1971) and Wang et al. (1975) have stressed the frequent asymmetry of the hyperplasia, that is, the degree of enlargement of the various glands may differ greatly (Fig. 22). In this situation, when an adenoma is present, examination of other glands reveals that they are of approximately normal size and appearance, 25–50 mg in average weight, and histologically normal. However, histological criteria are not absolute. The amount of fat found in a normal gland is a function of age (Roth, 1971), gradually increasing with advancing decades. In older persons the absence of significant numbers of fat cells in addition to the presence of uniform chief cells is evidence of hyperplasia. Such distinctions are more difficult to make in younger patients, in whose glands the absence of fat cells has little significance and need not imply hyperplasia. The older criterion of adenoma versus hyperplasia, namely, finding a rim of normal tissue around the tumor nodule in an adenoma ("encapsulation," Fig. 23), may not be found (Roth, 1971). Moreover, compression of tissue around an area of hyperplasia may give also the appearance of a capsule ("pseudoencapsulation") (Roth, 1971).

Accordingly, it is difficult to use histological criteria to reconcile the opposing viewpoints and to determine the frequency of multiple-gland disease. However, inasmuch as these different views of the pathology of hyperparathyroidism have led to different approaches in surgical management of patients, i.e., extensive surgical ablation versus limited extirpation (see Section III, F), careful follow-up evaluation of patients may prove revealing.

We favor the view that an abnormality limited to a single gland is the more common. Of the 525 new cases operated on at the Massachusetts General Hospital between 1932 and 1973, in 424 a single gland (adenoma) only was excised (Wang et al., 1975). In only three patients was the assessment subsequently recognized clinically to be incorrect and a second operation required because of persistent hypercalcemia. These patients proved to have multiple-gland involvement. There are, therefore, many accumulated symptom-free patient years after removal of a single gland. It will be essential in the future, however, to measure both blood calcium and parathyroid hormone levels at intervals in patients who have had a single gland removed to eliminate occult recurrence of hyperparathyroidism. If a high frequency of the latter was found to be present, this might lead to many symptomatic patients years later. On the other hand, studies seem necessary in those patients with subtotal parathyroidectomy to detect borderline or definite hypoparathyroidism, the principal clinical concern with extensive resection.

Parathyroid carcinoma is estimated to be found in approximately 3% of patients. The series of Paloyan *et al.* (1973) indicated an overall incidence of 2%, whereas Wang and Cope (Table III) currently report an incidence of 3%. On gross inspection, carcinoma of the parathyroid is characterized by the adherence of glandular tissue to surrounding structures. Histological criteria of Schantz and Castleman (1973) include the presence of

TABLE III

Frequency of Symptoms in Primary Hyperparathyroidism

	Study								Total cases with symptom
	Gordan *et al.*	Hellström and Ivemark	Wilson *et al.*	Pyrah *et al.*	Forland *et al.*	Wang	Aurbach *et al.*	Watson	
Year:	1962	1962	1964	1966	1968	1971	1973	1974	
No. of cases:	104	138	41	68	20	431	57	100	959
Symptoms Skeletal									
Skeletal pain:	—	28	2	11	1	93	5	13	153
%:		(20.3)	(4.9)	(16.2)	(5)	(22.6)	(8.8)	(13)	(16)
Renal colic:	76	101	27	27	11	238	12	47	539
%:	(73.1)	(73.2)	(65.9)	(39.7)	(55)	(57.6)	(21.1)	(47)	(56.5)
GI peptic ulcer:	7	15	4	1	2	74	10	12	125
%:	(6.7)	(10.9)	(9.8)	(1.5)	(10)	(17.9)	(17.5)	(12)	(14)
Pancreatic:	1	1	4	—	1	13	—	—	20
%:	(1.0)	(0.7)	(9.8)		(5)	(3.1)			(2.1)
Neuro-muscular:	—	—	—	—	2	8	14/16	—	24
%:					(10)	(1.9)	(88)		(5.1)
Psychiatric (depression):	—	11	—	—	1	4	11	2	29
%:		(8.0)			(5)	(1.0)	(19.3)	(2)	(3)
Constitutional fatigue, lethargy:	—	28	8	—	—	12	14	—	62
%:		(20.3)	(19.5)			(2.9)	(24.6)		(6.5)
Arthralgias:	—	See "Skeletal Pain"	—	—	—	3	6	—	9
%:						(0.7)	(10.5)		(0.9)
Hypertension:	30	14	—	2	9	6	—	4	65
%:	(28.8)	(10.1)		(2.9)	(45)	(1.6)		(4)	(6.8)
No symptoms:	11	—	—	0	0	4	—	8	23
%:	(10.6)			(0)	(0)	(1.0)		(8)	(24)

nuclear mitotic figures (normally none are seen in an entire section), fibrosis, and capsular or blood-vessel invasion (Fig. 25). Analysis of the data of Schantz and Castleman (1973) and of Wang *et al.* (1975) indicates that many carcinomas of the parathyroid often grow slowly, i.e., are relatively benign. If the involved parathyroid gland is removed without capsular rupture, long-term follow-up has generally shown no evidence of recurrence (Wang *et al.*, 1975), although there are reports of metastases before initial operation (Holmes *et al.*, 1969). When the

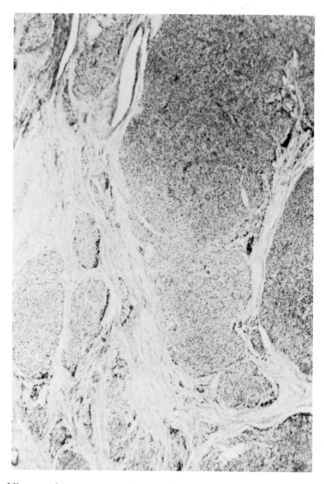

Fig. 25. Microscopic appearance of a parathyroid carcinoma, showing large islands of dense neoplastic chief cells separated by dense bands of connective tissue and occasional mitotic figures. (Courtesy of the Department of Pathology, Massachusetts General Hospital.)

parathyroid carcinoma does become metastatic, spread is usually to the lymphatics on the side of the neck where the original tumor developed (Wang *et al.*, 1975). Hematogenous spread (distant metastases) is less commonly seen; once hematogenous, parathyroid carcinoma localizes most frequently in the lung, but also in liver and bone (Holmes *et al.*, 1969). Of 50 cases reviewed by Holmes *et al.* (1969), 46 of the carcinomas were hyperfunctioning and 4 carcinomas were not associated with excessive parathyroid hormone secretion. Key features of these cases were the marked severity of hypercalcemia (greater than 14 mg/100 ml in 75% of cases) and a low overall cure rate (20% 7-year survival) (Holmes *et al.*, 1969). It was emphasized that survival is improved if capsular rupture at initial surgery is avoided. The poorer overall survival reported by Holmes *et al.*, in their cases collected largely from the literature, compared with the experience from one institution (Wang *et al.*) probably reflects the reporting of more serious cases as distinct from those in which the diagnosis is made on the basis of the microscopic criteria alone.

In the last several decades there has been increasing awareness of the hereditary aspects of hyperparathyroidism and the association of familial hyperparathyroidism with other well-defined, associated hereditable endocrine disorders. Several hundred families with familial hyperparathyroidism have been reported (Steiner *et al.*, 1968). Estimates of incidence suggest several thousand kindreds in the United States alone in which there is a genetic transmission of hyperparathyroidism and/or other endocrine tumors. In the personal experience of the authors within the last 5 years at the Massachusetts General Hospital, there have been 26 kindreds with one form of hereditary multiple endocrine disorders (MEN-I) and 4 kindreds with another form (MEN-II) newly detected.

Many features of these hereditary multiple-neoplasia syndromes remain obscure. At the present time, it is difficult to determine the natural history and true incidence of hereditary endocrinopathy in the general population; it is also difficult to determine the association of one discrete type of endocrine tumor with other types, the etiology of the syndromes, and the most efficient method for, and long-term result of, screening asymptomatic family members for preclinical disease.

Two basic syndromes are recognized, which are genetically distinct from one another (Fig. 26). The first, now termed multiple-endocrine-neoplasia type I, consists primarily of tumors of the parathyroid, pituitary, and pancreas; the second entity, termed multiple-encocrine-neoplasia type II, consists of medullary carcinoma of the thyroid, adrenal tumors (pheochromocytoma), and, again, tumors of the parathyroids.

Historically, the first report of association of two types of endocrine tumor in one patient dates from the report of Erdheim in 1903, in which a

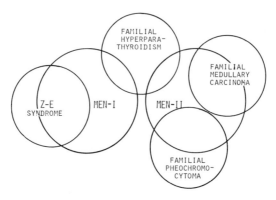

Fig. 26. Diagram to illustrate spectrum of hereditary disorders involving primary hyper-parathyroidism. The two multiple-endocrine-neoplasia syndromes (MEN-I and MEN-II) are genetically distinct, inasmuch as certain elements of one syndrome never occur in the other. Familial hyperparathyroidism is common to both. This syndrome, as well as the other disorders indicated, occurs not only as part of the multiple-neoplasia syndromes, but also as separate familial disorders.

pituitary tumor responsible for acromegaly was seen in association with parathyroid tumors. Cushing and Davidoff (1927) reported a patient with pituitary tumor, parathyroid tumors, and a pancreatic tumor. Rossier and Dressler in 1939 suggested that there might be a familial incidence of these multiple endocrine tumors. Wermer (1954) was the first to define the genetic aspects of the multiple endocrinopathies. He described a pattern that featured pituitary, pancreatic, and parathyroid tumors. Wermer correctly deduced that the high frequency with which one or more of these tumors was seen in family members from affected kindreds was compatible with an autosomal dominant inheritance. Further definition of several clinical features was documented in a report by Ballard *et al.* (1964) of 85 cases of what has been subsequently recognized as multiple-endocrine-neoplasia type-I-syndrome; they observed that 20–40% of patients with the Zollinger–Ellison syndrome have the multiple-endocrine-neoplasia syndrome.

The alternate syndrome, that of multiple-endocrine-neoplasia type II, was first reported as a suspected separate clinical entity by Sipple (1961). Schimke and Hartmann (1965), Schimke *et al.* (1968), and Steiner *et al.* (1968) all noted the linkage between pheochromocytoma and medullary carcinoma of the thyroid as originally described by Sipple, plus the additional features of parathyroid tumors and mucosal neuromas (see Chapter 2 for review). Steiner *et al.* (1968) deduced an autosomal dominant pattern of inheritance in a total of 29 families who exhibited pheochromocytoma, medullary carcinoma of the thyroid, and hyper-parathyroidism, and suggested nosological distinctions. They suggested the term multiple-endocrine-neoplasia type II (MEN-II) for the disorder involving the thyroid and adrenal, inasmuch as tumors of the pituitary and pancreas, common in the alternate endocrinopathy (which was then re-named endocrine-neoplasia-type-I syndrome, or MEN-I), were absent from the kindreds with thyroid and adrenal tumors.

It is particularly pertinent to decide whether the Zollinger–Ellison syn-drome (Ellison and Wilson, 1964; Fox *et al.*, 1974), familial medullary carcinoma of the thyroid (Williams, 1966; Block *et al.*, 1967), familial pheochromocytoma (Steiner *et al.*, 1968), and familial hyperparathyroidism (Marx *et al.*, 1973) can occur as entities separate from MEN-I or MEN-II. It is obviously important with regard to questions concerning the etiology and genetic features of the syndromes, as well as clinical management, to determine whether familial syndromes exist in which only one type of endocrine tumor is present. For example, it is at present still unclear whether all family members in a kindred, in which Zollinger-Ellison syndrome occurs in one individual, should be screened lifelong for other than gastrointestinal disease, i.e., features of multiple-endocrine-neoplasia type I. Unfortunately, it is impossible to predict accurately the hereditary linkages of different endocrine glands at present.

Most of the earlier reports involved a survey of kindreds over a limited time, although it was clear that there was occasionally a long delay (decades) in the appearance of the clinical manifestations of associated endocrine features. In addition, only recently have specific immunoassays for gastrin, calcitonin, parathyroid hormone, insulin, growth hormone, and prolactin and tests for catecholamine production and excretion been applied as screening tests. In the studies of Melvin *et al.* (1971) it was demonstrated that application of routine assays for calcitonin and parathyroid hormone at periodic intervals in asymptomatic individuals from kindreds with MEN-II syndrome can lead to the detection of medul-lary carcinoma and hyperparathyroidism before the onset of clinical symptoms. Hence, the actual frequency of multiple endocrine disorders in a given kindred or group of kindreds could, in earlier published reports, be easily underestimated. With the routine application of sensitive screening tests it should soon be possible to determine, as seems likely in one family with hyperparathyroidism recently reported (Goldsmith *et al.*, 1976), whether many kindreds have a single, rather than multiple, hereditary endocrine disorder.

Several explanations, none completely satisfactory, have been offered to explain the etiology of these syndromes. There have been speculations based on the observations of Pearse (1968) that the etiology underlying the multiple-endocrine-neoplasia syndromes involves a primary dysplasia of neuroectoderm (Weichert, 1970). Pearse (1976) reviewed and discussed the hypothesis that cells originally of neural-crest origin migrate widely during embryogenesis. The cells can be recognized by their histochemical characteristics (Amine Precursor Uptake plus Decarboxylation, hence the name APUD). Parafollicular cells of the thyroid, adrenal medullary cells, and cells in multiple sites in the gastrointestinal tract arise from the APUD series (Pearse, 1976). A neural-crest origin of parathyroid cells and of the cells of the anterior pituitary gland (growth hormone or prolactin-secreting) has not been regarded as likely. The theory of Weichert (1970), therefore, that primitive neural-crest cells migrate into and become the cell of origin of the hormones involved in hypersecretion, is not presently verifiable by embryological and histological evidence. Such a theory could not account for the clustering of pituitary and pancreatic neoplasia only in kindreds with the MEN-I syndrome and a similar, apparent segregation of parafollicular-cell and adrenal medullary tumors in the MEN-II syndrome. If a common cell type with ultimate dysplasia were the explanation, all endocrine tumors seen in the hereditary syndromes might be expected to appear in an affected kindred.

An additional explanation for the syndrome is that an initial overproduction of cne hormone leads to a compensatory response of another endocrine organ with hyperplasia and, eventually, neoplasia. Vance *et al.* (1969) offered the hypothesis that nesidioblastosis, or hypertrophy of pancreatic islet cells, led to overproduction of insulin and glucagon, which, in turn, stimulated excessive calcitonin release and, ultimately, parathyroid hyperplasia. Similar speculations have involved a stimulus/response association with medullary carcinoma and parathyroid hyperplasia in MEN-II.

The studies of Melvin *et al.* (1971) established, by serial testing of asymptomatic members of a large kindred with MEN-II syndrome, that elevated blood levels of parathyroid hormone (indicating hyperplasia) with normal blood levels of calcitonin were seen in some patients, whereas, in others, elevated calcitonin levels (medullary carcinoma) were associated with normal parathyroid hormone levels. These results are consistent with an independent appearance of the discrete forms of endocrine neoplasia. Thus, although a genetic pattern consistent with autosomal dominant inheritance of these syndromes has been demonstrated, a single, basic developmental defect explaining the peculiar linkage of some endocrine-gland tumors in the multiple-endocrine-neoplasia syndromes has so far eluded detection.

C. Clinical Manifestations

Most of the signs and symptoms of hyperparathyroidism reflect known pathophysiologic consequences of hypercalcemia (Tables III and IV). It is difficult to estimate accurately at present the true incidence of these complications, since many patients, now being discovered, have their hyperparathyroidism corrected surgically at a time when they are asymptomatic. In addition, a number of the important symptoms that are generally accepted as manifestations of primary hyperparathyroidism (particularly articular, neuromuscular, and certain gastrointestinal manifestations) were not appreciated in the earlier studies and hence were not reported.

Table IV gives the relative frequency of occurrence of renal involvement, bone involvement, and combinations of these diseases together. In the last decade and earlier, kidney involvement, particularly recurrent nephrolithiasis, was reported in 60–70% of patients (Krementz et al., 1967; Yendt and Gagne, 1968). The incidence of kidney involvement is less frequent today but is still the most frequent manifestation of primary hyperparathyroidism. Skeletal involvement, particularly osteitis fibrosa cystica, is seen much less frequently than before. Several groups have noted that hyperparathyroid patients with severe bone disease usually do not develop renal-stone disease and vice versa. Peacock (1975) has provided one explanation for this apparent paradox. He studied intestinal calcium absorption in 111 patients with primary hyperparathyroidism. Sixty-three of the 111 patients had renal-stone disease. The calcium absorption (fraction of dose absorbed per hour) in the group of "stone-formers" was higher (range 0.8 to 2.4) than in the hyperparathyroid patients without stones (0.3 to 1.5); in normal subjects, the average was 0.6. Thus, despite some overlap, most of the hyperparathyroid patients in whom stones formed had high rates of intestinal calcium absorption. Peacock reasoned that the increased throughput of calcium might protect against skeletal losses and predispose to renal calculi secondary to hypercalciuria.

1. Renal

The pathophysiologic effects of excessive parathyroid hormone on the kidney in patients with primary hyperparathyroidism can be considered in two broad categories: anatomic and functional. Under the category of anatomic defects is the occurrence of nephrolithiasis or nephrocalcinosis; under functional defects are included a spectrum of tubular and glomerular disorders that result from the deleterious effects of sustained hypercal-

Joel F. Habener and John T. Potts, Jr.

TABLE IV

Primary Hyperparathyroidism and Frequency of Skeletal and/or Renal Manifestation

Author	Year	No. of patients studied	Skeletal only No. pts.	(%)	Renal only No. pts.	(%)	Skeletal and renal No. pts.	(%)	Patients without manifestations No. pts.	(%)
Norris	1946	314	191	(61)	17	(5)	101	(32)	5	(2)
Albright and Reifenstein	1948	64	11	(17)	28	(44)	24	(38)	1	(2)
Hellström and Ivemark	1962	138	17	(12)	76	(55)	43	(31)	2	(1)
Chamberlin et al.	1963	32	1	(3)	20	(63)	7	(22)	4	(6)
Dent	1964	125	27	(22)	73	(58)	11	(9)	14	(11)
Wilson et al.	1964	41	5	(12)	27	(66)	10	(24)	—	—
Pyrah et al.	1966	68	17	(25)	26	(38)	20	(29)	3	(4)
Lloyd	1968	138	28	(20)	81	(59)	10	(7)	19	(14)
Forland et al.	1968	20	8	(40)	1	(5)	3	(15)	8	(40)
Total		940	305	(32)	349	(37)	229	(24)	56	(6)

Total patients with skeletal manifestations and total patients
with renal manifestations, with the inclusion of three studies not listed above

		No. of Patients Studied (%)	Skeletal		Renal	
		940	534	(57)	578	(62)
Gordan et al.	1962	107	22	(21)	85	(79)
Wang	1971	431	93	(22)	238	(55)
Watson	1974	100	47	(47)	13	(13)
Total		1578	696	(44)	914	(58)

cemia and/or excessive concentrations of parathyroid hormone, or both. Several observers, including Albright and Reifenstein (1948) and Hellström and Ivemark (1962), observed that patients with nephrocalcinosis usually do not have nephrolithiasis; similarly, patients with nephrolithiasis usually do not have nephrocalcinosis. In addition, nephrocalcinosis is most commonly seen in patients with severe primary hyperparathyroidism, particularly those with osteitis fibrosa cystica (Hellström and Ivemark, 1962).

The tables (III and IV) of the general incidence of clinical symptoms listed above show the frequency with which renal manifestations of one type or the other are seen in the large series of hyperparathyroidism that have been reported. Although frank osteitis fibrosa cystica and other severe complications of hyperparathyroidism are not seen as frequently as in former years, presumably reflecting milder forms of hyperparathyroidism detected in recent years, the overall incidence of nephrolithiasis remains quite high. In the report of Purnell *et al.* (1971) of patients with presumptive hyperparathyroidism but without symptoms at the time the diagnosis was established, the incidence of nephrolithiasis detectable radiographically was still 32%. It is not clear whether this high incidence of nephrolithiasis will continue to be found as more patients with hyperparathyroidism are detected with continued use of screening procedures in an unselected ambulatory population.

Hellström and Ivemark also noted (1962) that the presence of renal calcifications, whether nephrocalcinosis or nephrolithiasis, predisposes to superimposed urinary-tract infections. This complication may further aggravate irreversible impairment of renal function. This vicious circle of stone formation, infection, and further deterioration of renal function may partly explain the increased incidence of hypertension in association with hyperparathyroidism referred to elsewhere. Nephrocalcinosis in patients with hyperparathyroidism is also associated with discrete defects in renal tubular function (Morris *et al.*, 1972).

Despite the long clinical interest in hyperparathyroidism, there is relatively little information on the composition of the renal calculi. Melick and Henneman (1958), mentioning 10 patients with hyperparathyroidism in whom stone analyses were performed, reported that three of the calculi were calcium phosphate, one was calcium oxalate, five were mixtures of calcium phosphate and oxalate, and two were mixtures of magnesium ammonium phosphate and calcium phosphate and were stones of infected alkaline urines. Several stones from hyperparathyroid patients analyzed by Prien and Prien (1968) contained a mixture of calcium oxalate and calcium phosphate. Therefore, stones of alkaline urine are not the only stones found in hyperparathyroidism. Of course, working with such a small number of patients, it is possible that the stones had nothing to do with the hyperparathyroidism, and were only coincidentally discovered in the course of diagnostic procedures. Unfortunately, stone analyses have not been included in reports of large numbers of patients. One important report (McGeown, 1961) does document that the incidence of renal calculi decreases in patients whose hyperparathyroidism is successfully treated, confirming the general impression of the benefit of treatment.

A variety of renal functional abnormalities has been reported in hyperparathyroidism, even in the absence of detectable nephrocalcinosis and/or nephrolithiasis (Hellström and Ivemark, 1962; Thoren and Werner, 1969), and include elevation of blood urea nitrogen and serum creatinine, reflecting modest-to-marked reduction in glomerular filtration rate. Numerous renal tubular defects have also been described, particularly compromise of proximal tubular function with a reduction in net acid secretion (renal tubular acidosis of the proximal, or type I, category) (Morris *et al.*, 1972), aminoaciduria, glycosuria, and decrease in urinary concentrating capacity. These overall defects occur in a continuous spectrum of severity, and are influenced by anatomic changes in the kidney, such as calcium deposition and bacterial infection. In the latter category, more severe degrees of compromise of total renal function occur, often leading to further reduction of glomerular filtration rate. More-subtle types of tubular defects involving compromise of proximal tubular function and urinary concentrating ability may be found in the absence of roentgenographically demonstrable renal calcification or evidence of infection (Hellström and Ivemark, 1962; Epstein, 1968a; Morris *et al.*, 1972). The difficulty in estimating the true incidence of more-subtle tubular disorders involves the lack of detailed assessment of proximal and distal tubular function in most reported series of patients with hyperparathyroidism. The inability to excrete acid at normal rates (proximal RTA) is rather common in primary hyperparathyroidism, resulting in hyperchloremic acidosis and mild reduction in serum bicarbonate (Wills and McGowan, 1964; Epstein, 1968a, b; L. W. Gold *et al.*, 1973; Palmer *et al.*, 1974).

It was noted (Epstein, 1968a, b) that hypercalcemia per se produced experimentally (Richet *et al.*, 1963) or in disease states associated with hypercalcemia due to causes other than hyperparathyroidism, such as carcinoma and acute vitamin D intoxication (Heinemann, 1965; Verbanck, 1965), is usually associated with mild alkalosis rather than acidosis (Section III, E). Hence, Wills and McGowan (1964) and Palmer *et al.* (1974) found that hyperchloremia and/or mild reduction in serum bicarbonate serves to distinguish hyperparathyroidism from other causes of hypercalcemia.

The distinctions, however, are often subtle. Coe (1974), in a study of 13 patients, failed to detect a significant departure from normal in either serum chloride or serum bicarbonate levels. A lack of clear discrimination between nonparathyroid versus parathyroid-related hypercalcemic patients with hyperparathyroidism with regard to plasma chloride was also noted by Palmer *et al.* (1974); they made the interesting suggestion, however, that a discriminant value could be adduced when the tendency in hyperparathyroidism toward hyperchloremia and hypophosphatemia was combined by expressing a ratio of chloride to phosphate. Palmer *et al.* (1974), in this ratio analysis, found that the chloride-to-phosphate ratio ranged from 32 to 80% in hyperparathyroidism. Ninety-six percent of patients have a ratio of higher than 33%, whereas the ratio of chloride to phosphate ranged from 17 to 32% in those with hypercalcemia from other causes, with 92% having a ratio of less than 30.

In studies by Morris (1968, 1969) and Morris *et al.* (1971, 1972), close similarities were found in the abnormalities in renal function in patients with primary hyperparathyroidism and in patients with hereditary fructose intolerance. A patient with hereditary fructose intolerance and surgically induced hypoparathyroidism failed to respond to fructose administration, evidenced by the characteristic fall in bicarbonate reabsorption, until exogenous parathyroid hormone was administered. These findings are consistent with an effect of parathyroid hormone on the acidification process in the proximal tubule.

A reversibility of the defects in concentrating ability has been documented after surgical correction of hyperparathyroidism (Edvall, 1958; Epstein, 1968a); improvement in renal acidosis has also been noted in patients in whom this pattern was seen before surgical correction of the hyperparathyroidism (Gold *et al.*, 1973; Coe, 1974). Gold *et al.* (1973) also suggested a possible relationship between phosphate depletion and renal bicarbonate wasting. In studies in phosphate-depleted dogs, proximal renal tubular defects similar to those seen in hyperparathyroidism were noted, despite normal circulating levels of parathyroid hormone. Thus, phosphate repletion might account in part for the restoration of normal proximal tubular bicarbonate and acid handling after successful parathyroid surgery.

There are other reports of improvement after operation in renal tubular and glomerular dysfunction (Hellström and Ivemark, 1962; Epstein, 1968a; Purnell *et al.*, 1971, 1974), although in one brief report (Britton *et al.*, 1971) a more pessimistic view was presented with regard to the reversibility of renal functional abnormalities after surgical correction of hyperparathyroidism. Perhaps the degree of reversibility of the renal tubular disorders is related to the severity and/or the chronicity of the hyperparathyroidism. Severe hyperparathyroidism of long duration, as opposed to milder forms of the disease, would be more likely to produce irreversible damage to the renal tubules by way of nephrocalcinosis and chronic infection.

2. Skeletal

It is difficult to assess the clinical significance, frequency, etiology, and prognosis of skeletal disease in hyperparathyroidism. These difficulties arise because of the differences in clinical presentation and pathophysiologic changes in the skeleton seen in various patients with hyperparathyroidism and because of the changed pattern of skeletal disease in hyperparathyroidism. Present information suggests that the pathognomonic form of severe skeletal disease in hyperparathyroidism, osteitis fibrosa cystica, is declining in relative frequency and that a subtle, yet nonetheless often severe, form of skeletal disease, simple diffuse osteopenia resembling osteoporosis, is being seen more often. In a significant number of patients with hyperparathyroidism, osteopenia appears in an asymptomatic form (see Chapter 6, Volume I).

Bone disease sufficiently severe to produce symptoms has been reported in approximately 15% of patients in several reviews of the clinical manifestations of hyperparathyroidism compiled before 1970 (Table III). The incidence of symptomatic and radiologically evident osteitis fibrosa cystica, however, at present is much lower than was characteristic of the clinical picture of hyperparathyroidism several decades ago (Lloyd, 1968).

In an analysis of 138 cases of primary hyperparathyroidism, Hellström and Ivemark (1962) noted that in the two decades of 1930 through 1949, 53% of patients had symptomatic, generalized osteitis fibrosa cystica confirmed by radiological examination, whereas in the decade 1950–1960 only 20% were so afflicted. The relative incidence of radiologically demonstrable osteitis fibrosa cystica in the decade 1961–1970 is even lower. For example, in the review of Aurbach et al. (1973), only 9% of 57 patients seen between 1965 and 1973 had skeletal pain or evidence of osteitis fibrosa cystica.

Moreover, in the present era, patients with primary hyperparathyroidism who have pain referable to the axial skeleton are most likely to present with findings of diffuse spinal rarefaction indistinguishable from that of senile or postmenopausal osteoporosis rather than the findings of osteitis fibrosa. The degree of osteopenia may be severe. Of 319 patients with surgically proved primary hyperparathyroidism seen at the Mayo Clinic over a 3-year period in this decade, 14 (4.4%) had diffuse osteopenia of the spine with evidence of vertebral crush fractures (Dauphine et al., 1975). None of the 14 patients presented with a chief complaint of back pain. In none of the 319 patients, however, was there unequivocal roentgenographic evidence of osteitis fibrosa cystica. The patients with primary hyperparathyroidism demonstrated a statistically higher incidence of diffuse osteopenia of the spine and of vertebral crush fractures (Dauphine *et al.*, 1975) compared with a group of age- and sex-matched control patients with degenerative lumbar-disc disease. In a recent report of 87 patients with primary hyperparathyroidism, Genant *et al.* (1975) found roentgenographic manifestations of osteopenia of the spine in 21% and of the hands in 36% of the patients. Evidence of osteitis fibrosa (subperiosteal resorption of the phalanges) was noted in only 8% of the same patients.

This changing pattern of frequency of involvement of the skeleton has not been adequately explained. Radiological evidence of the characteristic skeletal disorder osteitis fibrosa cystica manifested by subperiosteal resorption, bone cysts, fractures, and deformities is not commonly found in patients at the time that the diagnosis of hyperparathyroidism is made, even though there may be a long history of renal and other complications of the disease (Gleason and Potchen, 1967) (Figs. 27 and 28). In most patients seen in the present decade, even with long-standing primary hyperparathyroidism, conventional roentgenological techniques demonstrate no abnormalities of the skeleton. Patients who do have evidence of skeletal involvement, when tested by more-refined techniques to assess content of bone mineral, more often show a diffuse osteopenia rather than the classic changes of osteitis fibrosa cystica.

Quantitative analyses by microradiography, however, indicated an average fivefold increase in the rate of bone turnover in all patients when they are compared with age-matched control subjects (Jowsey, 1966). In a later study, Jowsey and Riggs (1968) used quantitative microradiographic analysis to compare both resorptive and formative surfaces in biopsies obtained from 20 hyperparathyroid patients and 20 age-matched normal subjects. Although two-thirds of the patients with hyperparathyroidism had no visible roentgenological abnormalities, all biopsy specimens showed evidence of increased bone resorption and bone formation compared with the controls. Patients with hyperparathyroidism showed values of 14.1 ± 1.2 and 3.06 ± 0.42, and normal subjects showed values of 3.0 ± 0.26 and 1.72 ± 0.22, respectively, for percentages of resorptive versus formative surfaces of bone. An estimate of total bone porosity, that is, the nonmineralized versus mineralized areas, revealed a porosity index or percentage of $74.8 \pm 2.4\%$ in hyperparathyroidism and $26.3 \pm 1.9\%$ for age-matched controls.

In addition to the microscopic evidence of increased bone turnover in many patients with primary hyperparathyroidism, evidence of decreased

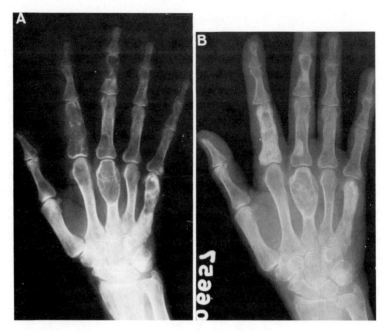

Fig. 27. Hand films of patient with hyperparathyroidism and severe osteitis fibrosa cystica (A) before and (B) after removal of parathyroid adenoma. Cystic destruction of bone, subperiosteal resorption, and a pathologic fracture of the 2nd proximal phalanx are evident. Some remineralization has occurred since the parathyroidectomy. (Courtesy of the Department of Radiology, Massachusetts General Hospital.)

bone density has been found by various sensitive bone densitometric techniques: [125]I bone densitometry (Forland *et al.,* 1968), X-ray spectrophotometry (Dalén and Hjern, 1974), and photon absorptiometric analyses (Pak *et al.,* 1975). Forland *et al.* (1968) found low or distinctly abnormal bone mineral density as determined by ^{125}I densitometry of a middle phalanx in 15 of 20 patients with primary hyperparathyroidism; conventional radiological techniques revealed abnormalities in only four of these.

Dalén and Hjern (1974) found a mean decrease in density of from 5 to 10% at various skeletal sites in 10 patients with hyperparathyroidism by spectrophotometry, but no roentgenological evidence of disease. In the 30 patients with hyperparathyroidism studied by Pak *et al.* (1975) with photon absorptiometric analysis, bone density was reduced in 10. These authors, incidentally, noted that bone density was lower in 7 of 11 postmenopausal women but reduced in only 2 of 13 men and 1 of 6 premenopausal women. It was suggested that estrogen deficiency characteristic of the menopause

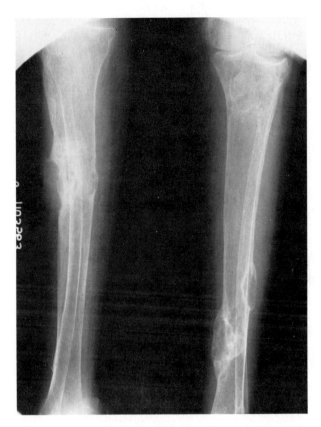

Fig. 28. Radii and ulnae of a patient with primary hyperparathyroidism. Severe osteopenia, increased trabeculation, and large areas of cystic degeneration are evident. (Courtesy of the Department of Radiology, Massachusetts General Hospital.)

contributes to the development of osteopenia by sensitizing bone to the action of parathyroid hormone; it was not possible, however, to compare results in the postmenopausal women with normal subjects of the same age.

Thus, although osteitis fibrosa cystica is infrequent in hyperparathyroidism, increased skeletal activity and mild-to-moderate decline in bone mineral density is not infrequent.

Although the explanation of the changing pattern of bone disease remains unclear, certain issues seem pertinent. It is useful to consider the dual actions of parathyroid hormone on bone. The hormone mobilizes calcium from the skeleton, perhaps principally through the process of stimulation of osteocytic osteolysis (Bélanger, 1965) and the activation of preexisting osteoclasts. This action of the hormone is rapid in onset (within 1 hour); the increased mineral release ceases within several hours when injected hormone disappears from the circulation (Parsons *et al.*, 1971; Robinson *et al.*, 1972). Such an action might lead to simple reduction in bone mass.

The second action of the hormone in bone involves a series of longer term events, which results in extensive remodeling of the bone. These chronic effects involve stimulation of bone cells, particularly the osteoclasts and osteoblasts, increased DNA and protein synthesis, and changes not only in bone mineral but also dissolution of bone matrix and increased activity of enzymes, such as collagenase, concerned with matrix destruction. These effects are relatively slow; for example, 22–26 hours are needed to see increased numbers of osteoclasts (Bingham *et al.*, 1969). Once induced, the effects appear to last for many hours, even after injected hormone disappears from the circulation. Widespread proliferation of osteoclasts might be the prelude to clinical development of osteitis fibrosa cystica.

Rasmussen and Bordier (1973) have emphasized that the long-term administration of parathyroid hormone to animals or moderately severe hyperparathyroidism in man leads to a secondary rise in the size of the osteoblast pool, which tends to reestablish relative skeletal balance. This results in increased numbers of bone remodeling units, but still resorptive processes may be predominant over formative processes, and an overall loss in skeletal mass ensues. They speculate that these effects of parathyroid hormone may lead to diffuse bone loss without classic osteitis fibrosa. Indeed, examination by microradiography of bone specimens from patients with hyperparathyroidism lacking evidence of osteitis fibrosa cystica indicates signs of increased osteocytic osteolysis (Bélanger, 1965). Many enlarged osteocytic lacunae, resembling small resorptive cavities, are detected; the lacunae are surrounded by areas of reduced mineral density.

Using precise and quantitative morphometric techniques on iliac bone biopsy specimens, Meunier *et al.* (1973) have evaluated periosteocytic lacunae size and osteoclastic resorptive surfaces in 40 patients with primary hyperparathyroidism and 62 control subjects. They found highly significant differences in these parameters between the hyperparathyroid and control groups; the percentages of total surfaces of trabecular bone involved by osteoclastic resorption were $9.1\% \pm 5\%$ for hyperparathyroid patients compared with $3.2\% \pm 0.9\%$ for control subjects. Mean surface areas of osteocytic lacunae were 65.6 ± 8.5 μm^2 and 50.6 ± 5.2 μm^2 in hyperparathyroid and normal subjects, respectively.

Some interesting observations were made by Bordier *et al.* (1973) made regarding correlations among the values found for serum immunoreactive PTH levels, serum calcium levels, and the degree of osteocytic osteolysis and osteoclast numbers (bone biopsies) in patients with primary hyperparathyroidism. There was a strongly positive correlation between serum calcium levels and the degree of osteocytic osteolysis over a wide range of serum calcium values and serum parathyroid hormone levels. They found that much higher levels of immunoreactive PTH are necessary to increase the numbers of osteoclasts. It is attractive to speculate that the increased bone turnover and consequent hypercalcemia found in patients with hyperparathyroidism who lack evidence of extensive bone remodeling or osteitis fibrosa cystica reflect the predominance of the action of parathyroid hormone to promote osteocytic osteolysis rather than osteoclast proliferation.

None of these observations seems adequate to explain the failure to detect osteitis fibrosa and extensive changes in bone remodeling in many present-day patients with primary hyperparathyroidism, despite greatly increased blood concentrations of parathyroid hormone and long duration of disease. Even the recognition of a dual action of the hormone on the skeleton with the possibility that either action, if predominant, will result in a distinctive clinical pattern of bone disease does not explain why one type of bone lesion rather than another is predominant, despite apparent similarities in duration and severity of disease. Other than the report of Bordier et al. (1973), there are few data concerning absolute PTH levels in blood and the presence or type of bone disease. It is possible that compensatory mechanisms or modifying influences, such as production of calcitonin, operate in response to the challenge of hypercalcemia. Some factor relating to calcium absorption, either content (Albright and Reifenstein, 1948; Dent, 1962) or efficiency of intestinal calcium absorption (Peacock, 1975), or the levels of active metabolites of vitamin D or phosphate balance, or extracellular fluid concentrations of phosphate may in some way influence the occurrence of osteitis fibrosa cystica in hyperparathyroidism. The observation of Peacock (1975) concerning differences in efficiency of absorption may prove important on further analysis.

Jowsey has reported that in all but 4 of 20 hyperparathyroid patients in whom bone biopsies were examined by microradiographic and other histological techniques there were definite features of osteomalacia (Jowsey, 1968), with widening of osteoid seams. The administration of inorganic phosphate to patients with primary hyperparathyroidism will sometimes restore skeletal balance completely (Rasmussen and Bordier, 1973). Phosphate administration leads to a rise in plasma phosphate, a fall in plasma calcium, and a positive calcium and skeletal balance with little change in urinary hydroxyproline excretion (an index of the rate of bone resorption). Most studies of the effects of phosphate have been short term, and the positive skeletal balance induced by phosphate administration may be a transient rather than a sustained change in skeletal balance. Overall, there are too little data on compensatory mechanisms for a critical analysis, and the pathogenesis of osteitis fibrosa remains unclear.

Clinically, a number of features of the bone disease, whether osteitis fibrosa cystica or simple osteopenia, are of importance in evaluating the symptoms of the patient, in providing diagnostic clues to the presence of the disease, or in helping to assess need for surgical treatment and the response of the patient following surgical correction of the hyperparathyroidism. When severe osteitis fibrosa cystica develops, the loss of bone mass may result in marked deformities and fractures; pain is then often quite severe and is localized. Radiological examinations and study by bone biopsy then often help to establish the diagnosis. Histological examination of bone specimens from patients with severe osteitis fibrosa cystica reveals a number of changes that collectively define the presence of parathyroid overactivity. These are a reduction in the number of trabeculae, an increase in multinucleated osteoclasts seen in scalloped areas on the surface of the bone (Howship's lacunae), and a marked replacement of normal cellular and marrow elements by fibrovascular tissue (Fig. 29).

In approximately 20% of patients with primary hyperparathyroidism, routine roentgenograms show abnormalities of the skeleton. In advanced stages of the disease there is evidence of erosion of the outer cortical surfaces and haversian canals of bone, demineralization of bones, localized destructive lesions, and calcification of fibrocartilage and of some soft tissues. In milder forms of osteitis fibrosa of the skeleton, visible changes may be limited to subperiosteal resorption or erosion of the outer cortical surfaces of bone usually seen first in the phalanges (Dent, 1962; Gleason and Potchen, 1967; Steinbach et al., 1961).

The most important roentgenograms for the diagnosis of generalized osteitis fibrosa are those of the hands in the posteroanterior view (Steinbach et al., 1961). In the majority of patients with roentgenographically demonstrable bone lesions, subperiosteal erosion of the radial aspect of the middle phalanges is seen (Fig. 30). In minimal disease the erosion may be limited to the cortical surfaces near the phalangeal base or proximal to its head at the transitional zone between the wide end and the slender shaft. The normal smooth outer surface at first loses the sharp demarcation from the surrounding soft tissues. Later, areas of destruction are seen to alternate with normal-appearing bone and may produce spicules of bone located perpendicular to the cortical surface. Detectable regions of subperiosteal resorption may also be detected at the acromioclavicular joint, symphysis pubis, and sacroiliac joints. Subperiosteal resorption, when found, is diagnostic of hyperparathyroidism; its occurrence appears to be a unique result of the action of excesses of parathyroid hormone.

As discussed earlier, diffuse undermineralization of bone, or osteopenia, is seen frequently in primary hyperparathyroidism. Osteopenia due to osteitis fibrosa usually differs from that due to senile or postmenopausal osteoporosis in that it is not homogeneous (Doyle, 1966; Steinbach et al., 1961). Bone of diminished density alternates with bone of apparently normal density, producing a mottled, or "punched out," appearance most apparent in the calvaria but also visible in other bones (Fig. 31).

Occasionally in patients with primary hyperparathyroidism, evidence of osteosclerosis may be manifested on roentgenograms by either a diffuse (Genant et al., 1975) or localized (Ellis and Hochstim, 1960; Templeton et al., 1962; Aitken et al., 1964; Eugenidis et al., 1972) increase in skeletal mineral density. It should be noted that although osteosclerosis is seen in 5 to 20% of patients with secondary hyperparathyroidism (Chapter 2) (Kaye et al., 1960; Zimmerman, 1962; Valvassori and Pierce, 1964; Doyle, 1966; A. I. Katz et al., 1969; Meema et al., 1974), its occurrence is rare in adult primary hyperparathyroidism. In contrast, children with primary hyperparathyroidism, a rare event in itself, commonly develop intense osteosclerosis particularly of the metaphyseal regions of the skeleton, and particularly in rapidly growing bones (Dresser, 1933; Adam and Ritchie, 1954; Lloyd et al., 1965).

Detection of loss of the lamina dura of the teeth is also helpful diagnostically, but is found less frequently than subperiosteal resorption. In one series of 67 patients with classic bone disease, the lamina dura was missing in 83% of those examined and present in the remainder (Rosenberg and Guralnick, 1962). In hyperparathyroidism the lamina dura is thinner than that presumed to result from disuse in normal teeth lacking opposing occlusion. In one study, despite biochemical evidence of healing 3 months following removal of parathyroid adenomas, no regain of the lamina dura was found on roentgenograms (Silverman et al., 1962). Rosenberg and Guralnick (1962) also described 10 patients in whom giant-cell granuloma (or epulis) was the presenting manifestation of hyperparathyroidism.

Two types of cystic lesions may be detected in patients with hyperparathyroidism and osteitis fibrosa cystica: true bone cysts and "brown tumors." These lesions appear similar on roentgenograms, but, in fact, represent quite different pathologic processes and evolve differently following surgical correction of the disease. A true bone cyst consists of a fluid-filled cavity lined with fibrous tissue; such cysts often occur subperiosteally (Figs. 27, 28, 29a). "Brown tumors" are composed of poorly

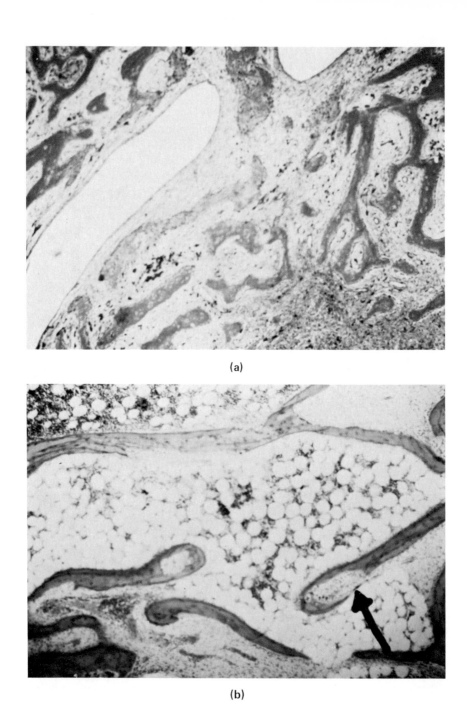

(a)

(b)

Fig. 29. Microscopic appearance of osteitis fibrosa cystica in bone from an iliac-crest biopsy. (a) Extensive replacement of marrow with fibrovascular tissue; cystic cavities are evident. Osseous trabeculae showed evidence of both osteoclastic resorption and areas of osteoblastic bone formation. (b) Classic appearance of dissecting osteitis within lamellar bone of trabeculae; several areas of fibrous replacement of marrow are evident. (c) Higher

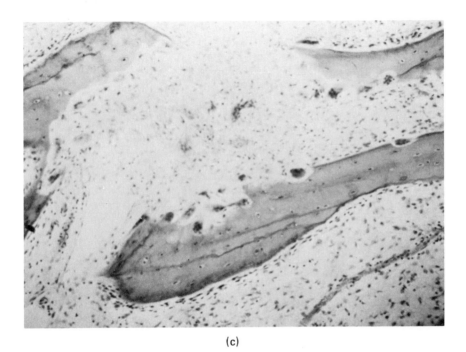

(c)

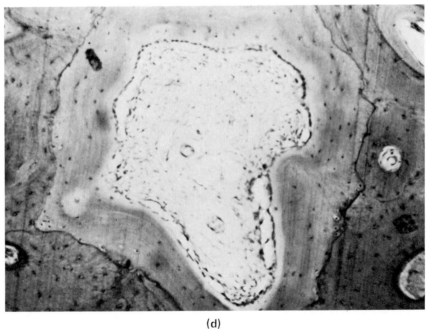

(d)

magnification of dissecting osteitis showing multinucleated osteoclasts resorbing bone. (d) Osteone in cortical bone after parathyroidectomy, showing marked bone formation; innermost concentric circle of bone is unmineralized. Dark line represents calcification front; this osteomalacia is due to formation of matrix that is occurring faster than the process of mineralization. (Courtesy of the Department of Pathology, Massachusetts General Hospital.)

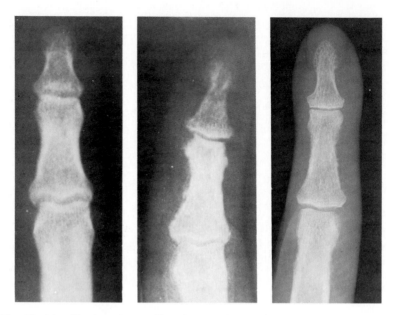

Fig. 30. Magnification of X-ray film of normal finger (left) and finger from two patients with primary hyperparathyroidism (middle and right) to emphasize typical features. The abnormal fingers show decreased demineralization in the phalangeal tuft (middle) and subperiosteal bone resorption (middle and right). (Modified from Potts and Deftos, 1974.)

mineralized woven bone, including osteoblasts and osteoclasts. These latter lesions are often referred to as osteoblastomas or osteoclastomas (Boyd, 1961; Golden and Canary, 1968). After surgical correction of the hyperparathyroidism the brown tumors disappear as they are repaired by ossification. True bone cysts, however, do not ossify and remain evident on subsequent examination (Riddick and Reiss, 1962). In addition to resolution of brown tumors, the other radiological changes, indicative of increased bone resorption, clearly resolve following adequate treatment.

The major unsettled issue regarding skeletal manifestations is the frequency, specific relation to hyperparathyroidism, and reversibility (post-parathyroidectomy) of the diffuse osteopenia attributed to many patients with the disease. A definite causal relationship between hyperparathyroidism and diffuse osteopenia requires further study. It will be important to document in prospective studies whether there is indeed a pattern of progressive decrease in bone mineral density detectable by quantitative techniques and whether there is improvement in bone density after parathyroidectomy. This type of analysis seems particularly necessary, since osteoporosis, unrelated to hyperparathyroidism, is frequently

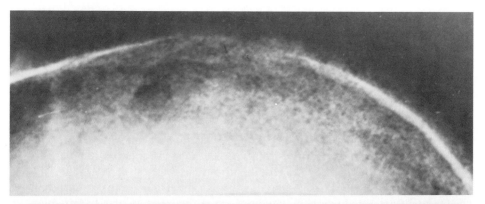

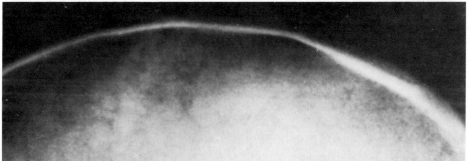

Fig. 31. Magnification of skull X-ray film from a patient with primary hyperparathyroidism (top) and of a normal subject (bottom) to emphasize the appearance of areas of localized resorption. (Courtesy of the Department of Radiology, Massachusetts General Hospital; from Potts and Deftos, 1974.)

seen in older patients. In patients with a documented decline in bone mineral density, application of the quantitative morphometric techniques of Meunier *et al.* (1973) may help to establish the parathyroid etiology of the osteopenia by definite histological changes. If the osteopenia in such patients is not reversed after parathyroidectomy but its progression is simply slowed, it will become even more important to detect early evidence of progressive osteopenia in patients with hyperparathyroidism to prevent progression of skeletal weakening to the point of pathologic fractures.

3. Neuromuscular and Neuropsychiatric

Muscle weakness and atrophy were described in several of the original cases of severe hyperparathyroidism (Recklinghausen, 1891; Hirschberg, 1889; Mandl, 1926). Since that time, reports have occasionally appeared stressing the occurrence of neuromuscular disorders (Vicale, 1949; Lemann and Donatelli, 1964). Recently, pathophysiologic features of neuromuscular involvement in hyperparathyroidism have been studied in more detail (Aurbach et al., 1973; Patten et al., 1974). Patten and associates have described the pattern of signs and symptoms of neuromuscular involvement in patients with severe primary hyperparathyroidism. Symptoms include weakness and easy fatiguability, particularly in proximal musculature. Muscles of the lower extremity were usually involved more frequently than those of the upper extremity, but both upper and lower limb weakness can be detected. Patients frequently complain of difficulty in climbing stairs, stepping up on curbstones, or arising from a chair. Atrophy may be detectable in involved muscle groups on physical examination, and definable weakness may be seen in the hamstrings, gluteus, psoas, deltoid, and biceps muscle groups. Electromyographic examination revealed multiple abnormalities, including both short duration/low amplitude motor unit potentials. and abnormally high amplitude/long duration polyphasic potentials. Motor-nerve conduction velocities were found to be normal. Definite sensory abnormalities were infrequent. Detailed histological and electron microscopic examination of muscle biopsy tissue from affected muscle groups revealed characteristic changes, resembling those seen in experimental denervation. Atrophy of type II muscle fibers was most frequently seen, but atrophy of type I muscle fibers was also detected. Inflammatory changes were usually minimal or absent.

Blood levels of serum glutamic-oxaloacetic transaminase, creatinine phosphokinase, and aldolase were uniformly all normal. Patten et al. (1974) emphasized that the overall findings are consistent with a neuropathic rather than a myopathic origin of the neuromuscular disease. Patten and associates (1974) have also stressed that in certain of the affected subjects the muscle weakness may be so profound that an initial diagnosis of amyotrophic lateral sclerosis, muscular dystrophy, or other serious neuromuscular disorders of an irreversible character was entertained before recognition of the presence of hypercalcemia and hyperparathyroidism. Improvement in symptoms of muscle weakness, as well as reversal of atrophy, was noted in all patients after successful parathyroid surgery and correction of the hyperparathyroidism.

Other reports have documented neuromuscular defects considered to be myopathic in patients with primary hyperparathyroidism (Frame et al., 1968; Cholod et al., 1970). However, the changes found on muscle biopsy were principally those of atrophy. Evidence for myositis, e.g., neutrophilic cellular infiltration, was detected in the muscle biopsy specimens from one patient described by Frame et al. (1968). Subsequent review of this report indicates that the electromyographic abnormalities were typical of those reported by Patten *et al.* (1974) in their more extensive study, i.e., polyphasic potentials in proximal muscle groups of the upper and lower extremities. As in the experience of Patten *et al.* (1974), the patients studied by Frame *et al.* and Cholod *et al.* showed disappearance of clinical symptoms, improvement in muscular atrophy, and a return of electromyographic pattern to normal after correction of the hyperparathyroidism.

The incidence of this neuromyopathic syndrome in primary hyperparathyroidism is still unknown. Analyses before the last 5 years were based on clinical examination of patients with hyperparathyroidism detected because of other signs and symptoms of primary hyperparathyroidism. Difficulties in determination of the true incidence of neuromyopathy in primary hyperparathyroidism are further compounded by the increasing frequency with which totally asymptomatic hyperparathyroidism is being detected on routine annual physical examinations (Purnell *et al.*, 1974). Neuromyopathic changes may turn out to be relatively frequent complications of the more severe forms of hyperparathyroidism. Wide variations have been reported in the apparent incidence of mild to severe neuromuscular complications in primary hyperparathyroidism. Early reviews when more severe forms of disease were seen often had reported neuromuscular symptoms in a high percentage of patients. Vicale (1949) and Lemann and Donatelli (1964) found muscle weakness and easy fatiguability in 70–80% of cases. Others such as Gutman *et al.* (1934) and Karpati and Frame (1964) reported a lower incidence of 25–30%. Most striking, however, in the quite recent prospective study of Patten *et al.* (1974) was that 14 of 16 patients showed manifestations of neuromyopathic involvement. Furthermore, several of the patients described in the later report had weakness, fatiguability, and other neuromuscular symptoms as their presenting symptoms. Hence, more detailed neurologic examination may reveal a much higher incidence of this complication than previously suspected.

In addition to the neuromyopathic manifestations of hyperparathyroidism, mental disturbances and impairment of function of the higher central nervous system are frequently seen (Henson, 1966; Petersen, 1968). Mental depression, personality changes, psychomotor retardation, memory impairment, and, occasionally, overt psychosis may occur (Lehrer and Levitt, 1960; Hockaday *et al.*, 1966; Petersen, 1968). Mental obtundation and coma may be observed (Wilson *et al.*, 1964). These neuropsychiatric disturbances are thought to be due to the hypercalcemia per se rather than to any direct effects of parathyroid hormone (Petersen, 1968). Characteristic electroencephalographic abnormalities have been described in hypercalcemia of many causes (Moure, 1967; Allen *et al.*, 1970). In some instances, the patient experiences multiple and vague complaints that can often be mistaken for psychoneurosis (Petersen, 1968).

In the experience of the authors, subtle depressive states are common manifestations of even mild primary hyperparathyroidism. Often the patient and/or physician is unaware of the depression and it is only after removal of the parathyroid adenoma that the degree of discomfort that existed before surgery is recognized. On the other hand, such vague symptoms may not be related to any metabolic abnormality, and improvement after surgery may result from psychological effects of surgery alone and cannot necessarily be attributed to correction of hyperparathyroidism per se. Mild depression and vague constitutional complaints are difficult to assess and probably cannot alone serve as an indication for surgery.

4. Gastrointestinal

a. Peptic Ulcer Disease. Peptic ulcer disease is seen in primary hyperparathyroidism with such high frequency that most investigators believe that the ulcer disease is causally related to the hyperparathyroidism. Gastrointestinal symptoms including epigastric pain and vomiting are commonly present. Some of the earliest clinical reports of hyperparathyroidism mentioned these symptoms (Gold, 1928; Barr *et al.*, 1929; Boyd *et al.*, 1929; Rogers, 1946) and since then the coincidence of peptic ulcers and hyperparathyroidism has been frequently analyzed (Howard *et al.*, 1953 — 12.7%; Hellström, 1954 — 11.5%; St. Goar, 1957 — 8.8%; Moses, 1958 — 8.8%; Hellström, 1959 — 11.5%; Keating, 1961 — 15.5%; Wilder *et al.*, 1961 — 28.1%; C. Ellis and D. M. Nicoloff, 1968 — 30.5%).

On the other hand, some authors have questioned whether the frequency of ulcer disease in primary hyperparathyroidism is actually higher than it is in the general population (Ostrow *et al.*, 1960). Barreras (1973), however, in a review of peptic ulcer disease in patients with primary hyperparathyroidism in 10 reported series found an incidence of proved ulcer disease in 131 of 928 cases, an overall incidence of 14.2% (range 7.7–30.5%). When consideration was given to the fact that in many patients studies of the gastrointestinal tract were not performed even in the presence of upper intestinal symptoms, Barreras concluded that the incidence of peptic ulcer disease, based on clinical and historical evidence, is probably close to 30%. The prevalence of peptic ulcer disease in the general adult population without hyperparathyroidism is reported as low as 2–3% in the United States (U.S. Public Health Service, 1960) to as high as 5–10% (Ostrow *et al.*, 1960), or a maximum 7.8% in Great Britain (Doll *et al.*, 1950).

These conclusions concerning a truly increased frequency of peptic ulcer disease in primary hyperparathyroidism are supported by the cumulative experience at the Massachusetts General Hospital. In the series of 431 cases of hyperparathyroidism reviewed in 1972 (Dent *et al.*, 1972) epigastric symptoms at the time of evaluation were present in 43%; 17% of these patients had proved peptic ulceration, and approximately 5% had already undergone operation for ulcer disease when their parathyroid disease was first diagnosed. Some of the patients with peptic ulcer disease, particularly those with severe symptoms and multiple ulcers, turn out to have Zollinger–Ellison syndrome (Zollinger and Ellison, 1955) or the multiple-endocrine-neoplasia syndrome, type I, with gastrin-producing tumors or diffuse hyperplasia of the pancreatic islet cells. These patients, however, constitute a small minority of patients with hyperparathyroidism and peptic ulcers; most have no recognized abnormalities of the endocrine pancreas.

The etiological basis for the increased incidence of ulcer disease in hyperparathyroidism may be due to increased gastrin secretion, and, hence, gastric-acid production, induced by the hypercalcemia (Barreras, 1973). Studies in hyperparathyroidism have demonstrated the existence in some patients of both increased basal acid secretion (Dent *et al.*, 1972; Patterson *et al.*, 1969; Ward *et al.*, 1964) and elevated serum immunoreactive gastrin (Dent *et al.*, 1972; McGuigan *et al.*, 1974). Following parathyroidectomy, the excessive acid production, hypergastrinemia, and peptic ulcer symptoms usually return to normal (Dent *et al.*, 1972; Barreras and Donaldson, 1967; Wilder *et al.*, 1961; McGuigan *et al.*, 1974). The administration of calcium either orally (Levant *et al.*, 1973) or by intravenous infusion (Reeder *et al.*, 1970; Donegan and Spiro, 1960) increases gastric acid production and serum gastrin levels in normal subjects, as well as in patients with the Zollinger–Ellison syndrome (Trudeau and McGuigan, 1969; Passaro *et al.*, 1972). Intragastric calcium perfusion has also been reported to increase acid secretion by as much as threefold without any change in serum immunoreactive gastrin levels (Holtermuller *et al.*, 1974), suggesting that calcium can cause gastric hypersecretion by a direct effect on the parietal cell. It has also been shown that in hypoparathyroid patients, there is no production of gastric acid until the serum calcium level rises above 7 mg% (Donegan and Spiro, 1960). Whether parathyroid hormone itself exerts any direct effects on gastrin secretion or acid production is not certain, although it was suggested that gastrin release may follow infusions of bovine parathyroid hormone in the absence of hypercalcemia (W. S. Hughes *et al.*, 1971) and that injections of parathyroid extracts per se increase basal acid output (Donegan and Spiro, 1960).

The weight of the evidence indicates that increased gastrin secretion and hyperacidity in hyperparathyroidism are due to the hypercalcemia and not to direct effects of the parathyroid hormone on gastrin production or on acid production per se.

Two further points should be stressed about the association between hyperparathyroidism and ulcer disease. The first, stressed elsewhere in analysis of frequency of signs and symptoms in hyperparathyroidism, is that estimates of incidence of ulcer disease in hyperparathyroidism might well be revised downward from the estimates of Barreras (1973), the latter derived from retrospective surveys of symptomatic cases; estimates of incidence of gastrointestinal complications in asymptomatic hyperparathyroidism have not been made. Secondly, the ulcer disease does seem to improve after successful cure of the hyperparathyroidism. Even in the Zollinger–Ellison syndrome, it has been reported that the hyperacidity, elevated gastrin levels, and peptic ulcer symptoms may be reversed acutely by parathyroidectomy (Dent *et al.*, 1972). However, long-term follow-up of some of these patients revealed ultimate recurrence of the Zollinger–Ellison syndrome despite the persistence of normal parathyroid function (J. E. Fischer, personal communication, 1976). The results do serve to emphasize, however, the close relationship between hyperparathyroidism and gastric acid production.

b. Pancreatitis. Pancreatitis occurs with a statistically significant frequency, at least in conjunction with symptomatic primary hyperparathyroidism. Cope *et al.* (1957), in their description of two patients with pancreatitis and hyperparathyroidism, were the first to suggest an association, and proposed that pancreatitis occasionally may be a diagnostic clue to the presence of hyperparathyroidism. Subsequently, Mixter *et al.* (1962) described 62 cases of pancreatitis occurring in primary hyperparathyroidism, an incidence of about 12%. In an extension of this series, the appearance of pancreatitis was the primary diagnostic clue to the presence of otherwise unrecognized hyperparathyroidism in 3% of 431 cases of surgically proved cases (Wang, 1971). The incidence of pancreatitis is higher in instances of hypercalcemic crisis occurring as an acute complication of hyperparathyroidism (Kleppel *et al.*, 1965). In one study, 19 of 56 cases (34%) of patients with "acute parathyroid intoxication" were found to have hemorrhagic pancreatitis (Fink and Finfrock, 1961).

Five types of pancreatitis associated with hyperparathyroidism have been described: (1) acute, (2) acute postoperative (after any operation in patients who have unsuspected hyperparathyroidism), (3) recurrent, (4) chronic with pain, and (5) chronic without pain (Mixter *et al.*, 1962). The most common type is chronic with pain. Pancreatic insufficiency with steatorrhea complicating the chronic pancreatitis of primary hyperparathyroidism was also described (Warshaw *et al.*, 1968). Asymptomatic pancreatic calcifications may be the only clue to the presence of pancreatitis (Mixter *et al.*, 1962; Eversman *et al.*, 1967), and an attack of acute pancreatitis may occasionally occur as a serious complication just after parathyroidectomy for hyperparathyroidism. Therefore, it seems reasonable to suggest that a careful scrutiny of the abdominal roentgenograms for the presence of pancreatic calcifications should be made before patients with primary hyperparathyroidism undergo surgery.

Although the association of pancreatitis and hyperparathyroidism is well documented, the basis for it is unknown. Some authors have suggested that the hyperparathyroidism develops in response to pancreatitis (Paloyan *et al.*, 1967a), whereas most others have suggested that the hypercalcemia per se associated with the hyperparathyroidism predisposes to the development of pancreatitis (Edmondson *et al.*, 1952; Mixter *et al.*, 1962). Pancreatitis is known to occur with hypercalcemia caused by disorders other than hyperparathyroidism. Another suggestion was that calcium salts are deposited in pancreatic cells and ducts and that these deposits lead to obstruction and injury (Edmondson *et al.*, 1952). This explanation of the pathogenesis of pancreatitis is supported by the observations that pancreatic calcifications are present in more than half of the cases of pancreatitis seen in association with hyperparathyroidism, although pancreatic calcifications are often seen in the absence of pancreatitis and vice versa. Other explanations for the pancreatic injury include increased calcium-dependent conversion of trypsinogen to trypsin (Haverback *et al.*, 1960) and possibly a direct toxic effect of parathyroid hormone on the pancreas (Hueper, 1927).

At least two mechanisms, clearly speculative, have been proposed by which pancreatitis might lead to stimulation of the parathyroid glands, and both imply that the development of a sustained period of hypocalcemia is the factor leading to parathyroid hyperfunction. First, calcium deficiency per se, secondary to pancreatic exocrine insufficiency and ensuing malabsorption of vitamin D and calcium, could result in chronic stimulation and hyperplasia of the parathyroids and eventually lead to autonomous hyperfunction due to development of an adenoma (Davies *et al.*, 1956; Plough and Kyle, 1957; Dreiling *et al.*, 1962). Second, some have called attention to the alpha-cell hyperplasia of the pancreatic islets that results in excessive secretion of pancreatic glucagon known to occur in chronic pancreatitis (Wacjner, 1965). The hyperglucagonemia could lead to hypocalcemia (by mechanisms unknown) and then to secondary parathyroid hyperplasia (Paloyan et al., 1967b). On the other hand, it is possible that there is a reactive secretion of glucagon, secondary to hypercalcemia or hyperparathyroidism, not associated with pancreatitis (Paloyan et al., 1967a,b). Neither of these explanations proposed for the genesis of hyperparathyroidism in patients with pancreatitis has substantive supporting data; the authors conclude that, most likely, the hyperparathyroidism causes the pancreatitis, not the reverse.

Regardless of the nature of the pathogenetic interrelationships between pancreatitis and hyperparathyroidism, awareness of this association has several practical consequences. The diagnosis of hyperparathyroidism should be considered in patients with pancreatitis, particularly those in whom there is no predisposing factor present such as alcoholism or hyperlipidemia (Type II) (Snodgrass, 1970). Conversely, one should be aware of the possible development of pancreatitis as a complication of hyperparathyroidism, particularly in parathyroid crisis. It is well documented that both acute and chronic pancreatitis (the latter due to malabsorption) may cause a decrease in serum calcium concentration to deceptively normal or even low levels in hyperparathyroidism. Thus, the findings of even a normal level of serum calcium in the face of pancreatitis may be a clue to the concomitant existence of primary hyperparathyroidism (Mixter et al., 1962).

5. Articular

Several articular and periarticular disorders are recognized in association with primary hyperparathyroidism (Bywaters et al., 1963; Wang et al., 1969; Grahame et al., 1971; McCarty, 1975). These disorders include, either singly or in combination, chondrocalcinosis with or without acute attacks of pseudogout, juxtaarticular erosions, subchondral fractures, traumatic synovitis, calcific periarthritis, and urate gout. There have also been some confusing reports concerning the association of ankylosing spondylitis and primary hyperparathyroidism.

The most distinctive disorder generally recognized is that of chronic chondrocalcinosis characterized by the deposition of calcium pyrophosphate dihydrate (CPPD) crystals in the articular cartilages and menisci (chondrocalcinosis) (McCarty and Haskin, 1963) and occasionally by the occurrence of acute attacks of arthritis (pseudogout), associated with CPPD in the synovial space, usually within polymorphonuclear leukocytes.

In 1958, Zitnan and Sitaj first described the highly distinctive form of articular calcifications and named it "chondrocalcinosis polyarticularis familiaris." The clinical syndrome of acute arthritic attacks was subsequently recognized by McCarty *et al.* (1962) and was termed "pseudogout." The etiologies of chondrocalcinosis are diverse, but certain metabolic abnormalities such as hemochromatosis, diabetes mellitus, or hyperparathyroidism appear to be present in many cases. The incidence of chondrocalcinosis in primary hyperparathyroidism is reported to be from 7.5 to 18% (McCarty, 1966; Dodds and Steinbach, 1968). Recent studies using sensitive radioimmunoassays for parathyroid hormone have indicated that the frequency of this association may be even higher. Elevated concentrations of immunoreactive parathyroid hormone were found in the sera of 10 (38%) of 26 patients (Phelps and Hawker, 1973) and in 59% of 28 patients (McCarty *et al.*, 1974) with chondrocalcinosis. Somewhat unexpectedly, in the latter study, elevated levels of serum parathyroid hormone were also found in approximately 60% of 21 control patients with osteoarthritis and no signs of chondrocalcinosis. The serum calcium values were normal in all but two of the patients in both groups, casting some doubt about the discriminant value of the abnormal levels of serum immunoreactive parathyroid hormone.

Occasionally, the finding of chondrocalcinosis may provide the initial clue to the diagnosis of subclinical hyperparathyroidism (Wang *et al.*, 1969). It should be noted that acute arthritis of pseudogout occasionally develops immediately after parathyroidectomy, even in the absence of a preceding history of arthritic symptoms (Bilezikian *et al.*, 1973).

The diagnosis of chondrocalcinosis is best made by radiological identification of characteristic CPPD deposits in articular cartilages (Fig. 32). Finely detailed roentgenograms are helpful in detecting small or faint deposits (Parlee *et al.*, 1967; McCarty, 1975). The diagnosis of pseudogout occurring as acute arthritic attacks is established by the finding of CPPD crystals in aspirates of joint fluid. These rhomboidal crystals are characteristically located within polymorphonuclear leukocytes in the joint fluid and show weak positive birefringence under polarized light (Phelps *et al.*, 1968).

It may at times be difficult to differentiate the polyarthritis of urate gout from that of pseudogout, particularly since the two forms of arthritis may coexist in the same patient with primary hyperparathyroidism (Grahame *et al.*, 1971). Hyperuricemia is frequently seen in primary hyperparathyroidism (Mintz *et al.*, 1961) and attributed to decreased renal clearance of urates. Approximately 20% of patients with pseudogout and hyperparathyroidism have hyperuricemia, a factor that may further confuse the diagnosis (Scott *et al.*, 1964; McCarty, 1975). Examination of the synovial fluid in gouty arthritis per se usually shows negatively birefringent needle-shaped urate crystals within polymorphonuclear leukocytes. In addition, differences in the clinical manifestations of the two disorders

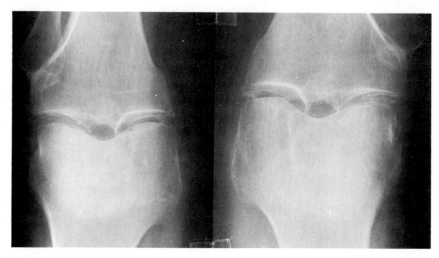

Fig. 32. Radiographic appearance of chondrocalcinosis in articular cartilages of the knee. (Courtesy of Dr. S. M. Krane.)

may be helpful in establishing the correct diagnosis. Acute or subacute self-limited attacks of arthritis lasting for a day to a few weeks and involving one or more axial or appendicular joints are characteristic of both pseudogout and gout, but the attacks in pseudogout tend to be much less severe than they are in gout. Large joints, for example, the knee, are more likely to be affected in pseudogout, and the small joints are affected in gout. The effectiveness of colchicine in ameliorating the symptoms in pseudogout is usually much less than it is in gout.

Apart from chondrocalcinosis, a form of degenerative osteoarthritis has been described in conjunction with primary hyperparathyroidism (Bywaters *et al.,* 1963). It has been proposed that the articular manifestations develop secondary to the bone disease. Crush lesions of articular bone occur in hyperparathyroidism leading to a traumatic type of synovitis manifested by effusion and disability. In some cases of this disorder, the roentgenographic appearance may mimic that of rheumatoid arthritis but can usually be differentiated from rheumatoid involvement by the finding of calcification in the synovial membrane and articular cartilages, a feature not seen in rheumatoid arthritis (Bywaters *et al.,* 1963).

Bunch and Hunder (1973) reported finding three cases of hyperparathyroidism with ankylosing spondylitis. The concurrence of these two diseases in the same patient appears to be three or more times greater than that expected by chance alone. In another study of 50 patients with ankylosing spondylitis, serum immunoreactive parathyroid hormone levels were elevated compared with the levels in a group of control patients (Fairney *et al.*, 1975). However, the data were pooled, and the existence of other disorders such as vitamin D deficiency and/or malabsorption were not screened for. Blood calcium levels were normal. This interesting reported association requires confirmation and further analysis.

There also are reports of avulsion of tendons, particularly of the quadriceps, occurring spontaneously without trauma in patients with hyperparathyroidism, associated with ectopic calcification (E. T. Preston, 1972; F. S. Preston and Adicoff, 1962).

It is clear that multiple manifestations of articular disease are seen with clinically severe hyperparathyroidism; certain disorders, such as pseudogout, are so frequently associated with parathyroid disorders that the presence of the former should indeed raise diagnostic suspicion of the latter.

6. Cardiovascular

There is evidence that hypertension may occur more frequently in hyperparathyroidism, particularly with elderly patients, than in the general population (Hellström, 1950, 1954; Hellström *et al.*, 1958). Hellström *et al.* (1958) found that 70% of 105 patients with hyperparathyroidism had hypertension during the course of their disease. The severity of the hypertension correlated with the extent of renal involvement; severe renal damage was present in 81% of the patients with severe hypertension, but in only 32% of those with minimal hypertension. Hypertension contributed to the immediate cause of death in 7 of the 105 cases. In these cases impairment of renal function preceded the development of hypertension, indicating that renal disease led to the hypertension rather than the reverse; there was no evidence of any direct vasopressor effects of the hormone. In some cases, hypertension developed after parathyroidectomy. Britton *et al.* (1971) observed that of 19 patients with hyperparathyroidism and hypertension, in only one did the blood pressure return to normal after operation. An additional 17 patients became hypertensive after surgery.

Hence, on the basis of (1) the above information and, particularly, (2) the high frequency of essential hypertension, at least in the United States, where it occurs in 20% of the adult population (U.S. Public Health Service, 1964), and (3) the increasing frequency of detection of asymptomatic hyperparathyroidism, it must be concluded that random association of the two diseases might be expected. The presence of hypertension per se (in the absence of MEN-II) should not serve as an indication for surgery in the expectation of reversal of hypertension.

7. Other Manifestations and Complications

Skin necrosis, which may be found in patients with hypercalcemia of any cause, has also been found in hyperparathyroidism (D. C. Anderson *et al.*, 1968). Calcification of the cornea (band keratopathy) is occasionally a manifestation of hypercalcemia of whatever cause (Cogan *et al.*, 1948). It is not commonly found in primary hyperparathyroidism when serum phosphorus levels are low and renal function maintained. If hyperphosphatemia develops, usually because of renal failure or due to excessive calcium intake, then this abnormality may be seen grossly or in more subtle degrees on slit-lamp examination.

There are special complications and/or considerations pertinent to the occurrence of hyperparathyroidism in specific types of patients. In one review of pregnancy in women with hyperparathyroidism during the period of gestation, it was found that 20 normal infants were delivered from 21 women (Ludwig, 1962). However, in that same group of mothers, there were an additional 19 cases of spontaneous abortion, stillbirth, neonatal death, and tetany, and one instance of permanent hypoparathyroidism in the infant. Ludwig (1962) suggested on the basis of these data that surgical exploration should be performed when hyperparathyroidism is diagnosed during pregnancy.

Hyperparathyroidism does occur, although infrequently, in children. By 1966 there were reports of 30 proved cases of childhood primary hyperparathyroidism (Nolan *et al.*, 1960; Reinfrank and Edwards, 1961; Rajasuriya *et al.*, 1964; Lloyd *et al.*, 1965; Chaves-Carballo and Hayles, 1966; Steendijk, 1971). Most of the affected children were in adolescence. The disorder is particularly rare in patients below age 10 (Nolan *et al.*, 1960). In many of the reported cases, hypercalcemia was severe and bone disease prominent. Other symptoms may be even more nonspecific than in adults. Most of the cases came to medical attention because of the development of changes in school performance or in personality, and the majority were found to have bone and/or joint symptoms. Eighteen of 22 reported cases had overt skeletal disease (Rajasuriya *et al.*, 1964; Lloyd *et al.*, 1965; Steendijk, 1971), whereas only 6 had renal stones. Five of these patients presented with joint symptoms that mimicked either gout or rheumatoid arthritis. In some instances, skeletal roentgenograms revealed evidence of rickets that had healed after parathyroidectomy. Growth failure, however, was not commonly observed in these patients. The serum calcium levels of the children with primary hyperparathyroidism were unusually high, with the average between 14 and 16 ng per 100 ml. In the case of the 13-year-old girl reported by Reinfrank and Edwards (1961), the preoperative serum calcium level was an astounding 21.8 mg per 100 ml. It is likely that with the use of screening procedures that more instances will be found of hyperparathyroidism in children. The serum levels of calcium and phosphorus will have to be interpreted with respect to normals for that age. Cross-sectional data for normal children have been collected and used for this purpose (Goldsmith *et al.*, 1973).

It should also be noted that, in hyperparathyroidism generally, spontaneous infarction of a parathyroid adenoma may occur (Howard *et al.*, 1953), which could produce remission of the hyperparathyroidism; such reports are rare, however. In other instances, acute hypercalcemia has been found after hemorrhage into a parathyroid adenoma or cyst (De-Groote, 1969). These patients may complain of pain in the neck and present themselves with a tender neck mass.

D. Diagnosis

1. General Considerations

Primary hyperparathyroidism is most often searched for in patients with otherwise unexplained hypercalcemia, recurrent kidney stones, peptic-ulcer disease, pancreatitis, chondrocalcinosis, or, in rarer instances, with symptoms and/or signs of osteitis fibrosa. Blood calcium measurements may lead to detection of hypercalcemia in patients with vague constitutional complaints, lethargy and weakness, gastrointestinal symptoms, atypical arthritis, and myopathy, or as a result of multiphasic routine blood testing in asymptomatic subjects.

Hypercalcemia is the most invariant manifestation of hyperparathyroidism. In fact, without definite hypercalcemia, there is almost never a justification for surgical exploration. Repeated measurements of plasma calcium should be made in patients with suspected hypercalcemia (normal range in most centers is 8.6 to 10.4 mg per 100 ml or an even narrower range). It is important to eliminate errors or misinterpretations due to altered concentrations of blood proteins, venous stasis during collection of blood (Krull *et al.*, 1969), or unsuspected variation in a given laboratory's range of normal. One may detect either a sustained hypercalcemia or a pattern of high normal blood calcium values alternating with occasional slightly elevated values.

It is the latter pattern of blood calcium values that is a focus of special interest; the hypercalcemia of mild hyperparathyroidism may occasionally present a subtle or intermittent pattern and thus confuse the interpretation. Careful scrutiny of reports of "normocalcemic hyperparathyroidism" (Yendt and Gagné, 1968; Wills *et al.*, 1969; Wills, 1971) reveals that the patients were, in fact, frankly hypercalcemic, albeit mildly, at some times in their course, representative of the mild or subtle pattern of hypercalcemia. At other times these same patients had calcium values in the high normal range. Such patients could more correctly be described, therefore, as having "intermittent hypercalcemia." Repeated estimations of fasting blood calcium in normal individuals reveal a pattern of values that vary up or down by 0.5 to 1.0 mg per 100 ml, centered around an average value of 9.5 mg per 100 ml, i.e., in the mid-normal range. Patients with the pattern of intermittent hypercalcemia, suspected of having hyperparathyroidism, typically show all values to be at least in the upper 25% of the normal range, 10.0 mg per 100 ml or greater, with some samples just above the upper limit of normal.

Some workers have presented data on a group of patients whom they believe represent true "normocalcemic hyperparathyroidism," meaning consistently mid-normal values of blood calcium. These patients, many of whom were recurrent stone-formers, were operated on and found to have normal parathyroids grossly and by light microscopy. Abnormalities in gland histology by electron microscopy were reported; the patients' clinical courses subsequently were marked by a reduction in frequency of stones (Shieber *et al.*, 1971). There may well prove to be patients in this category, but until there is much wider experience in other centers, the authors stress caution in accepting the concept of truly normocalcemic hyperparathyroidism.

The variable causes and clinical course of recurrent nephrolithiasis make it difficult to invoke clinical improvement, even over a period of several years, to support the view that hyperparathyroidism was the cause of the nephrolithiasis when all calcium values are well within the normal range, and the parathyroids are found at surgery and by light microscopy to be normal grossly. A decreased renal tubular reabsorption of phosphate is seen in patients with idiopathic hypercalciuria (Melick and Henneman, 1958), most of whom do not appear to have or go on to develop hyperparathyroidism; hence, occasional hypophosphatemia in stone-formers cannot be used to support the concept of normocalcemic hyperparathyroidism. One must be reluctant to consider patients as having primary hyperparathyroidism in the presence of persistent normocalcemia, unless as observed by Reiss and Canterbury (1975), there is known malabsorption or renal failure to modify the calcium-elevating effects of excessive PTH secretion.

The serum inorganic-phosphorus level in primary hyperparathyroidism is usually low but may be normal, especially in patients with abnormal renal function. Even in primary hyperparathyroidism, serum phosphate levels may rise when glomerular filtration rates fall to very low levels. Detection of hypophosphatemia can be useful but is less specific than hypercalcemia, particularly in light of reports that severe hypercalcemia of any cause may lower serum phosphorus by altering renal tubular handling of phosphate (Eisenberg, 1965; Schussler *et al.*, 1972). Blood samples should be obtained in the morning, under fasting conditions, since after eating there may be a sharp fall in blood phosphorus levels.

Hypercalciuria is also commonly seen in hyperparathyroidism with hypercalcemia. However, since parathyroid hormone reduces calcium clearance, the urinary excretion of calcium is lower in patients with hyperparathyroidism than in patients with equivalent degrees of hypercalcemia of nonparathyroid cause (Nordin and Peacock, 1969; Dent and Harper, 1962).

Blood alkaline phosphatase and urinary hydroxyproline excretion (Kivirikko, 1970) are usually elevated only when there is remarkable bone involvement. Renal involvement can be reflected by a decreased concentrating ability, by specific tubular defects such as tubular acidosis, and, finally, by frank renal failure with the chemical findings of azotemia (Epstein, 1968a). Other electrolyte abnormalities such as the finding of a mild hyperchloremic acidosis, as described earlier, may also be of diagnostic value.

2. Special Tests

Over the years a number of special tests have been proposed to aid in establishing the diagnosis of hyperparathyroidism. Many of these tests are not as useful as was originally hoped. Principal difficulties in diagnosis arise in patients with recurrent stones but without convincing evidence of hypercalcemia; the special tests are often either inapplicable in this situation or misleading. Efforts have been made to quantitate the effect of parathyroid hormone on reduction in tubular phosphate reabsorption and increase in urinary phosphate clearance, but have not proved to be successful (Strott and Nugent, 1968). Many factors such as intrinsic renal disease, dietary phosphate intake, and the physiological diurnal variation in phosphate excretion interfere with the interpretation of phosphate clearance. Measurements utilizing calcium infusion to suppress parathyroid secretion and reduce phosphate clearance (Kyle *et al.*, 1962) were undertaken before it was realized that the parathyroid glands are responsive to changes in blood calcium levels even in primary hyperparathyroidism (Murray *et al,*, 1972).

If special tests of renal phosphorus handling are to be used, appropriate caution must therefore be observed in interpretation. Several convenient indices of phosphate excretion by the kidneys may be determined (Goldsmith, 1969). Because of the diurnal variation in renal phosphate handling and the fluctuations in plasma phosphate after meals, 24-hour urine collections should not be used for determinations of phosphate clearance; short periods of collection in the morning during fasting give more reproducible results.

Phosphate clearance is determined by standard techniques involving simultaneous measurements of urinary and blood phosphate and creatinine concentrations; usually urine samples are collected over a 1–4-hour period. Normal subjects have a phosphate clearance of 10.8 ± 2.7 ml per min. Increases of 50% or greater above this figure have been detected in some patients with hyperparathyroidism. The ratio of phosphate clearance to creatinine clearance indicates the percent of filtered phosphate excreted. The tubular resorption of phosphate can be calculated from the phosphate clearance and the glomerular filtration rate, the latter usually determined by creatinine clearance (see Chapter 2, Volume I).

In normal subjects, the tubular resorption of phosphate exceeds 85%; in some patients with hyperparathyroidism, but unfortunately also in other subjects as well, tubular resorption of phosphate is lower. It is essential to control phosphate intake in such studies, as renal tubular phosphate transport, with or without excessive parathyroid effect, will vary with extremes of oral phosphate intake (Chapter 2, Volume I). Low phosphate intake leads to increased tubular reabsorption. It is critical that measurements of phosphate clearance be considered quantitatively with respect to serum levels.

Thiazide diuretics in the usual doses of 1–2 gm daily of chlorothiazide or its equivalent can produce sustained hypercalcemia in patients with hyperparathyroidism and borderline calcium values (see Chapter 6). Such a response is not usually seen in normal subjects. Although thiazide diuretics may produce transient elevations of blood calcium in normal subjects, normocalcemia returns in a few days despite continued administration. Thiazide administration, therefore, has been suggested as a provocative test for the presence of hyperparathyroidism (Duarte *et al.*, 1971).

Glucocorticoid administration has been useful in distinguishing the hypercalcemia of hyperparathyroidism from that associated with sarcoidosis, multiple myeloma, vitamin D intoxication, and some malignant diseases with osseous metastases (Dent, 1962; Dent and Watson, 1966). In the latter diseases, doses of hydrocortisone of 100 mg per day for 10 days result in a lowering of the serum calcium to normal levels, whereas calcium levels typically do not fall in primary hyperparathyroidism. Patients with hypercalcemia due to sarcoidosis occasionally have failed to respond within 10 days to prednisone or to cortisone at doses less than 150 mg (cortisone) daily (J. Anderson *et al.*, 1954; Phillips and Fitzpatrick, 1956;

McSwiney and Mills, 1956; Winnacker *et al.*, 1968). Hydrocortisone has usually been the glucocorticoid used for the calcium-suppression test. There may be false positive results in hyperparathyroidism, usually when severe skeletal disease is present (Gwinup and Sayle, 1961; Boonstra and Jackson, 1965).

3. Radioimmunoassay for Parathyroid Hormone

a. Primary Hyperparathyroidism. Before considering the diagnostic uses of the parathyroid hormone immunoassay, it is useful to review the pathophysiology of parathyroid hormone secretion in hyperparathyroidism. In primary hyperparathyroidism the mechanisms involved in the normal control of secretion of hormone must be abnormal by definition, since patients have inappropriately high levels of the circulating hormone despite concomitant hypercalcemia. Although the complexities of hormone metabolism, discussed earlier, introduce the possibility that increased hormone levels in the circulation could be due, at least in part, to prolonged metabolic clearance, all evidence indicates that abnormal secretion of hormone is the predominant causative factor in the pathogenesis of primary hyperparathyroidism.

In the past, the hypothesis had been advanced that the abnormal pattern of secretion is due to autonomous secretion, which is independent of blood calcium (Reiss and Canterbury, 1969). This concept was challenged by Murray *et al.* (1972), who showed, in 13 patients with parathyroid adenomas and one with parathyroid carcinoma, that hormone secretion was responsive to alterations in blood calcium by infusions of EDTA and/or calcium. The findings indicated that hormone production by these tumors was not autonomous (Figs. 33 and 34). Because hormone secretion does respond to changes in serum calcium, one must conclude that the defect in control of hormone production is a mechanism more subtle than simple autonomy.

Two types of defect in secretion control might explain the abnormality. One is that higher than normal levels of serum calcium are necessary to suppress hormone production, a "set-point" error (Fig. 35). Alternatively, a small fractional amount of hormone secretion may be totally autonomous, that is, independent of the blood calcium concentration (Fig. 36). In the former instance, the secretion of hormone in patients with hyperparathyroidism would be suppressed, but at higher concentrations of serum calcium than in normal subjects (Fig. 35). In the latter situation, the large mass of parathyroid tissue characteristic of hyperparathyroidism might result in an exaggeration of nonsuppressible secretion due to the increased number of cells per se and thus result in secretion of a sufficiently excessive amount of hormone to produce a state of hyper-

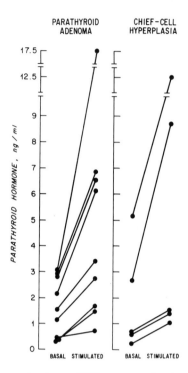

Fig. 33. Maximal increase in plasma PTH concentration in peripheral venous plasma stimulated by EDTA infusion in 13 patients with primary hyperparathyroidism due to either parathyroid adenoma or chief-cell hyperplasia. Suppression of hormone concentration was seen during calcium infusion in these same patients. (Modified from Potts and Deftos, 1974.)

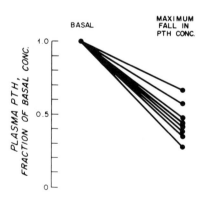

Fig. 34. Decrease in PTH concentration after calcium infusion in patients with primary hyperparathyroidism. (From Potts and Deftos, 1974.)

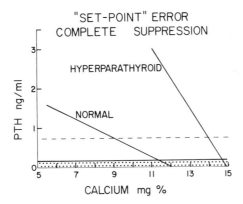

Fig. 35. Diagram depicting hypothesis of "set-point" error to explain physiological mechanism of abnormality in control of hormone secretion in primary hyperparathyroidism. Ordinate represents plasma parathyroid hormone concentration, and abscissa, plasma calcium. Hyperparathyroid individuals show steeper slopes of response, owing to large mass of tissue. Complete suppression of hormone output occurs at abnormally high calcium level. Dashed line represents upper limit of normal PTH concentration. PTH values within shaded area are below limits of assay detection.

parathyroidism (Fig. 36). Some experimental evidence is available at present in support of the first mechanism, that of a "set-point error," based on analyses of hormone release *in vitro* from adenomas (Habener, 1978).

Several lines of evidence lend credence to the possibility that non-suppressible secretion plays a role in the abnormal secretion of parathyroid hormone. Gittes and Radde (1966) found that transplantation of several normal parathyroids into a single rat, thus considerably increasing the total mass of parathyroid tissue in the animal, could produce hypercalcemia and a state of hyperparathyroidism. Later studies by Targovnik *et al.* (1971), done *in vitro,* showed that it was not possible to completely inhibit the output of hormone by normal bovine glands maintained in organ culture. Convincing evidence for incomplete suppression of hormone secretion was obtained by Mayer (1973) and Mayer *et al.* (1976) in studies carried out *in vivo.* These workers demonstrated, by radioimmunoassay, sustained secretion of small amounts of hormone into parathyroid gland venous effluent in calves made hypercalcemic for up to 40 hours by infusion of calcium. It is not known, however, whether the component of the hormone secreted by the gland during maximum suppression by calcium consists entirely of intact hormone or in part of biologically active or inactive fragments of the hormone. Mayer *et al.* (1976) reported that at least a fraction of the hormone secreted under

Joel F. Habener and John T. Potts, Jr.

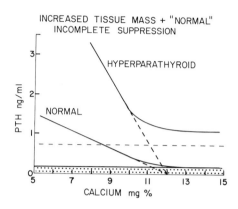

Fig. 36. Diagram of an alternative hypothesis to explain secretory defect in primary hyperparathyroidism (see Figs. 12 and 13). Hypothesis requires that a small amount of hormone secretion persists despite elevated calcium. In the normal parathyroid, this secretion is small and insignificant. In hyperparathyroidism, greatly increased tissue mass leads to persistent secretion of hormone above normal range (dashed line). Note slopes of both normal and hyperparathyroid extrapolate to same calcium value (12 mg%). PTH values within shaded area are below limits of assay detection.

conditions of calcium suppression consists of intact hormone. Combining the evidence of Mayer *et al.* (1976) and Gittes and Radde (1966), one could conclude that the concept of nonsuppressible secretion by an increased mass of tissue may be important in the pathophysiology of primary hyperparathyroidism. Certain evidence, however, discussed below in connection with catheterization localization studies, suggests that normal glands may be completely suppressed with chronic hypercalcemia of a duration of weeks to months.

Hence, it is clear that further study is required to definitively analyze the nature of the pathophysiologic defect in hormone production in hyperparathyroidism.

b. General Diagnostic Use. The development of a specific radioimmunoassay sufficiently sensitive to detect circulating human parathyroid hormone has provided, for the first time, a specific test for parathyroid function. Assay procedures are now widely available in referral centers and special commercial diagnostic laboratories. There have been and continue to be, however, numerous problems with the application and interpretation of the assay, accounted for by the heterogeneity of plasma parathyroid hormone.

There is general agreement that the principal form of immunoreactive hormone detected in blood is a large fragment, biologically inert, that comprises the middle and carboxyl-terminal two-thirds of the peptide; the biologically active amino-terminal end has been removed from this prominent circulating fragment. Whether the peripheral cleavage represents an activation step, rather than metabolic degradation, and whether the amino-terminal active portion is delivered to receptors or reenters the circulation is at present unknown (as discussed in earlier sections). What is clear is that there is only a low concentration of intact hormone in blood relative to the quantity of the metabolically inert middle and carboxyl-terminal fragment (the concentration of amino-terminal fragment, if any, must also be relatively low). Hence, most laboratories have found that antisera that recognize the carboxyl half of the hormone are most useful in detecting immunoreactive hormone in blood. Assays based on such antisera, even though they are not detecting biologically active forms of hormone, do correlate with physiological and clinical indices of parathyroid secretory activity.

Most antisera are made against intact bovine parathyroid hormone, and each antibody recognizes different regions of the polypeptide. Inasmuch as there is a preponderance, in plasma, of fragments corresponding to the carboxyl half of the molecule, and the antisera used have reactive sites against both amino-terminal and carboxyl-terminal determinants of the intact hormone used as tracer, plasma samples added in progressively larger doses do not always displace tracer from antibody as well as does intact hormone (Fig. 37). This is because of the much more effective competition exerted by intact hormone in displacement of tracer from the predominant antibodies (Fig. 9A).

The problems of measurement thus include nonparallelism of assay response due to heterogeneity of recognition sites of antibodies present with each animal immunized, and different quantities of fragments versus intact hormone in each patient sample. Since human and bovine hormone differ in amino acid sequence, the cross-reaction between the bovine and human peptides varies from one antiserum to another, which introduces yet another variable in the measurement of human hormone.

The solution to these measurement problems chosen by most laboratories has been to select as the reference standard a pool composed of a mixture of serum or plasma from patients with hyperparathyroidism. By this device, one provides a standardized mixture of intact hormone and fragments. Since there is a high concentration of fragments in the standard, nonparallel responses in the assay between standard and unknown are greatly minimized; quantitation of hormone is more accurate and reproducible. One then determines, for each antiserum used, the range of the concentration found in normal subjects expressed as the displacement of radioactive hormone tracer from antibody produced by fractions of the blood from the normal patient compared to the displace-

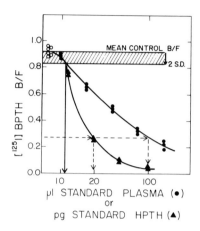

Fig. 37. Radioimmunoassay dose–dilution curves relating amounts of either standard plasma pooled from several patients with primary hyperparathyroidism (●) or a highly purified, chemically defined standard solution of intact human parathyroid hormone (▲) to the bound/free ratio of ^{125}I-labeled bovine PTH tracer. Note that the two curves are not parallel. Thus, for identical decreases in the bound/free ratio of from 0.82 to 0.25 (actually measured in the assay), the necessary amount of pooled-plasma standard solution is 10 times more (10 or 100 μl) than the necessary amount of HPTH standard solution (10 to 20 μl).

ment given by equivalent fractions of the plasma standard from patients with hyperparathyroidism (μl equivalents per ml of blood). For example, if a patient has a high concentration of hormone, the response given by 1000 μl of the patient's serum may, for example, equal that of 300 μl of the standard hyperparathyroid serum (300 μl Eq/ml). If in a second patient there is a much lower concentration of hormone, 1000 μl of this patient's blood may give a response equivalent to that of only 100 μl of standard hyperparathyroid serum (100 μl Eq/ml).

By use of arbitrarily chosen plasma standards, consisting of pooled blood from subjects with hyperparathyroidism, the variation introduced by individual differences from patient to patient in the relative content of different fragments is minimized. The problem of difference in cross-reaction between human and bovine hormone is minimized by expressing activity in the bovine assay in terms of units of human hormone. The difference between antisera from one laboratory and others is minimized by determination of normal range in each laboratory from arbitrary but reproducible values (units of plasma standard) for many normal subjects with each antiserum used. It is not possible to compare the sensitivity and standardization of assays used in different laboratories because of the problems discussed above and the resultant need to use an arbitrary plasma standard as reference for calculation of a normal range. Although it would be clearly helpful, there have not yet been reports that deal with careful analysis of frequency of false positive and false negative results.

Despite these problems, when appropriate precautions are observed, the immunoassay for parathyroid hormone is quite helpful in the diagnostic evaluation of patients with hypercalcemia and hypocalcemia, particularly concerning the assigning of a role to parathyroid excess or deficiency. The assay is especially useful in making the distinction between hypercalcemia of primary hyperparathyroidism and that of nonparathyroid origin. In patients with hypercalcemia not caused by parathyroid disease, concentrations of parathyroid hormone are usually undetectable because parathyroid gland secretion is suppressed.

In agreement with the findings of Berson and Yalow (1971) and Arnaud *et al.* (1971a), we find overlap in the basal concentration of hormone found in some subjects with proven hyperparathyroidism and that found in some normal subjects.

The discrimination between normal and hyperparathyroid subjects can be improved by considering the concentration of parathyroid hormone as a function of serum blood calcium concentration (Arnaud *et al.*, 1971b) (Fig. 38). A given parathyroid hormone concentration that would be

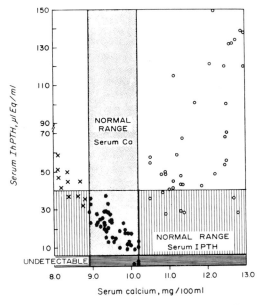

Fig. 38. Serum human ^{125}I-PTH as function of serum calcium in normal subjects (●), hypocalcemic patients (X), and patients with surgically proved primary hyperparathyroidism (o) and serum ^{125}I-PTH values less than 150 μl Eq/ml (correlation coefficient, r, for normal subjects = 0.569, $p < 0.0001$). (From Arnaud *et al.*, 1971b).

normal on an absolute basis is clearly elevated in the face of an elevated calcium level; hypercalcemia results in undetectable levels of hormone in subjects with normal parathyroids. As explained in the preceding section, the output of parathyroid hormone by a parathyroid adenoma is not autonomous with respect to serum calcium. Hence, if calcium concentration is quite high, hormone production may be somewhat lowered, leading to a concentration not readily distinguishable, without reference to the calcium level, from a normal value. Whether the hormone values include a proportion of active hormone that is higher in hyperparathyroid than in normal subjects is unknown at present.

This problem of partial overlap in assay values between normal subjects and those with hyperparathyroidism is probably related to the heterogeneity of circulating hormone.

c. *Location of Abnormal Parathyroid Tissue.* Because of the small size of the parathyroid glands, even when hyperplastic or neoplastic, and because of their variable position and the complex anatomy of the neck, localization of abnormal parathyroid tissue at surgery is often difficult and tedious. For this reason, several methods have been devised to attempt preoperative localization of abnormal parathyroid tissue. Roentgenographic examination of the esophagus during barium swallow can reveal an indentation on the esophagus caused by pressure from a large parathyroid gland (Stevens and Jackson, 1967). The selective uptake or differential concentration of selenium-labeled methionine by parathyroid tissue, detected by scanning the neck, has been used, but with limited success (Potchen *et al.*, 1967). These procedures suffer from the limitation that they are nonspecific; nonparathyroid tumors or thyroid tissue may give false positive results.

Recently, a new approach in localization was introduced. The procedure involves use of venous sampling of veins in the neck and mediastinum in combination with radioimmunoassay and selective arteriography (H. Eisenberg *et al.*, 1974). The initial procedure of venous sampling and radioimmunoassay involved collection of blood from the jugular and innominate vessels (Reitz *et al.*, 1969). This technique, while useful, failed to detect the site of abnormal tissue in a considerable number of patients.

Detection of the site of the abnormal glands was based on finding a higher concentration of hormone (compared to all other sites) in the venous sample obtained near the site of drainage of the abnormal gland into the general circulation. Dilution of parathyroid-hormone-rich effluent blood with numerous other tributaries in the jugular and innominate veins, however, blunted the gradient in immunoassayable hormone in many patients to background levels.

Studies by Doppman and Hammond (1970) and by Eisenberg *et al.*

(1974) showed that selective sampling of the thyroid venous plexus (the superior, middle, and inferior thyroid veins) leads to a high frequency of localization because there is less dilution of parathyroid-effluent blood. These studies indicated that although paired superior, middle, and inferior thyroid veins constitute an anatomic plexus, thyroid venus effluent drains ipsilaterally.

In a report of 33 patients suspected of having hyperparathyroidism (Powell *et al.*, 1972), venous samples were obtained by catheter from the small veins of the thyroid plexus. In all patients in whom a single cervical adenoma was subsequently found at surgery, a marked unilateral gradient in hormone concentration was seen in the small thyroid veins on the side of the neoplasm. Samples taken from the contralateral thyroid veins were found to have a hormone concentration no higher than the peripheral level, i.e., there was no hormone gradient, confirming the roentgenologic observations that thyroid venous blood drains ipsilaterally. In addition, the findings indicated that the normal parathyroid glands were probably suppressed by the hypercalcemia caused by the parathyroid adenoma (Fig. 39). At least, within the limitations of assay discrimination, a gradient could not be detected in veins draining the normal parathyroids. In

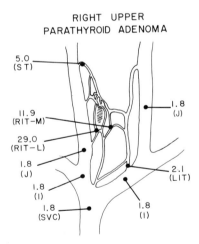

RIGHT UPPER
PARATHYROID ADENOMA

Fig. 39. Tracings made from a thyroid venogram, showing the results of radioimmunoassay of PTH on samples from the sites indicated. The PTH is elevated in samples taken from the right inferior thyroid veins, suggesting an adenoma on the right side. There is a small gradient in right ST, but note absence of gradient in LIT; this pattern, unilateral gradient, points to a single abnormal gland as opposed to hyperplasia. I, innominate vein; J, jugular vein; SVC, superior vena cava; ST, superior thyroid vein; LIT, left inferior thyroid vein; RIT, right inferior thyroid vein. (From D. Powell, personal communication, 1972, cited in Habener and Potts, 1976c.)

patients who had abnormal parathyroid tissue on both sides of the neck (i.e., hyperplasia), however, gradients in hormone concentration were found on both sides of the thyroid venous plexus.

Selective arteriography has proved useful, in particular when the gradient in immunoassayable hormone is found in the inferior thyroid vein or in the thymic vein (H. Eisenberg *et al.*, 1974). In such situations, experience indicates that the drainage into the inferior thyroid vessel can come not only from an abnormal gland located in the neck, but also by drainage upward from a gland within the mediastinum. In these situations, injection into the inferior thyroid artery on the indicated side often reveals the parathyroid tumor by the detection of its vascular bed or "blush" (Fig. 40).

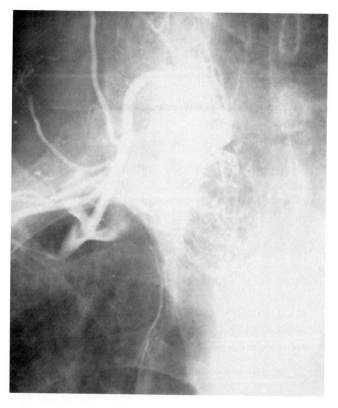

Fig. 40. Radio-contrast arteriogram of right cervical circulation in a patient with severe hyperparathyroidism. Note markedly increased vascularity in the localized area, indicating the presence of a large parathyroid adenoma. (Courtesy of the Department of Radiology, Massachusetts General Hospital.)

Since the expertise necessary to catheterize thyroid veins or perform selective arteriography is not available in many centers, the angiographic techniques are recommended only for patients in whom previous neck surgery has failed to locate hyperfunctioning parathyroid tissue or in patients who present special diagnostic problems. In the latter category, for example, are patients with recent history of malignancy in whom the question of hyperparathyroidism arises (see Chapter 6).

E. Differential Diagnosis

1. General

Hypercalcemia is one of the more common diagnostic problems in medicine (Goldsmith, 1966; Boonstra and Jackson, 1965). Although malignant neoplasms with or without skeletal metastases and primary hyperparathyroidism are probably the leading causes of hypercalcemia in adults, other etiologies must be considered in the differential diagnosis. The correct diagnosis can be made in many patients after a careful history and physical examination and the use of several routine radiological procedures and laboratory tests. In many instances there may be obvious manifestations of the responsible disease state, such as widespread malignant disease, thyrotoxicosis, or a history of excessive ingestion of vitamin D. Quite frequently, however, the underlying cause for the hypercalcemia is not obvious and one must embark on a detailed evaluation of the patient. First, however, it is essential to ensure that true hypercalcemia exists. This generally requires several repeated determinations of the serum calcium level over a period of a few days. Patients with mild degrees of hyperparathyroidism, for example, may have levels of calcium that fluctuate in the range from high normal to slightly elevated, and it takes several determinations to establish a truly convincing pattern of hypercalcemia.

It is important to emphasize that hyperparathyroidism is characteristically a chronic disorder; historical information or clinical evidence of the chronicity of a disorder in calcium metabolism such as recurrent renal calculi, chronic peptic ulcer disease, documented hypercalcemia many months earlier, or evidence of renal stone usually favors the diagnosis of hyperparathyroidism rather than malignancy, as has been pointed out by Lafferty (1966). On the other hand, if hypercalcemia has been detected only recently without other historical features of chronicity, the search for other causes of hypercalcemia must be particularly thorough.

As mentioned earlier, most laboratories determine total calcium values, which includes both free or ionized calcium and protein-bound calcium.

The serum calcium value must be interpreted in relation to serum protein concentrations, inasmuch as only an abnormality in non-protein-bound calcium reflects an abnormality in calcium metabolism. A rough guide is to adjust the total serum calcium by 0.8 mg% for each gram of serum proteins above or below normal before deciding that a given level of total calcium is truly abnormal.

The serum alkaline phosphatase may be elevated in several conditions that produce hypercalcemic states. Procedures used to determine the origin of the various alkaline phosphatase isoenzymes are discussed in Chapter 3, Volume 1. A substantially elevated total alkaline phosphatase in the absence of radiologically evident bone disease is an unusual occurrence in primary hyperparathyroidism. Hyperphosphatasia under these circumstances is more consistent with metastatic malignancy or sarcoidosis with hepatic involvement. Serum chloride and bicarbonate values may be helpful; a mild hyperchloremic acidosis favors the diagnosis of primary hyperparathyroidism, whereas metabolic alkalosis would suggest malignancy, hypervitaminosis D, or milk/alkali syndrome. Persistent azotemia in the well-hydrated patient may point to renal damage secondary to long-standing hypercalcemia and suggests the chronicity of the hypercalcemia. Additional tests might include a sedimentation rate and serum protein electrophoresis or immunoelectrophoresis, which, if abnormal, may point to multiple myeloma or other non-parathyroid-related disorders. These parameters are usually normal in uncomplicated primary hyperparathyroidism. Fraser *et al.* (1971) have claimed high usefulness for a multivariant analysis of serum phosphorus, alkaline phosphatase, bicarbonate, and urea for the differential diagnosis of hypercalcemia. The diagnosis by this simple analysis in their hands coincided in 197 of 218 cases of hypercalcemia with the diagnosis reached after a long period of detailed clinical investigation.

Roentgenological procedures that should be undertaken in patients with hypercalcemia include plain films of the lungs, hands, skull, and abdomen (often with IVP) to search for, respectively, pulmonary sarcoidosis or malignancy, subperiosteal resorption, enlargement of the sella turcica, and renal calculi or renal tumor. If occult malignancy is suspected, then, in addition to an intravenous pyelogram, a complete gastrointestinal series plus a bone scan and/or skeletal survey should be performed.

2. Malignancy

Hypercalcemia is a frequent complication of malignant disease. The elimination of malignancy as the underlying cause of hypercalcemia can be one of the most difficult problems in differential diagnosis, particularly when one considers the possibility of pseudohyperparathyroidism or ectopic production of hypercalcemic factors by malignant tumors. The patient's medical history, as well as physical and laboratory findings, are helpful in the differentiation. If a patient with hypercalcemia has a history of vague complaints and recurrent symptoms extending over several years before the evaluation, it is much less likely that occult malignant disease is responsible; if malignancy is the cause of the hypercalcemia, definite clinical evidence of the primary or metastatic lesions would be uncovered by careful evaluation of the patient. Lafferty (1966) has emphasized that the hypercalcemia of malignancy ("pseudohyperparathyroidism") is usually manifested by a rapid, fulminant course with severe symptoms and relatively severe hypercalcemia, often >12 mg per 100 ml (see Chapter 6).

Hypercalcemia complicating malignancy usually results from one of two basic processes: (a) osteolytic metastases, more commonly seen in carcinoma of the breast, kidney, lung, or thyroid (Omenn et al., 1969) or (b) true pseudohyperparathyroidism, defined by Lafferty (1966) as a syndrome involving hypercalcemia in the absence of osteolytic metastases, resulting from the elaboration, by tumors of nonparathyroid tissue, of a humoral agent causing hypercalcemia. Pseudohyperparathyroidism seems due to ectopic production of parathyroid hormone or excessive production of humoral substances chemically distinct from parathyroid hormone. Evidence (Seyberth et al., 1976) has pointed to prostaglandins as potential mediating agents in some cases of pseudohyperparathyroidism. This subject of malignancy and hypercalcemia is discussed in detail in Chapter 6.

3. Sarcoidosis

Abnormalities in calcium metabolism including hypercalcemia, hypophosphatemia, hyperphosphatasia, and hypercalciuria are relatively frequent accompaniments of sarcoidosis (Winnacker et al., 1968), and may mimic those of primary hyperparathyroidism. Difficulty in establishing a diagnosis may result particularly when other manifestations of sarcoidosis such as hepatomegaly, lymphadenopathy, skin lesions, hyperglobulinemia, and respiratory symptoms are minimal or absent. Several reports have appeared of patients ultimately proven to have sarcoidosis who have undergone neck explorations because of erroneously suspected primary hyperparathyroidism (Klatskin and Gordon, 1953; Solomon and Channick, 1960; Dent, 1962; Dent and Watson, 1966). The situation is further complicated by the occasional occurrence of both sarcoidosis and primary hyperparathyroidism in the same patient (Burr et al., 1959; Dent, 1962; Dent and Watson, 1966).

Goldstein et al. (1971) surveyed the reported incidence of hypercalcemia in sarcoidosis. The frequency of hypercalcemia varied quite widely; estimates ranged from 0.7 to 63% with most series between 10 and 20%. The frequency of hypercalcemia was usually highest in those studies that included many patients examined before corticosteroid therapy was widely used in treatment. It seems probable, therefore, that corticosteroids, which are known to lower serum calcium in sarcoidosis (Dent, 1956), have altered the incidence of hypercalcemia. Usually hypercalcemia is mild, but levels may occasionally be as high as 18–20 mg per 100 ml (Citron, 1954; M. Ellis and Wilson, 1958).

The levels of serum inorganic phosphorus in patients with sarcoidosis, although typically normal, may occasionally be low. In fact, one report suggested that hypophosphatemia may be more common than hypercalcemia in sarcoidosis (Putkonen et al., 1965). Serum alkaline phosphatase levels are frequently elevated, the result of hepatic rather than bone involvement by sarcoid granulomata. The excretion of urinary calcium is more often elevated, inasmuch as hypercalciuria was reported in from 29 to 36% of patients with sarcoidosis (Basset, 1964; James, 1964). Prolonged hypercalcemia and hypercalciuria in sarcoidosis can lead to urolithiasis, nephrocalcinosis, and occasionally to renal failure.

The pathogenesis of the disturbances in calcium metabolism that are seen in sarcoidosis is generally regarded as due to an enhanced sensitivity to vitamin D (Bell et al., 1964). Patients with sarcoidosis are unusually sensitive to vitamin D either administered exogenously in small doses (Nelson, 1949; Larsson et al., 1952) or formed endogenously by exposure to ultraviolet light (Taylor et al., 1963).

Although in the review of Goldstein et al. (1971) no seasonal variation in hypercalcemia (attributed to higher vitamin D levels secondary to increased sunlight in summer) was found, it seems possible that the increased use of glucocorticoids may have blunted the effects of sunlight. In our experience in the management of patients with severe sarcoidosis and hypercalcemia not receiving glucocorticoids, hypercalcemia worsens in the summer. In one patient, the coexistence of vitiligo seemed to enhance the sensitivity to sunlight. Severe hypercalcemia appeared abruptly in June and July during several successive summers despite careful precautions to minimize exposure of skin. The hypercalcemia abated spontaneously during the winter months. Thus, it is advisable to instruct patients who have hypercalcemic sarcoidosis to avoid exposure to sunlight.

It has been observed that the changes in values of serum, urine, and fecal calcium in hypercalcemic sarcoidosis closely resemble those found in vitamin D intoxication (Henneman et al., 1956). In addition, these abnormalities in calcium metabolism are rapidly corrected by treatment with glucocorticoids as in true vitamin D intoxication (Dent, 1956). Although some workers believe that the ameliorative effects of corticosteroids are due to a direct action on sarcoid granulomas in bone (J. Anderson *et al.*, 1954), most have interpreted the hypocalcemic effects of glucocorticoids as due to an antagonism of vitamin D action. No correlation has been found between hypercalcemia and granulomatous involvement of the skeleton; many patients with demonstrable bone disease do not have hypercalcemia (Mather, 1957). Indeed, in our experience hypercalcemia is more likely to occur in patients with pulmonary sarcoidosis. Furthermore, decreased fecal calcium is almost a constant finding in sarcoidosis (Winnacker *et al.*, 1968), an observation consistent with the known major action of vitamin D to increase intestinal calcium absorption.

On the other hand, several lines of evidence indicate that even though there is increased sensitivity to vitamin D in sarcoidosis, increased intestinal calcium absorption is not the sole basis for the abnormalities of calcium metabolism. Several lines of evidence suggest the existence of excessive skeletal turnover. Metabolic balance studies carried out in patients with sarcoidosis have indicated that hypercalcemia and hypercalciuria can persist in the absence of increased intestinal calcium absorption (Hunt and Yendt, 1963); hypercalciuria has been observed in patients who have normal serum and fecal calcium (Hendrix, 1966). Henneman *et al.* (1956) found that the levels of urinary calcium occasionally exceeded calcium intake during carefully performed balance studies. The negative calcium balances observed in these patients can only be attributed either singly or in combination to decreased accretion or increased resorption of bone mineral or to decreased renal tubular resorption of calcium.

The latter seems unlikely since there is no convincing evidence that vitamin D exerts any direct effect on the renal handling of calcium. Thus, it appears that hypercalcemia, hypercalciuria, or both, of sarcoidosis are a result of an unusual sensitivity of bone and intestine to the actions of vitamin D. The metabolic basis of the enhanced sensitivity to vitamin D is unknown. One might speculate, however, that one or more defects may exist in the metabolism of vitamin D to its active hydroxylated metabolites (increased conversion of vitamin D to 1,25-dihydroxycholecalciferol or decreased destruction of 1,25-dihydroxycholecalciferol or, alternatively, that receptor sites in bone and intestine are unusually responsive to the dihydroxy vitamin. One report did establish that 25-OHD levels per se were not abnormal in two patients who had hypercalcemic sarcoidosis (Bell and Sinha, 1977).

In these patients in whom the clinical signs and symptoms associated with hypercalcemia were not sufficient to distinguish between the diagnosis of primary hyperparathyroidism and sarcoidosis, one or more of several laboratory tests will help to establish the correct diagnosis. An elevated or even a detectable level of serum immunoreactive parathyroid hormone strongly suggests the diagnosis of hyperparathyroidism. In a study of 26 unselected patients with sarcoidosis, 6 of whom had hypercalcemia, serum immunoreactive parathyroid hormone was undetectable or low in 19 (Cushard et al., 1972). Of the seven with normal levels, five had been treated with corticosteroids at the time of the study. These data indicate that most patients with sarcoidosis have functional hypoparathyroidism. The increased intestinal absorption of calcium presumably leads to a suppression of parathyroid hormone secretion.

As discussed previously, the cortisone suppression test is useful in distinguishing between hypercalcemic sarcoidosis and hyperparathyroidism (Dent, 1956). The hypercalcemia of hyperparathyroidism is usually unaffected, whereas that due to sarcoidosis (as well as that due to vitamin D excess) is corrected by administration of cortisone. Only rarely will the hypercalcemia of hyperparathyroidism respond to corticosteroids.

A careful examination of the chest roentgenograms may help to establish the diagnosis of hypercalcemic sarcoidosis. Although hilar adenopathy is the classic-opathy finding [stage I in the international classification (Siltzbach et al., 1974)], it is now evident that a more subtle pattern of diffuse fibroreticular infiltrate in the peripheral lung fields may be present in the absence of detectable hilar adenopathy, so-called stage II disease (Siltzbach et al., 1974). Evaluation of pulmonary function also may prove helpful when the roentgenographic changes are equivocal. The authors have seen several patients in whom the diagnosis of sarcoidosis was at first unsuspected (chest roentgenograms initially read as negative), but the presence of a low serum immunoreactive parathyroid hormone level and a low chloride/phosphorus ratio in the serum argued against hyperparathyroidism and led to further studies including pulmonary function studies. The finding of low carbon monoxide diffusion and hypoxemia on exercise eventually revealed the presence of sarcoidosis rather than hyperparathyroidism, and unnecessary neck exploration was avoided.

In addition to the special tests of parathyroid hormone assay and cortisone suppression, other laboratory determinations may be useful in differentiating these two diseases. Although hypophosphatemia occurs, an elevated or normal fasting serum phosphorus level is more consistent with sarcoidosis than with hyperparathyroidism. The finding of a mild hyperchloremia (plasma chloride above 102 mEq per liter) is more consistent with hyperparathyroidism than sarcoidosis. An elevated sedimentation rate and/or hypergammaglobulinemia is not found in uncomplicated hyperparathyroidism. A definitive procedure, whenever possible, is to establish a histological diagnosis by biopsy of liver or lymph node; a positive Kveim test is also of value (Siltzbach *et al.,* 1974). It has also been emphasized that, in addition to sarcoidosis, other types of chronic granulomatous disease such as tuberculosis (Shai *et al.,* 1972) or berylliosis (Tepper *et al.,* 1961) can cause hypercalcemia.

4. Thyrotoxicosis

Severe and symptomatic hypercalcemia is a rare complication of thyrotoxicosis. However, mild elevations of serum calcium have been reported in as many as 23% of patients with hyperthyroidism (Rose and Boles, 1953; Bryant *et al.,* 1964). The cause of hypercalcemia in hyperthyroidism appears to be secondary to increased bone resorption, probably owing to direct effects of thyroxine and triiodothyronine on the skeleton (Aub *et al.,* 1929; Laake, 1955; Krane *et al.,* 1956; Adams *et al.,* 1967; Adams and Jowsey, 1967; Krane and Goldring, 1976) (see Chapter 4).

The turnover of calcium by the skeleton is increased by thyroid hormone (Krane *et al.,* 1956). Adams and Jowsey (1967) found that the serum calcium in 10 hyperthyroid patients averaged 0.5 mg% higher than in a group of matched normal control subjects. The serum protein concentrations in these patients tended to be lower than normal, indicating that the serum ionized calcium was significantly elevated. Serum inorganic phosphorus levels were high and urinary clearance decreased, suggesting that parathyroid hormone secretion was suppressed. Castro *et al.* (1975) have reported finding that serum parathyroid hormone levels are low in patients with hyperthyroidism and hypercalcemia. Suppression of parathyroid hormone in these patients might be expected to lead to hypercalciuria, a finding often seen in patients with thyrotoxicosis. Patients with thyrotoxicosis are more sensitive than are normal persons to the hypercalcemic effects of parathyroid hormone (M. T. Harrison *et al.,* 1964; Bouillon and DeMoor, 1974). Epstein (1968b) emphasized that patients with thyrotoxicosis who develop severe hypercalcemia may have concomitant hyperparathyroidism, inasmuch as the hypercalcemia of uncomplicated thyrotoxicosis is usually mild. The patient reported by Epstein *et al.* (1958), with a serum calcium of 15 mg per 100 ml, later proved to have a parathyroid adenoma (Baxter and Bondy, 1966). Breuer and McPherson (1966) described 17 patients with thyrotoxicosis and concomitant parathyroid adenomas.

The diagnosis of hyperthyroidism usually offers no difficulties, because, in most cases, it is the thyrotoxicosis rather than the hypercalcemia that brings the patient to the physician. However, particularly in the elderly, the signs of thyrotoxicosis may be minimal. During the treatment of a patient with thyrotoxicosis and hypercalcemia, repeated determinations of serum calcium should be made. If the serum calcium does not return toward normal as the thyrotoxicosis is brought under control, another cause for the hypercalcemia, such as hyperparathyroidism, should be suspected.

5. Adrenal Insufficiency

Hypercalcemia can occasionally occur in adrenal insufficiency, most often in acute adrenal failure (Loeb, 1932; Leeksma *et al.*, 1957; Walser *et al.*, 1963). At least part of the hypercalcemia can be attributed to hemoconcentration and resultant hyperproteinemia. Walser *et al.* (1963) produced adrenal insufficiency in dogs and found that the plasma ionized calcium was normal. They concluded that three alterations combined to produce hypercalcemia: the elevated plasma protein concentration associated with hemoconcentration; an increase in filtrable calcium complexes, especially calcium citrate; and an increase in the affinity of plasma protein for calcium, explained as a consequence of hyponatremia and low plasma ionic strength. Excessive amounts of a nonfiltrable complex of calcium and phosphate, formed either *in vivo* or *in vitro* was also found. The increased calcium concentration of the plasma is not dependent on increased intestinal absorption of calcium, inasmuch as it occurs on a calcium-free diet.

Although it is reasonable to propose that the loss of the antivitamin D effect of glucocorticoids in adrenal insufficiency could predispose to hypercalcemia, there is little evidence to support this contention (see Chapter 3). In any event, particularly in acute adrenal failure, hypercalcemia is usually only a transient phenomenon, and blood calcium levels return to normal with adrenal-hormone replacement therapy.

6. Vitamin D Intoxication

The chronic ingestion of large doses of vitamin D can produce hypercalcemia. The mode of action of excessive doses of the vitamin is twofold: to promote increased bone resorption and excessive gastrointestinal absorption of calcium (Kodicek, 1967). Usually the ingestion of doses in excess of 100,000 units of vitamin D_2 or D_3 for several months is necessary for this complication to occur. However, in certain cases, hypercalcemia may develop after only a few weeks of excessive vitamin D ingestion.

Vitamin D intoxication may occur as a complication of treatment of patients with hypoparathyroidism (see Chapter 3) and with intestinal malabsorption. Despite long periods of stable control on a given replacement dose of the vitamin, hypercalcemia may suddenly develop without obvious explanation. The diagnosis in self-induced intoxication is usually established by uncovering a history of excessive vitamin D intake. The presence of a high level of serum phosphorus and the presence of a mild metabolic alkylosis rather than acidosis supports the diagnosis of hypervitaminosis D rather than hyperparathyroidism. Hypophosphatemia, however, occasionally is found, rendering this differential point not always useful. The recent development of competitive binding assays for vitamin D and some of its metabolites should be helpful in establishing the diagnosis of vitamin D toxicity (Belsey *et al.,* 1971; Haddad and Chyu, 1971).

It should be emphasized in considering vitamin D intoxication in the differential diagnosis of hypercalcemia that the hypercalcemia may persist for weeks to months after vitamin D ingestion is stopped. Excessive quantities of the vitamin are stored in the liver and fat depots and are released slowly (Habener and Potts, unpublished data). Glucocorticoids are of value not only to confirm the diagnosis through acute suppression of hypercalcemia (cortisone suppression test) but also for treatment that may prevent irreversible renal damage.

7. *Hypervitaminosis A*

Excessive ingestion of vitamin A should be considered in the differential diagnosis of hypercalcemia, although the disorder is seen infrequently. Elevations in the serum calcium to 12–14 mg per 100 ml with associated symptoms of fatigue and anorexia have been reported in patients who have taken chronically 10–20 times the recommended minimum daily requirement (5000 IU) in the mistaken belief of benefit (Katz and Tzagournis, 1972; Frame *et al.,* 1974). In addition to symptoms attributable to the hypercalcemia, these patients frequently manifest myalgias and pronounced diffuse bone pain. Skeletal roentgenograms may be normal but occasionally may show multiple sites of distinct, smooth periosteal calcifications along the shafts of the phalanges and metacarpals (Caffey, 1951). This unusual roentgenographic appearance strongly suggests the diagnosis of hypervitaminosis A. A finding of increased levels of vitamin A in the serum (often twice the upper limit of normal), as well as elicitation of a history of excessive ingestion of the vitamin, confirms the diagnosis of hypervitaminosis A.

Although recent evidence suggests that vitamin A is a secretagogue for parathyroid hormone (see Chapter 2) the hypercalcemia of vitamin A intoxication is thought to result primarily from a direct effect of the vitamin on the skeleton via osteoclastic bone resorption (Jowsey and Riggs, 1968), allegedly through the release of lysosomal enzymes from bone cells. Studies of effects on calcium absorption, if any, have not been reported. Cessation of ingestion of the vitamin usually leads to prompt amelioration of the symptoms and healing of the skeleton. Occasionally, if hypercalcemia and other symptoms persist despite withdrawal, administration of corticosteroids as in the treatment of vitamin D intoxication proves helpful (doses equivalent to 100–200 mg of cortisone daily).

8. Administration of Thiazide Diuretics

Administration of diuretics of the benzothiadiazine class (Goodman and Gilman, 1970) to patients with high rates of bone turnover, including those with hyperparathyroidism (Parfitt, 1969; Duarte et al., 1971), juvenile osteoporosis (Parfitt, 1969), or hypoparathyroidism treated with high doses of vitamin D (Parfitt, 1972) results in appearance or aggravation of hypercalcemia. This effect appears to be unique to the benzothiadiazine (thiazide) diuretics such as chlorothiazide, hydrochlorothiazide, and chlorthalidone and is not usually seen with other classes of diuretics such as furosemide, ethacrynic acid, or mercurials. Although thiazides have been reported to increase serum calcium concentration significantly in normal individuals, the degree of calcium elevation is small (Seitz and Jaworski, 1964; Stote et al., 1972). Thus, thiazide-induced hypercalcemia implies that an underlying disorder of calcium metabolism exists. The controlled administration of thiazide diuretics has even been proposed as a provocative test for the diagnosis of subclinical primary hyperparathyroidism (van der Sluys Veer et al., 1965). This test, however, has not been used widely because of lack of specificity.

Adams et al. (1970) have reported that the administration of chlorothiazide (1 gm per day) in conjunction with phosphate depletion was useful in detecting the presence of primary hyperparathyroidism in patients with idiopathic hypercalciuria, a disorder characterized by hypercalciuria, recurrent renal calculi, and hypophosphatemia (Melick and Henneman, 1958). Adams et al. (1970) found that 8 of 19 patients with idiopathic hypercalciuria developed frank hypercalcemia when treated with chlorothiazide plus a low-phosphate diet. Of the five of the eight patients who underwent neck exploration, four had parathyroid adenomas and one had "normal glands" but responded to subtotal parathyroidectomy. A sixth patient who failed to develop hypercalcemia had a diagnosis of primary chief-cell hyperplasia of the parathyroid glands. Thus, the use of thiazide diuretics may be of value in detection of occult hyperparathyroidism in certain patients, particularly those with recurrent kidney stone disease and equivocal hypercalcemia.

Although a part of the hypercalcemic effects of thiazides can be accounted for by contraction of the extracellular fluid volume and hemoconcentration, sustained hypercalcemia probably arises from actions of the drug on both kidney and bone (Popovtzer et al., 1975; Brickman et al., 1972). The acute administration of thiazides increases urinary calcium excretion (Popovtzer et al., 1975), but chronic therapy results in a decrease in calcium in the urine (Lamberg and Kuhlback, 1959; Seitz and Jaworski, 1964; Duarte and Bland, 1965; Parfitt, 1972). The latter effect is the basis for the use of these diuretics to lower calcium excretion in idiopathic hypercalciuria (Nassim and Higgins, 1965; Yendt *et al.*, 1966). The acute hypercalciuric and chronic hypocalciuric actions of thiazides on the kidney may be secondary to the effects of the diuretics on sodium excretion inasmuch as renal tubular resorption of the two cations appears to be coupled; hypercalciuria accompanies the acute natriuretic response, and the chronic effect of lowering of urinary calcium excretion may reflect the enhancement of proximal tubular resorption of both sodium and calcium in response to sodium depletion (Epstein, 1968a). As discussed below, however, the hypocalciuric effects of thiazide diuretics on the kidney appear to require the presence of parathyroid hormone (Parfitt, 1972).

Two lines of evidence suggest a skeletal action of the drug. The first is that anephric patients maintained on hemodialysis also show a hypercalcemic response to hydrochlorothiazide administration in doses of 200 mg per day for 2–4 weeks (Koppel *et al.*, 1970). The second is that hypercalcemic response (both ionized and total calcium) to short-term chlorothiazide infusion has been observed in normal subjects and patients with hyperparathyroidism when urinary excretion of calcium (and sodium) was markedly increased (Popovtzer *et al.*, 1975). This hypercalcemic response appears to require parathyroid hormone inasmuch as the serum calcium levels of hypoparathyroid patients did not rise during chlorothiazide infusion alone but did when parathyroid extract was infused along with the chlorothiazide. On the other hand, the hypercalcemic response to thiazides administered chronically to patients with postoperative hypoparathyroidism treated with high doses of vitamin D does not appear to require parathyroid hormone (Parfitt, 1972). Parfitt studied the effect of thiazide administration (chlorothiazide 2 gm per day or equivalent) for 7 days in seven patients with hypoparathyroidism on vitamin D, one hypoparathyroid patient on calcium infusion, and seven patients with idiopathic hypercalciuria and apparently normal parathyroid function. In the group of hypoparathyroid patients taking vitamin D, urinary calcium excretion fell by only 11%. In the hypoparathyroid patient not receiving vitamin D, neither urinary nor plasma calcium changed significantly. In the control group of patients, urinary calcium fell by 44% and plasma total calcium corrected for protein concentration did not change. He concluded from these studies that (1) the hypocalciuric effect of thiazides requires the presence of parathyroid hormone, (2) thiazides enhance the action of parathyroid hormone on bone and kidney, (3) vitamin D can replace parathyroid hormone in the interaction in bone but not in kidney, and (4) the hypercalcemic effect of thiazides in hypoparathyroidism is due to increased release of calcium from bone and requires the presence of pharmacologic doses of vitamin D.

A special point of clinical importance should be emphasized. Given the frequency of use of thiazides in hypertensive subjects, one can conclude that if a patient on thiazides has been hypercalcemic for at least several weeks since thiazides were started, the patient is not a normal subject with a drug reaction, but rather has primary hyperparathyroidism or some other underlying skeletal disorder. Thiazides should be stopped in these patients because the apparent degree of severity of the hypercalcemia is exaggerated by their use. Inasmuch as the degree of hypercalcemia in patients with hyperparathyroidism is a factor in judging whether surgery is mandatory, the additive effect of thiazides should be eliminated by use of other agents for control of hypertension.

9. Prolonged Immobilization

Generalized immobilization of a patient may rarely lead to hypercalcemia, particularly in patients with high rates of bone turnover, such as those with Paget's disease (see Chapter 5). Immobilization may also cause hypercalcemia and osteopenia in young patients at a stage of rapid growth and higher bone turnover rates (Winters et al., 1966). The hypercalcemia and associated hypercalciuria resolve when the patient becomes ambulatory (see Chapter 6, Volume I).

a. Hemodialysis. Hypercalcemia may occur in renal disease as a complication of secondary hyperparathyroidism, particularly in subjects undergoing chronic hemodialysis or renal transplantation (Freeman et al., 1967; Segal et al., 1968). The pathophysiology and management of this disorder are discussed in Chapter 2. However, it should also be kept in mind that primary hyperparathyroidism and hypercalcemia may lead to chronic renal disease and that the hypercalcemia may persist even after renal function has been compromised.

10. Milk–Alkali Syndrome (Burnett's Syndrome)

In this syndrome, hypercalcemia and renal failure occur as a complication of ingestion of large amounts of calcium in some form, usually milk or absorbable antacids (Burnett et al., 1949). The disorder is less prevalent because, in the treatment of peptic ulcers, the nonabsorbable antacids have replaced soluble alkali such as sodium carbonate or bicarbonate or calcium carbonate (Lotz, 1964). The hypercalcemia commonly results in structural damage to the kidney and progressive impairment of renal function; hence, hypercalciuria may not be observed at the time of diagnosis (McMillan and Freeman, 1965). Renal failure is often, but not invariably, present; it has been established that hypercalcemia precedes the onset of renal damage. The latter can result after only a short course of therapy with soluble alkali and calcium (Ivanovich *et al.*, 1967). Calcium carbonate can elevate serum calcium within days in normal individuals, if taken in sufficient quantities. Although the diagnosis is suggested when hypercalcemia coexists with a history of ingestion of excessive calcium and/or alkali, it should be kept in mind, in view of the high incidence of ulcer disease in hyperparathyroidism (Kyle, 1954), that a "milk–alkali syndrome" may coexist with hyperparathyroidism.

11. Idiopathic Hypercalcemia of Infancy

This is a rare syndrome characterized by hypercalcemia, often in association with multiple congenital facial and cardiovascular lesions (Garcia *et al.*, 1964; Coleman, 1965; Wiltse *et al.*, 1966). The cause of the hypercalcemia is unknown; hypersensitivity to vitamin D has been postulated (Wiltse *et al.*, 1966). The distinctive clinical features and age distribution of the syndrome make it unlikely to be a problem in the differential diagnosis of most cases of hypercalcemia (Chapter 7).

F. Treatment

1. General

Once the presumptive diagnosis of primary hyperparathyroidism has been made, surgical removal of the diseased parathyroid glands is the indicated treatment, at least traditionally. At times a decision may be made to defer surgery, however. This is particularly true when asymptomatic hypercalcemia is discovered in an elderly patient or when the risk of surgery for other reasons is too great. Too little is known about the natural history of hyperparathyroidism to recommend surgery automatically, particularly in older patients, if there are no signs or symptoms definitely attributable to hyperparathyroidism (Purnell *et al.*, 1971, 1974). One may elect simply to observe the patient carefully if hypercalcemia is mild (Purnell *et al.*, 1974).

Attempts to evaluate the natural history of hyperparathyroidism and to define clear-cut, objective criteria for surgical treatment of the disease are receiving considerable attention. The results of detailed observations on the course of asymptomatic hyperparathyroidism have been reported by Purnell *et al.* (1971, 1974). Criteria recommended for surgical intervention include (1) a mean serum calcium concentration greater than 11.0 mg per 100 ml, (2) roentgenographic evidence of bone disease (osteitis fibrosa or advanced osteoporosis), (3) decreased renal function (glomerular filtration rate less than 60 ml/min), (4) progressive, active renal lithiasis or pyelonephritis in association with renal lithiasis, and (5) uncontrolled gastrointestinal complications, including peptic ulcer. In the absence of these abnormalities, the patients were observed carefully at intervals, some for more than 5 years (Purnell et al., 1974). Operations have been performed on some patients because of the progression of complications, and on others because the patients or their physicians did not elect to continue observation without surgery. The number of patients at the end of 5 years still in the nonoperative group was 58% (Purnell et al., 1974). The authors are in full agreement with this approach and have a similar independent study in progress. Many questions remain unanswered at this time, as discussed above, for example, whether simple osteopenia can be due to hyperparathyroidism and whether progressive loss of bone will cease once the hyperparathyroidism is surgically corrected. The extent and reversibility of deterioration of renal function (in the absence of renal calcification) is likewise unsettled (see discussion above).

If the question of a relationship of vague constitutional symptoms to hypercalcemia is raised, it may be useful to evaluate the symptomatic response following the temporary lowering of blood calcium. Since serum phosphate in most patients with hyperparathyroidism is low, it may be useful to administer sodium or potassium phosphate in doses containing 1 to 2 gm of phosphate phosphorus daily. Serum calcium usually falls several milligrams/100 ml; improvement, if any, in constitutional complaints can then serve as a guide to surgery. Phosphate therapy may sometimes be employed chronically in patients deemed poor operative risks. However, complications such as metastatic calcification may develop during phosphate therapy especially if serum phosphate is allowed to rise above normal and hypercalcemia persists.

Another and entirely different indication for medical therapy develops when a patient without previous medical history of disorders related to calcium metabolism presents with severe hypercalcemia. When the etiology is unknown, a curable disease such as primary hyperparathyroidism must be considered. Under the circumstances, it is critical to lower blood calcium rapidly to safe levels so that diagnostic studies can be performed and a potentially curable disorder can be treated definitively. If the diagnosis seems likely, surgical extirpation of the diseased parathyroid glands is desirable as soon as possible (Reinfrank and Edwards, 1961; Anglem, 1966).

After rehydration has been accomplished, it is now agreed that the most effective mode of emergency medical therapy is intravenous infusion of sodium chloride, 4–5 liters daily, plus administration of potent natriuretic agents such as furosemide. The use of thiazide diuretics, however, should be avoided (see p. 116). This mode of therapy can be undertaken only if renal function is adequate; strict records of intake and output and avoidance of fluid overload must be observed. Depletion of sodium, magnesium, and potassium must be watched for. Several grams of calcium may be excreted daily, resulting in rapid lowering of blood calcium. The beneficial effects result from the close coupling of sodium and calcium transport in the proximal tubule; natriuresis leads to calciuresis.

Intravenous phosphate is effective in lowering calcium (Goldsmith and Ingbar, 1966), but widespread metastatic calcification is believed by some to be a potential hazard if used when calcium is high. Mithramycin given as a single intravenous dose of 25 to 50 μg per kg may lower calcium to normal within several days (Ryan *et al.*, 1971); this approach serves as an alternate therapy if the saline/furosemide regimen cannot be applied. These and other approaches to medical management are discussed in detail in Chapter 6.

2. Management Issues in Hereditary Endocrinopathies

Many practical clinical implications are evident in the chronic management of patients with familial hyperparathyroidism and/or multiple-endocrine-neoplasia syndromes (Section III, B). As experience with the practicability, true diagnostic value, and reliability of the immunoassays and related clinical chemical procedures accumulates, it is becoming clear that appropriate screening procedures can be developed to permit early detection of hyperplasia and/or neoplasia of endocrine tissue in members of the kindred. The thyroid and pancreatic lesions are usually malignant, and, therefore, early detection may clearly affect survival. The pituitary tumors may be subject to control via noninvasive treatments such as proton-beam therapy (Kjellberg and Kliman, 1974); if undetected until late in the evolution of gland enlargement, irreversible consequences such as impairment of vision and other complications secondary to the space-occupying lesion may occur.

It is appreciated that immunoassays for growth hormone and prolactin may prove helpful as screening procedures. Because many patients with multiple-endocrine-neoplasia type I have chromophobe tumors not involved in overproduction of growth hormone, pituitary insufficiency or complications of tumor growth may be the presenting symptoms. In a review by Ballard *et al.* (1964), acromegaly in association with eosinophilic hyperplasia in the pituitary was found in only 27% of the 55 cases involving abnormality of the pituitary. It is now appreciated that many pituitary tumors, even when small, are associated with excessive prolactin secretion or rarely actual amenorrhea and galactorrhea (Daughaday, 1974) rather than acromegaly or excessive growth-hormone secretion.

The familial medullary carcinoma is clearly multifocal in origin, requiring total thyroidectomy (Melvin *et al.*, 1971). As noted in Chapter 4, calcitonin assays have proved uniquely useful not only in screening for subclinical disease (Melvin *et al.*, 1972) but also in chronic management (Goltzman *et al.*, 1974). When pheochromocytoma is detected in familial cases, in over 50% of patients there is bilateral adrenal disease, in contrast with only 5% bilateral involvement in nonfamilial cases (Steiner *et al.*, 1968); more extensive exploration of the adrenals is required, therefore, in familial cases. Melvin *et al.* (1972) pointed to the high incidence of Cushing's syndrome in MEN-type-II syndrome; the etiology appears to be principally ectopic ACTH production from the medullary carcinoma. Hence, an ectopic thyroidal source of ACTH production rather than primary adrenal or pituitary pathology should be carefully considered in any patient with MEN-II and suspected Cushing's syndrome.

Recognition of the presence of Zollinger–Ellison syndrome leads to special management decisions; total rather than subtotal gastrectomy leads to improved long-term survival, even despite the occurrence of metastases of the pancreatic, gastrin-producing tumors (Fox *et al.*, 1974a, b). Primary surgical attack on the pancreas is not employed because of the high incidence of multifocal, inoperable pancreatic carcinoma (Fox *et al.*, 1974a,b). In the cumulative experience summarized by Fox and associates, the 10-year survival in 137 patients treated by total gastrectomy was 42%. In 130 patients with subtotal gastrectomy, survival was 52% at 1 year but only 18% at 10 years. In the patients with total gastrectomy, 73 patients had liver metastases at the time of gastric surgery; survival was 68% at 1 year, 42% at 5 years, and 30% at 10 years. In sharp contrast, of the 54 patients with subtotal gastrectomy and metastases at the time of original surgery, survival figures were bleak: 44% survived 1 year, 7% survived 5 years, and none survived 10 years. As noted by Fox *et al.* (1974a,b) and Friesen (1967, 1968), the results seem to imply, at least indirectly, some feedback from the stomach on the growth of gastrinomas of the pancreas. In the summary of Fox and associates (1974a,b), actual regression of metastases was shown or implied in 9 patients with total gastrectomy, but in only 2 with subtotal gastrectomy. Death in the patients with only subtotal gastrectomy was directly attributable to growth of pancreatic metastases in 50%. On the other hand, the nature and predictability of the gastric feedback concept is still unclear since ultimate cause of death in patients even with presumed total gastrectomy was still attributable to growth of the pancreatic tumor and metastases in many of the group who failed to survive beyond 10 years.

However, despite the morbidity and chronic management difficulties encountered in the more radical surgery, total gastrectomy is clearly the procedure of choice in management of patients with Zollinger–Ellison syndrome.

3. Surgical Treatment

Parathyroid exploration should only be undertaken by a surgeon experienced in neck procedures and with the help of an experienced pathologist. There are many critical decisions regarding management that can be best made only during the course of the operation. The subsequent course of the operation may be modified by results of histological examination of frozen sections of the parathyroid tissue excised. The procedure followed by Cope (1960) and Wang *et al.* (1975) and Purnell *et al.* (1974) is to identify an abnormal gland, remove it, and then to search for at least one additional gland. If the second gland is normal both grossly and histologically, a single adenoma is most likely. Cope (1960) and Wang *et al.* (1975) recommend removal of the single gland. In the experience of Cope and Wang, the occurrence of a "double" adenoma is rare. On the other hand, based on a different interpretation of the usual pathology in hyperparathyroidism, some surgeons recommend identification of and usually subtotal resection of all glands (Paloyan *et al.*, 1973). Long-term evaluation of the experience in various centers will be required to definitively resolve these controversies concerning optimal approach to surgical management.

The surgical procedures followed with primary hyperplasia of the parathyroid glands are more complex. Once a diagnosis of hyperplasia has been established, all agree that it is necessary to identify each of the glands. It is usually recommended that most of the glands be totally removed and that one or two glands be partially excised, care being taken to leave an intact blood supply to the remaining gland fragments.

Other special problems are sometimes seen. There are documented cases of the presence of five or six glands (Wang, 1976), as well as unusual locations for an adenoma arising in one of the usual four glands. If no abnormalities are found in the glands identified in the neck, mediastinal exploration must be undertaken. When parathyroid carcinoma is encountered, it is important that the tissues be widely excised and care should be taken to avoid rupture of the capsule to prevent local seeding of the tumor. Recognition that an enlarged gland may be malignant is sometimes suggested by a thick capsule and adherence to surrounding tissues (Schantz and Castleman, 1973).

4. Postoperative management

Many issues arise in the management of patients in the days and weeks after parathyroid surgery. Adequacy of the surgery as well as the function of residual normal tissue is most effectively evaluated by serial determinations of plasma calcium and phosphate values on successive days after neck exploration. Albright and Reifenstein (1948) carefully documented the rate of change in serum calcium levels after successful parathyroid surgery, such as removal of a single adenoma. Their observations, made nearly 30 years ago, have continued to prove valuable in the postoperative management of patients. Serum calcium usually falls by several milligrams per 100 ml within the first 24 hours after surgery. Thereafter, calcium values fall typically to subnormal values in the range of 8 to 8.5 mg per 100 ml over a period of 3 to 4 days. The nadir of the serum calcium is usually reached in about 4 or 5 days, and then there is return to normal or to the lower level of normal. Albright and Reifenstein (1948) demonstrated, however, great individual variation in this pattern of response. Furthermore, they observed that in patients with high serum alkaline phosphatase levels and other evidence of osteitis fibrosa there was a more profound fall to values often less than 7 mg per 100 ml; the nadir in serum calcium was not reached for as long as 5 to 50 days after operation, presumably reflecting continued uptake of calcium and phosphate by bone in excess of that released. The abrupt reduction in levels of parathyroid hormone in the circulation results in a cessation of excessive bone resorptive processes, whereas stimulation of new bone formation persists. Serial bone biopsies taken and examined after parathyroidectomy have shown a marked osteoblastic response manifested by the deposition of large amounts of osteoid in areas previously involved by osteoclastic resorption (Fig. 41). Osteoid is apparently laid down much faster than it is mineralized, resulting in a histological picture resembling that seen in osteomalacia. Hence, for several weeks to months after operation, reparative processes in the skeleton may be limited by the availability of calcium and phosphorus from the circulation. Greatly accelerated uptake of calcium and phosphate by the skeleton is probably the major factor contributing to the prolonged hypocalcemia (and hypophosphatemia) often seen in the postoperative period. Such findings are most pronounced in those patients who have the most severe bone disease.

The factors controlling the extent and time course of the fall in serum calcium after successful parathyroid surgery have never been critically assessed. This comes about largely because of the lack of effective means, such as repetitive analyses by parathyroid hormone immunoassays, to accurately measure the rate of secretion of hormone day by day by the residual parathyroid tissue, particularly biologically active hormone (as distinct from inactive fragments). The classic view has been that, in the situation in which one gland (an adenoma) has been removed, the persistence of hypocalcemia for some days reflects lack of hormone, since the other three normal glands are functionally inactive and must recover. As noted by Wang *et al.* (1975) the gross appearance of the normal glands in patients with a single adenoma differs in several respects from that of a gland involved with (chief cell) hyperplasia, regardless of size. The normal gland is relatively avascular and yellow-tan whereas the hyperplastic gland is hyperemic and therefore redder. On the other hand, histological sections of such normal glands examined by light microscopy show no evidence of cellular atrophy.

Examination by electron microscopy of tissue from adenomas, hyperplastic glands (whether primary or secondary), and normal glands does reveal differences. The majority of cells from normal glands exposed to chronic hypercalcemia show changes that have been interpreted (Roth, 1971) as indicating reduced or absent secretory activity. The granular endoplasmic reticulum is composed of dispersed sacules spread throughout the cytoplasm; in addition, the Golgi apparatus is usually small. There is a relative lack of secretory granules and vesicles. The appearance of cells from adenomas or hyperplastic glands, in which a high level of activity is presumed, shows different features. There are complex Golgi structures, large numbers of secretory vesicles, and an increased quantity and organization of the granular endoplasmic reticulum. These changes have been interpreted as consistent with a high rate of cellular activity (Black and Utley, 1968; Black and Haff, 1970; Roth, 1971). On the other hand, Roth (1971) pointed out that even within normal glands there are a small number of cells whose appearance is consistent with active hormone secretion. The histological studies, therefore, do suggest that there is a low level of overall cellular activity in the normal glands at the time of parathyroid surgery in hyperparathyroidism; the relatively inactive state of most cells in the normal glands reflects their long-term exposure to hypercalcemia.

Data that permit direct assessment of the secretory activity, if any, of the normal glands as a function of long-standing hypercalcemia are minimal. There are two types of evidence. Mayer *et al.* (1976) recently showed that, in the normal animal, induction of sustained hypercalcemia for periods of as long as 40 hours is associated with continued secretion of hormone at a low level. These findings are consistent with observations (Roth, 1971) of continued cellular activity in remaining normal glands in patients with parathyroid adenomas. On the other hand (Bilezikian *et al.*, 1973; Powell *et al.*, 1973), samples taken from the venous drainage of normal glands at the time of localization studies show no increase over peripheral blood in immunoassayable hormone, in contrast to the high gradients detected in the effluent from the affected, hyperfunctioning gland. The absence of a gradient from the normal glands indicates that

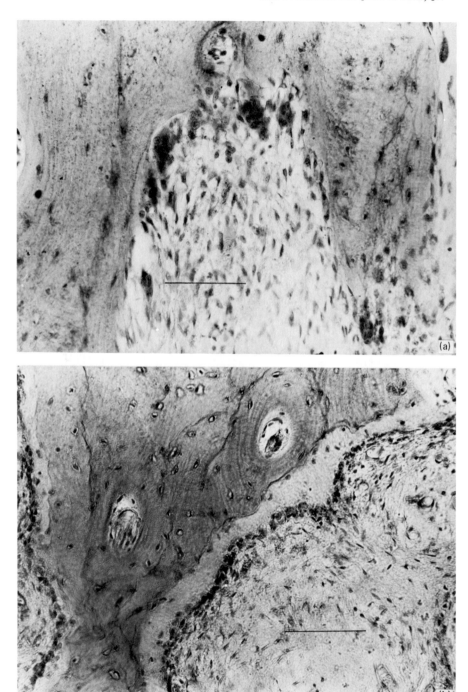

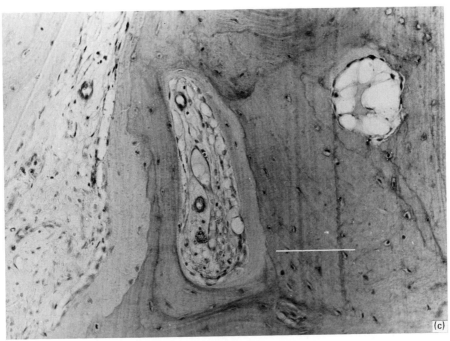

Fig. 41. Serial photomicrographs of bone biopsies of the tibia taken during and after removal of a parathyroid adenoma. (*a*) Day of parathyroidectomy, (*b*) 7 days, and (*c*) 35 days after surgery. At time of surgery (*a*) typical histological findings of osteitis fibrosa cystica are evident. There is marked fibroblastic proliferation with several large, multinucleotoid osteoclasts adjacent to the surface of laminar bone. These findings are indicative of active bone resorption. By 7 days after parathyroidectomy (*b*) the histological findings have changed completely. A large seam of unmineralized osteoid has appeared adjacent to the mineralized bone, which, in turn, is lined by a continuous row of osteoblasts. These findings indicate the rapid formation of new bone. Osteoid is being laid down faster than the process of mineralization, resulting in a histological picture similar to that seen in osteomalacia. Considerable poorly mineralized osteoid is still evident by 35 days after surgery (*c*). The patient was severely hypocalcemic (serum calcium values of 5.1–5.5) during this time, requiring the intermittent intravenous administration of calcium chloride with ingestion of large amounts of calcium glycerol phosphate to prevent tetany.) The photomicrographs, provided by Dr. S. M. Krane, were retaken by the Department of Pathology, Massachusetts General Hospital, from the original histological preparations from case No. 8 described by Albright and Reifenstein (1948). H & E stain of partially decalcified tissues. Magnification, 300× (horizontal bar = 300 μm).

their functional activity in long-standing hyperparathyroidism and hypercalcemia must be low or absent, whereas the normal glands in normocalcemic cows have a high output of hormone readily detectable by selective sampling of the gland effluent (Mayer *et al.*, 1976).

The interpretation that seems most reasonable from these data is that the normal parathyroid glands in the presence of a functioning adenoma have a negligible rate of hormone secretion. Presumably, the rapid fall in serum calcium after the removal of the abnormal, hyperactive gland reflects the delay required for resumption of normal rates of secretory activity by the residual, suppressed parathyroid glands. Eventually, it should become possible to obtain frequent measurements of plasma parathyroid hormone using techniques that measure exclusively the biologically active, intact hormonal molecule, and thereby obtain useful data concerning the basal level of activity of the normal parathyroid glands before correction of the hyperparathyroidism and the time course of recovery of the suppressed glands after operation.

Failure of the serum calcium level to fall below 10 mg per 100 ml in the first 2 or 3 postoperative days is usually a sign of inadequate surgery (Cope et al., 1961; Cope, 1966). When multiple glands are hyperplastic and at least one hyperfunctioning gland has eluded detection by the surgeon, the usual fall in blood calcium to subnormal levels does not occur, owing to the continued secretion of a greater than normal level of parathyroid hormone.

Regardless of whether the failure to correct hyperparathyroidism surgically is due to failure to remove either any or all of the involved abnormal parathyroid tissue, it is recommended (Wang and Cope, 1977) that reexploration be deferred because of the technical difficulties encountered in examining the recently explored tissues of the neck. In view of the chronicity of hyperparathyroidism, except in the rare occasions when severe hypercalcemia is present, several months should be allowed to elapse before the decision is made to reexplore. The use of special localization techniques, such as venous catheterization and/or angiography, may be of use in localization of the remaining abnormal tissue.

Wang and Cope (1977) emphasize that the need for additional surgery is as high as 5–10% in reported series. They note that, when reexploration is performed, the residual abnormal tissue is still found within the neck in at least 3 of 4 cases. Hence, it is not usually advisable to explore the mediastinum prior to reexploration of the neck, except when review of previous operative findings provides proof by histological examination of at least four glands within the neck or, alternatively, when there is direct angiographic localization of a tumor within the mediastinum. In the 71 cases referred to the Massachusetts General Hospital for reexploration between 1926 and 1975, the missing gland was found within the neck in 82% of the patients; in only 18% was a sternotomy required to reach an abnormal gland (Wang and Cope, 1977).

The opposite problem in postoperative management, the occurrence of protracted postoperative hypocalcemia, varies greatly in frequency depending on the presence or absence of associated medical complications and the type of surgical approach used. The problem can best be considered with regard to the cause of protracted postoperative hypocalcemia. Hypocalcemia may be due to inadequate residual parathyroid tissue, that is, true hypoparathyroidism, either temporary or permanent. Hypocalcemia may also be caused by failure of systemic tissue to respond to adequate levels of circulating parathyroid hormone, for example, severe hypomagnesemia, chronic renal failure, severe bone disease with large mineral deficits in the skeleton, malabsorption or other causes of vitamin D lack, and, rarely, intraoperative pancreatitis. The problem is considered in greater detail in Chapter 3.

It would seem obvious that the frequency of hypocalcemia is influenced by the philosophy and technique of surgery. In patients in whom all four glands are biopsied or subtotally resected, there is a greater risk of temporary or permanent hypoparathyroidism. Inadequate survival of functioning parathyroid tissue or delay in recovery of normal glands occurs more frequently than it does in the alternate approach stressed by Cope and Wang and associates (Cope et al., 1961; Cope, 1966; Wang et al., 1975), in which only the abnormal gland is removed (in the case of single-gland disease) and biopsy is undertaken of only one of the remaining, presumably normal, parathyroid glands. Apart from the type of surgical approach undertaken at the initial operation, problems in patients who are subjected to reexploration can occur and can easily lead to hypoparathyroidism. In the experience of Wang and colleagues, several patients, who had reoperations for persistent hyperparathyroidism after previous exploratory surgery and in whom a single abnormal gland was removed in toto at the second operation, developed permanent hypoparathyroidism. Although it was not established either by surgical notes or by pathology reports, all of the normal parathyroid glands must have been removed or have had their vascular supply compromised during the surgical procedures. As a result of this experience, Wang and colleagues favor, in reexploration, only a subtotal resection of the abnormal gland when it is not possible to identify (and prove by histological examination of a biopsy specimen) at least one additional normal gland.

A clue to the onset of permanent hypoparathyroidism is often provided by serial determinations of blood phosphate as well as calcium. Normally, after correction of hyperparathyroidism, persistent hypophosphatemia due to rapid repair of bone mineral deficits occurs. When hypoparathyroidism is present, hyperphosphatemia occurs as a consequence of the loss of parathyroid action on renal phosphate clearance, an effect that predominates over skeletal uptake of phosphate.

Oral calcium supplementation may suffice as treatment for mild symptomatic hypocalcemia in the postoperative period. Because intestinal absorption of calcium is reasonably efficient for several days after parathyroidectomy (Albright and Reifenstein, 1948), addition to the diet of several grams of elemental calcium per 24 hours (given as any of several preparations, plus liberal use of milk as tolerated) will often lead to a lessening of the symptoms of increased neuromuscular irritability. The presence of Chvostek's sign may be helpful to monitor the success of oral therapy. If hypocalcemia is severe and/or continues, intravenous calcium is necessary to avoid serious consequences of tetany, laryngo-spasm, and convulsions. Solution of calcium (gluconate or chloride) at a concentration of 1 mg/ml may be administered in 5% dextrose/water. The rate and duration of intravenous calcium therapy are determined by the severity of symptoms and the response to therapy detected by monitoring both blood calcium levels and signs of neuromuscular irritability. A rate of infusion of 0.5 to 2 mg/kg/hour or 30 to 100 ml/hour of the 1 mg/ml solution will usually suffice to relieve symptoms. In most instances, parenteral therapy will be required for only a few days. If the requirement for parenteral calcium continues for more than 4 or 5 days, replacement therapy with vitamin D (or its analogues) and/or oral calcium should be initiated as detailed in Chapter 3.

If true hypoparathyroidism is present, 10 days or longer may be re-quired for the calcium-raising action of large doses of vitamin D plus oral calcium to take effect (Albright and Reifenstein, 1948) (see Chapter 3). The recent finding that 1α-hydroxycholecalciferol or 1,25-dihy-droxycholecalciferol can raise serum calcium to normal within 24 hours after initiation of treatment indicates that use of these rapidly acting derivatives of vitamin D is preferred regardless of whether the hypocal-cemia is permanent or transient (Kooh et al., 1975; Neer et al., 1975).

Postoperative hypocalcemia is a frequent occurrence in patients who have primary hyperparathyroidism and coexistent chronic renal failure and/or vitamin D deficiency or malabsorption. The nature of the underly-ing defects in calcium homeostasis, particularly impairment of normal vitamin D metabolism (impaired renal 1-hydroxylation of 25-OHD) and direct impairment of efficiency of intestinal calcium absorption, is re-viewed in Chapter 2. In our experience over the last 5 years, patients with severe renal failure, despite the presence of general hyperplasia of all parathyroid glands, have difficulty in maintaining a normal serum calcium when the bulk of hyperplastic tissue has been removed. This difficulty arises even though the residual parathyroid tissue continues to provide concentrations of circulating hormone well above the upper limit of nor-mal. The management of such patients is similar to the approach used in true hypoparathyroidism.

Significant magnesium depletion and resulting severe hypomagnesemia occasionally appear in patients with primary hyperparathyroidism (Harmon, 1956; Barnes *et al.,* 1957; Agna and Goldsmith, 1958; Potts and Roberts, 1958; Sutton, 1970). The hypomagnesemia per se may be responsible for persistent and refractory hypocalcemia, and, unless magnesium levels are restored to normal, it may be difficult if not impossible to correct postoperative hypocalcemia. The hypocalcemia associated with magnesium depletion is thought to arise from a magnesium-sensitive blockade of the peripheral responsiveness to parathyroid hormone (Estep *et al.,* 1969) and/or to an impairment of the secretion of parathyroid hormone from the residual parathyroid gland (Anast *et al.,* 1975; Singer *et al.,* 1975). Repletion of magnesium leads to a prompt restoration of the normal secretory activity of the parathyroids. The origin of the hypomagnesemia in hyperparathyroidism is not entirely understood. It is believed that in the face of severe and protracted loss of bone mineral in patients with osteitis fibrosa cystica, a deficiency in total-body magnesium develops as a result of chronic loss of magnesium, along with calcium, phosphate, and other mineral ions, from bone. Bulger and Gausmann (1933) observed a negative balance in primary hyperparathyroidism with osteitis fibrosa, followed by a reversal after correction of the hyperparathyroidism. Although in normal subjects, parathyroid hormone acts at the level of the kidney to promote magnesium reabsorption as well as calcium reabsorption (MacIntyre *et al.,* 1963), in patients with hyperparathyroidism renal magnesium loss contributes to the magnesium depletion (Barnes *et al.,* 1957). Excessive filtered loads of magnesium due to skeletal breakdown predominate over renal conservation effects (analogous to findings with calcium excretion). Sutton (1970) also described several patients with hyperparathyroidism in whom there was true renal wasting of magnesium, that is, abnormally high magnesium clearance.

Whatever the cause, detection of hypomagnesemia may provide a clue to a readily reversible cause of protracted hypocalcemia that is not due to hypoparathyroidism. Magnesium deficiency may complicate the postoperative course of parathyroid surgery and may be another factor in the genesis of tetany, independent of hypocalcemia (Barnes *et al.,* 1957; Potts and Roberts, 1958), and should therefore be promptly corrected whenever detected. $MgCl_2$ is sufficiently soluble to be effective by mouth, but preparations of this compound are not widely available, and oral repletion is slower. Accordingly, repletion should usually be parenteral. The extent of total-body magnesium deficiency may well be as great as 150–200 mEq. Inasmuch as the depressant effect of magnesium on central and peripheral neural function is not seen below 4 mEq/liter (normal range is 1.5–2.0 mEq/liter), magnesium replacement can be accomplished rapidly. A dose as great as 100 mEq/kg can be given over 8–12 hours if severe hypomagnesemia is detected, provided renal function is not impaired (Shils, 1969). The magnesium is given either as an intravenous infusion over 8–12 hours or in divided doses intramuscularly ($MgSO_4$ USP is the preparation normally used, available as a 20% solution, 200 mg or 8 mEq/ml, or as a more concentrated 50% solution). If hypocalcemia is due to hypomagnesemia, blood calcium usually returns to normal within 24–48 hours, together with normal rates of parathyroid hormone secretion and/or peripheral response to the hormone (Anast *et al.*, 1975; Singer *et al.*, 1975). If in doubt, a guide to the correction of the magnesium deficit is the restoration of normal rates of excretion of Mg, i.e., excretion of 70–90% of the administered dose (Shils, 1969) when the intracellular deficit is corrected.

ACKNOWLEDGMENT

We would like to express our appreciation to Elise Hauenstein for her excellent secretarial assistance.

REFERENCES

Abe, M., and Sherwood, L. M. (1972). *Biochem. Biophys. Res. Commun.* **48,** 396.
Adam, A., and Ritchie, D. (1954). *J. Bone Joint Surg., Br. Vol.* **37,** 257.
Adams, P. [H.], and Jowsey, J. (1967). *Endocrinology* **81,** 735.
Adams, P. [H.], Jowsey, J., Kelly, P. J., Riggs, B. L., Kinney, V. R., and Jones, J. D. (1967). *Q. J. Med.* **36,** 1.
Adams, P. [H.], Chalmers, T. M., Hill, L. F., and Truscott, B. McN. (1970). *Br. Med. J.* **4,** 582.
Agna, J. W., and Goldsmith, R. E. (1958). *N. Engl. J. Med.* **258,** 222.
Agus, Z. S., Gardner, L. B., Beck, L. H., and Goldberg, M. (1973). *Am. J. Physiol.* **224,** 1143.
Aitken, R. E., Kerr, J. L., and Lloyd, H. M. (1964). *Am. J. Med.* **37,** 813.
Albright, F., and Reifenstein, E. C., Jr. (1948). "The Parathyroid Glands and Metabolic Bone Disease: Selected Studies." Williams & Wilkins, Baltimore, Maryland.
Albright, F., Aub, J. C., and Bauer, W. (1934). *J. Am. Med. Assoc.* **102,** 1276.
Allen, E. M., Singer, F. R., and Melamed, D. (1970). *Neurology* **20,** 15.
Anast, C. S., Mohs, J. M., Kaplan, S. L., and Burns, T. W. (1972). *Science* **177,** 606.
Anast, C. S., Winnacker, J. C., Forte, L. R., and Burns, T. R. (1975). *Proc. 57th Annu. Meet., Am. Endocr. Soc.* A-47, p. 74.
Anderson, D. C., Stewart, W. K., and Piercy, D. M. (1968). *Lancet* **2,** 323.
Anderson, J., Dent, C. E., Harper, C., and Philpot, G. R. (1954). *Lancet* **2,** 720.
Anglem, T. J. (1966). *Surg. Clin. North Am.* **46,** 727.
Arnaud, C. D., Sizemore, G. W., Oldham, S. B., Fischer, J. A., Tsao, H. S., and Littledike, E. T. (1971a). *Am. J. Med.* **50,** 630.
Arnaud, C. D., Tsao, H. S., and Littledike, T. (1971b). *J. Clin. Invest.* **50,** 21.
Aub, J. C., Bauer, W., Heath, C., and Ropes, M. (1929). *J. Clin. Invest.* **7,** 97.
Aurbach, G. D. (1959). *J. Biol. Chem.* **234,** 3179.

Aurbach, G. D., Keutmann, H. T., Niall, H. D., Tregear, G. W., O'Riordan, J. L. H., Marcus, R., Marx, S. J., and Potts, J. T., Jr. (1972). *Recent Prog. Horm. Res.* **28,** 353.
Aurbach, G. D., Mallette, L. E., Patten, B. M., Heath, D. A., Doppman, J. L., and Bilezikian, J. P. (1973). *Ann. Intern. Med.* **79,** 566.
Ball, J. H., Kaminsky, N. I., Hardman, J. G., Broadus, A. E., Sutherland, E. W., and Liddle, G. W. (1972). *J. Clin. Invest.* **51,** 2124.
Ballard, H. S., Frame, B., and Hartsock, R. J. (1964). *Medicine (Baltimore)* **43,** 481.
Barnes, B. A., Krane, S. M., and Cope, O. (1957). *J. Clin. Endocrinol. Metab.* **17,** 1407.
Barnicot, N. A. (1948). *J. Anat.* **82,** 233.
Barr, D. P., Bulger, H. A., and Dixon, H. H. (1929). *J. Am. Med. Assoc.* **92,** 951.
Barreras, R. F. (1973). *Gastroenterology* **64,** 1168.
Barreras, R. F., and Donaldson, R. M., Jr. (1967). *N. Engl. J. Med.* **276,** 1122.
Basset, G. (1964). *Bull. Mem. Soc. Med. Hop. Paris* **115,** 583.
Bates, W. K., McGowen, J., and Talmage, R. V. (1962). *Endocrinology* **71,** 189.
Bauer, W., and Federman, D. D. (1962). *Metab., Clin. Exp.* **11,** 21.
Baxter, J. D., and Bondy, P. K. (1966). *Ann. Intern. Med.* **65,** 429.
Bélanger, L. F. (1965). *In* "The Parathyroid Glands: Ultrastructure, Secretion, and Function" (P. J. Gaillard, R. V. Talmage and A. M. Budy, eds.), p. 53. Univ. of Chicago Press, Chicago, Illinois.
Bell, N. H., Gill, J. R., Jr., and Bartter, F. C. (1964). *Am. J. Med.* **36,** 500.
Bell, N. H., and Sinha, T. K. (1977). *In* "Vitamin D: Biochemical, Chemical, and Clinical Aspects Related to Calcium Metabolism" (A. W. Norman, K. Schaefer, J. W. Coburn, H. F. DeLuca, O. Fraser, H. G. Gregoleit, and D. V. Herrath, eds.), p. 747. Walter de Gruyter, Berlin, New York.
Belsey, R., DeLuca, H. F., and Potts, J. T., Jr. (1971). *J. Clin. Endocrinol. Metab.* **33,** 554.
Benson, R. C., Jr., Riggs, B. L., Pickard, B. M., and Arnaud, C. D. (1974). *J. Clin. Invest.* **54,** 175.
Berson, S. A., and Yalow, R. S. (1968). *J. Clin. Endocrinol. Metab.* **28,** 1037.
Berson, S. A., and Yalow, R. S. (1971). *Am. J. Med.* **50,** 623.
Berson, S. A., Yalow, R. S., Aurbach, G. D., and Potts, J. T., Jr. (1963). *Proc. Natl. Acad. Sci. U.S.A.* **49,** 613.
Biddulph, D. M. (1972). *Endocrinology* **90,** 1113.
Biddulph, D. M., and Gallimore, L. B., Jr. (1974). *Endocrinology* **94,** 1241.
Bilezikian, J. P., Doppman, J. L., Shimkin, P. M., Powell, D., Wells, S. A., Heath, D. A., Ketcham, A. S., Monchik, J., Mallette, L. E., Potts, J. T., Jr., and Aurbach, G. D. (1973). *Am. J. Med.* **55,** 505.
Bingham, P., Brazell, I. A., and Owen, M. (1969). *J. Endocrinol.* **45,** 387.
Black, W. C., III, and Haff, R. C. (1970). *Am. J. Clin. Pathol.* **53,** 565.
Black, W. C., III, and Utley, J. R. (1968). *Am. J. Clin. Pathol.* **49,** 761.
Block, M. A., Horn, R. C., Jr., Miller, J. M., Barrett, J. L., and Brush, B. E. (1967). *Trans. Am. Surg. Assoc.* **85,** 101.
Blum, J. W., Hunziker, W., Binswanger, U., and Fischer, J. A. (1975), *Program/Abstracts, 57th Annu. Meetg. Endocrine. Soc.,* Abstract No. 46, p. 73.
Blum, J. W., Mayer, G. P., and Potts, J. T., Jr. (1974). *Endocrinology* **95,** 84.
Boonstra, C. E., and Jackson, C. E. (1965). *Ann. Intern. Med.* **63,** 468.
Boonstra, C. E., and Jackson, C. E. (1971). *Am. J. Clin. Pathol.* **55,** 523.
Bordier, P. J., Arnaud, C. [D.], Hawker, C., Tun Chot, S., and Hioco, D. (1973). *Clin. Aspects Metab. Bone Dis., Proc. Int. Symp., 1972.* Int. Congr. Ser., No. 270, p. 222–228. Excerpta Medica, Amsterdam. (ICS No. 270.)
Bouillon, R., and De Moor, P. (1974). *J. Clin. Endocrinol. Metab.* **38,** 999.
Boyd, J. D., Milgram, J. E., and Stearns, G. (1929). *J. Am. Med. Assoc.* **93,** 684.

Boyd, W. (1961). "Pathology," p. 1027. Lea & Febiger, Philadelphia, Pennsylvania.

Breuer, R. I., and McPherson, H. T. (1966). *Arch. Intern. Med.* **118**, 310.

Brewer, H. B., Jr., and Ronan, R. (1970). *Proc. Natl. Acad. Sci. U.S.A.* **67**, 1862.

Brewer, H. B., Jr., Fairwell, T., Ronan, R., Sizemore, G. W., and Arnaud, C. D. (1972). *Proc. Natl. Acad. Sci. U.S.A.* **69**, 3585.

Brewer, H. B., [Jr.], Fairwell, T., Ronan, R., Rittel, W., and Arnaud, C. (1975). *In* "Calcium-Regulating Hormones" (R. V. Talmage, M. Owen, and J. A. Parsons, eds.), Int. Congr. Ser. No. 346, p. 23. Excerpta Med., Found., Amsterdam.

Brickman, A. S., Massry, S. G., and Coburn, J. W. (1972). *J. Clin. Invest.* **51**, 945.

Britton, D. C., Thompson, M. H., Johnson, I. D. A., and Fleming, L. B. (1971). *Lancet* **2**, 74.

Bryant, L. R., Wulsin, J. H., and Altemeier, W. A. (1964). *Ann. Surg.* **159**, 411.

Buckle, R. M., Aurbach, G. D., and Potts, J. T., Jr. (1969). *In* "Protein and Polypeptide Hormones" (N. Margolies, ed.), Int. Congr. Ser. No. 161, p. 389. Excerpta Med. Found., Amsterdam.

Bulger, H. A., and Gausmann, F. (1933). *J. Clin. Invest.* **12**, 1135.

Bunch, T. W., and Hunder, G. G. (1973). *J. Am. Med. Assoc.* **225**, 1108.

Burnett, C. H., Commons, R. R., Albright, F., and Howard, J. E. (1949). *N. Engl. J. Med.* **240**, 787.

Burr, J. M., Farrell, J. J., and Hills, A. G. (1959). *N. Engl. J. Med.* **261**, 1271.

Bywaters, E. G. L., Dixon, A. St. J., and Scott, J. T. (1963). *Ann. Rheum. Dis.* **22**, 171.

Caffey, J. (1951). *Am. J. Roentgenol. Radium Ther.* [N. S.] **65**, 12.

Candlish, J. K., and Taylor, T. G. (1970). *J. Endocrinol.* **48**, 143.

Canterbury, J. M., and Reiss, E. (1972). *Proc. Soc. Exp. Biol. Med.* **140**, 1393.

Canterbury, J. M., Levey, G. S., and Reiss, E. (1973). *J. Clin. Invest.* **52**, 524.

Canterbury, J. M., Bricker, L. A., Levey, G. S., Kozlovskis, P. L., Ruiz, E., Zull, J. E., and Reiss, E. (1975). *J. Clin Invest.* **55**, 1245.

Care, A. D., Sherwood, L. M., Potts, J. T., Jr., and Aurbach, G. D. (1966). *Nature (London)* **209**, 55.

Castro, J. H., Genuth, S. M., and Klein, J. (1975). *Metab., Clin. Exp.* **24**, 839.

Chamberlin, J. A., Nicholas, H. O., and Hanna, E. (1963). *Surgery* **53**, 719.

Chang, H. Y. (1951). *Anat. Rec.* **111**, 23.

Charbon, G. A. (1968). *Eur. J. Pharmacol.* **3**, 275.

Chase, L. R., and Aurbach, G. D. (1967). *Proc. Natl. Acad. Sci. U.S.A.* **56**, 518.

Chase, L. R., and Aurbach, G. D. (1968). *Science* **159**, 545.

Chase, L. R., Fedak, S. A., and Aurbach, G. D. (1969). *Endocrinology* **84**, 761.

Chaves-Carballo, E., and Hayles, A. B. (1966). *Am. J. Dis. Child.* **112**, 553.

Cholod, E. J., Haust, M. D., Hudson, A. J., and Lewis, F. N. (1970). *Am. J. Med.* **48**, 700.

Chu, L. L. H., MacGregor, R. R., Anast, G. S., Hamilton, J. W., and Cohn, D. V. (1973a). *Endocrinology* **93**, 915.

Chu, L. L. H., MacGregor, R. R., Liu, P. I., Hamilton, J. W., and Cohn, D. V. (1973b). *J. Clin. Invest.* **52**, 3089.

Chu, L. L. H., Huang, W. Y., Hamilton, J. W., and Cohn, D. V. (1975). *Program, 57th Annu. Meet., Am. Endocr. Soc., New York, 1975.* Abstract No. 41, p. 71.

Citron, K. M. (1954). *Proc. R. Soc. Med.* **47**, 507.

Coe, F. L. (1974). *Arch. Intern. Med.* **134**, 262.

Cogan, D. G., Albright, F., and Bartter, F. C. (1948). *Arch. Ophthalmol.* **40**, 624.

Cohn, D. V., MacGregor, R. R., Chu, L. L. H., Kimmel, J. R., and Hamilton, J. W. (1972). *Proc. Natl. Acad. Sci. U.S.A.* **69**, 1521.

Coleman, E. N. (1965). *Arch. Dis. Child.* **40**, 535.

Collip, J. B. (1925). *J. Biol. Chem.* **63**, 395.

Cope, O. (1960). *Am. J. Surg.* **99**, 394.

Cope, O. (1966). *N. Engl. J. Med.* **274**, 1174.

Cope, O., Culver, P. J., Mixter, C. G., and Nardi, G. L. (1957). *Ann. Surg.* **145**, 857.

Cope, O., Barnes, B. A., Castleman, B., Mueller, G. C. E., and Roth, S. I. (1961). *Ann. Surg.* **154**, 491.

Copp, D. H., and Davidson, A. G. F. (1961). *Proc. Soc. Exp. Biol. Med.* **107**, 342.

Cushard, W. G., Jr., Bercovitz, M., Canterbury, J. M., and Reiss, E. (1971). *J. Clin. Invest.* **50**, No. 6, Abstr. No. 76, p. 23a.

Cushard, W. G., Jr., Simon, A. B., Canterbury, J. M., and Reiss, E. (1972). *N. Engl. J. Med.* **286**, 395.

Cushing, H., and Davidoff, L. M. (1927). *In* "The Pathological Findings in Four Autopsied Cases of Acromegaly, with a Discussion of Their Significance," Rockefeller Inst. Med. Res., New York. Monogr. No. 22.

Dalén, N., and Hjern, B. (1974). *Acta Endocrinol. (Copenhagen)* **75**, 297.

Daughaday, W. H. (1974). *In* "Textbook of Endocrinology" (R. H. Williams, ed.), 5th ed., p. 31. Saunders, Philadelphia, Pennsylvania.

Dauphine, R. T., Riggs, B. L., and Scholz, D. A. (1975). *Ann. Intern. Med.* **83**, 365.

Davies, D. R., Dent, C. E., and Willcox, A. (1956). *Br. Med. J.* **2**: 113.

Deftos, L. J., Goodman, D. A., Engelman, K., and Potts, J. T., Jr. (1971). Metab., Clin. Exp. **20**, 428.

DeGroote, J. W. (1969). *J. Am. Med. Assoc.* **208**, 2160.

Dent, C. E. (1956). *Br. Med. J.* **1**, 230.

Dent, C. E. (1962). *Br. Med. J.* **2**, 1419.

Dent, C. E. (1964). Cited as personal communication in Pyrah *et al.* (1966).

Dent, C. E., and Harper, C. M. (1962). *Lancet* **1**, 559.

Dent, C. E., and Watson, L. (1966). *Br. Med. J.* **1**, 646.

Dent, R. I., James, J. H., Wang, C. A., Deftos, L. J., Talamo, R., and Fischer, J. E. (1972). *Ann. Surg.* **176**, 360.

Dodds, W. J., and Steinbach, H. L. (1968). *Am. J. Roentgenol., Radium Ther. Nucl. Med.* [N. S.] **104**, 884.

Doll, R., Jones, F. A., and Buckatzsch, M. M. (1950). "Occupational Factors in the Aetiology of Peptic Gastric and Peptic Duodenal Ulcers. *Med. Res. Counc. (G. B.), Spec. Rep. Ser.* **SRS-276.**

Donegan, W. L., and Spiro, H. M. (1960). *Gastroenterology* **38**, 750.

Doppman, J. L., and Hammond, W. G. (1970). *Radiology* **95**, 603.

Doyle, F. H. (1966). *Br. J. Radiol.* **39**, 161.

Dreiling, D. A., Mazure, P. A., Cohen, N., Moskovitz, H., Todaro, R. T., and Paulino-Netto, A. (1962). *Am. J. Dig. Dis.* **7**, 112.

Dresser, R. (1933). *Am. J. Roentgenol. Radium Ther.* [N. S.] **30**, 596.

Duarte, C. G., and Bland, J. H. (1965). *Metab., Clin. Exp.* **14**, 899.

Duarte, C. G., Winnacker, J. L., Becker, K. L., and Pace, A. (1971). *N. Engl. J. Med.* **284**, 828.

Dufresne, L. R., Andersen, R., and Gitelman, H. J. (1971). *Clin. Res.* **19**, 529.

Edmondson, H. A., Beine, C. J., Homann, R. E., Jr., and Wertman, M. (1952). *Am. J. Med.* **12**, 34.

Edvall, C. A. (1958). *Acta Chir. Scand., Suppl.* **229.**

Eisenberg, E. (1965). *J. Clin. Invest.* **44**, 942.

Eisenberg, H., Pallotta, J., and Sherwood, L. M. (1974). *Am. J. Med.* **45**, 810.

Ellis, C., and Nicoloff, D. M. (1968). *Arch. Surg. (Chicago)* **96**, 114.

Ellis, K., and Hochstim, R. J. (1960). *Am. J. Roentgenol. Radium Ther. Nucl. Med.* [N. S.] **83**, 732.

Ellis, M., and Wilson, S. (1958). *J. Tenn. State Med. Assoc.* **51**, 283.

Ellison, E. H., and Wilson, S. D. (1964). *Ann. Surg.* **160**, 512.

Epstein, F. H. (1968a). *Am. J. Med.* **45**, 700.

Epstein, F. H. (1968b). *Ann. Intern. Med.* **68**, 490.

Epstein, F. H., Freedman, L. R., and Levitin, H. (1958). *N. Engl. J. Med.* **258**, 782.

Erdheim, J. (1903). *Beitr. Pathol. Anat.* **33**, 158.

Estep, H. L., Martinez, G. R., and Jones, D. (1969). *Program, 51st Annu. Meet., Am. Endocr. Soc., 1969.* Abstract No. 145.

Eugenidis, N., Olah, A. J., and Haas, H. G. (1972). *Radiology* **105**, 265.

Eversman, J. J., Farmer, R. G., and Brown, C. H. (1967). *Arch. Intern. Med.* **119**, 605.

Fairney, A., Wojtuleski, J., and Hart, F. D. (1975). *In* "Calcium-Regulating Hormones" (R. V. Talmage, M. Owen, and J. A. Parsons, eds.), Int. Congr. Ser. No. 346, p. 72. Excerpta Med. Found., Amsterdam.

Fang, V. S., and Tashjian, A. H., Jr. (1972). *Endocrinology* **90**, 1177.

Fawcett, C. P., Powell, A. E., and Sachs, H. (1968). *Endocrinology* **83**, 1299.

Fink, W. J., and Finfrock, J. D. (1961). *Am. Surg.* **27**, 424.

Finkelstein, J. W., Roffwarg, H. P., Boyar, R. M., Kream, J., and Hellman, L. (1972). *J. Clin. Endocrinol. Metab.* **35**, 665.

Fischer, J. A., Oldham, S. B., Sizemore, G. W., and Arnaud, C. D. (1971). *Horm. Metab. Res.* **3**, 223.

Fischer, J. A., Blum, J. W., and Binswanger, U. (1973). *J. Clin. Invest.* **52**, 2434.

Fischer, J. A., Binswanger, U., and Dietrich, F. M. (1974). *J. Clin. Invest.* **54**, 1382.

Forland, M., Strandjord, N. M., Paloyan, E., and Cox, A. (1968). *Arch. Intern. Med.* **122**, 236.

Fox, P. S., Hofmann, J. W., Decosse, J. J., and Wilson, S. D. (1974a). *Ann. Surg.* **180**, 558.

Fox, P. S., Hofmann, J. W., Wilson, S. D., and Decosse, J. J. (1974b). *Surg. Clin. North Am.* **54**, 395.

Frame, B., Heinze, E. G., Block, M. A., and Manson, G. A. (1968). *Ann. Intern. Med.* **68**, 1022.

Frame, B., Jackson, C. E., Reynolds, W. A., and Umphrey, J. E. (1974). *Ann. Intern. Med.* **80**, 44.

Fraser, P., Healy, M., Rose, N., and Watson, L. (1971). *Lancet* **1**, 1314.

Freeman, R. M., Lawton, R. L., and Chamberlain, M. A. (1967). *N. Engl. J. Med.* **276**, 1113.

Friesen, S. R. (1967). *Surgery* **62**, 609.

Friesen, S. R. (1968). *Ann. Surg.* **168**, 483.

Gaillard, P. J. (1955). *Exp. Cell Res., Suppl.* **3**, 154.

Gaillard, P. J. (1961). *Proc. K. Ned. Akad. Wet., Ser. C* **64**, 119.

Garabedian, M., Holick, M. F., DeLuca, H. F., and Boyle, I. T. (1972). *Proc. Nat. Acad. Sci. U.S.A.* **69**, 1673.

Garcia, R. E., Friedman, W. E., Kaback, M. M., and Rowe, R. D. (1964). *N. Engl. J. Med.* **271**, 117.

Genant, H. K., Baron, J. M., Straus, F. H., II, Paloyan, E., and Jowsey, J. (1975). *Am. J. Med.* **59**, 104.

Gittes, R. F., and Radde, I. C. (1966). *Endocrinology* **78**, 1015.

Gleason, D. C., and Potchen, E. J. (1967). *Radiol. Clin. North Am.* **5**, 277.

Gold, E. (1928). *Mitt. Grenzgeb. Med. Chir.* **41**, 63.

Gold, L. W., Massry, S. G., Arieff, A. I., and Coburn, J. W. (1973). *J. Clin. Invest.* **52**, 2556.

Golden, A., Jr., and Canary, J. J. (1968). *In* "Endocrine Pathology" (J. M. Bloodworth, ed.), p. 181. Williams & Wilkins, Baltimore, Maryland.

Goldhaber, P., Stern, B. D., Glimcher, M. J., and Chao, J. (1968). *In* "Parathyroid Hormone and Thyrocalcitonin (Calcitonin) (R. V. Talmage, L. F. Bélanger, and I. Clark, eds.), Int. Congr. Ser. No. 159, p. 182. Excerpta Med. Found., Amsterdam.

Goldsmith, R. E., Sizemore, G. W., Chen, I.-W., Zalme, E., and Altemeier, W. A. (1976). *Ann. Intern. Med.* **84**, 36.

Goldsmith, R. S. (1966). *N. Engl. J. Med.* **274**, 674.

Goldsmith, R. S. (1969). *N. Engl. J. Med.* **281**, 367.

Goldsmith, R. S., and Ingbar, S. H. (1966). *N. Engl. J. Med.* **274**, 1.

Goldsmith, R. S., Furszyfer, J., Johnson, W. J., Fournier, A. E., Sizemore, G. W., and Arnaud, C. D. (1973). *J. Clin. Invest.* **52**, 173.

Goldstein, R. A., Israel, H. L., Becker, K. L., and Moore, C. F. (1971). *Am. J. Med.* **51**, 21.

Goltzman, D., Potts, J. T., Jr., Ridgway, E. C., and Maloof, F. (1974). *N. Engl. J. Med.* **290**, 1035.

Goltzman, D., Peytremann, A., Callahan, E. [N.], Tregear, G. W., and Potts, J. T., Jr. (1975). *In* "Calcium-Regulating Hormones" (R. V. Talmage, M. Owen, and J. A. Parsons, eds.), Int. Congr. Ser. No. 346, p. 172. Excerpta Med. Found., Amsterdam.

Goltzman, D., Peytremann, A., Callahan, E. N., Segre, G. V., and Potts, J. T., Jr. (1976). *J. Clin. Invest.* **57**, 8.

Goodman, D. B. P., Rasmussen, H., DiBella, F., and Guthrow, C. E., Jr. (1970). *Proc. Natl. Acad. Sci. U.S.A.* **67**, 652.

Goodman, L. S., and Gilman, A., eds. (1970). "The Pharmacological Basis of Therapeutics" 4th ed. Macmillan, New York.

Gordan, G. S., Eisenberg, E., Loken, H. F., Gardner, B., and Hayashida, T. (1962). *Recent Prog. Horm. Res.* **18**, 297.

Grahame, R., Sutor, D. J., and Mitchener, M. B. (1971). *Ann. Rheum. Dis.* **30**, 597.

Greenwald, I. (1911). *Am. J. Physiol.* **28**, 103.

Gutman, A. B., Swenson, P. C., and Parsons, W. B. (1934). *J. Am. Med. Assoc.* **103**, 87.

Gwinup, G., and Sayle, B. (1961). *Ann. Intern. Med.* **55**, 1001.

Habener, J. F. (1976). *Polypept. Horm.: Mol. Cell. Aspects, Ciba Found. Symp. No. 41*, p. 197.

Habener, J. F. (1978). *J. Clin. Invest.* **62**,

Habener, J. F., and Potts, J. T., Jr. (1976a). *Endocrinology* **98**, 209.

Habener, J. F., and Potts, J. T., Jr. (1976b). *Handb. Physiol., Sect. 7: Endocrinol.* **7**, 313, (ed.), American Physiological Society, Bethesda, Maryland.

Habener, J. F., and Potts, J. T., Jr. (1976c). *In* "Hormones in Human Blood: Detection and Assay" (H. N. Antoniades, ed.), Chapter 36. Harvard Univ. Press, Cambridge, Massachusetts.

Habener, J. F., and Potts, J. T., Jr. (1977). *In* "Handbuch der inneren Medizin: klinische Osteologie" (H. Bartelheimer and F. Kuhlencordt, eds.), Vol. VI, Part 1. Springer-Verlag, Berlin and New York (in press).

Habener, J. F., Powell, D., Murray, T. M., Mayer, G. P., and Potts, J. T., Jr. (1971a). *Proc. Natl. Acad. Sci. U.S.A.* **68**, 2986.

Habener, J. F., Singer, F. R., Deftos, L. J., Neer, R. M., and Potts, J. T., Jr. (1971b). *Nature (London), New Biol.* **232**, 91.

Habener, J. F., Kemper, B., Potts, J. T., Jr., and Rich, A. (1972a). *Science* **178**, 630.

Habener, J. F., Segre, G. V., Powell, D., Murray, T. M., and Potts, J. T., Jr. (1972b). *Nature (London) New Biol.* **238**, 152.

Habener, J. F., Kemper, B., Potts, J. T., Jr., and Rich, A. (1973a). *Endocrinology* **92**, 219.

Habener, J. F., Tregear, G. W., van Rietschoten, J., Hamilton, J. W., Cohn, D. V., and Potts, J. T., Jr. (1973b). *Clin. Res.* **21**, 493 (abstr.).

Habener, J. F., Tregear, G. W., Stevens, T. D., Dee, P. C., and Potts, J. T., Jr. (1974a). *Endocr. Res. Commun.* **1**, 1.

Habener, J. F., Kemper, B. W., Potts, J. T., Jr., and Rich, A. (1974b). *Endocr. Res. Commun.* **1,** 239.

Habener, J. F., Kemper, B., and Potts, J. T., Jr. (1975a). *Endocrinology* **97,** 431.

Habener, J. F., Kemper, B., Potts, J. T., Jr., and Rich, A. (1975b). *Biochem. Biophys. Res. Commun.* **67,** 1114.

Habener, J. F., Kemper, B., Potts, J. T., Jr., and Rich, A. (1975c). *J. Clin. Invest.* **56,** 1328.

Habener, J. F., Mayer, G. P., Dee, P. C., and Potts, J. T., Jr. (1976a). *Metab., Clin. Exp.* **24,** 385.

Habener, J. F., Potts, J. T., Jr., and Rich, A. (1976b). *J. Biol. Chem.* **251,** 3893.

Habener, J. F., Stevens, T. D., Tregear, G. W., and Potts, J. T., Jr. (1976c). *J. Clin. Endocrinol. Metab.* **42,** 520.

Haddad, J. G., and Chyu, K. J. (1971). *J. Clin. Endocrinol. Metab.* **33,** 992.

Hamilton, J. W., MacGregor, R. R., Chu, L. L. H., and Cohn, D. V. (1971a). *Endocrinology* **89,** 1440.

Hamilton, J. W., Spierto, F. W., MacGregor, R. R., and Cohn, D. V. (1971b). *J. Biol. Chem.* **246,** 3224.

Hamilton, J. W., Niall, H. D., Jacobs, J. W., Keutmann, H. T., Potts, J. T., Jr., and Cohn, D. V. (1974). *Proc. Natl. Acad. Sci. U.S.A.* **71,** 653.

Hamilton, J. W., Huang, D. W. Y., Chu, L. L. H., MacGregor, R. R., and Cohn, D. V. (1975). *In* "Calcium-Regulating Hormones" (R. V. Talmage, M. Owens, and J. A. Parsons, eds.), Int. Congr. Ser. No. 346, p. 40. Excerpta Med. Found., Amsterdam.

Harmon, M. (1956). *Am. J. Dis. Child.* **91,** 313.

Harris, E. D., and Sjoerdsma, A. (1966). *J. Clin. Endocrinol. Metab.* **26,** 358.

Harrison, H. E., and Harrison, H. C. (1963). *Am. J. Physiol.* **205,** 107.

Harrison, M. T., Harden, R. M., and Alexander, W. D. (1964). *J. Clin. Endocrinol. Metab.* **24,** 214.

Haussler, M. R., Boyce, D. W., Littledike, E. T., and Rasmussen, H. (1971). *Proc. Natl. Acad. Sci. U.S.A.* **68,** 177.

Haverback, B. J., Dyce, B., Bundy, H., and Edmondson, H. A. (1960). *Am. J. Med.* **29,** 424.

Heath, D. A., Palmer, J. S., and Aurbach, G. D. (1972). *Endocrinology* **90,** 1589.

Heersche, J. N. M. (1969). *Proc. K. Ned. Akad. Wet., Ser. C Biol. Med.* **72,** 578.

Heersche, J. N. M., and de Voogd van der Straaten, W. (1965). *Proc. K. Ned. Akad. Wet., Ser. C* **68,** 277.

Heinemann, H. O. (1965). *Metab., Clin. Exp.* **14,** 1137.

Hellman, D. E., Au, Y. W., and Bartter, F. C. (1965). *Am. J. Physiol.* **209,** 643.

Hellström, J. (1950). *Acta Chir. Scand.* **100,** 391.

Hellström, J. (1954). *Acta Endocrinol. (Copenhagen)* **16,** 30.

Hellström, J. (1959). *Acta Chir. Scand.* **116,** 207.

Hellström, J., and Ivemark, B. I. (1962). *Acta Chir. Scand., Suppl.* **294,** p. 1.

Hellström, J., Birke, G., and Edvall, C. A. (1958). *Br. J. Urol.* **30,** 13.

Hendrix, J. Z. (1966). *Ann. Intern. Med.* **64,** 797.

Henneman, P. H., Dempsey, E. F., Carroll, E. L., and Albright, F. (1956). *J. Clin. Invest.* **35,** 1229.

Henson, R. A. (1966). *J. R. Coll. Physicians, Lond.* **1,** 41.

Herrmann-Erlee, M. P. M., and van der Meer, J. M. (1974). *Endocrinology* **94,** 424.

Herrmann-Erlee, M. P. M., Heersche, J. N. M., Hekkelman, J. W., Gaillard, P. J., Tregear, G. W., Parsons, J. A., and Potts, J. T., Jr. (1976). *Endocr. Res. Commun.* **3,** 21.

Hirschberg, K. (1889). *Beitr. Pathol. Anat.* **6,** 513.

Hockaday, T. D. R., Keynes, W. M., and McKenzie, J. K. (1966). *Br. Med. J.* **1,** 85.

Holick, M. F., Schnoes, H. K., and DeLuca, H. F. (1971). *Biochemistry* **10,** 279.

Holmes, E. C., Morton, D. L., and Ketcham, A. S. (1969). *Ann. Surg.* **169**, 1969.

Holtermuller, K. H., Goldsmith, R. S., Sizemore, G. W., and Go, V. L. W. (1974). *Gastroenterology* **67**, 1101.

Holtrop, M. E., and Weinger, J. M. (1972). In "Calcium, Parathyroid Hormone and the Calcitonins" (R. V. Talmage and P. L. Munson, eds.), Int. Congr. Ser. No. 243, p. 365. Excerpta Med. Found, Amsterdam.

Howard, J. E., Follis, R. H., Jr., Yendt, E. R., and Connor, T. B. (1953). *J. Clin. Endocrinol. Metab.* **13**, 997.

Huang, D. W.-Y., Chu, L. L. H., Hamilton, J. W., MacGregor, R. R., and Cohn, D. V. (1975). *Arch. Biochem. Biophys.* **166**, 67.

Hueper, W. (1927). *Arch. Pathol. Lab. Med.* **3**, 14.

Hughes, M. R., Brumbaugh, P. F., Haussler, M. R., Wergedal, J. E., and Baylink, D. J. (1975). *Science* **190**, 578.

Hughes, W. S., Hawker, C. D., Brooks, F. P., and Utiger, R. D. (1971). *Clin. Res.* **18**, 607.

Humbel, R. E., Bosshard, H. R., and Zahn, H. (1972). *Handb. Physiol. Sect. 7: Endocrinol.* **1**, 111. (R. O. Greep and E. B. Astwood, eds.).

Hunt, B. J., and Yendt, E. R. (1963). *Ann. Intern. Med.* **59**, 554.

Ivanovich, P., Fellows, H., and Rich, C. (1967). *Ann. Intern. Med.* **66**, 917.

Jacobs, J. W., Kemper, B., Niall, H. D., Habener, J. F., and Potts, J. T., Jr. (1974). *Nature (London)* **249**, 155.

James, D. G. (1964). *Acta Med. Scand.* **176**, Suppl. 425, 203.

Jowsey, J. (1966). *Am. J. Med.* **40**, 485.

Jowsey, J. (1968). In "Parathyroid Hormone and Thyrocalcitonin (Calcitonin)" (R. V. Talmage, L. F. Bélanger, and I. Clark, eds.), Int. Congr. Ser. No. 159, p. 137. Excerpta Med. Found., Amsterdam.

Jowsey, J., and Riggs, B. L. (1968). *J. Clin. Endocrinol. Metab.* **28**, 1833.

Karpati, G., and Frame, B. (1964). *Arch. Neurol. (Chicago)* **10**, 387.

Katz, A. I., Hampers, C. L., and Merrill, J. P. (1969). *Medicine (Baltimore)* **48**, 333.

Katz, C. M., and Tzagournis, M. (1972). *Metab., Clin. Exp.* **21**, 1171.

Kaye, M. B., Pritchard, J. E., Halpenny, G. W., and Light, W. (1960). *Medicine (Baltimore)* **39**, 159.

Keating, F. R., Jr. (1961). *J. Am. Med. Assoc.* **178**, 547.

Keiser, H. R., Gill, J. R., Sjoerdsma, A., and Bartter, F. C. (1964). *J. Clin. Invest.* **43**, 1073.

Kemper, B., Habener, J. F., Potts, J. T., Jr., and Rich, A. (1972). *Proc. Natl. Acad. Sci. U.S.A.* **69**, 643.

Kemper, B., Habener, J. F., Mulligan, R. C., Potts, J. T., Jr., and Rich, A. (1974a). *Proc. Natl. Acad. Sci. U.S.A.* **71**, 3731.

Kemper, B., Habener, J. F., Rich, A., and Potts, J. T., Jr. (1974b). *Science* **184**, 167.

Kemper, B., Habener, J. F., Ernst, M. D., Potts, J. T., Jr., and Rich, A. (1976a). *Biochemistry* **15**, 15.

Kemper, B., Habener, J. F., Potts, J. T., Jr., and Rich, A. (1976b). *Biochemistry* **15**, 20.

Keutmann, H. T., Aurbach, G. D., Dawson, B. F., Niall, H. D., Deftos, L. J., and Potts, J. T., Jr. (1971). *Biochemistry* **10**, 2779.

Keutmann, H. T., Dawson, B. F., Aurbach, G. D., and Potts, J. T., Jr. (1972). *Biochemistry* **11**, 1973.

Keutmann, H. T., Barling, P. M., Hendy, G. N., Segre, G. V., Niall, H. D., Aurbach, G. D., Potts, J. T., Jr., and O'Riordan, J. L. H. (1974). *Biochemistry* **13**, 1646.

Keutmann, H. T., Niall, H. D., O'Riordan, J. L. H., and Potts, J. T., Jr. (1975). *Biochemistry* **14**, 1842.

Keutmann, H. T., Niall, H. D., Jacobs, J. W., Barling, P. M., Hendy, G. N., O'Riordan, J.

L. H., and Potts, J. T., Jr. (1975b). *In* "Calcium-Regulating Hormones" (R. V. Talmage, M. Owen, and J. A. Parsons, eds.), Int. Congr. Ser. No. 346, Excerpta Med. Found., Amsterdam. p. 9.

Kivirikko, K. I. (1970). *Int. Rev. Connect. Tissue Res.* **5**, 93.

Kjellberg, R. N., and Kliman, B. (1974). *Proc. R. Soc. Med.* **67**, 32.

Klatskin, G., and Gordon, M. (1953). *Am. J. Med.* **15**, 484.

Kleeman, C. R., Rockney, R. E., and Maxwell, M. H. (1958). *Clin. Invest.* **37**, 907 (abstr.).

Kleeman, C. R., Bernstein, D., Rockney, R., Dowling, J. T., and Maxwell, M. H. (1961). *In* "The Parathyroids" (R. O. Greep and R. V. Talmage, eds.), p. 353. Thomas, Springfield, Illinois.

Kleppel, N. H., Goldstein, M. H., and LeVeen, H. H. (1965). *J. Am. Med. Assoc.* **192**, 224.

Knox, F. G., and Lechene, C. (1975). *Am. J. Physiol.* **229**, 1556.

Knox, F. G., Haas, J. A., and Lechene, C. (1975). *Program/Abstr. Int. Workshop Phosphate,* 1975.

Kodicek, E. (1967). *Proc. Nutr. Soc.* **26**, 67.

Kooh, S. W., Fraser, D., DeLuca, H. F., Holick, M. F., Belsey, R. E., Clark, M. B., and Murray, T. M. (1975). *N. Engl. J. Med.* **293**, 840.

Koppel, M. H., Massry, S. G., Shinaberger, J. H., Hartenblower, D. L., and Coburn, J. W. (1970). *Ann. Intern. Med.* **72**, 895.

Kraintz, L., Kraintz, F. W., and Talmage, R. V. (1965). *Proc. Soc. Exp. Biol. Med.* **120**, 118.

Krane, S. M. (1970). *Int. Encycl. Pharmacol. Ther.* Section 51, vol. I: Pharmacology of the Endocrine System and Related Drugs: Parathyroid Hormone, Thyrocalcitonin and Related Drugs. p. 19.

Krane, S. M., and Goldring, S. R. (1978). *In* "The Thyroid" (S. C. Werner and S. H. Ingbar, eds.), Harper, New York.

Krane, S. M., Brownell, G. L., Stanbury, J. B., and Corrigan, H. (1956). *J. Clin. Invest.* **35**, 874.

Krementz, E. T., Race, J. L., Sternberg, W. H., and Hawley, W. D. (1967). *Ann. Surg.* **165**, 681.

Krull, G. H., Muller, H., Leijnse, B., and Gerbrandy, J. (1969). *Lancet* **2**, 174.

Kunin, A. S., and Krane, S. M. (1965). *Endocrinology* **76**, 343.

Kuo, J. F., and Greengard, P. (1969). *Proc. Natl. Acad. Sci. U.S.A.* **64**, 1349.

Kyle, L. H. (1954). *N. Engl. J. Med.* **251**, 1035.

Kyle, L. H., Canary, J. J., Mintz, D. H., and de Leon, A. (1962). *J. Clin. Endocrinol. Metab.* **22**, 52.

Laake, H. (1955). *Acta Med. Scand.* **151**, 229.

Lafferty, F. W. (1966). *Medicine (Baltimore)* **45**, 247.

Laitinen, O. (1967). *Endocrinology* **80**, 815.

Lamberg, B. A., and Kuhlback, B. (1959). *Scand. J. Clin. Lab. Invest.* **11**, 351.

Larsson, L. G., Liljestrand, A., and Wahlund, H. (1952). *Acta Med. Scand.* **143**, 280.

Lassiter, W. E., Gottschalk, C. W., and Mylle, M. (1963). *Am. J. Physiol.* **204**, 771.

Lawson, D. E. M., Fraser, D. R., Kodicek, E., Morris, H. R., and Williams, D. H. (1971). *Nature (London)* **230**, 228.

Leeksma, C. H. W., De Graeff, J., and De Cock, J. (1957). *Acta Med. Scand.* **156**, 455.

Lehrer, G. M., and Levitt, M. F. (1960). *J. Mt. Sinai Hosp., N.Y.* **27**, 10.

Lemann, J., and Donatelli, A. A. (1964). *Ann. Intern. Med.* **60**, 447.

Levant, J. A., Walsh, J. H., and Isenberg, J. I. (1973). *N. Engl. J. Med.* **289**, 555.

Levi, J., Massry, S. G., Coburn, J. W., Llach, F., and Kleeman, C. R. (1974). *Metab., Clin. Exp.* **23**, 323.

Lloyd, H. M. (1968). *Medicine (Baltimore)* **47**, 53.

Lloyd, H. M., Aitken, R. E., and Ferrier, T. M. (1965). *Br. Med. J.* **2**, 853.

Loeb, R. F. (1932). *Science* **76**, 420.

Lotz, M., Ney, R., and Bartter, F. C. (1964). *Trans. Assoc. Am. Physicians* **77**, 281.

Ludwig, G. D. (1962). *N. Engl. J. Med.* **267**, 637.

MacGregor, R. R., Chu, L. L. H., Hamilton, J. W., and Cohn, D. V. (1973). *Endocrinology* **92**, 1312.

MacIntyre, I., and Robinson, C. J. (1969). *Ann. N.Y. Acad. Sci.* **162**, 865.

MacIntyre, I., Boss, S., and Troughton, V. A. (1963). *Nature (London)* **198**, 1058.

McCarty, D. J., [Jr.] (1966). *Mod. Trends Rheumatol.* **1**, 287.

McCarty, D. J., [Jr.] (1975). *Bull. Rheum. Dis.* **25**, 804.

McCarty, D. J., Jr., and Haskin, M. E. (1963). *Am. J. Roentgenol.* **90**, 1248.

McCarty, D. J., Jr., Kohn, N. N., and Faires, J. S. (1962). *Ann. Intern. Med.* **56**, 711.

McCarty, D. J., [Jr.], Silcox, D. C., Coe, F., Jacobelli, S., Reiss, E., Genant, H., and Ellman, M. (1974). *Am. J. Med.* **56**, 704.

McGeown, M. G. (1961). *Lancet* **1**, 586.

McGuigan, J. E., Colwell, J. A., and Franklin, J. (1974). *Gastroenterology* **66**, 269.

McMillan, D. E., and Freeman, R. B. (1965). *Medicine (Baltimore)* **44**, 485.

McSwiney, R. R., and Mills, I. H. (1956). *Lancet* **2**, 862.

Mandl, F. (1926). *Arch. Klin. Chir.* **143**, 1.

Marcus, R., and Aurbach, G. D. (1969). *Endocrinology* **85**, 801.

Martin, T. J., Greenberg, P. B., and Melick, R. A. (1972). *J. Clin. Endocrinol. Metab.* **34**, 437.

Marx, S. J., Powell, D., Shimkin, P. M., Wells, S. A., Ketcham, A. S., McGuigan, J. E., Bilezkan, J. P., and Aurbach, G. D. (1973). *Ann. Intern. Med.* **78**, 371.

Mather, G. (1957). *Br. Med. J.* **1**, 248.

Mayer, G. P. (1970). *In* "Parturient Hypocalcemia" (J. J. Anderson, ed.), p. 177. Academic Press, New York.

Mayer, G. P. (1973). *Program, 55th Annu. Meet., Am. Endocr. Soc., 1973.* p. A-160.

Mayer, G. P. (1974). *Program, 56th Meet., Am. Endocr. Soc., 1974* p. A-181.

Mayer, G. P., Ramberg, C. F., Jr., and Kronfeld, D. S. (1968). *Dairy Sci.* **49**, 1288.

Mayer, G. P., Ramberg, C. F., and Kronfeld, D. S. (1969). *Clin. Orthop. Relat. Res.* **62**, 79.

Mayer, G. P., Habener, J. F., and Potts, J. T., Jr. (1976). *J. Clin. Invest.* **57**, 678.

Meema, H. E., Oreopoulos, D. G., Rabinovich, S., Husdan, H., and Rapoport, A. (1974). *Radiology* **110**, 513.

Melick, R. A., and Henneman, P. H. (1958). *N. Engl. J. Med.* **259**, 307.

Melvin, K. E. W., Miller, H. H., and Tashjian, A. H., Jr. (1971). *N. Engl. J. Med.* **285**, 1115.

Melvin, K. E. W., Tashjian, A. H., Jr., and Miller, M. H. (1972). *Recent Prog. Horm. Res.* **28**, 399.

Meunier, P., Vignon, G., Bernard, J., Edouard, C., and Courpron, P. (1973). *Clin. Aspects Metab. Bone Dis., Proc. Int. Symp., 1972* Int. Congr. Ser. No. 270, p. 215.

Milhaud, G., Perault-Staub, L. D., and Perault-Staub, A. M. (1971). *Eur. J. Clin. Biol. Res.* **16**, 451.

Mintz, D. H., Canary, J. J., Carreon, G., and Kyle, L. H. (1961). *N. Engl. J. Med.* **265**, 112.

Mixter, C. G., Jr., Keynes, W. M., and Cope, O. (1962). *N. Engl. J. Med.* **266**, 265.

Moroz, L. A., and Krane, S. M. (1963). *J. Clin. Invest.* **42**, 958.

Morris, R. C., Jr. (1968). *J. Clin. Invest.* **47**, 1648.

Morris, R. C., Jr. (1969). *N. Engl. J. Med.* **281**, 1405.

Morris, R. C., Jr., McSherry, E., and Sebastian, A. (1971). *Proc. Natl. Acad. Sci. U.S.A.* **68**, 132.

Morris, R. C., Jr., Sebastian, A., and McSherry, E. (1972). *Kidney Intern.* **1**, 322.

Moses, A. M. (1958). *J. Mt. Sinai Hosp., N.Y.* **25**, 339.

Moure, J. M. B. (1967). *Arch. Neurol. (Chicago)* **17**, 34.

Murray, T. M., Peacock, M., Powell, D., Monchik, J. M., and Potts, J. T., Jr. (1972). *Clin. Endocrinol.* **1,** 235.

Nassim, J. R., and Higgins, B. A. (1965). *Br. Med. J.* **1,** 675.

Neer, R. [M.], Berman, M., Fisher, L., and Rosenberg, L. E. (1967). *J. Clin. Invest.* **46,** 1364.

Neer, R. M., Holick, M. F., DeLuca, H. F., and Potts, J. T., Jr. (1975). *Metab., Clin. Exp.* **24,** 1403.

Nelson, C. T. (1949). *J. Invest. Dermatol.* **13,** 81.

Niall, H. D., Keutmann, H. [T.], Sauer, R., Hogan, M. [L.], Dawson, B. [F.], Aurbach, G. [D.], and Potts, J. [T.], Jr. (1970). *Hoppe-Seyler's Z. Physiol. Chem.* **351,** 1586.

Niall, H. D., Sauer, R. T., Jacobs, J. W., Keutmann, H. T., Segre, G. V., O'Riordan, J. L. H., Aurbach, G. D., and Potts, J. T., Jr. (1974). *Proc. Natl. Acad. Sci. U.S.A.* **71,** 384.

Nichols, G., Jr., Flanagan, B., and Woods, J. H. (1965). *In* "The Parathyroid Glands: Ultrastructure, Secretion and Function" (P. J. Gaillard, R. V. Talmage, and A. M. Budy, eds.), p. 243. Univ. of Chicago Press, Chicago, Illinois.

Nicholson, T. F., and Shepherd, G. W. (1959). *Cand. J. Biochem. Physiol.* **37,** 103.

Nolan, R. B., Hayles, A. B., and Woolner, L. B. (1960). *Am. J. Dis. Child.* **99,** 622.

Nordin, B. E. C., and Peacock, M. (1969). *Lancet* **2,** 1280.

Nordin, B. E. C., Peacock, M., and Wilkinson, R. (1972). *In* "Calcium, Parathyroid Hormone and the Calcitonins" (R. V. Talmage and P. L. Munson, eds.), Int. Congr. Ser. No. 243. p. 263. Excerpta Med. Found., Amsterdam.

Nordin, B. E. C., Marshall, D. H., Peacock, M., and Robertson, W. G. (1975). *In* "Calcium-Regulating Hormones" (R. V. Talmage, M. Owen, and J. A. Parsons, eds.), Int. Congr. Ser. No. 346. p. 239. Excerpta Med. Found., Amsterdam.

Norris, E. H. (1946). *Arch. Path.* **42,** 261.

Oldham, S. B., Fischer, J. A., Capen, C. C., Sizemore, G. W., and Arnaud, C. D. (1971). *Am. J. Med.* **50,** 650.

Olson, E. B., Jr., DeLuca, H. F., and Potts, J. T., Jr. (1972). *In* "Calcium, Parathyroid Hormone and the Calcitonins" (R. V. Talmage and P. L. Munson, eds.), Int. Congr. Ser. No. 243, p. 241. Excerpta Med. Found., Amsterdam.

Omdahl, J., Holick, M., Suda, T., Tanaka, Y., and DeLuca, H. F. (1971). Biochemistry **10,** 2935.

Omenn, G. S., Roth, S. J., and Baker, W. H., Jr. (1969) *Cancer* **24,** 1004.

O'Riordan, J. L. H., Page, J., Kerr, D. N. S., Walls, J., Moorehead, J., Crockett, R. E., Franz, H., and Ritz, E. (1970). *Q. J. Med.* **39,** 359.

Ostrow, J. D., Blanshard, G., and Gray, S. J. (1960). *Am. J. Med.* **29,** 769.

Pak, C. Y. C., Stewart, A., Kaplan, R., Bone, H., Notz, C., and Browne, R. (1975). *Lancet* **2,** 7.

Palmer, F. J., Nelson, J. C., and Bacchus, H. (1974). *Ann. Intern. Med.* **80,** 200.

Paloyan, E., Lawrence, A. M., Straus, F. H., II, Paloyan, D., Harper, P. V., and Cummings, D. (1967a). *J. Am. Med. Assoc.* **200,** 757.

Paloyan, E., Paloyan, D., and Harper, P. V. (1967b). *Metab., Clin. Exp.* **16,** 35.

Paloyan, E., Paloyan, D., and Pickleman, J. R. (1973). *S. Clin. North Am.* **53,** 211.

Pappenheimer, A. M., and Wilens, S. L. (1935). *Am. J. Pathol.* **11,** 73.

Parfitt, A. M. (1969). *N. Engl. J. Med.* **281,** 55.

Parfitt, A. M. (1972). *J. Clin. Invest.* **51,** 1879.

Parlee, D. E., Freundlich, I. M., and McCarty, D. J., Jr. (1967). *Am. J. Roentgenol., Radium Ther. Nucl. Med.* [N. S.] **99,** 688.

Parsons, J. A., Neer, R. M., and Potts, J. T., Jr. (1971). *Endocrinology* **89,** 735.

Parsons, J. A., and Potts, J. T., Jr. (1972). *Clin. Endocrinol. Metab.* **1,** 33.

Parsons, J. A., Reit, B., and Robinson, C. J. (1973). *Endocrinology* **92,** 454.

Parsons, J. A., and Robinson, C. J. (1968). *In* "Parathyroid Hormone and Thyrocalcitonin (Calcitonin)" (R. V. Talmage, L. F. Bélanger, and I. Clark, eds.), Int. Congr. Ser. No. 159, p. 329. Excerpta Med. Found., Amsterdam.

Parsons, J. A., Rafferty, B., Gray, D., Reit, B., Zanelli, J. M., Keutmann, H. T., Tregear, G. W., Callahan, E. N., and Potts, J. T., Jr. (1975). *In* "Calcium Regulating Hormones" (R. V. Talmage, M. Owen, and J. A. Parsons, eds.), Int. Congr. Ser. No. 346, p. 33. Excerpta Med. Found., Amsterdam.

Passaro, E., Jr., Basso, N., and Walsh, J. H. (1972). *Surgery* **72,** 60.

Patt, H. M., and Luckhardt, A. B. (1942). *Endocrinology* **31,** 384.

Patten, B. M., Bilezikian, J. P., Mallette, L. E., Prince, A., Engel, W. K., and Aurbach, G. D. (1974). *Ann. Intern. Med.* **80,** 182.

Patterson, M., Wolma, F., Drake, A., and Ong, H. (1969). *Arch. Surg. (Chicago)* **99,** 9.

Peacock, M. (1975). *In* "Calcium-Regulating Hormones" (R. V. Talmage, M. Owen, and J. A. Parsons, eds.), Int. Congr. Ser. No. 346, p. 78. Excerpta Med. Found., Amsterdam.

Peacock, M., and Nordin, B. E. C. (1968). *J. Clin. Pathol.* **21,** 353.

Peacock, M., Robertson, W. G., and Nordin, B. E. C. (1969). *Lancet* **1,** 384.

Pearse, A. G. E. (1968). *Calcitonin, Proc. Symp. Thyrocalcitonin C Cells, 1967.* p. 98.

Pearse, A. G. E. (1976). *In* "Peptide Hormones" (J. A. Parsons, ed.), p. 33. Macmillan, New York.

Peck, W. A., Carpenter, J., Messinger, K., and De Bra, D. (1973). *Endocrinology* **92,** 692.

Petersen, P. (1968). *J. Clin. Endocrinol. Metab.* **28,** 1491.

Peytremann, A., Goltzman, D., Callahan, E. N., Tregear, G. W., and Potts, J. T., Jr. (1975). *Endocrinology* **97,** 1270.

Phelps, P., and Hawker, C. D. (1973). *Arthritis Rheum.* **16,** 590.

Phelps, P., Steele, A. D., and McCarty, D. J., Jr. (1968). *J. Am. Med. Assoc.* **203,** 508.

Phillips, R. W., and Fitzpatrick, D. P. (1956). *N. Engl. J. Med.* **254,** 1216.

Plough, I. C., and Kyle, L. H. (1957). *Ann. Intern. Med.* **47,** 590.

Popovtzer, M. M., Subryan, V. L., Alfrey, A. C., Reeve, E. B., and Schrier, R. W. (1975). *J. Clin. Invest.* **55,** 1295.

Potchen, E. J., Watts, J. G., and Awwad, H. K. (1967). *Radiol. Clin. North Am.* **5,** 267.

Potts, J. T., Jr. (1976). *In* "Peptide Hormones" (J. A. Parsons, ed.), p. 119. Macmillan, New York.

Potts, J. T., Jr., and Deftos, L. J. (1974). *In* "Duncan's Diseases of Metabolism" (P. K. Bondy and L. E. Rosenberg, eds.), p. 1225. Saunders, Philadelphia, Pennsylvania.

Potts, J. T., Jr., and Roberts, B. (1958). *Am. J. Med. Sci.* **235,** 206.

Potts, J. T., Jr., Keutmann, H. T., Niall, H. D., and Tregear, G. W. (1971). *Vitam. Horm. N.Y.* **29,** 41.

Potts, J. T., Jr., Habener, J. F., Segre, G. V., Niall, H. D., Tregear, G. W., Keutmann, H. T., and Powell, D. A. (1973). *Clin. Aspects Metab. Bone Dis., Proc. Int. Symp., 1972.* p. 208.

Powell, D., Shimkin, P. M., Doppman, J. L., Wells, S., Aurbach, G. D., Marx, S. J., Ketcham, A. S., and Potts, J. T., Jr. (1972). *N. Engl. J. Med.* **286,** 1169.

Powell, D., Murray, T. M., Pollard, J. J., Cope, O., Wang, C. A., and Potts, J. T., Jr. (1973). *Arch. Intern. Med.* **131,** 645.

Preston, E. T. (1972). *J. Am. Med. Assoc.* **241,** 406.

Preston, F. S., and Adicoff, A. (1962). *N. Engl. J. Med.* **266,** 968.

Prien, E. L., and Prien, E. L., Jr. (1968). *Am. J. Med.* **45,** 645.

Purnell, D. C., Smith, L. H., Scholz, D. A., Elveback, L. R., and Arnaud, C. A. (1971). *Am. J. Med.* **50,** 670.

Purnell, D. C., Scholz, D. A., Smith, L. H., Sizemore, G. W., Black, B. M., Goldsmith, R. S., and Arnaud, C. A. (1974). *Am. J. Med.* **56,** 800.

Putkonen, T., Hannuksela, M., and Halme, H. (1965). *Acta Med. Scand.* **177,** 327.

Pyrah, L. N., Hodgkinson, A., and Anderson, C. K. (1966). *Br. J. Surg.* **53,** 245.
Raisz, L. G., and O'Brien, J. E. (1963). *Am. J. Physiol.* **205,** 816.
Raisz, L. G., Brand, J. S., Au, W. Y. W., and Niemann, I. (1968). *In* "Parathyroid Hormone and Thyrocalcitonin (Calcitonin)" (R. V. Talmage, L. F. Bélanger, and I. Clark, eds.), Int. Congr. Ser. No. 159. p. 370. Excerpta Med. Found., Amsterdam.
Raisz, L. G., Brand, J. S., Klein, D. C., and Au, W. Y. W. (1969). *In* "Progress in Endocrinology" (C. Gaul, ed.), Int. Congr. Ser. No. 184, p. 696. Excerpta Med. Found., Amsterdam.
Raisz, L. G., Holtrop, M. E., and Simmons, H. A. (1973). *Endocrinology* **92,** 556.
Rajasuriya, K., Peiris, O. A., Ratnaike, V. T., and de Fonseka, C. P. (1964). *Am. J. Dis. Child.* **107,** 442.
Randall, R. V., and Keating, F. R., Jr. (1958). *Trans. Assoc. Am. Physicians* **71,** 77.
Rasmussen, H. (1959). *Endocrinology* **65,** 517.
Rasmussen, H., and Bordier, P. (1973). *N. Engl. J. Med.* **289,** 25.
Rasmussen, H., and Bordier, P. (1974). "The Physiological and Cellular Basis of Metabolic Bone Disease." Williams & Wilkins, Baltimore.
Rasmussen, H., and Tenenhouse, A. (1970). *In* "Biochemical Actions of Hormones" (G. Litwak, ed.), p. 365. Academic Press, New York.
Rasmussen, H., Sze, Y.-L., and Young, R. (1964). *J. Biol. Chem.* **239,** 2852.
Rasmussen, H., Pechet, M., and Fast, D. (1968). *J. Clin Invest.* **47,** 1843.
Rasmussen, H., Wong, M., Bikle, D., and Goodman, D. B. P. (1972). *J. Clin. Invest.* **51,** 2502.
Recklinghausen, F., von (1891). *In* "Festschr. Rudolph Virchow Seinem 71 Geburtstage." p. 1.
Reeder, D. D., Jackson, B. M., Ban, J., Clendinnen, B. G., Davidson, W. D., and Thompson, J. C. (1970). *Ann. Surg.* **172,** 540.
Reinfrank, R. F., and Edwards, T. L., Jr. (1961). *J. Am. Med. Assoc.* **178,** 468.
Reiss, E., and Canterbury, J. M. (1969). *N. Engl. J. Med.* **280,** 1381.
Reiss, E., and Canterbury, J. M. (1975). *In* "Calcium-Regulating Hormones" (R. V. Talmage, M. Owen, and J. A. Parsons, eds.), Int. Congr. Ser. No. 346, p. 66. Excerpta Med. Found., Amsterdam.
Reitz, R. E., Pollard, J. J., Wang, C. A., Fleischli, D., Cope, O., Murray, T., Deftos, L. J., and Potts, J. T., Jr. (1969). *N. Engl. J. Med.* **281,** 348.
Reitz, R. E., Mayer, G. P., Deftos, L. J., and Potts, J. T., Jr. (1971). *Endocrinology* **89,** 932.
Richet, G., Ardaillou, R., Amiel, C., and Lecestre, M. (1963). *J. Urol. Nephrol.* **69,** 373.
Riddick, F. A., Jr. (1967). *Med. Clin. North Am.* **81,** 871.
Riddick, F. A., Jr., and Reiss, E. (1962). *Ann. Intern. Med.* **56,** 183.
Riggs, L. B., Arnaud, C. D., Reynolds, J. C., and Smith, L. H. (1971). *J. Clin. Invest.* **50,** 2079.
Robinson, C. J., Rafferty, B., and Parsons, J. A. (1972). *Clin. Sci.* **42,** 235.
Rodan, S. B., and Rodan, G. A. (1974). *J. Biol. Chem.* **249,** 3068.
Rogers, H. M. (1946). *J. Am. Med. J. Assoc.* **130,** 22.
Rose, E., and Boles, R. S., Jr. (1953). *Med. Clin. North Am.* **37,** 1715.
Rosenberg, E. H., and Guralnick, W. C. (1962). *Oral Surg., Oral Med., Oral Pathol.* **15,** Suppl. 2, 84.
Rossier, P. H., and Dressler, M. (1939). *Schweiz. Med. Wochenschr.* **69,** 985.
Roth, S. I. (1962). *Arch. Pathol.* **73,** 495.
Roth, S. I., and Schiller, A. L. (1976). *Hndb. Physiol., Sect. 7: Endocrinol.* **7,** 281.
Roth, S. I. (1971). *Am. J. Med.* **50,** 612.
Rubin, R. P. (1970). *Pharmacol. Rev.* **22,** 389.

Rude, R. K., Oldham, S. B., and Singer, F. R. (1976). *Clin. Endocrinol. Oxford* **5**, 209.

Russell, R. G. G., Casey, P. A., and Fleisch, H. (1968). *Calcif. Tissue Res., Suppl. p. 54.*

Ryan, W. G., Schwartz, J. B., and Northrop, G. (1971). *J. Am. Med. Assoc.* **213**, 1153.

St. Goar, W. T. (1957). *Ann. Intern. Med.* **46**, 102.

Samiy, A. H., Hirsch, P. F., Ramsay, A. G., Giordano, C., and Merrill, J. P. (1960). *Endocrinology* **67**, 266.

Samiy, A. H., Hirsch, P. F., and Ramsay, A. G. (1965). *Am. J. Physiol.* **208**, 73.

Sauer, R. T., Niall, H. D., Hogan, M. L., Keutmann, H. T., O'Riordan, J. L. H., and Potts, J. T., Jr. (1974). *Biochemistry* **13**, 1994.

Schantz, A., and Castleman, B. (1973). *Cancer* **31**, 600.

Schimke, R. N., and Hartmann, W. H. (1965). *Ann. Intern. Med.* **63**, 1027.

Schimke, R. N., Hartmann, W. H., Prout, T. E., and Rimoin, D. L. (1968). *N. Engl. J. Med.* **279**, 1.

Schussler, G. C., Verso, M. A., and Nemoto, T. (1972). *J. Clin. Endocrinol. Metab.* **35**, 497.

Scott, J. T., Dixon, A. St. J., and Bywaters, E. G. L. (1964). *Br. Med. J.* **1**, 1070.

Segal, A. J., Miller, M., and Moses, A. M. (1968). *Ann. Intern. Med.* **68**, 1066.

Segre, G. V., Niall, H. D., Habener, J. F., and Potts, J. T., Jr. (1974). *Am. J. Med.* **56,**

Segre, G. V., Habener, J. F., Powell, D., Tregear, G. W., and Potts, J. T., Jr. (1972). *J. Clin. Invest.* **51**, 3163.

Segre, G. V., Niall, H. D., Habener, J. F., and Potts, J. T., Jr. (1974). *Am. J. Med.* **56,** 774.

Seitz, H., and Jaworski, Z. F. (1964). *Can. Med. Assoc. J.* **90**, 414.

Seyberth, H. W., Segre, G. V., Hamet, P., Sweetman, B. H., Potts, J. T., Jr., and Oates, J. A. (1976). *Trans. Assoc. Am. Physicians* **89**, 92.

Shai, F., Baker, R. K., Addrizzo, J. R., and Wallach, S. (1972). *Endocrinology* **34**, 251.

Sherwood, L. M., and Abe, M. (1972). *J. Clin. Invest.* **51**, 88a.

Sherwood, L. M., Potts, J. T., Jr., Care, A. D., Mayer, G. P., and Aurbach, G. D. (1966). *Nature (London)* **209**, 52.

Sherwood, L. M., Mayer, G. P., Ramberg, C. F., Kronfeld, D. S., Aurbach, G. D., and Potts, J. T., Jr. (1968). *Endocrinology* **83**, 1043.

Sherwood, L. M., Rodman, J. S., and Lundberg, W. B. (1970). *Proc. Natl. Acad. Sci. U.S.A.* **67**, 1631.

Shieber, W., Birge, S. J., Avioli, L., and Teitelbaum, S. L. (1971). *Arch. Surg. (Chicago)* **103**, 299.

Shils, M. E. (1969). *Medicine (Baltimore)* **48**, 61.

Siltzbach, L. E., James, D. G., Neville, E., Turiaf, J., Battesti, J. P., Sharma, O. P., Hosoda, Y., Mikami, R., and Odaka, M. (1974). *Am. J. Med.* **57**, 847.

Silverman, R., and Yalow, R. S. (1973). *J. Clin. Invest.* **52**, 1958.

Silverman, S., Gordan, G., Grant, T., Steinbach, H., Eisenberg, E., and Manson, R. (1962). *Oral Surg., Oral Med., Oral Pathol.* **15**, 426.

Singer, F. R., Segre, G. V., Habener, J. F., and Potts, J. T., Jr. (1975). *Metab., Clin. Exp.* **24**, 139.

Sipple, J. H. (1961). *Am. J. Med.* **31**, 163.

Slatopolsky, E., Caglar, S., Pennell, J. P., Taggart, D. D. Canterbury, J. M., Reiss, E., and Bricker, N. S. (1971). *J. Clin. Invest.* **50**, 492.

Snodgrass, P. J. (1974). "Harrison's Principles of Internal Medicine," p. 1568. 7th ed. M. M. Wintrobe *et al.*, eds. McGraw-Hill, New York.

Solomon, R. B., and Channick, B. J. (1960). *Ann. Intern. Med.* **53**, 1232.

Steendijk, R. (1971). *Clin. Orthop. Relat. Res.,* **77**, 247.

Steinbach, H. L., Gordan, G. S., Eisenberg, E., Crane, J. T., Silverman, S., and Goldman, L. (1961). *Am. J. Roentgenol., Radium Ther. Nucl. Med.* [N. S.] **86**, 329.

Steiner, A. L., Goodman, A. D., and Powers, S. R. (1968). *Medicine (Baltimore)* **47**, 371.

Stevens, A. C., and Jackson, C. E. (1967). *Am. J. Roentgenol., Radium Ther. Nucl. Med.* [N. S.] **99**, 222.

Stote, R. M., Smith, L. H., Wilson, D. M., Dube, W. J., Goldsmith, R. S., and Arnaud, C. D. (1972). *Ann. Intern. Med.* **77**, 587.

Strott, C. A., and Nugent, C. A. (1968). *Ann. Intern. Med.* **68**, 188.

Suh, S. M., Tashjian, A. H., Matsuo, N., Parkinson, D. K., and Fraser, D. (1973). *J. Clin. Invest.* **52**, 153.

Sutton, R. A. L. (1970). *Br. Med. J.* **1**, 529.

Talmage, R. V., and Elliott, J. R. (1956). *Endocrinology* **59**, 27.

Talmage, R. V., and Elliott, J. R. (1958). *Fed. Proc., Fed. Am. Soc. Exp. Biol.* **17**, 160 (abstr.).

Talmage, R. V., Kraintz, F. W., and Buchanan, G. D. (1955). *Proc. Soc. Exp. Biol. Med.* **88**, 600.

Tanaka, Y., Frank, H., and DeLuca, H. F. (1973). *Science* **181**, 564.

Targovnik, J. H., Rodman, J. S., and Sherwood, L. M. (1971). *Endocrinology* **88**, 1477.

Taylor, R. L., Lynch, H. J., Jr., and Wysor, W. G., Jr. (1963). *Am. J. Med.* **34**, 221.

Templeton, A. W., Jaconette, J. R., Jr., and Ormond, R. S. (1962). *Radiology* **78**, 955.

Tepper, L. B., Hardy, H. L., and Chamberlain, R. I. (1961). *In* "Toxicity of Beryllium Compounds" (E. Browning, ed.), p. 63. Elsevier, Amsterdam.

Thorén, L., and Werner, I. (1969). *Acta Chir. Scand.* **135**, 395.

Toverud, S. U., and Munson, P. L. (1965). *Ann. N.Y. Acad. Sci.* **64**, 336.

Tregear, G. W., van Rietschoten, J., Greene, E., Keutmann, H. T., Niall, H. D., Reit, B., Parsons, J. A., and Potts, J. T., Jr. (1973). *Endocrinology* **93**, 1349.

Trudeau, W. L., and McGuigan, J. E. (1969). *N. Engl. J. Med.* **281**, 862.

U.S. Public Health Service (1960). "U.S. National Health Survey: Peptic Ulcers Reported in Interviews." USPHS, Washington, D.C.

U.S. Public Health Service (1964). U.S. National Center for Health Statistics: "Heart Disease in Adults: United States 1960–62," PHS Publ. No. 1000, Ser. 11, No. 6. USPHS, Washington, D.C.

Vaes, G. (1968). *Nature (London).* **219**, 939.

Valvassori, G. E., and Pierce, R. H. (1964). *Radiology* **82**, 385.

Vance, J. E., Stoll, R. W., Kitabchi, A. E., Williams, R. H., and Wood, F. C., Jr. (1969). *J. Am. Med. Assoc.* **207**, 1679.

van der Sluys Veer, J., Birkenhäger, J. C., and Smeenk, D. (1965). *Ned. Tijdschr. Geneeskd.* **109**, 1795.

Verbanck, M. (1965). *Acta Clin. Belg., Suppl.* **1**:1–130.

Vicale, C. T. (1949). *Trans. Am. Neurol. Assoc.* **74**, 143.

Wacjner, G. (1965). *Bibl. Gastroenterol.* **7**, 179.

Walser, M. (1961). *J. Clin. Invest.* **40**, 723.

Walser, M., Robinson, B. H. B., and Duckett, J. W. (1963). *J. Clin. Invest.* **42**, 456.

Walsh, D. A., and Ashby, C. D. (1973). *Recent. Prog. Horm. Res.* **29**, 329.

Wang, C. A. (1971). *Adv. Surg.* **5**, 109.

Wang, C. A. (1976). *Ann. Surg.* **183**, 271.

Wang, C. A., and Cope, O. (1977). *In* "Rhoad's Textbook of Surgery: Principles and Practice" (J. D. Hardy, ed.). Lippincott, Philadelphia, Pennsylvania, p. 727.

Wang, C. A., Miller, L. M., Weber, A. L., and Krane, S. M. (1969). *Am. J. Surg.* **117**, 558.

Wang, C. A., Potts, J. T., Jr., and Neer, R. M. (1975). *In* "Calcium-Regulating Hormones" (R. V. Talmage, M. Owen, and J. A. Parsons, eds.), Int. Congr. Ser. No. 346, p. 82. Elsevier, Amsterdam.

Ward, J. T., Adesola, A. A., and Welbourn, R. B. (1964). *Gut* **5**, 173.

Warshaw, A. L., Heizer, W. D., and Laster, L. (1968). *Ann. Intern. Med.* **68,** 161.

Watson, L. (1974). *Clinics Endocrinol. Metab.* **3,** 215.

Weichert, R. F., III (1970). *Am. J. Med.* **49,** 232.

Wermer, P. (1954). *Am. J. Med.* **16,** 363.

Wesson, L. G., Jr., and Lauler, P. D. (1959). *Proc. Soc. Exp. Biol. Med.* **101,** 235.

Wilder, R. M. (1929). *Endocrinology* **13,** 231.

Wilder, W. T., Frame, B., and Haubrich, W. S. (1961). *Ann. Intern. Med.* **55,** 885.

Williams, E. D. (1966). *J. Clin. Pathol.* **19,** 114.

Wills, M. R. (1971). *Lancet* **1,** 849.

Wills, M. R., and McGowan, G. K. (1964). *Br. Med. J.* **1,** 1153.

Wills, M. R., Pak, C. Y. C., Hammond, W. G., and Bartter, F. C. (1969). *Am. J. Med.* **47,** 384.

Wilson, R. E., Bernhard, W. F., Polet, H., and Moore, F. D. (1964). *Ann. Surg.* **159,** 79.

Wiltse, H. E., Goldbloom, R. B., Antia, A. U., Ottesen, O. E., Rowe, R. D., and Cooke, R. E. (1966). *N. Engl. J. Med.* **275,** 1157.

Winickoff, R., and Aurbach, G. D. (1970). *Program, 52nd Annu. Meet., Am. Endocr. Soc., June 1970.* Abstract No. 17, p. 45.

Winnacker, J. L., Becker, K. L., and Katz, S. (1968). *N. Engl. J. Med.* **278,** 427.

Winters, J. L., Kleinschmidt, A. G., Jr., Frensilli, J. J., and Sutton, M. (1966). *J. Bone Joint Surg.* **48,** 1182.

Wong, E. T., and Lindall, A. W. (1973). *Proc. Natl. Acad. Sci. U.S.A.* **70,** 2291.

Wong, G. L., and Cohn, D. V. (1975). *Proc. Natl. Acad. Sci. U.S.A.* **72,** 3167.

Woodhead, J. S., O'Riordan, J. L. H., Keutmann, H. T., Stoltz, M. L., Dawson, B. F., Niall, H. D., Robinson, C. J., and Potts, J. T., Jr. (1971). *Biochemistry* **10,** 2887.

Yendt, E. R., and Gagné, R. J. A. (1968). *Can. Med. Assoc. J.* **98,** 331.

Yendt, E. R., Gagné, R. J. A., and Cohanim, M. (1966). *Am. J. Med. Sci.* **251,** 449.

Zimmerman, H. B. (1962). *Am. J. Roentgenol., Radium Ther. Nucl. Med.* [N. S.] **88,** 1152.

Zitnan, D., and Sitaj, S. (1958). *Bratisl. Lek. Listy* **28,** 217.

Zollinger, R. M., and Ellison, E. H. (1955). *Ann. Surg.* **142,** 709.

Zull, J. E., and Repke, D. W. (1972). *J. Biol. Chem.* **247,** 2183.

2

Renal Osteodystrophy

LOUIS V. AVIOLI

I. Introduction 149
II. Pathogenesis of Renal Osteodystrophy 151
    A. Malabsorption of Calcium 151
    B. Alterations in Vitamin D Metabolism 153
    C. Secondary Hyperparathyroidism 160
    D. Acidosis 165
III. Clinical and Radiological Correlates 166
IV. Soft Tissue Calcification 177
V. Dialysis Bone Disease 183
VI. The Nature of the Bone Lesions 187
    A. Histological Manifestations 187
    B. Biochemical Defects 191
VII. Therapeutic Management 195
    A. Dietary Factors 195
    B. Vitamin D 197
    C. Vitamin D Metabolites and Synthetic Analogues 198
    D. Parathyroidectomy 201
    E. Transplantation 203
References 205

I. INTRODUCTION

Chronic renal failure is characterized by profound alterations in the orderly biochemical and physiological sequelae that normally condition cellular integrity and metabolic homeostasis. A multiplicity of factors including retained "uremic toxins" contributes to the metabolic and hormonal imbalances. The kidney is an important site of degradation of many

Copyright © 1978 by Academic Press, Inc.
All rights of reproduction in any form reserved
ISBN 0-12-068702-X

polypeptide hormones, including insulin (Rubenstein and Spitz, 1968), glucagon (Nahara and Williams, 1957), and oxytocin and vasopressin (Walter and Bowman, 1973). Basal levels of plasma aldosterone (Walter and Cooke, 1973; Read *et al.*, 1973) and growth hormone (Samaan and Freeman, 1970; Wright *et al.*, 1968) are increased while those of somatomedin, Lewy and New, 1975; Schwalbe *et al.*, 1977), testosterone (Lim and Fang, 1975), and thyroid hormone (Silverberg *et al.*, 1973) may be decreased. Although serum free cortisol levels are usually normal, the plasma half-life of this steroid is prolonged in uremia and its secretion episodic (Bacon *et al.*, 1973; Mishkin *et al.*, 1972). These acquired alterations in hormonal degradation and secretion, together with defective cellular responsivity to hormone stimulation, ultimately result in growth disturbances (Lewy and New, 1975) and derangements in electrolyte, acid–base, lipid, and carbohydrate metabolism (DeFronzo *et al.*, 1973; Bilbrey *et al.*, 1974). The kidney functions as a biological filter for potentially toxic metabolic waste products and also serves as a pivotal control system of extracellular electrolyte water and acid–base metabolism. In addition to this important role of controlling the "sea within us," the kidney serves to regulate mineral and skeletal metabolism via a complex tubular system, which normally reabsorbs over 95% of the filtered calcium and facilitates the excretion of 85–95% of the filtered inorganic phosphorus (see Chapter 2, Volume I). In addition to its excretory role, the kidney also serves to metabolically inactivate parathyroid hormone and calcitonin and to condition the enzymatic formation of 1,25-dihydroxycholecalciferol [$1,25\text{-}(OH)_2D_3$], the most potent biologically active metabolite of vitamin D.

In 1883, R. C. Lucas of Guy's Hospital first described "rickets" in adolescents with chronic renal disease. It subsequently has been demonstrated repeatedly that chronic renal failure is attended by an acquired impairment of intestinal calcium absorption, secondary hyperparathyroidism, and defective maturation of both osteoid and mineral moieties of skeletal tissue. Although some of these derangements in mineral metabolism are occasionally reversed temporarily by chronic hemodialysis, they are usually refractory to dialytic therapy and may actually progress in an accelerated fashion during treatment. Disordered mineral metabolism in renal failure results in osteopenia (See Chapter 6, Volume I), fracture, ectopic calcification, and sustained hyperparathyroidism, all of which present a frustrating therapeutic challenge. So-called "renal osteodystrophy" subsequently becomes resistant to vitamin D therapy in that the requirement of the vitamin to produce an effective sustained biological response is increased when compared to dosages used in other nonuremic malabsorptive, rachitic or osteomalacic disorders.

II. PATHOGENESIS OF RENAL OSTEODYSTROPHY

A. Malabsorption of Calcium

Chronic renal failure is characterized by a marked impairment in the intestinal absorption of calcium (Ca) (Genuth *et al.*, 1969; Liu and Chu, 1943; Coburn *et al.*, 1973; Parker *et al.*, 1974; Brickman *et al.*, 1974c; Ogg, 1968; Recker and Saville, 1971; Charnard *et al.*, 1974). Patients with end-stage renal failure are also unable to adapt to alterations in dietary Ca and, as a consequence, develop large fecal Ca losses during periods of malnutrition or compromised Ca intake as may occur with low-protein dietary regimens (Coburn *et al.*, 1973; Parker *et al.*, 1974) (Fig. 1). Alterations in Ca absorption are ususaly detectable when serum creatinine values are greater than 2.5 ml/100 ml (Coburn *et al.*, 1973), although an inverse correlation between the blood urea nitrogen (BUN) level and Ca absorption has been reported for patients with BUN levels between 25 and 150 mg/100 ml (Recker and Saville, 1971). The intestinal defect in Ca absorption appears restricted to those vitamin D-dependent active or carrier-mediated Ca transport sites in the duodenal and upper jejunum (Parker *et al.*, 1974; Brickman *et al.*, 1974c), which also serve to mediate

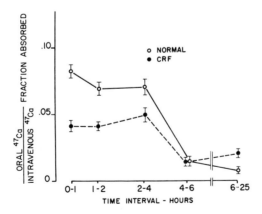

Fig. 1. Fraction of ^{47}Ca absorbed at successive time intervals in normal subjects ($n = 31$) and in patients with stable chronic renal failure ($n = 30$). ^{47}Ca was administered with 200 mg of stable calcium carrier as the gluconate salt to fasting subjects. Results are expressed as mean ± 1 S.E. (From Brickman *et al.*, 1974c.)

the intestinal adaptation to diets deficient in calcium (Avioli, 1972). More distal non-vitamin D-dependent sites where calcium absorption is primarily passive (Avioli, 1972) are apparently functionally intact (Brickman *et al.*, 1974c), since uremic patients can absorb Ca normally when dietary calcium intake is augmented to 4–10 gm/day (Clarkson *et al.*, 1966, 1973), and a direct relation obtains between calcium balance (i.e., retained calcium) and calcium intake (Kopple and Coburn, 1973). The intestinal malabsorption of Ca observed in patients with end-stage renal disease is resistant to vitamin D therapy (Liu and Chu, 1943; Dent *et al.*, 1961) unaltered by chronic intermittent hemodialysis (Genuth *et al.*, 1969; Brickman *et al.*, 1974a, 1974b; Messener *et al.*, 1969), and ultimately unrelated to the skeletal pathology, since the progression of the osteodystrophic bone lesions is not attended by further deterioration of the intestinal absorption of calcium (Ogg, 1968).

The specific pathogenesis and exact nature of the intestinal Ca transport defect in the chronic uremic state is still uncertain. There is mounting evidence that renal insufficiency not only directly affects cellular Ca transport parameters (Gonick *et al.*, 1974; Ritz, 1970; Kessner and Epstein, 1965; Baerg *et al.*, 1970; McDermott *et al.*, 1974), but also results in derangements in vitamin D metabolism with defective production of 1,25-$(OH)_2D_3$ (Brumbaugh *et al.*, 1974; Avioli *et al.*, 1968; Piel *et al.*, 1973) (see Chapter 5, Volume I). Since 1,25-$(OH)_2D_3$ functions primarily to regulate intestinal absorption of calcium, acquired alterations in its production by the diseased kidney obviously play a major role in initiating and perpetuating the intestinal malabsorption of Ca. In this regard it should be emphasized that Ca absorption can be reduced even further when uremic patients are subjected to nephrectomy (Oettinger *et al.*, 1974). The specific intestinal transport defect resulting from defective renal production of 1,25-$(OH)_2D_3$ in uremic man is still virtually unknown since vitamin D-activated intestinal ATPase (Avioli, 1972; Kowarski and Schachter, 1973) and mitochondrial (Avioli, 1972; Russell and Avioli, 1974) activities as well as intestinal cellular proliferation (McDermott *et al.*, 1974; Birge and Alpers, 1973) and calcium-binding protein synthesis (Avioli, 1972; Avioli *et al.*, 1969b; Helmke *et al.*, 1974; Piazolo *et al.*, 1972) are all reportedly defective in the chronic uremic state. Moreover, reports of raised serum calcitonin levels in patients with chronic renal failure (Heynen and Franchimont, 1974) and calcitonin inhibition of vitamin D-induced intestinal calcium absorption (Olson *et al.*, 1972) should also be considered.

Derangements in protein, amino acid, and mitochondrial metabolism and ATPase activity in non-vitamin D-dependent tissues have been well established in the chronic uremic state and attributed to one or more retained uremic toxins (Avioli, 1972; Shear, 1969; Schreiner, 1975; Scribner and Babb, 1975; Olsen and Bassett, 1951). The possibility obtains, therefore, that uremic toxins per se may impose certain conditioned alterations in the established orderly sequence of intestinal cell multiplication, maturation, and in the translational and transcriptional processes normally regulating intestinal protein synthesis. Synthesized proteins could possibly be structurally or catalytically unable to effect the translocation of Ca^{2+} across the intestinal cell. That vitamin responsiveness and metabolism is probably unaltered early in the course of uremia is reflected in reports of normal intestinal Ca absorption in patients with serum creatinine less than 2.5 mg/100 ml (Coburn et al., 1973) and other reports citing the cure of the bone lesions of patients with early renal failure by treatment with vitamin D alone in doses similar to those used to cure nutritional rickets (Stanbury et al., 1969). As the uremic state advances, each of the aforementioned non-vitamin D-related derangements in Ca^{2+} transport and net intestinal absorption could obtain albeit with varying degrees of severity. Increments in intestinal luminal K^+ concentrations in uremic patients with secondary hyperaldosteronism would further compromise calcium absorption since K^+ does interfere with Ca^{2+} transport (Schachter, 1963). With progressive decrease in functioning renal mass, the additional insult imposed by decreased $1,25-(OH)_2D_3$ production must obviously contribute to the intestinal malabsorption of calcium and observed "resistance" to vitamin D therapy. Regardless of the cause, the calcium malabsorption attending the clinical course of patients with chronic renal failure, especially those with restricted dietary intakes, adds another insult to calcium homeostasis by providing an additional stimulus to parathyroid hyperplasia, elevated circulating parathyroid hormone levels, and progressive skeletal demineralization.

B. Alterations in Vitamin D Metabolism

It has been demonstrated with biological assay techniques that vitamin D activity (i.e., anti-rachitic activity) in the serum of untreated patients with chronic uremia is lower than that observed in either a well-fed healthy population or in malnourished individuals with terminal cachexia (Lumb et al., 1971; Ritz and Jantzen, 1969). In addition, patients with acute, rapidly progressive (Bell and Bartter, 1964) or terminal uremia (Lumb et al., 1971) require a greater intake of vitamin D and higher levels of assayable anti-rachitic activity for biological effectiveness than do normal individuals. This well-recognized phenomenon of vitamin D resistance in renal failure has been variably attributed to uremic toxins interfering with the normal production of the biologically active 1,25-

(OH)$_2$D$_3$ vitamin D$_3$ metabolite, or to the response of the end organs (i.e., bone and intestine) to these metabolites. Following the hepatic conversion of vitamin D$_3$ to 25-OHD$_3$ (see Chapter 5, Volume I), this metabolite is deposited in adipose tissue and muscle. 25-OHD$_3$, which circulates with a biological half-life of 12 days (Haddad and Rojanasathit, 1976), is also further hydroxylated by the kidney to either 1,25-dihydroxycholecalciferol [1,25-(OH)$_2$D$_3$] or 24,25-dihydroxycholecalciferol [24,25-(OH)$_2$D$_3$] by a carbon monoxide sensitive mitochondrial system requiring reduced pyridine nucleotide and molecular oxygen for maximal activity (Ghazarian and DeLuca, 1974; Henry and Norman, 1974).

A number of observations made either in intact animals or from renal homogenates, isolated renal mitochondria, or proximal tubular preparation are consistent with the view that the control of 1,25-(OH)$_2$D$_3$ production by the kidney is indeed complex with intracellular concentrations of calcium, inorganic phosphate, cyclic AMP, as well as parathyroid hormone, prolactin, calcitonin, and pH all functioning as controlling factors (Fraser and Kodicek, 1973; Bikle and Rasmussen, 1974, 1975; Spanos *et al.*, 1976; Lee *et al.*, 1977; Bikle *et al.*, 1975; Tanaka *et al.*, 1973). Preliminary observations are consistent with the view that the conversion of 25-OHD$_3$ to either 1,25-(OH)$_2$D$_3$ or 24,25-(OH)$_2$D$_3$ is regulated by a sensitive servo-control mechanism modulated by circulating calcium, parathyroid hormone, calcitonin, and the inorganic phosphate content of renal cortical cells. A theory coordinating some of these varied experimental observations would hold that hypocalcemia acts as a stimulus for parathyroid hormone secretion; the latter, either directly or by depleting renal cortical inorganic phosphate concentration (or both) (Gray *et al.*, 1977), stimulates the hydroxylation of 25-OHD$_3$ to 1,25-(OH)$_2$D$_3$, which in turn completes the negative feedback loop of hormonal control by stimulating the intestinal absorption and bone resorption of calcium (Fig. 2). As a consequence, the circulating ionized calcium level is raised to normal and parathyroid hormone secretion returns to the basal state. On the other hand, hypercalcemia, while decreasing the rate of parathyroid hormone release, also stimulates calcitonin release from the parafollicular cells of the thyroid gland. In accordance with this unified homeostatic hypothesis, a rise in circulating calcitonin levels, either directly or indirectly by increasing renal cortical inorganic phosphate concentration (or both), results in a suppression of 1,25-(OH)$_2$D$_3$ production, a decrease in both bone resorption and intestinal calcium absorption, a return of the ionized calcium to normal, and a gradual reduction in calcitonin secretion by the thyroid gland.

Although this theory is attractive and supported by a number of observations, it must still be entertained with moderation, since there are

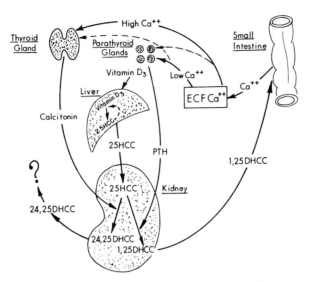

Fig. 2. Proposed interrelationship between vitamin D_3 and its metabolites (25-hydroxycholecalciferol) (25-HCC), 1,25-dihydroxycholecalciferol (1,25-DHCC), 24,25-dihydroxycholecalciferol (24,25-DHCC), parathyroid hormone (PTH), calcitonin, and calcium homeostasis. Dotted lines represent inhibition of either calcitonin or parathyroid hormone release by hypocalcemia and hypercalcemia, respectively, and the substrate (25-HCC) inhibition of enzymatic hydroxylation in the liver. (Reproduced from Metabolism 22:507, 1973, with permission of the authors and publishers.

additional observations supporting the thesis that parathyroid hormone in high concentrations not only *suppresses* the renal conversion of 25-OHD$_3$ to 1,25-(OH)$_2$D$_3$ but also enhances the conversion of 25-OHD$_3$ to 24,25-(OH)$_2$D$_3$ (Galante *et al.,* 1972). In addition, in studies with cell-free suspension of biologically active renal tubules, parathyroid hormone and extracellular calcium ion concentration were observed to exert no regulatory effect upon either the renal tubular consumption of 25-OHD$_3$ or production of 1,25-(OH)$_2$D$_3$ (Shain, 1972). It has also been demonstrated that 1,25-(OH)$_2$D$_3$ also plays an integral role in the renal metabolism of 25-OHD$_3$, since 1,25-(OH)$_2$D$_3$ administration to animals reduces the renal production of 1,25-(OH)$_2$D$_3$ and stimulates the production of 24,25-(OH)$_2$D$_3$ (Tanaka and DeLuca, 1974a). In contrast, 24,25-(OH)$_2$D$_3$ appears to exert no effect on the conversion of 25-OHD$_3$ to 1,25-(OH)$_2$D$_3$. 24,25-(OH)$_2$D$_3$ is also formed in extrarenal tissue since circulating levels are relatively normal in anephric subjects (Haddad *et al.,* 1977). 1,25-(OH)$_2$D$_3$ once synthesized by the kidney is also degraded to a metabolite with unknown biological activity (Kumar *et al.,* 1976). 24,25-(OH)$_2$D$_3$ is also further metabolized by the kidney to 1,24,25-trihydroxy-vitamin D$_3$

[1,24,25-(OH)$_3$D$_3$] (Fig. 3) (Kleiner-Bossaller and DeLuca, 1974). Evidence has also been produced demonstrating the formation of 1,24,25-(OH)$_3$D$_3$ from either 25-OHD$_3$ or 1,25-(OH)$_2$D$_3$. 1,24,25-(OH)$_3$D$_3$ is reportedly 60% as active as vitamin D$_3$ in curing rickets in animals and is less active on a weight basis than 1,25-(OH)$_2$D$_3$ in stimulating and sustaining the intestinal absorption of calcium and bone resorption (Holick *et al.,* 1973a). Presently, 1,24,25-(OH)$_2$D$_3$ is considered to exert its biological activity preferentially on promoting the intestinal absorption of calcium.

1,25-(OH)$_2$D [i.e., 1,25-(OH)$_2$D$_2$ + 1,25-(OH)$_2$D$_3$] normally circulates with a biological half-life of 24 hours at concentrations of 25 to 33 pg/ml in adults and 49-66 pg/ml in children (Brumbaugh *et al.,* 1974; Haussler *et al.,* 1976; Eisman *et al.,* 1976). This vitamin D$_3$ derivative is "the" metabolic or hormonal form of vitamin D$_3$ that controls the intestinal transport of calcium, since it is some 4 to 13 times as effective as vitamin D$_3$ and over twice as effective as 25-OHD$_3$ in this regard (Avioli and Haddad, 1973). Unlike 25-OHD$_3$, 1,25-(OH)$_2$D$_3$ has a minimal effect on the renal tubular reabsorption of phosphate (Editorial, 1974) and directly

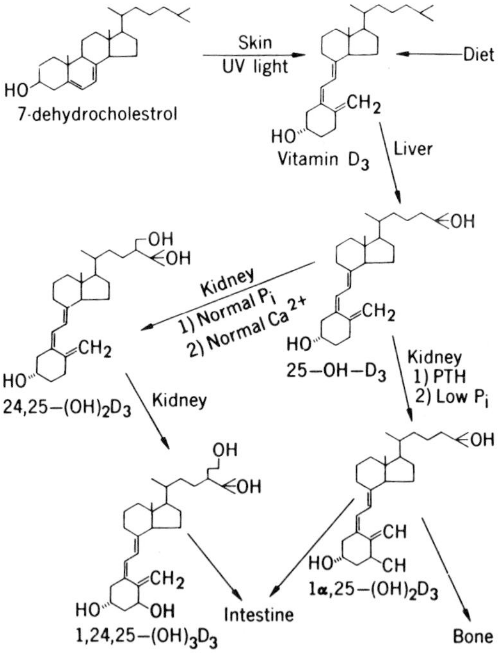

Fig. 3. Schematic representation of the effect of calcium (Ca^{2+}), inorganic phosphate (P$_i$), and parathyroid hormone (PTH) on the metabolism of 25-hydroxycholecalciferol (25-OHD$_3$). (Submitted by H. F. DeLuca.)

stimulates jejunal phosphate absorption (Chen *et al.*, 1974; Tanaka and DeLuca, 1974b). 1,25-$(OH)_2D_3$ also possesses significant bone resorptive properties with an *in vitro* effectiveness some 100 times that of the parent 25-$(OH)D_3$ (Raisz *et al.*, 1972a). The preferential accumulation of 1,25-$(OH)_2D_3$ in the nucleus of bone cells and the subcellular skeletal distribution pattern of other vitamin D_3 metabolites suggest a mechanism of 1,25-$(OH)_2D_3$ action in bone similar to that proposed for the control of calcium translocation across the intestinal cell.

The manner in which 1,25-$(OH)_2D_3$ exerts control over the biomolecular events that precede and condition the intestinal absorption of calcium is still uncertain. Preliminary observations suggest that the diol or triol metabolites are initially bound to specific cytosol proteins prior to their incorporation into nuclear receptor sites, where they ultimately effect either the transcriptional processes directly or regulate the release or transport of nuclear-derived RNA (Brumbaugh and Haussler, 1973, 1974; Chen and DeLuca, 1973). Alternatively, it has been shown that 1,25-$(OH)_2D_3$ acts in the intestine by a process that does not involve the retrieval of genetic information and that new protein synthesis is only essential for the conversion of 25-OHD_3 to 1,25-$(OH)_2D_3$ by the kidney (Tsai *et al.*, 1973). The fact that *de novo* stimulated protein synthesis may not be essential for the intestinal response to 1,25-$(OH)_2D_3$ does not mitigate against the theory that the action of the vitamin D metabolites on the intestine is mediated ultimately by transport proteins or enzymes. The metabolites may still theoretically function in this regard by activating certain protein precursors within the cell.

1,25-$(OH)_2D_3$ may also be considered a trophic substance for the intestinal mucosa, since vitamin D_3 stimulates intestinal mucosal growth as well as protein synthesis. Since the turnover time of intestinal mucosa is estimated at 30–40 hours, changes in cell size, cell migration rate, and villus size probably make significant contributions to intestinal transport activation. Both DNA synthesis and mucosal cell migration along the villus are significantly accelerated by vitamin D_3 treatment (Birge and Alpers, 1973). A comparison between intestinal epithelial cell turnover and the time course of intestinal localization and action of 1,25-$(OH)_2D_3$ also suggests that both are regulated at a molecular rather than cellular level. By accelerating cell proliferation and migration, vitamin D metabolites may be effectively altering the ratio of mature and undifferentiated cells with respect to the total mucosal cell population. Since the enzyme content of mucosal cells undergoes dramatic evolution with maturation, an acceleration of mucosal cell migration following 1,25-$(OH)_2D_3$ stimulation may result in increased activation of particular proteins or enzymes as well as overall increase in the intestinal absorptive surface. In fact, the observed response of the intestine to $1,25\text{-}(OH)_2D_3$ may reflect the reaction of functionally intact systems to a stimulus and/or nonspecific unrelated increments in both protein synthesis and in the number of intestinal mucosal cells capable of transporting calcium.

Studies with radioactive isotopic forms of vitamin D_3 (Avioli et al., 1968; Piel et al., 1973; Gray et al., 1974) and $25\text{-}OHD_3$ (Piel et al., 1973; Gray et al., 1974; Mawer et al., 1973) in subjects with renal failure, anephric animals (Gray et al., 1971; Hill et al., 1971), and in animals with experimentally induced chronic renal failure (Avioli et al., 1969a, Van Stone et al., 1977), have stressed the loss of renal parenchyma rather than the loss of renal excretory function as the primary cause for the malabsorption of calcium. It appears logical to assume that a reduction in functional renal mass would result in decreased $1,25\text{-}(OH)D_3$ synthesis, and a subsequent reduction in the intestinal mucosa concentration of $1,25\text{-}(OH)_2D_3$. Results demonstrating that small doses of $1,25\text{-}(OH)_2D_3$ augment calcium absorption and raise the serum calcium of uremic man (Henderson et al., 1974a; Brickman et al., 1974a,b) are consistent with this hypothesis, as is the failure of intermittent hemodialysis (Genuth et al., 1969; Brickman et al., 1974a and b) Messener et al., 1969) to reverse the calcium malabsorption and intestinal response to vitamin D. The observation that reduction in intestinal calcium absorption becomes apparent only when glomerular filtration rates reach levels of 25–30 ml/min (Lumb et al., 1971; Schaefer et al., 1968) is also consistent with the hypothesis that calcium malabsorption may result, in part, from defective $1,25\text{-}(OH)_2D_3$ production due to hyperphosphatemia [also progressive when glomerular filtration rates fall below 20–30 ml/min (Goldman et al., 1974)]. Progressive increments in the phosphate concentration of renal cortical cells similar to that reported for muscle phosphate in patients with glomerular filtration rates less than 30 ml/min (Mioni et al., 1973) may possibly suppress the renal mitochondrial hydroxylation of $25\text{-}OHD_3$ to $1,25\text{-}(OH)_2D_3$ (Tanaka et al., 1973).

In addition, alterations in the metabolism of vitamin D or its hydroxylated metabolites may result in the accumulation of structurally related abnormal metabolites (Avioli et al., 1968; Piel et al., 1973; Hartenbower et al., 1977; Gray et al., 1974), which compete with $1,25\text{-}(OH)_2D_3$ for receptor sites in the cytosol or nucleus of specific target organs. Moreover, tissue $1,25\text{-}(OH)_2D_3$ receptor sites may exhibit a relative rather than an absolute specificity for diol and triol vitamin D-related sterols and as such are readily available to $25\text{-}OHD_3$ and vitamin D_3 as well (Brumbaugh and Haussler, 1973, 1974; Tsai and Norman, 1973). Demonstrated in vitro effectiveness of vitamin D (Corradino, 1974) and $25\text{-}OHD_3$ (Olson and DeLuca, 1969) on calcium transport and in vivo intestinal responses to dihydrotachysterol (Kaye and Sagar, 1972; Kaye, 1969), a compound that when hydroxylated by the liver is structurally similar to 1,25-$(OH)_2D_3$ (Fig. 4) (DeLuca, 1973), support this contention. It may also be premature to assume that negative feedback hormonal and ionic control mechanisms for 25-OHD_3 and 1,25-$(OH)_2D_3$ generation by the liver and kidney, respectively, are intact in the uremic subject (Ghazarian *et al.*, 1973; Henry and Norman, 1974; Fraser and Kodicek, 1973; Bikle and Rasmussen, 1974, 1975; Bikle *et al.*, 1975; Tanaka *et al.*, 1973). Although in theory, the attendant hypocalcemia and resultant secondary hyperparathyroidism observed in patients with chronic renal insufficiency should compensate for the decrease in 1,25-$(OH)_2D_3$ production anticipated by the progressive hyperphosphatemia and loss of renal mass, this is obviously not the case since circulating 1,25-$(OH)_2D$ [i.e., 1,25-$(OH)_2D_3$ + 1,25-$(OH)_2D_2$] levels are decreased in uremic patients (Brumbaugh *et al.*, 1974).

When quantitated in untreated uremic patients, plasma 25-OHD_3 levels are normal or low (Offermann *et al.*, 1974; Eastwood *et al.*, 1976; Bayard *et al.*, 1973) and a significant direct correlation observed between osteomalacia calcium and 25-OHD_3 plasma concentrations (Eastwood *et al.*, 1976; Bayard *et al.*, 1973). Since 25-OHD_3 is effective in raising serum calcium in the anephric state (Pavlovitch *et al.*, 1973; Counts *et al.*, 1975), it appears well established that the renal conversion of 25-OHD_3 to 1,25-

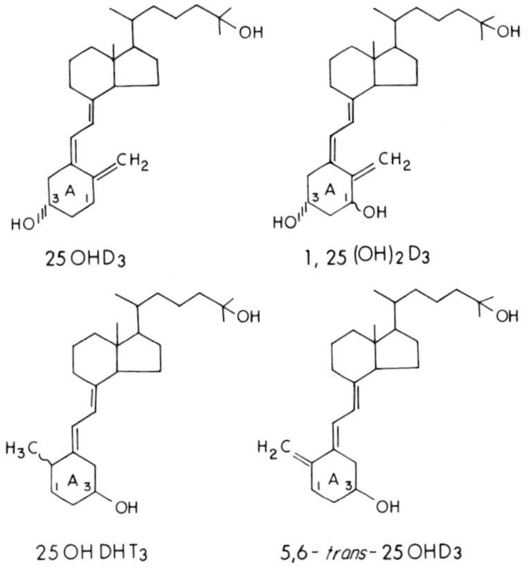

Fig. 4. Structural similarities between 25-hydroxycholecalciferol (25-OHD_3), 1,25-dihydroxycholecalciferol [1,25-(OH_2D_3)], 25-hydroxydihydrotachysterol$_3$, (25-OHDHT$_3$), and 5,6-*trans*-25-hydroxy-cholecalciferol (5,6-*trans*-25-OHD_3).

$(OH)_2D_3$ is not an obligatory step for its biological effect on bone or intestine. In fact, the osteomalacia observed in untreated uremic hypocalcemic patients with hyperphosphatasia (Cochran *et al.*, 1973) may result, at least in part, from the decreased biological availability of $25\text{-}OHD_3$ (Bayard *et al.*, 1973; Eastwood *et al.*, 1976). Although the cause for decreased circulating $25\text{-}OHD_3$ in patients with advanced renal failure has been attributed primarily to poor nutrition and inadequate sunlight exposure, it should be emphasized that the circulating anti-rachitic activity of serum obtained from uremic patients is still lower than that of malnourished sedentary patients with terminal cachexia (Ritz and Jantzen, 1969). The intestinal absorption of vitamin D_3 is normal in uremic patients (Avioli *et al.*, 1968), and circulating $25\text{-}OHD_3$ levels ultimately increase following vitamin D_3 feeding (DeLuca, 1973).

These observations are reminiscent of documented alterations of vitamin D_3 metabolism of individuals on anti-convulsant therapy with low circulating $25\text{-}OHD_3$ levels (Jubiz *et al.*, 1977; Hahn *et al.*, 1972, 1975), an effect attributed to a malfunctioning hepatic microsomal cytochrome *P*-450 enzyme system (Hahn *et al.*, 1974). Such may also be the case in patients with chronic renal failure on normal or marginally low vitamin D intakes since, as reported previously for glutethimide (Greenwood *et al.*, 1973) and Dilantin and phenobarbital (Hahn *et al.*, 1975), hepatic microsomal cytochrome *P*-450 metabolic pathways are also impaired by uremia (Leber and Schutterle, 1972). Finally, one must acknowledge reports that vitamin D metabolites other than $25\text{-}OHD_3$ generated at extrarenal sites are biologically activated by the kidney (Garabedian *et al.*, 1974), and that trace metals that may, in fact, accumulate in either nontreated or dialyzed renal patients (Alfrey and Smythe, 1975) may impair the renal hydroxylation of $25\text{-}OHD_3$ to $1,25\text{-}(OH)_2D_3$ (Feldman and Cousins, 1973).

C. Secondary Hyperparathyroidism

Since the association between renal disease and bone disease was first reported in 1883 (Lucas, 1883), it has been well established that progressive renal failure in both children and adults is attended by elevations in circulating parathyroid hormone (PTH) (Reiss *et al.*, 1969; Berson and Yalow, 1966; Stanbury and Lumb, 1962, 1966; Kaye *et al.*, 1960; Parfitt, 1969a; Roof *et al.*, 1974; Katz *et al.*, 1969). Histological analysis of parathyroid glands obtained from uremic subjects reveals increments in the absolute number of parathyroid cells early in the course of the disease. Subsequently, with further compromise in renal excretory parameters, an increasing number of cells assume the secretory phase of their functional cycle (Thiele *et al.*, 1974; Roth and Marshall, 1969). Thus, not only do the size and number of parathyroid cells increase, but each hyperplastic cell is capable of producing abnormally greater amounts of PTH when stimulated (Parfitt, 1969a). The "secondary hyperparathyroidism" observed in uremic patients can be considered to represent progressive cellular and biomolecular adaptative responses of the parathyroid glands to chronic and sustained stimulations, the most important of which is the tendency toward hypocalcemia. Whether or not the calcium control of PTH release is mediated via alterations in glandular ATP (Dufresne *et al.*, 1972) or specific pepidases (Fischer *et al.*, 1972) is presently uncertain. Eventually the total mass of functioning parathyroid tissue may assume such large proportions that, despite acquired or induced hypercalcemia with levels as high as 12–13 mg/100 ml, PTH secretion continues at an excessive rate (Fig. 5). This relative autonomous secretory state has often been considered to represent a form of "tertiary hyperparathyroidism" (CPC, 1972).

The resultant sustained elevations in circulating PTH not only distorts normal skeletal remodeling and maturational processes (Holtrop *et al.*, 1974; Kaye *et al.*, 1960; Eugenidis *et al.*, 1972; Kalu *et al.*, 1970), but also most probably contributes to the glucose intolerance (Moxley *et al.*, 1974; DeFronzo *et al.*, 1973) and acidosis (Muldowney *et al.*, 1970, 1971, 1972) of uremic patients. Preliminary observations suggest that elevations in plasma PTH may also function to control the anemia of the uremic subject, since PTH acts as a secretagogue for erythropoietin production by the kidney (Rodgers *et al.*, 1974). Although hypocalcemia (or a tendency thereto) is the primary stimulus to parathyroid gland hyperplasia and PTH release (see Chapter 1), elevations in circulating vitamin A levels, which may be quite significant in patients with chronic renal disease (Smith and Goodman, 1971), may ultimately prove contributory in this regard, since vitamin A directly stimulates the glandular release of PTH (Chertow *et al.*, 1974). Moreover, since renal degradation may normally account for 50–60% of the metabolic clearance rate of PTH (Martin *et al.*, 1977; Hruska *et al.*, 1973), progressive loss of functioning renal tissue must also contribute to the sustained elevations in plasma PTH.

Since both vitamin D-dependent and vitamin D-independent intestinal calcium absorption is impaired in uremia (Avioli, 1972), the resultant propensity toward hypocalcemia obviously contributes to parathyroid overactivity characteristic of uremic patients. However, intestinal dysfunction cannot account for the elevations of plasma PTH of patients with early renal failure (Reiss *et al.*, 1969) (Fig. 6), since the intestinal absorption of calcium is reportedly normal in uremic patients with serum

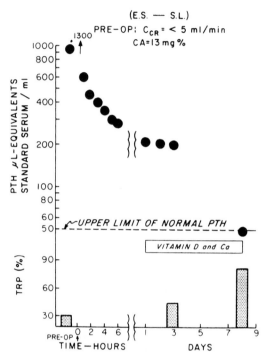

Fig. 5. Autonomous renal "tertiary hyperparathyroidism" in a patient with a creatinine clearance (C_{cr}) less than 5 ml/min and hypercalcemia. Note that despite a serum calcium of 13 mg%, circulating parathyroid hormone values are approximately *26 times* normal values and the tubular resorption of phosphate (%TRP) less than 30. PTH levels decreased following subtotal parathyroid surgery and plateaued at levels *4 times* normal. At this time appropriate therapy with vitamin D and calcium (Ca) resulted in a suppression of PTH to normal and a subsequent rise in %TRP. (From Reiss *et al.*, 1969. With the permission of the authors and publisher).

creatinine levels less than 2.5 mg/100 ml (Coburn *et al.*, 1973) or with glomerular filtration rates greater than 25–30 ml/min (Lumb *et al.*, 1971; Schaefer *et al.*, 1968).

Bricker (1972) and associates, in advocating the "trade off hypothesis" concept, have accumulated considerable data in defense of their premise that the secondary hyperparathyroidism seen in early renal failure reflects an adaptation of the biological control system governing the maintenance of external phosphorus balance (Slatopolsky *et al.*, 1971, 1972; Reiss *et al.*, 1970). Dietary phosphorus intake usually averages 800–900 mg/day and the efficiency of phosphate absorption by the intestine is a function of the dietary intake with 60–70% absorbed on a normal intake and maximal absorption (up to 90%) achieved on very low intakes (see Chapter 2 Volume

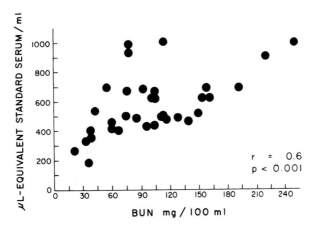

Fig. 6. The relationship between circulating parathyroid hormone (expressed as μl equivalents on the ordinate) and blood urea nitrogen (BUN). The correlation is direct with $p <$ 0.001. Normal values of PTH are less than 50 in this assay system (see Fig. 5). Note the significant elevations in PTH in patients with BUN values between 15 and 45 mg/100 ml. (From Reiss and Canterbury, 1970. With the permission of the authors and publisher.)

I). Unlike the well-documented control of calcium absorption described earlier, there is no known effective physiological mechanism governing the intestinal absorption of phosphate, although 1,25-(OH)$_2$D$_3$ may be effective in this regard (Editorial, 1974; Chen *et al.*, 1974; Brickman *et al.*, 1977; Tanaka and DeLuca, 1974a). The control of phosphate economy in man is achieved primarily by variation in renal excretion with parathyroid hormone playing a major regulatory role (Knox *et al.*, 1973). It is reasoned that in the early stages of renal failure, patients on unrestricted phosphate intakes tend toward hyperphosphatemia, the latter, in turn, effecting a transient fall in the ionized calcium and a stimulated release of PTH. The subsequent rise in circulating PTH promotes a greater degree of phosphaturia by the remaining intact nephrons, and a normalization of circulating phosphate levels (Bricker, 1972; Slatopolsky *et al.*, 1971). According to this hypothesis, secondary hyperparathyroidism evolves early in the course of uremia as nephrons are progressively lost in order to permit residual nephrons to maintain normophosphatemia. Direct correlations noted between circulation of PTH and inorganic phosphate in uremic patients (Fig. 7) are consistent with this hypothesis.

A necessary corollary to this hypothesis is that the greater the rate of phosphate excretion per nephrons required (as may be the case in individuals on high protein diets), the greater the degree of secondary hyperparathyroidism. The intestinal absorption of phosphate is slightly lower in uremic patients than in individuals with normal renal function (Liu and

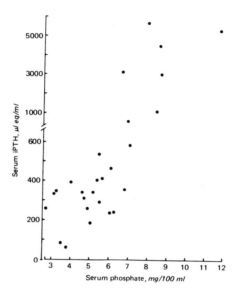

Fig. 7. Relationship between parathyroid hormone (PTH) and inorganic phosphate in patients with renal failure. (From Bordier *et al.*, 1975. With the permission of the authors and publisher.)

Chu, 1943; Kopple and Coburn, 1973; Sherman *et al.*, 1918) for reasons that are poorly understood, although elevations in circulating calcitonin observed in end-stage renal disease (Heynen and Franchimont, 1974) may be contributory (Tanzer and Navia, 1973). Despite a tendency toward phosphate malabsorption, uremic patients do absorb a significant amount of dietary phosphate and in fact develop hyperphosphatemia when glomerular filtration rates fall below 25–30 ml/min (Goldman *et al.*, 1954). At this level of renal dysfunction, the remaining functioning viable nephrons are unable to maintain normophosphatemia despite circulating PTH levels 10–20 times normal. The relationship between dietary phosphate and excessive parathyroid hormone is again illustrated by a form of nutritional secondary hyperparathyroidism that develops in horses fed rations containing an excess of phosphorus in proportion to the amount of calcium (Joyce *et al.*, 1971), and the demonstration by Reiss *et al.* (1970) that oral phosphorus administration initiates a highly sensitive calcium-mediated stimulus for PTH secretion in normal individuals. Although serum inorganic phosphate may be a major determinant of the degree of secondary hyperparathyroidism, other factors appear essential, since there is also evidence that parathyroid hormone may not be required for phosphate homeostasis in renal failure (Swenson *et al.*, 1975; Popovtzer *et al.*, 1972).

D. Acidosis

In 1965, Goodman *et al.* noted that, despite stable plasma bicarbonate levels, patients with chronic renal acidosis excreted less acid in their urine than could be accounted for by established intrarenal metabolic buffering processes. They suggested that bone acted as a buffer via the gradual dissolution of alkaline bone salts, stimulated by the extracellular acidosis (Lemann *et al.*, 1965). Subsequently, Lemann *et al.* (1966), utilizing classic metabolic balance techniques during periods of NH_4Cl loading, showed that the negative calcium balance (i.e., -185 mEq) obtained during the period of induced acidosis was consistent with this hypothesis, since 193 mEq of the acid load had not been excreted in the urine despite normal serum bicarbonate levels. They concluded that bone mineral (i.e., calcium) served as an important buffer reservoir in chronic metabolic acidosis. These latter observations were confirmed by Reidenberg *et al.* (1966) in man and by Kaye (1974a) in animals with chronic uremia. The conclusions are also consistent with the demonstration of low carbonate content of bone, obtained from patients with chronic renal failure (Pellegrino and Biltz, 1965; Kaye *et al.*, 1970b) and histological increments in bone resorption of animals with NH_4Cl-induced acidosis (Barzel and Jowsey, 1969) as well as with those reports documenting significant osteopenia in individuals on keotgenic diets (Mazess, 1970). In fact, changes in bone carbonate attending metabolic acidosis are sufficiently large to account for the postulated buffering capacity of bone in uremic acidosis (Burnell, 1971; Lemann *et al.*, 1966; Reidenberg *et al.*, 1966).

Despite the fact that the accumulated data are all consistent with a deleterious effect of acidosis on the integrity of osseous tissue, there is presently no concrete evidence that uremic acidosis leads to a dissolution of bone in a manner similar to that observed when bone is placed in test tubes containing acid solutions. In fact, bone specimens obtained from uremic patients release *less calcium in vitro* when subjected to acidifying solutions (Kaye *et al.*, 1970a). Acidosis decreases renal tubular calcium reabsorption (Lemann *et al.*, 1967), alters collagen turnover (Finlayson *et al.*, 1964), favors hydroxyapatite formation in bone from the less crystalline amorphous calcium phosphate (ACP) precursors (Termine, 1972), and interfere with $1,25(OH)_2D$ production (Lee *et al.*, 1977). In addition to these considerations, it should be noted that when bone turnover is accelerated and bone resorption predominates (as is the case in patients with end-stage renal disease), the conversion of the complex skeletal hydroxyapatite crystal to circulating Ca^{2+} and PO_4^{-3} results in a stoichiometric removal of H^+ from the extracellular fluids (Kildeberg *et al.*, 1969). Thus, accelerated bone destruction per se may in fact serve as a biological buffer for H^+. Finally, all previous observations made in nonuremic subjects or animals relating either dietary (i.e., ketogenic diets) or NH_4Cl-induced osteopenia to increased bone resorption may simply represent the sequence

Acidosis→hypercalciuria→increased PTH release→increase bone resorption

since induced elevations in urinary calcium observed in patients with normal glomerular filtration rates result in elevations in circulating PTH (Wachman and Bernstein, 1970; Coe et al., 1973).

III. CLINICAL AND RADIOLOGICAL CORRELATES

Despite some authors who note no correlation between renal pathology and the type and incidence of the associated osteodystrophy (Hampers et al., 1969; Fournier et al., 1971), patients with chronic pyelonephritis, polycystic kidneys, and obstructive uropathy appear more predisposed to symptomatic skeletal disease than are those with chronic glomerulonephritis or renal vascular disease (Kaye et al., 1960; Ellis and Paert, 1973; Bergdahl and Boquist, 1973). In addition, whereas osteomalacic osteodystrophy is frequent in Europe, it is reportedly less common in the United States (Lumb et al., 1971) and Australia (Ireland et al., 1969). This discrepancy may stem from regional variations in sunlight exposure, dietary habits, and vitamin D supplementation, all of which condition the vitamin D status of individuals (Haddad and Kyung, 1971; Preece et al., 1975; Stamp et al., 1972; Ingham et al., 1973; Arnaud et al., 1977).

The frequency of symptoms referable to the musculoskeletal system in patients with renal failure is variable. Siddiquai and Kerr (1971) and Katz et al. (1969) report incidences of 4% and 10%, respectively, of uremic patients with symptomatic osteodystrophy. Others report greater frequencies of bone pain in chronically uremic patients (Stanbury et al., 1960) with as many as 100% symptomatic after 4 to 5 years of intermittent hemodialysis (Kerr et al., 1969). Although disabling symptoms are rare, many uremic patients are suprisingly stoic to skeletal fractures (Katz et al., 1969). They may in turn experience significant arthralgias, particularly in the knees and shoulders (Kerr et al., 1969), not infrequently associated with pseudogout (Ritz et al., 1971). The perplexing wide variations in the incidence of symptomatic bone disease in the population of patients with end-stage renal disease may be related to longevity and the nature of the pathological process. Certainly those patients who live longer with renal failure are more likely to develop osteodystrophy than those who expire shortly after the diagnosis has been established (O'Riordan et al., 1970; Ingham et al., 1973). Moreover, patients with severe osteomalacia are more likely to have symptomatic bone disease than are those with a predominance of osteitis fibrosa (Ellis and Peart, 1973).

Although many uremic patients with histologically documented bone disease (Katz et al., 1969; Kleeman et al., 1969; Cohen et al., 1970), especially those with a predominance of osteomalacia (Stanbury, 1966; Ingham et al., 1973), have normal skeletal radiographs, there are often correlative roentgenographic changes, particularly associated with moderate and severe osteitis fibrosa (Katz et al., 1969; Cohen et al., 1970; Greenfield, 1972; Stanbury, 1966; DeVeber et al., 1970; Pendras, 1969). Approximately 50% of patients with histological evidence of increased osteoclastic activity demonstrate subperiosteal resorption (Katz et al., 1969; Greenfield, 1972), a radiological sign considered pathognomonic for excess circulating parathyroid hormone (Fig. 8). When detectable, osteitis fibrosa indicates advanced stages of "secondary hyperparathyroidism" since histologically, the extent of osteoclastosis and osteitis fibrosa is a reliable index of the mass of parathyroid tissue (Stanbury et al., 1969; Ellis and Peart, 1973; Ritz et al., 1971). The frequency with which radiological changes are detected relates directly to the duration of uremic and/or dialysis treatment (Kerr et al., 1969; Ritz et al., 1971; Ingham et al., 1973). An objective radiological study of subperiosteal erosions, fractures, and periarticular and vascular calcifications in 135 dialyzed patients revealed that the four lesions progressed at different rates wlth calcification of the dorsalis pedis artery the earliest detectable lesion (Tatler et al., 1973). Improved radiological diagnosis of bone mineral loss has been obtained using fine-grained industrial film (Meema et al., 1972). This technique, as well as more recently developed photon absorptiometry (Meema et al., 1972; Griffiths et al., 1973) methods, offers significantly greater detection sensitivity over routine radiographs, which are able to demonstrate only a 40% or greater change in bone mineral (Lachman, 1955; Wray et al., 1963).

Subperiosteal resorption when apparent is best observed in the small tubular bones of the hands or feet (Fig. 8) and the medial margin of the proximal tibia (Massry et al., 1969). This lesion is also frequently associated with resorption of the distal ends of the clavicles (Fig. 9), phalangeal tufts (Fig. 10), and sites of muscle insertions such as the ischial tuberosities (Cohen et al., 1970). The skull often has a mottled, ground-glass appearance (Fig. 11) (Massry et al., 1969; Greenfield, 1972); rarely the lamina densa is resorbed and large cystic-like "brown-tumors" appear. These lesions, which contain numerous giant cells histologically and are solid and brown due to hemosiderin deposition, are commonly noted radiologically in the innominate and long bones (Fig. 12), phalanges (Fig. 13), metacarpals, ribs, and skull (Fig. 14) (Katz et al., 1969). Not in-

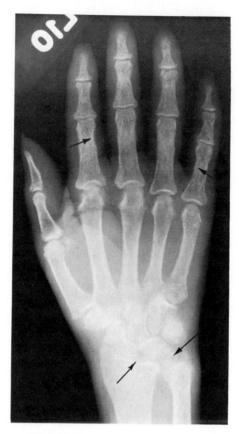

Fig. 8. Subperiosteal resorption in the proximal phalanges of a patient with chronic renal disease as noted by the arrows. Also note the associated finding of chondrocalcinosis (i.e., pseudogout) in the wrist joint space (arrows).

frequently periosteal bone formation may also be marked (Meema *et al.*, 1974; Heath and Martin, 1970).

Despite *in vivo* densinometric studies reporting decreased bone mass in renal failure (Ritz *et al.*, 1971), histological osteoporosis and diffuse radiographic osteopenia are unusual (Kaye *et al.*, 1960; Garner and Ball, 1966; Duursma *et al.*, 1972). In fact, "osteosclerosis" may be the most common skeletal abnormality in patients with long-standing renal disease (Kaye *et al.*, 1960; Haust *et al.*, 1964) and increased bone density is most common in patients younger than 50 years of age, particularly children (Haust *et al.*, 1964). As osteosclerosis does not result in fractures, visible

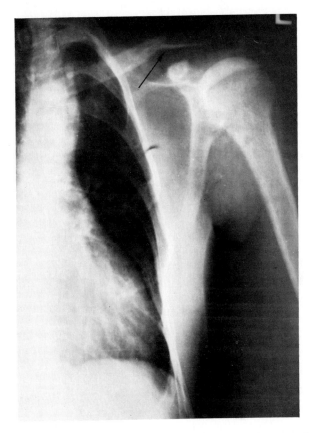

Fig. 9. Resorption of the distal end of the left clavicle (arrow) in a patient with renal insufficiency and secondary hyperparathyroidism.

deformities, or bone pain, it is frequently overlooked (Jowsey *et al.*, 1969). There is a predisposition for the axial rather than the appendicular skeleton producing the characteristic "rugger jersey" sign (Stanbury and Lumb, 1966; Kaye *et al.*, 1960; Agus and Goldberg, 1972). This distinctive roentgenographic picture is the result of horizontal bands of increased bone density alternating with relatively less dense bands of bone (Fig. 15). Osteosclerosis can also be seen as increased density with generalized coarsening of the trabecular pattern. When osteosclerosis develops in long tubular bones, the process involves the metaphysis and occasionally the epiphysis with sparing of diaphyseal regions (Katz *et al.*, 1969; Cohen *et al.*, 1970). Histologically, osteosclerotic trabeculae, often covered by

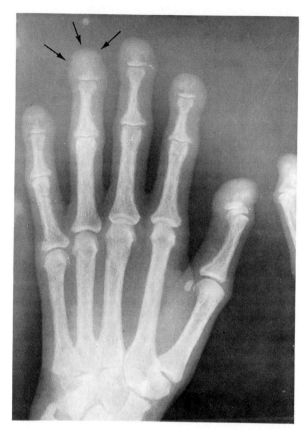

Fig. 10. Resorption of the distal phalanges of the hand in a patient with severe renal insufficiency and secondary hyperparathyroidism. The soft tissue response to the loss of skeletal tissue gives the appearance of clubbing of the fingers (i.e., "pseudoclubbing") as outlined by the arrows.

wide osteoid seams, usually contain sizable volumes of woven bone*, frequently separated by zones of decreased bone mass (Garner and Ball, 1966).

Although the pathogenesis of osteosclerosis is still uncertain and in some dialyzed patients ascribed to the use of fluoridated water in dialysis (Sreepada Rao and Friedman, 1975), it is probably primarily the result of excessive circulating parathyroid hormone (Eugenidis *et al.*, 1972; Kalu *et*

---

* "Woven" or nonlamellar bone is composed of randomly arranged collagen fibers of various diameters and is present only in pathological states except around tooth sockets, sites of tender insertions, or in neonates. The presence of woven collagen is a manifestation of rapid bone turnover as obtains in healing fractures, bone neoplasms, Paget's disease, and in osseous tissue stimulated by excessive parathyroid hormone (see Chapter 4, Volume I).

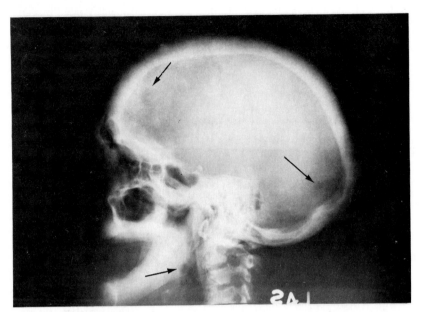

Fig. 11. Skull and mandible of an untreated patient with chronic renal failure. Note the combination of osteosclerosis and lytic lesions (arrows).

al., 1970). Most patients with osteosclerosis have roentgenographic and histological evidence of coincidental osteitis fibrosa with both processes progressing in tandem (Kaye *et al.,* 1960; Cohen *et al.,* 1970). However, although the calcium and phosphate content of the lumbar vertebrae increase with the duration of uremia (Kaye and Thibault, 1964), no consistent relationship between serum calcium and phosphate and bone mass has been demonstrated for individuals with chronic renal disease. In addition, despite claims that patients with a serum Ca × P product greater than 70 usually have osteitis fibrosa and those with lower Ca × P products have predominantly osteomalacia (Stanbury *et al.,* 1969), it is impossible to predict the histological pattern of osteodystrophy using this simple biochemical parameter (Ritz *et al.,* 1971; Garner and Ball, 1966). Although values for Ca × P generally bear no relationship to the associated osteomalacia and the rate of bone resorption (Potts *et al.,* 1969), serum levels of immunoassayable parathyroid hormone (Krempien *et al.,* 1972a; Ritz *et al.,* 1971) and urinary hydroxyproline (DeVeber *et al.,* 1970) often correlate with the osteitis fibrosa detected histologically. In addition, uremic patients with decreased total-body calcium measured by neutron activation tend to have predominantly osteomalacia, while osteitis fibrosa predominates in those with elevated whole-body calcium content (Denney *et al.,* 1973; Hosking and Chamberlain, 1973).

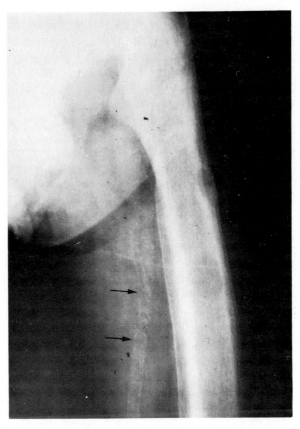

Fig. 12. Cystic lesions in the femur of a 35-year-old patient with chronic renal disease and secondary hyperparathyroidism. Also note the extensive arterial calcification (arrows).

Further attempts to establish interrelations of biochemical and morphometric findings in bone of uremic patients reveal significant correlations between serum alkaline phosphatase and osteoblastic surface area in both dialyzed and nondialyzed uremic patients (Duursma *et al.*, 1974). In nondialyzed patients the serum calcium concentrations can be directly correlated with the extent of bone mineralization and negatively correlated with the extent of osteoid tissue (Duursma *et al.*, 1974). There appears to be no correlation between serum calcium and total osteoid content of bone in dialyzed patients. Thus, only in nondialyzed patients does the serum calcium offer insight into the extent of bone covered with osteoid tissue (Duursma *et al.*, 1974). These correlations may prove useful clinically in individual cases or during group analysis but may prove hazardous when attempting to determine the progression of osteodys-

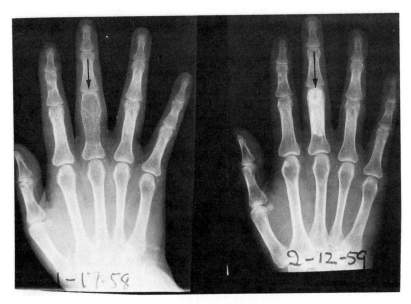

Fig. 13. Cystic lesion in the 3rd proximal phalanx (arrow) in a uremic patient before (1-17-58) and after (2-12-59) subtotal parathyroidectomy.

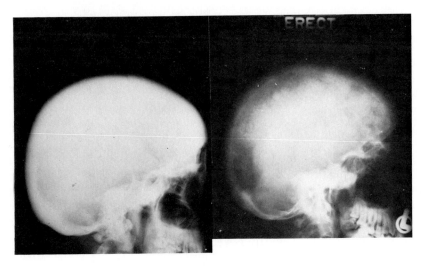

Fig. 14. Skeletal response to subtotal parathyroidectomy following vitamin D and calcium administration.

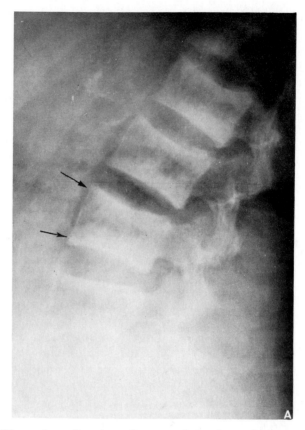

Fig. 15. "Rugger-Jersey" spine of a uremic patient with secondary hyper-parathyroidism (A). Classically a banded sclerosis (arrows) is noted initially localized to the inferior and superior portions of the vertebrae. The sclerosis ultimately advances to involve the entire vertebral body (B).

trophy in any one patient since, for example, over 30% of the circulating alkaline phosphatase seen in patients in intermittent hemodialysis with rising total alkaline phosphatase values represents the intestinal alkaline phosphatase isoenzyme rather than the heat-liable alkaline phosphatase isoenzyme produced by the osteoblast (DeBroe *et al.*, 1974) (see Chapter 3, Volume I). More specific heat-liabile alkaline phosphatase measurements appear to be quite useful in predicting the extent of osteitis fibrosa in patients with chronic renal failure both in cases with normal or elevated total alkaline phosphatase values (Sagar *et al.*, 1971) (see Chapter 3, Volume I).

Children with chronic renal failure develop osteodystrophic changes

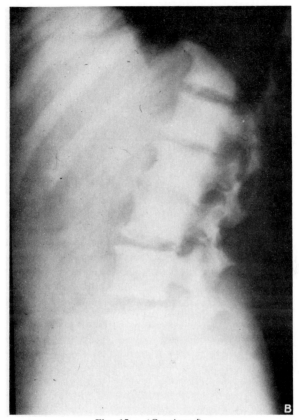

Fig. 15.   (*Continued*)

more frequently than adults (Stanbury, 1967; Mehls *et al.*, 1973; Krempien *et al.*, 1974). In addition to quantitative differences there are qualitative distinctions between adult and childhood uremic bone disease. In
children, uremic osteodystrophy is a disease of the growing skeleton and
as a consequence, striking abnormalities are found in the growth plates of
long bones (Mehls *et al.*, 1973). Generalized demineralization, although
unusual (Fine *et al.*, 1972), is often quite marked in the hands (Fig. 16). In
general, osteomalacia accompanies childhood renal failure more frequently than does osteitis fibrosa (Follis, 1950). In children with chronic
renal insufficiency, malnutrition, acidosis, osteodystrophy, and diminished somatomedin levels (Lewy and New, 1975; Schwalbe *et al.*, 1977)
all contribute to the growth retardation.

Whereas defective calcification of trabecular bone occurs in adult osteomalacia, in childhood osteomalacia or "renal rickets" there is insufficient mineralization of epiphyseal cartilage (Follis, 1950; Friis *et al.*,

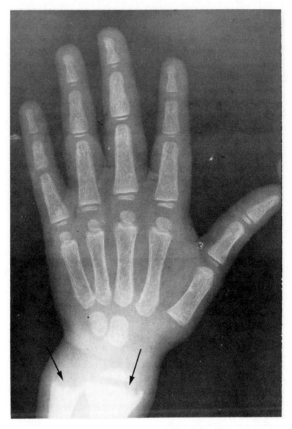

Fig. 16. Advanced skeletal demineralization in the hand of a child with chronic renal disease. Note the "renal rickets" with characteristic irregular wide "cup-shaped" epiphyses (arrows) and the soft tissue swelling at the wrist.

1968). The acquired defect in endochondrial calcification is characterized roentgenographically in children by thick, swollen, and irregular epiphyseal plates, loss of a distinct calcification zone, and cup-shaped epiphyses particularly prominent at the growing ends of long bones (Fig. 16). Subsequently, progression of the epiphyseal growth plate lesion leads to epiphyseolysis and "epiphyseal slipping" (Krempien *et al.,* 1974). In contrast to disturbances in areas of endochondrial calcification, sites of cancellous or trabecular bone (i.e., skull, pelvis, scapulae, vertebrae, and metaphyses of tubular bones) are more dense or sclerotic roentgenographically (Haust *et al.*, 1964). Although the epiphyseal changes of childhood renal rickets are radiologically similar, the subepiphyseal radiolucent area in the X ray does *not* represent the cartilage of the growth plate as in simple vitamin D-deficient nutritional rickets, where nonmineralized irregularly structured cartilage accumulates. In renal rickets this same subepiphyseal radiolucent area represents the zone of "primary spongiosa" transformed into low-mineral-content woven bone* under excessive parathyroid hormone stimulation (Mehls *et al.*, 1973). Whereas metaphyseal fibrosis occasionally develops into other forms of rickets, it is usually the rule in renal rickets (Stanbury, 1967). In addition, as children with renal rickets are generally older than those with nutritional rickets and consequently heavier and more ambulant, the skeletal deformities of uremic children tend to be more severe, often resulting in varus or valgus deformities of the lower extremities.

Serum calcium and phosphate levels of children with advanced renal insufficiency are comparable to those seen in adults (Fine *et al.*, 1972). Decreased osteoblastic activity and growth retardation are reflected in circulating alkaline phosphatase activity, which may be inappropriately low either for the stage of normal bone development and/or the extent of the attendant osteodystrophy (Fine *et al.*, 1972). In occasional circumstances children with minimal impairment (i.e., glomerular filtration rates > 40–50 ml/min) have serum phosphate values that are actually lower than normal. This seemingly paradoxical phenomenon, also reported for adults with early renal failure (Friis *et al.*, 1968), probably reflects the early development of secondary hyperparathyroidism and compensated phosphaturia (Bricker, 1972; Slatopolsky *et al.*, 1971, 1972; Reiss *et al.*, 1970).

IV. SOFT TISSUE CALCIFICATION

Soft tissue calcification is an increasingly frequent accompaniment of chronic renal disease and probably the major symptomatic complication of uremic osteodystrophy (Katz *et al.*, 1969). Both metastatic and dystrophic calcification occur in uremia (Parfitt, 1969b), the former a reflection of an abnormal chemical milieu resulting in mineral deposition in normal tissue while the latter represents soft tissue mineralization due to local changes in cellular structure. Uremic soft tissue calcification invariably contains calcium phosphate (Parfit, 1969b). Occasionally characteristic calcium oxalate crystals are evident under polarized light (Parfitt, 1969b). Contiguglia *et al.* (1973) and co-workers (LeGeros *et al.*, 1973) describe gross and histological differences between visceral and nonvisceral mineralization. Whereas visceral calcification is a whitish, solid

* See footnote cited earlier in this Section.

material, generally deposited as small nodules eliciting only a slight fibrotic response, nonvisceral mineralization is present as a liquid or semisolid and evokes an intense fibrotic reaction resulting in encapsulation of the calcified mass. X-ray diffraction analysis of metastatic calcification deposits reveals that nonvisceral and arterial calcifications are hydroxyapatite in nature whereas calcification in heart, lung, and skeletal muscle is characteristically an amorphous or microcrystalline compound (Termine, 1972; Contiguglia et al., 1973; LeGros et al., 1973).

Although DeVeber et al. (1970) find no biochemical parameter correlating with the incidence of soft tissue calcification in uremia, hyperphosphatemia or an increased Ca × P product are probably important components of this complication (Katz et al., 1969; Hampers et al., 1969; Pedras, 1969). The most advanced examples of soft tissue calcification usually accompany osteitis fibrosa (Katz et al., 1969; Hampers et al., 1969). In addition, therapeutic modalities such as vitamin D or calcium supplements may result in soft tissue calcification (Hampers et al., 1969; Stanbury, 1966; Pendras, 1969; Parfitt, 1969b) as may the correction of uremic acidosis (Parfitt, 1969b; Contiguglia et al., 1973). In decreasing order of frequency, uremic calcification appears in arteries, eyes, periarticular tissue, skin and subcutaneous tissue, and viscera (Parfitt, 1969b).

Between one-fourth (Ritz et al., 1971) and one-half (Friedman et al., 1969) of patients on maintenance hemodialysis develop X-ray evidence of arterial calcification (Fig. 17). Although rarely occurring in children (Parfitt, 1969b) arterial mineralization is the only type of soft tissue calcification commonly recognized during the life of a uremic patient. The abdominal aorta and its branches are the most common sites of metastatic calcification (Katz et al., 1969) while in the arteries of the limbs, the process usually begins above the wrists and ankles (Parfitt, 1969b) (Fig. 17). Arterial calcium deposition is almost always Monkeberg's in type involving the media of the vessel (Augus and Goldberg, 1972; Parfitt, 1969b). This may be due to uremic or hypertensive damage of medial elastin fibers resulting in dystrophic mineralization. Although gangrene has been a sequelae of this process (Pendras, 1969; Richardson et al., 1969; Friedman et al., 1969), due to intimal sparing it is a rare complication. However, difficulties may arise when dialysis shunts are prepared utilizing these vessels (Agus and Goldberg, 1972).

Corneal and conjunctival calcifications are the most common types of soft tissue mineralization occurring in dialysis patients (Parfitt, 1969b). The corneal lesions occur close to the corneal limbus in areas exposed by the interpalpebral fissure (Parfitt, 1969b). Cataracts are also noted in patients with advanced renal failure and attributed primarily to chronic hypocalcemia (Berlyne et al., 1972a). Patients with conjunctival calcifica-

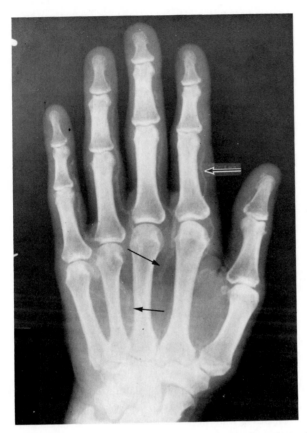

Fig. 17. Calcification of the digital arteries (arrows) in a uremic patient with secondary hyperparathyroidism. The sclerotic component of the osteodystrophy can be seen best in the proximal and distal phalanges.

tion characteristically demonstrate "granular conjunctivae" with acute injection and inflammation, the so-called "red eye" syndrome of renal failure (Ritz *et al.*, 1971; Berlyne, 1968; Parfitt, 1969b). The most striking examples of this 1971; Berlyne, 1968; Parfitt, 1969b). The most striking examples of this syndrome occur in patients with markedly elevated parathyroid hormone levels (Pendras, 1969). In contrast, band keratopathy as a manifestation of corneal calcification correlates poorly with the degree of secondary hyperparathyroidism or with other sites of soft tissue calcification (Katz *et al.*, 1968, 1969).

The periarticular tissue about small joints, the shoulder, and hand is most often involved by metastatic calcification (Fig. 18). Tumoral calcinosis around large joints (Fig. 19) was unusual prior to the era of chronic

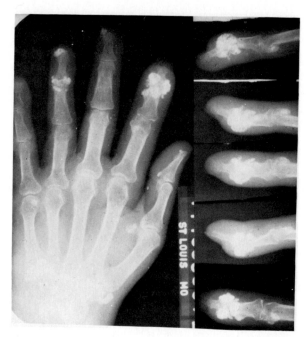

Fig. 18. Periarticular calcification in the hand of a uremic patient. (Courtesy of Dr. James Debnam.)

dialysis but now occurs with increasing frequency (Parfitt, 1969b; Mirahmadi *et al.*, 1973). These lesions, often incapacitating, contain hydroxyapatite crystals and appear clinically as a calcific tenosynovitis (Parfitt, 1969b) or an acute, aseptic periarthritic inflammatory arthritis (Mirahmadi *et al.*, 1973). As reported for patients with primary hyperparathyroidism and normal renal function (Grahame *et al.*, 1971), periarticular calcification has a complex relationship to hyperurecemia, as the signs and symptoms of gouty arthritis may sometimes be precipitated in uremia by excess uric acid (Parfitt, 1969b; Caner and Decker, 1964). Although the symptoms respond to colchicine (Caner and Decker, 1964) or phenylbutazone (Mirahmadi *et al.*, 1973), the inflammatory sequellae may result in a form of dystrophic calcification (Parfitt, 1969b). In dialyzed patients recurrent attacks of periarthritis due to hydroxyapatite deposits can be prevented by measures directed toward controlling the serum phosphate (Mirahmadi *et al.*, 1973).

When calcinosis cutis occurs it is often agonizing. Uremic patients, particularly those on dialysis, may also develop large deposits of dermal calcification resulting in severe pruritus (Hampers *et al.*, 1969). Histological examination of skin biopsies demonstrates mineral deposits, often

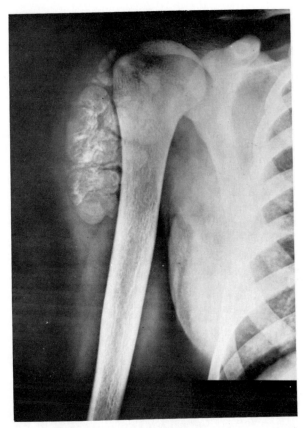

Fig. 19. Advanced soft tissue (muscle) calcification in a patient with chronic renal insufficiency.

extensive, in the dermal fibrous tissue along the hair follicles and in the sebaceous glands (Eisenberg and Bartholomew, 1963). Phosphate restriction and administration of large quantities of phosphate-binding agents may lead to disappearance of the lesions (Eisenberg and Bartholomew, 1963). In addition, as the pruritus is related to the severity of hyperparathyroidism, parathyroidectomy usually results in rapid relief (Katz *et al.*, 1969). Visceral calcification, an unusual clinical manifestation of renal disease, may portend serious consequences (Pendras, 1969). It occurs commonly in the lungs, kidneys, and heart and is rarely detected during life (Parfitt, 1969b). In one series only 12% of uremic patients who came to autopsy with nephrocalcinosis had antemortem X-ray evidence of renal calcification (Katz *et al.*, 1969).

Most nonuremic patients with diffuse pulmonary calcification have malignant neoplasms (Kaltreider *et al.*, 1969). When complicating renal disease, clinical manifestations of pulmonary mineralization (Fig. 20) are usually ominous, although significant regression has occurred during therapy (McLachlan *et al.*, 1968; Jacobs *et al.*, 1973; Neff *et al.*, 1974). Pathologically, the calcium deposition occurs in the alveolar septae and media of the pulmonary vessels (McLachlan *et al.*, 1968).

Cardiac calcification is also often undetected antemortem (Terman *et al.*, 1971). X-ray evidence of metastatic calcification or osteitis fibrosa may be absent and electrocardiographic change is often the only clue to diagnosis (Terman *et al.*, 1971). These patients may develop first degree heart block, intractable congestive heart failure, or die suddenly (Terman *et al.*, 1971). At autopsy, calcium deposits are noted in the atrial-ventricular or sinoatrial node or in the intraventricular septum, correlating to the type of conduction abnormality (Terman *et al.*, 1971). The calcium deposits are surrounded by myocardial fiber degeneration and fibrosis. Small myocardial vessels of uremic patients with cardiac mineralization are universally narrowed by calcium, which is first deposited in the internal elastic lamina extending subsequently into the media and intima (Terman *et al.*, 1971). Massive mineral deposition may also be seen in the superior mediastinum (Fig. 21). In some instances dystrophic mineral deposition has actually been localized to the parathyroid glands (Figs. 22 and 23) (Caldwell *et al.*, 1971). Proximal muscle weakness with associated calcification commonly develops in uremic patients, particu-

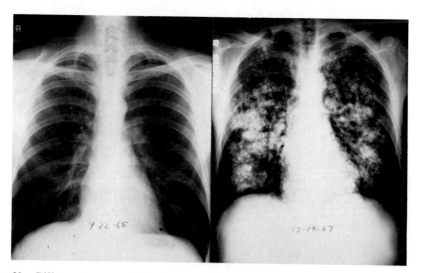

Fig. 20. Diffuse pulmonary calcification in a patient with advanced uremia. (Courtesy of Dr. Eduardo Slatopolsky.)

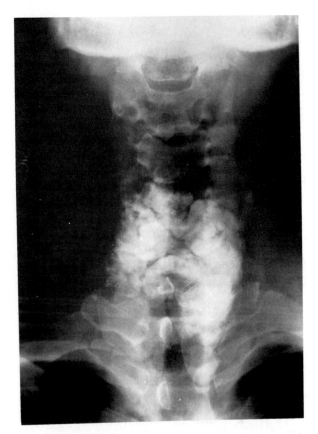

Fig. 21. Diffuse mediastinal calcification in a patient with advanced renal disease. (Courtesy of Dr. Shaul Massry.)

larly those on maintenance hemodialysis (Kerr *et al.,* 1969). Although some investigators (Siddiqui and Kerr, 1971) report normal muscle histology associated with abnormal enzyme activity, others (Goodhue *et al.,* 1972) find a noninflammatory ischemic myopathy with focal calcium deposits. Goodhue *et al.* (1972) attribute these changes to muscle ischemia due to luminal stenosis of arterioles with circumferential medial calcification and concentric fibrous intimal proliferation.

V. DIALYSIS BONE DISEASE

The advent of maintenance hemodialysis has not only prolonged the lives of vast numbers of uremic patients, but has also yielded a plethora of

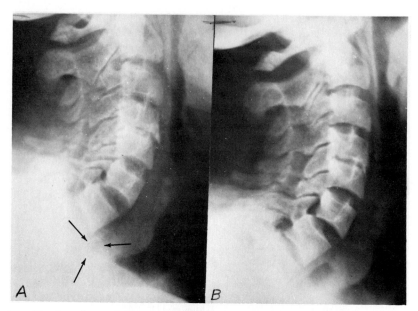

Fig. 22. Lamellar "onion skin" calcification of the parathyroid gland (arrow) in a uremic patient (arrows) before (A) and following (B) parathyroidectomy.

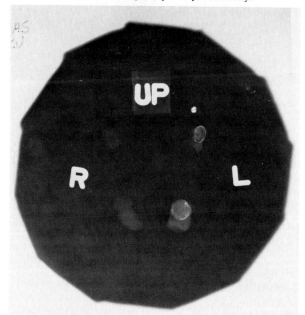

Fig. 23. *In vitro* radiograph of surgically removed parathyroid tissue from patient noted in Fig. 22. The glands were placed in a Petri dish in isotonic saline before the radiograph was obtained.

184

osteodystrophy. The clinical manifestations of bone disease were rare and overshadowed by renal failure in uremics prior to the introduction of maintenance hemodialysis (Ellis and Peart, 1973). Not only are symptoms of bone disease relatively more common among dialyzed patients but most of those who are symptomatic frequently sustain fractures (Kerr *et al.*, 1969; Cadnapaphornchai *et al.*, 1974; Parfitt *et al.*, 1972; Platts *et al.*, 1973). When nondialyzed patients with mild or moderate renal failure complain of skeletal pain or tenderness, osteomalacia is most often the dominant histological lesion. Presently more than 90% of patients treated longer than 2 years have radiological evidence of bone disease (Massry *et al.*, 1969; Cadnapaphornchai *et al.*, 1974; Calenoff and Norfray, 1973). Although dialysate calcium concentrations less than 6.0 ml/100 ml (Fournier *et al.*, 1971; Goldsmith and Johnson, 1973; Gerdon *et al.*, 1972; Goldsmith *et al.*, 1971) and magnesium concentrations less than 0.5 mEq/liter (Pletka *et al.*, 1974) can aggravate secondary hyperparathyroidism, the most significant factor in the persistence of renal hyperparathyroidism prior to the onset of overt vitamin D resistance may be the failure to control blood phosphate (Slatopolsky *et al.*, 1972; Parfitt *et al.*, 1971). Despite a plethora of potentially controllable factors, the longer the patient remains on maintenance hemodialysis, the larger the parathyroid glands tend to be (Pendras, 1969).

The persistence and/or the progression of secondary hyperparathyroidism undoubtedly plays a role in the genesis of dialysis (Genuth *et al.*, 1970). However, the extent of that role is controversial (Massry *et al.*, 1973; O'Riordan *et al.*, 1970; Henderson *et al.*, 1974b). Despite the greater incidence of overt bone disease in dialyzed patients, they may have lower levels of circulating parathyroid hormone than nondialyzed uremics (O'Riordan *et al.*, 1970). Furthermore, dialyzed patients with bone disease may have less immunoreactive parathyroid hormone than their counterparts without osteodystrophy (O'Riordan *et al.*, 1970), and bone disease of dialyzed patients may heal in the presence of persistently elevated parathyroid hormone (Ritz *et al.*, 1968). Some of these discrepancies may be explained by augmented skeletal responsiveness to parathyroid hormone in dialyzed patients (Massry *et al.*, 1969) and by bone remineralization due to mobilization of soft tissue calcification (Ritz *et al.*, 1968). However, the poor correlation between the degree of clinical osteodystrophy and circulating levels of parathyroid hormone persists. Other factors which may play a role in the genesis of dialysis osteopenia may be heparin (Avioli, 1975), and arterial venous shunting (Parfitt *et al.*, 1972), and the removal of a "bone-stimulating factor" from blood (Parfitt *et al.*, 1972). It should be noted in this regard that the bone disease and soft tissue calcification progress in patients on hemodialysis but not in those on peritoneal dialysis (Atkinson *et al.*, 1973; Cangiano *et al.*, 1972).

This seemingly paradoxical observation has been attributed to the removal of a substance (or substances) by peritoneal dialysis that normally inhibits the calcification of bone (Oreopoulos et al., 1974).

Reflecting the variable incidences of dialysis bone disease in different centers, investigators report a variety of roentgenographic changes. Whereas Cohen et al. (1970) note a very high incidence of subperiosteal resorption and osteosclerosis, Ritz et al. (1971) report that a ground-glass skull and "spongiosation of the compacta" of the phalanges are the two most common changes. Both Parfitt et al. (1972) and Doyle (1972) believe that dialysis bone disease roentgenographically resembles osteoporosis rather than osteitis fibrosa or osteomalacia. Unfortunately, sufficient supportive histological proof is lacking. Moreover, Ellis and Peart (1973) find that very few dialyzed patients develop osteoporosis and report normal total bone volume and decreased quantities of mineralized bone characteristic of the osteodystrophy of dialyzed patients. The degree of osteopenia and/or bone demineralization may be grossly underestimated when routine radiographs are used as the sole determinant of skeletal changes during dialysis. When skeletal mineral content is evaluated in the same group of individuals by a number of techniques, demineralization is detected in 77% by photon absorption measurements, and in 93% when neutron activation analysis is used as the detection device (Catto et al., 1973). In contrast only 15% of this same patient population demonstrated progressive demineralization radiographically (Catto et al., 1973). In selected instances a direct correlation has been reported between plasma alkaline phosphatase and the mineral content of the forearm as measured by direct photon absorptiometry (Stewart et al., 1973).

Pathological studies reflect the controversy concerning the nature of dialysis bone disease. There is little question that dialyzed patients have decreased rates of bone formation measured micromorphometrically (Jowsey et al., 1972; Sarnsethsiri et al., 1969). However, whereas both Krempien et al. (1972b) and Binswanger et al. (1973) find no quantitative differences in the bone of dialyzed and nondialyzed patients, others report both increased (Kerr et al., 1969; DeVeber et al., 1970; Sarnsethsiri et al., 1969) and decreased (Ritz et al., 1971) osteoid volumes and increased incidences of osteomalacia in dialyzed patients. Uremic patients dialyzed against a high fluoride containing dialysate appear particularly prone to develop osteomalacia (Ellis and Peart, 1973). In addition, both progression (Massry et al., 1973; Duursma et al., 1972) and regression (Ritz et al., 1971) of resorptive activity are noted on dialysis. Goldsmith and Johnson (1973) inversely correlate the degree of resorptive activity with the calcium concentration of the dialysate. Ritz et al. (1971) attribute this observation to the suppression of parathyroid activity by calcium and ascribe the increased bone osteoclastic activity of others to autonomous hyper-parathyroidism. Since there is actually no correlation between the "inter-dialytic" blood calcium level, circulating PTH, and radiographic osteitis fibrosa (Wills *et al.*, 1974), the intermittent nature of dialysis and fluctuation of plasma calcium during and between dialytic therapy must result in varied degrees of parathyroid autonomy and bone osteoclas-tosis. Although the incidence of osteitis fibrosa is higher in dialyzed pa-tients (DeVeber *et al.* 1970), it is less severe than that of nondialyzed individuals. Quantitative histological studies by Bishop *et al.* (1972) in dialyzed patients demonstrate progressive increments in mean osteoid area and unmineralized osteoid lamellae with no significant change in the os-teitis fibrosa component. There is also evidence that some dialyzed patients develop significantly more osteodystrophy in the cannulated than noncan-nulated limb (Parfitt *et al.*, 1972).

Similar to the osteodystrophic complications that attend maintenance hemodialysis, the incidence of soft tissue calcification is also quite vari-able. Whereas some groups observe mineralized soft tissue in 80% of their patients, others (Cohen *et al.*, 1970; Kaye, 1969) find it an unusual compli-cation, which when apparent, is transient and responsive to dialysis (Kaye, 1969). This response has been variably attributed to a suppression of the secondary hyperparathyroidism due to a prevention of the hypocal-cemic state and to a direct effect of heparin on extraskeletal mineral stores (Korz, 1971). However, whereas soft tissue calcification usually de-creases during dialysis, other forms of extraskeletal calcification, particu-larly that of the ocular and vascular systems, may progress (Massry *et al.*, 1969).

VI. THE NATURE OF THE BONE LESIONS

A. Histological Manifestations

Although the response of bones of uremic patients to parathyroid hor-mone is blunted (Parfitt, 1969a; Potts *et al.*, 1969; Massry *et al.*, 1974), much of the pathology of renal osteodystrophy is due to excess parathyroid hormone. The morphological effects of parathyroid hormone on skeletal tissue have been known since the early 1930s. Hunter and Turnball (1931) describe marrow fibrosis, woven bone formation*, in-creased osteoclastic activity with formation of Howship's lucunae, as well as an increase in the size and number of osteoblasts. In uremia the fraction of activated osteocytes in Haversian bone are also significantly

---

* See footnote in Section III.

increased and a direct correlation obtains between the size of the osteo-cytic lacunae and the level of circulating PTH (Krempien *et al.*, 1973). Parathyroid hormone not only stimulates osteoclastic activity and induces osteocytic osteolysis (see Chapter 1), but is a general stimulator of bone cell activity (Byers and Smith, 1971). Therefore, not only is bone resorption increased, but in the uncomplicated nonuremic hyperparathyroid state, new bone formation or apposition is often augmented (Wilde *et al.*, 1973) with the net bone mass reflecting the balance between formation and resorption.

Regardless of etiology, the histological hallmark of osteomalacia is an increase in the total volume and linear coverage of trabecular bone by inactive osteoid and failure of tetracycline uptake (Frost, 1969) at the calcification front.* The normal ability of bone to assume a tetracycline label, which binds to calcium molecules taking part in active mineralization, may identify those patients with increased osteoid and unimpaired mineralization (Kelley *et al.*, 1965). The calcification front may also be identified by a characteristic histological appearance when subjected to a variety of stains (Melvin *et al.*, 1970; Matrajt and Hioco, 1966). A unique feature of tetracycline uptake by uremic bone is the labeling of complete osteons in short periods to time. It is doubtful if this phenomenon represents increased bone formation but is probably a manifestation of defective mineralization, particularly the delay of maturation of amorphous calcium phosphate to its crystalline phase (Russel *et al.*, 1973; Rolle, 1969). The osteomalacic component of renal osteodystrophy is represented by a decrease in mineralized bone and an increase both in the number of unmineralized osteoid lamellae and the mean osteoid area (Figs. 24 and 25).

When associated primarily with a mineralization defect, most osteoid seams are lined by resting osteoblasts, flat cells having a membranous appearance, arranged in a linear pattern in apposition to osteoid. Active osteoblasts cover the majority of osteoid associated with states of increased bone collagen formation. These cells are columnar and suggest an active metabolic state (Merz and Schenk, 1970). The "hyperosteoidosis" of renal disease may not be only a product of deficient mineralization but also a manifestation of secondary hyperparathyroidism (Eugenidis *et al.*, 1972; Kalu *et al.*, 1970; Krempien *et al.*, 1972a). Notwithstanding the necessity of vitamin D for physiological calcification, the bones of uremic patients in the United States are probably more directly affected by the

---

* Fluorescent tetracycline markers of active mineralization are essential for the histological evaluation of bone formation of appositional rate. Net bone appositional rate can be determined by calculating the distance between two labels after the tetracycline has been administered sequentially at predetermined time (see Chapter 4, Volume I).

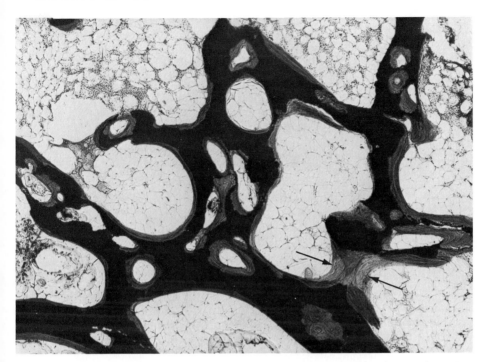

Fig. 24.   Undecalcified iliac crest bone biopsy obtained from a patient with chronic renal failure. The mineralized bone is black and unmineralized or poorly mineralized osteoid is gray. Note the extensive sheathing of all trabeculae with osteoid and an "osteoid bridge" (arrows) between mineralized segments of trabeculae (100×).

secondary hyperparathyroidism than by vitamin D resistance. Obviously when populations are routinely subjected to marginal sunlight exposure or decreased levels of dietary vitamin D (Haddad and Kyung, 1971; Stamp *et al.*, 1972), the occult osteomalacia may become the prominant aspect of osteodystrophy if and when these same individuals develop renal insufficiency (Figs. 24 and 25). Whereas abnormalities of vitamin D metabolism effect intestinal calcium transport and modify PTH activity on bone, there is no evidence of a lack of direct action of this vitamin on bone in most patients with renal failure, although some have a marked deficiency of tetracycline uptake at the mineralization front (Eastwood *et al.*, 1971). Although abnormal rates of metabolism and excretion of vitamin D have been documented to obtain in renal failure (Avioli *et al.*, 1968, 1969a; Piel *et al.*, 1973; Gray *et al.*, 1974; Mawer *et al.*, 1973), Bordier *et al.* (1973) and Fournier *et al.* (1972) fail to demonstrate osteomalacia in anephric patients. As renal parenchyma is necessary for the production of the highly active compound 1,25-dihydroxycholecalciferol (Ghazarian and

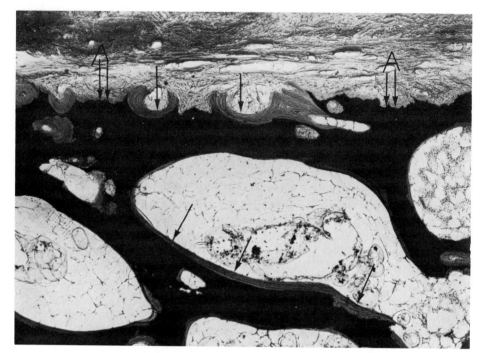

Fig. 25. Subperiosteal resorption (A double arrows) and the accumulation of osteoid tissue (single arrows) in a patient with chronic uremia. Bone biopsied specimen is undecalcified and obtained from the iliac crest (100×).

DeLuca, 1974; Henry and Norman, 1974; Fraser and Kodicek, 1973; Bikle and Rasmussen, 1974, 1975; Bikle *et al.*, 1975; Tanaka *et al.*, 1973), the importance of this metabolite in bone mineralization remains questionable. Observations of Bordier *et al.* (1973, 1978 and Pavlovitch *et al.* 1973), do suggest that 25-hydroxycholecalciferol may have a direct effect on bone in the uremic or relatively anephric state.

Osteitis fibrosa often precedes evidence of abnormal bone mineralization and indirect observations suggest that secondary hyperparathyroidism occurs prior to vitamin D resistance in uremia (Lumb *et al.*, 1971; Schaefer *et al.*, 1968; Reiss *et al.*, 1969; Bricker, 1972). Although there may be adequate or increased numbers of active osteoblasts lining osteoid seams in uremic bone, the rate of collagen formation per cell is usually decreased while the absolute rate of bone synthesis is elevated. This discrepancy is reflected in reports of increased (Kleeman *et al.*, 1969; Nichols *et al.*, 1969; Sherrard *et al.*, 1974), normal (Sherrard *et al.*, 1974; Kaye and Silverman, 1965), and decreased (Richardson *et al.*, 1969; Eastwood *et al.*, 1971; Jowsey *et al.*, 1969; Sherrard *et al.*, 1974; Kaye and Silverman, 1965) rates of bone accretion attending uremia. The pathogenesis of the variable bone accretion rates observed in uremic patients is unclear. It obviously depends on the degree of acquired resistance to PTH, intestinal malabsorption of calcium, and extent of hyperphosphatemia and vitamin D resistance.

Although Ritz *et al.* (1971) report good correlation between the levels of circulating PTH and histological parameters of osteitis fibrosa in patients on maintenance hemodialysis and argue against resistance to PTH, the calcemic response to PTH is suppressed in renal failure (Potts *et al.*, 1969; Massry *et al.*, 1973, 1974). This skeletal resistance to PTH may result in part from the attendant hyperphosphatemia that antagonizes PTH-induced bone resorption (Brand and Raisz, 1972) and/or a combination of impaired osteoclastic generation (Bordier *et al.*, 1975) and function (Jaworski *et al.*, 1975; Villanueva *et al.*, 1970). As measured microradiographically (Massry *et al.*, 1973) and biochemically (Potts *et al.*, 1969; Massry *et al.*, 1973) the responsivity of uremic bone to PTH varies inversely with the quantity of preexisting bone resorption. Since vitamin D therapy reportedly corrects the suppressed calcemic response to PTH in uremia (Stanbury *et al.*, 1969), resistance to PTH has also been ascribed by some to attendant abnormalities of vitamin D metabolism (Potts *et al.*, 1969; Agus and Goldberg, 1972; Agus and Goldberg, 1972). Although the rate of resorption per osteoclast is decreased in renal failure (Villanueva *et al.*, 1970; Jaworski *et al.*, 1975), the PTH-resistant state may also be due to the protective effect of osteoid tissue. Notwithstanding morphological evidence that osteoclasts are occasionally capable of resorbing nonmineralized bone (Garner and Ball, 1966), pathological situations wherein thick osteoid seams cover all potentially resorbable bone surfaces are highly resistant to the osteoclastic-stimulating effects of PTH (Jowsey, 1972).

B. Biochemical Defects

Although considerable attention has been focused on the abnormalities of parathyroid secretion and metabolism in uremia, calcium malabsorption and disordered metabolism of vitamin D, and changes in bone mineral content, relatively little information exists on the metabolism and fate of the organic bone matrix and the degree of bone crystal maturation (Termine, 1972) in patients with long-standing renal disease. Nichols *et al.* (1969, 1972) have demonstrated that both the metabolic activity of bone cells and collagen turnover are increased in virtually all patients with chronic renal insufficiency despite absence of bone disease by routine radiographic analysis. In addition, there have been reports of elevated plasma levels of free proline and hydroxyproline and the accumulation of a plasma peptide-bound proline moiety (Dubovsky *et al.*, 1965; Laitinen *et al.*, 1966; Kowalewski *et al.*, 1971) as well as histological evidence of osteoid accumulation and an increase in total bone mass in azotemic subjects (Garner and Ball, 1966).

The "osteosclerosis" usually encountered in terminal uremic states has been associated with an excess of unmineralized osteoid tissue and the replacement of lamellar bone by woven bone (see footnote, Section III) under the stimulus of abnormally high circulating parathyroid hormone levels (Eugenidis *et al.*, 1972; Kalu *et al.*, 1970). The "osteosclerosis" has also been attributed to a dialyzable "collagen-stimulating factor" (Handy *et al.*, 1969). Conversely, derangements in collagen metabolism in humans with end-stage renal disease and abnormally low values for urinary hydroxyproline have been attributed to a gradual replacement of collagen by elastin-like fibers that are relatively deficient in hydroxyproline (Finalyson *et al.*, 1964). Bone collagen is known to be degraded to hydroxyproline-containing peptides and free hydroxyproline both of which circulate in plasma and are subsequently excreted (Prockop and Kivirikko, 1967). Plasma-free hydroxyproline and urinary total hydroxyproline are commonly used as indices of collagen turnover. They both are increased by bone disease (Lee and Lloyd, 1964; Benoit *et al.*, 1963), growth (Klein and Teree, 1966), acromegaly (Lee and Lloyd, 1964), hyperthyroidism (Kivirikko *et al.*, 1965; Siersbaek-Nielsen *et al.*, 1971; Fink *et al.*, 1967), primary hyperparathyroidism (Klein *et al.*, 1962; Avioli and Prockop, 1967), and in the postpartum uterus undergoing involution (Klein, 1964). Attempts to evaluate bone collagen metabolism by an analysis of plasma or urinary hydroxyproline in patients with chronic renal failure (Dubovsky *et al.*, 1965; Laitinen *et al.*, 1966; Kowalewski *et al.*, 1971) are fraught with interpretive difficulties, since alterations in renal glomerular or tubular function per se affect hydroxyproline excretion (Benoit and Watten, 1968) and circulating levels of free hydroxyproline are normally conditioned by the state of hepatic and renal enzymatic activities (Avioli *et al.*, 1964; Efron *et al.*, 1965). Elevations in plasma levels of a hydroxyproline-containing protein (hyproprotein) have been observed in chronic uremia and correlated with alterations in skeletal metabolism (LeRoy and Sjoerdsma, 1965). These findings are also equivocal at best since the existence of a specific hyproprotein in plasma reflecting tissue collagen metabolism has been refuted (Bankowski *et al.*, 1970) and chemical studies of the human plasma complement component, Clq, reveal a structural similarity remarkably close to collagen and collagen-like proteins (Shelton *et al.*, 1972; Russell *et al.*, 1975).

Since attempts to define alterations in bone collagen metabolism in patients with chronic renal failure are indirect and the data thus derived difficult to interpret, animal models have been devised in order to study the pathogenesis of the skeletal defects that develop in the chronic uremic state. Early controlled studies by Krempien et al. (1972b) in animals with experimentally induced chronic uremia revealed a reduction of bone collagen synthesis which could not be attributed to the associated secondary hyperparathyroid state. Hahn and Avioli (1970) extracted the immature soluble collagen fractions from the bone and skin of uremic animals and demonstrated a significant *increase* in the soluble or immature collagen fraction and a *decrease* in the more mature highly cross-linked insoluble collagen fraction of bone (Pinnell and Martin, 1968; Bornstein, 1970) (see Chapter 1, Volume I), whereas the soluble and insoluble collagen fractions in the skin were unaltered. The results of these studies also suggested that uremia failed to alter bone cell uptake and release of free proline, a precursor of hydroxyproline in the collagen peptide, although collagen maturation was delayed. Studies in animals with progressive end-stage renal disease by Russell et al. (1973) and Russell and Avioli (1972) revealed that the advancing uremic state resulted in an acquired maturational defect in both mineral and collagen moieties in bone with accumulation of less crystalline amorphous calcium phosphate (Termine, 1972) and early forms of collagen. Subsequently, Russell et al. (1975) attributed (at least in part) the collagen maturation defects of chronic uremic animals to an acquired alteration of the quantitative relations between cross-links and aldehydric precursors (Pinnell and Martin, 1968; Bornstein, 1970; Siegel and Martin, 1970; Deshmukh and Nimni, 1969; Rojkind and Gutierrez, 1969; Tanzer et al., 1966; Rucker et al., 1969; Bailey et al., 1974; Mechanic and Tanzer, 1970; Mechanic et al., 1971; Mechanic, 1971) of bone collagen.

Since maturation and increased cross-linking of newly synthesized collagen precedes calcification in hard tissues (Mills and Bavetta, 1968; Uitto and Laitinen, 1968), the deranged maturational sequences in the bone and mineral acquired in experimentally induced renal failure were considered to represent altered cellular and/or enzymatic activities essential for the development of collagen. The progressive accumulation of less dense, more immature forms of bone collagen, which accumulate during the course of experimental chronic renal insufficiency, is reminiscent of the actions of β-aminoproprionitrile and D-penicillamine on collagen maturation (Bornstein, 1970; Siegel and Martin, 1970; Deshmukh and Nimni, 1969; Deshmukh et al., 1973). Uremic toxins may possibly function as inhibitors of the enzymatic activity (Gitelman, 1970). They might also act as thiosemicarbazides, which inhibit the formation of aldehydes in collagen, binding to preformed aldehydes (Rojkind and Gutierrez, 1969;

Tanzer *et al.*, 1966). The specific causal relationship between these documented alterations in the formation of collagen cross-links (Russell *et al.*, 1975), the crystallinization defect (Russell *et al.*, 1973; Russell and Avioli, 1972), and the chronic uremic state is still conjectural, although it is tempting to postulate the existence of one or more acquired alterations in those biochemical sequences that regulate the molecular metabolism of skeletal collagen as the fundamental cause for the observed defects. However, the accumulation of amorphous calcium phosphate within bone at the expense of crystalline apatite may be independent of the collagen maturational defect and due primarily to the increments in bone magnesium, which also characterizes the chronic uremic state in both man (Burnell *et al.*, 1974) and animals (Kaye, 1974b). The magnesium ion reportedly retards the formation of mature apatite in bone by stabilizing the precursor, relatively immature amorphous calcium phosphate phase (Termine, 1972). Should the animal uremic model prove to be an appropriate one for human renal osteodystrophy, the accumulated data would lend support to the hypothesis that chronic uremia in man leads to a panoply of biochemical and biophysical derangements in skeletal tissue, which renders it structurally unsound and physiologically unable to meet the homeostatic demands imposed upon it.

Although the data accumulated to date im the experimental animal uremic model incriminates a disorder of collagen metabolism in bone with resultant defective osteoid formation as a major component of the osteodystrophic skeletal lesion, the pathogenesis of this defect may be multifactorial since recent studies have also uncovered alterations in the cartilage metabolism of uremic animals, which is reminiscent of earlier observations made in vitamin D-deficient animals. In both pathological states there appears to be a shift in the normal rate of glycolytic versus pentose shunt activity with a concomitant alteration in the TCA cycle activity (Meyer and Kunin, 1969; Russell and Avioli, 1975). As such, the reduced glycolytic activity and diminished $^{14}CO_2$ production via the TCA cycle observed in cartilaginous tissue obtained from the epiphyses of uremic animals (Russell and Avioli, 1975) may be ascribable in part to the vitamin D "resistant," hyperphosphatemic state characteristic of the uremic syndrome. Since calcium mobilization in bone has been associated with intramitochondrial mineral deposits (Martin and Mathews, 1969), recent documentation of defective electron transport and oxidative phosphorylation of mitochondria obtained from the tissue of uremic animals (Russell and Avioli, 1974) also bears consideration. In the final analysis the biochemical defect(s) in bone, which are acquired in chronic renal disease may, in fact, prove to be much more complicated than previously anticipated. More definitive analysis of the interrelationship between acquired derangements in the metabolic activities of bone cells, carbohydrate metabolism, collagen maturation, mitochondrial function, mineral sequestration from extracellular fluids, and subsequent apatitic formation in bone is essential before the true biochemical and biophysical nature of the skeleton lesion can be appreciated.

VII. THERAPEUTIC MANAGEMENT

Choice of therapy for those derangements in mineral and skeletal metabolism that complicate the clinical course of patients with end-stage renal disease should be based on (1) an adequate appraisal of the bone disease by radiographic analysis and whenever possible localized iliac crest needle bone biopsy (which can be accomplished with ease in the out-patient ambulatory state); (2) measurements of circulating calcium phosphate, parathyroid hormone, and 25-hydroxycholecalciferol; (3) the presence or absence of soft tissue and/or vascular calcifications; (4) the degree of clinical disability such as nausea, vomiting, intractable pruritis, muscular weakness, bone pain, or pathological fractions; and (5) evaluation of the overall therapeutic approach to the chronic euremic state in each instance, including potential plans for either 1 long-term dialysis without renal transplantation or intermittent dialysis in preparation for transplantation surgery. It must be emphasized that for each patient, the therapeutic approach to the osteodystrophic skeletal disorder and derangements in mineral metabolism must be considered an adjunct to the overall management of the renal insufficiency.

A. Dietary Factors

Patients with chronic renal failure have elevated circulating vitamin A levels (Smith and Goodman, 1971; Kopple and Swendseid, 1975). Since vitamin A, either directly (Frame et al., 1974; Raisz, 1965; Jowsey and Riggs, 1968) or indirectly, by stimulating the glandular release of parathyroid hormone (Chertow et al., 1974), may potentiate the resorption of bone, multivitamin preparations that contain vitamin A should be avoided. In contrast to vitamin A, plasma levels of vitamin D and pyridoxine are low in uremic patients especially those undergoing maintenance hemodialysis (Kopple and Swendseid, 1975). It has also been suggested that the activity of pyridoxal kinase, an enzyme that catalyzes the phosphorylation of pyridoxine and its analogues, is inhibited in uremia (Jowsey and Riggs, 1968). As noted in Chapter 1, Volume I, both vitamin C and pyridoxine function are essential co-factors in the formation of the collagen molecule and its subsequent maturation (Hutton et al., 1967; Pinnell and Martin, 1968). It would seem appropriate, therefore, to ensure adequate intake of both water soluble vitamins by dietary supplementation if necessary, since water soluble vitamins tend to be low in diets of uremic patients (Dobbelstein et al., 1974; Pendras and Erickson, 1966). In this regard it should be noted that rigorous protein restriction (i.e., diets < 60 gm per day) may actually accentuate the propensity to both pyridoxine and vitamin C deficiency (Kopple and Swendseid, 1975; Sullivan and Eisenstein, 1970).

Calcium and phosphate intake should be carefully monitored, since progressive hyperphosphatemia and hypocalcemia exacerbate the secondary hyperparathyroid state (Bricker, 1972; Slatopolsky et al., 1971, 1972; Reiss et al., 1970). Dietary phosphate restriction and the addition of phosphate binding gels such as aluminum or magnesium hydroxide should be combined in order to ensure that the plasma phosphate remains in the 3–4 mg/100 range in nondialyzed patients. Aluminum-containing gels should not be prescribed indiscriminately, since hyperaluminemia may result (Berlyne et al., 1970) and aluminum intoxication may induce cerebral degeneration (Crapper et al., 1973), orbital bleeding, lethargy, and anorexia (Berlyne et al., 1972c). In dialysis patients, higher phosphate values (i.e., 4–5 mg/100 ml) are acceptable before dialytic treatment in order to prevent postdialytic hypophosphatemia. Phosphate-containing enemas should also be prescribed with caution in patients with chronic renal insufficiency, since hypocalcemia and tetany may result (Chesney and Haughton, 1974; Oxnard et al., 1974). Although rigorous control of dietary phosphate and the intestinal absorption of phosphate may prove quite effective in controlling the secondary hyperparathyroidism of uremic patients (Slatopolsky et al., 1972; Clarkson et al., 1972), hypophosphatemia should be avoided. Hemolytic anemia and somatic cell dysfunction (Klock et al., 1974), myopathy, and osteomalacia (Ludwig et al., 1967; Dent and Winter, 1974; Baker et al., 1974) have all been reported to attend the hypophosphatemic syndrome induced by phosphate restriction in man.

Dietary calcium should be monitored and supplemental, if necessary, to insure a total intake of approximately 1–1.5 gm per day. This intake may be essential to maintain circulating calcium levels between 9.0 and 10.0 mg%, levels that would retard the development of cataracts (Berlyne et al., 1972a) and the progression of secondary hyperparathyroidism. Calcium-containing compounds such as calcium gluconate (9% calcium), calcium carbonate (40% calcium), and calcium lactate (13% calcium) are all appropriate for supplementing the dietary intake. Proposed dietary regimens which include 4–10 gm of calcium per day (Clarkson et al., 1966,

1973) should be attempted with caution, especially in patients receiving vitamin D or one of its biologically active metabolites because severe hypercalcemia may develop and the metastatic calcification propagated (Counts *et al.*, 1975; Ginsburg *et al.*, 1973). Despite reports of progressive falls in plasma PTH in patients dialyzed against a calcium concentration of 8 mg/100 ml (Goldsmith *et al.*, 1971), the dialyzate calcium concentration should not exceed 6.5–7 mg/100 ml, since not only do higher concentrations accentuate the metastatic calcification process, especially in patients with significant hyperphosphatemia, but the skeletal response to concentrations of 8 mg/100 ml may in fact be negligible (Mirahmadl *et al.*, 1971). The decrease in serum magnesium observed in patients with uremia on oral calcium therapy is ascribed to a combination of decreased intestinal absorption and increased urinary loss (Popovtzer and Robinette, 1974).

B. Vitamin D

The judicious use of vitamin D and supplemental calcium has also been advocated to maintain the serum calcium at a level that effectively suppresses PTH secretion, thereby reducing the tendency toward skeletal demineralization. Frequent monitoring of serum calcium, phosphate, and PTH levels is mandatory during vitamin D therapy of hemodialyzed patients to avoid life-threatening hypercalcemia and excessive soft tissue calcification. Vitamin D therapy is perhaps most advantageous to patients with osteomalacia dominating the osteodystrophic skeletal pattern and children with "renal rickets" may respond with relatively small doses of 600–10,000 IU per day. In adults, the osteomalacia can be effectively established by evaluating undecalcified needle bone biopsy specimens, although the presence of severe generalized bone pain (Ingham *et al.*, 1974) and/or low circulating 25-hydroxycholecalciferol levels (Bayard *et al.*, 1973) are most consistent with extensive bone demineralization. If no apparent changes occur in 6–12 weeks of vitamin D therapy, as reflected in clinical improvement, a progressive rise in plasma calcium, or a gradual fall in plasma alkaline phosphatase and PTH, the daily dose of vitamin D should be *gradually* and *cautiously* increased. When continued vitamin D therapy results in a sustained circulating calcium in the range of 10.0–10.5 mg/100 ml without symptomatic improvement or an associated fall in plasma parathyroid hormone and/or alkaline phosphatase, subtotal parathyroidectomy should be considered the treatment of choice. Although vascular calcifications reportedly disappear and skeletal lesions heal when dialyzed patients are subjected to vitamin D therapy in doses of 1.2 million units per week (Verberckmoes *et al.*, 1975), this high dose vitamin D should not be attempted unless circulating phosphate levels are rigidly controlled (Verberckmoes *et al.*, 1975).

Not infrequently patients resistant to vitamin D in doses of 50,000–100,000 IU per day respond quite dramatically to dihydrotachysterol (DHT) (Dent *et al.*, 1961; Liu and Chu, 1943; Kaye and Sagar, 1972; Ahmed *et al.*, 1976; Kaye *et al.*, 1970a) in doses of 0.25–0.375 mg/day. DHT, like cholecalciferol, requires hepatic enzymatic hydroxylation in position 25 before it becomes biologically effective (Hallick and DeLuca, 1972). Chemically synthesized 25-hydroxydihydrotachysterol (25-OHDHT) is more potent and faster acting than dihydrotachysterol in the mobilization of bone mineral. It is also more antirichitic than dihydrotachysterol and more effective in promoting elevations of plasma calcium in hypoparathyroidism (Hallick and DeLuca, 1971; Hibberd and Norman, 1969). The biological effectiveness of 25-OHDHT may depend on its structural characteristics, since the *trans*-diene configuration of the dihydrotachysterol molecule (Fig. 4) confers a positional change in its 3-hydroxyl group so that it occupies a position sterically analogous to the 1-hydroxyl group in the *cis*-diene configuration of 1,25-$(OH)_2D_3$ (Fig. 4). Thus in the absence of further 1-hydroxylation by the kidney, 25-OHDHT might possess an affinity for intestinal or bone receptor sites equal to that of 1,25-$(OH)_2D_3$. This is undoubtedly an oversimplification because the A-ring geometry of the dihydrotachysterol differs substantially from vitamin D. However, such a closely related compound might be able to overcome strict stereochemical constraints by mass action. This theory is also compatible with the observed structural specificities for both the intestinal and bone receptor sites for a variety of biologically active "vitamin D_3-like" compounds. Those with side chains of vitamin D_3 or dihydrotachysterol may act preferentially on the intestine, whereas compounds with the side chain of vitamin D_2 (ergocalciferol) or dihydrotachysterol act preferentially to mobilize skeletal mineral (Hibberd and Norman, 1969).

C. Vitamin D Metabolites and Synthetic Analogues

Reports of vitamin D intoxication in the anephric uremic state (Counts *et al.*, 1975) and others citing a direct effect of 25-OHD on bone metabolism *in vitro* (Raisz *et al.*, 1972b; Reynolds, 1973; Reynolds *et al.*, 1974) and *in vivo* in the anephric state (Pavlovitch *et al.*, 1973) collectively suggest that this hydroxylated metabolite may prove useful in reversing renal osteodystrophy in man. Preliminary studies by Bordier *et al.* (1975) reveal that the osteomalacic component of the osteodystrophy of uremic man is less resistant to 25-OHD$_3$ (i.e., 30 to 200 μg/day) than to vitamin D_2

or D_3. Moreover, 25-OHD$_3$, in doses of 100 μg/day for a 6–12-month period, does effectively reverse the skeletal abnormalities of uremic patients undergoing intermittent hemodialysis with concomitant increments in intestinal calcium absorption and a decrease in circulating alkaline phosphatase and PTH (Teitelbaum *et al.*, 1976). Although 100-μg daily doses of 25-OHD$_3$ are still considerably higher than those required to heal dietary rickets or the osteomalacia attending malabsorption syndromes, they are much lower than those of vitamin D_2 or D_3 used unsuccessfully in azotemic osteodystrophy by others (Dent *et al.*, 1961).

1,25-(OH)$_2$D$_3$ has also been used successfully in vitamin D-resistant uremic patients with osteodystrophy (Henderson *et al.*, 1974a,b; Brickman *et al.*, 1972, 1974a,b; Silverberg *et al.*, 1975; Ahmed *et al.*, 1978) and improvements in bone mass (Silverberg *et al.*, 1975), calcium absorption (Brickman *et al.*, 1972) (Fig. 26), and a decrease in circulating PTH (Brickman *et al.*, 1974a,b) have been documented on doses of 1.0–2.7 μg per day. Although the potentially powerful bone resorbing activity of 1,25-(OH)$_2$D (Reynolds, 1973) would theoretically appear to modify any enthusiasm to treat uremic patients with relatively high doses for prolonged periods, limited long-term therapeutic trials with this agent are promising (Silverberg *et al.*, 1975; Henderson *et al.*, 1974a). In one instance a 14-year-old child given 0.68 μg daily for over 3 months demonstrated progressive healing of the skeletal lesions radiographically (detectable after 4 weeks of therapy) and a fall in alkaline phosphatase. This response was

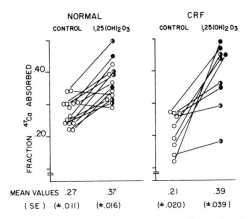

Fig. 26. The absolute fraction of radioactive calcium (^{47}Ca) absorbed when given with 200 mg calcium carrier in normal subjects and patients with chronic renal failure (CRF) before and after treatment with 1,25-dihydroxycholecalciferol [1,25-(OH)$_2$D$_3$]. Lines connect results in the same subject. Quantities of 1,25-(OH)$_2$D$_3$ given include 2.7 μg/day (●), 0.68 μg/day (○), and 0.14 μg/day (◐).

attended by a complete reversal of the secondary hyperparathyroidism and osteomalacic bone lesions noted on iliac crest biopsied specimens prior to the intervention of 1,25-$(OH)_2D_3$ therapy (Henderson *et al.*, 1974a). Of additional interest is the observation that during the 1,25-$(OH)_2D_3$ treatment period, muscular weakness also improved both clinically and by electromyographic testing (Henderson *et al.*, 1974a).

1,24,25-$(OH)_3D_3$, another vitamin D metabolite produced by the kidney, may also prove an effective therapeutic agent for osteodystrophic patients. Although it is less active on a weight basis than 1,25-$(OH)_2D_3$ in stimulating and sustaining intestinal calcium transport and bone calcium mobilization, it appears to exert its biological action primarily on the intestine (Holick *et al.*, 1973a). As such it may prove more effective than either 25-OHD_3 or 1,25-$(OH)_2D_3$ in reversing the skeletal defects, since each of these vitamin D_3 metabolites possesses significant bone resorptive activities (Reynolds, 1973; Reynolds *et al.*, 1974), an effect that would appear to delay the reversal of the accelerated PTH-induced bone resorption so characteristic of end-stage renal disease. To date no reported therapeutic trials with 1,24,25-$(OH)_3D_3$ have been attempted in uremic patients because of its limited availability.

Attempts to develop a compound with the unique properties of 1,25-$(OH)_2D_3$ led to the chemical synthesis of the 5,6-*trans* isomers of vitamin D_3 and 25-OHD_3 (Fig. 4). 5,6-*trans*-Vitamin D_3 exerts a biological effect on both the intestine and bone, whereas 5,6-*trans*-25-OHD_3 functions only to stimulate calcium absorption (Holick *et al.*, 1972). Short-term (8 days) therapeutic trials in uremic patients with 5,6-*trans*-vitamin D_3 are also promising, since doses of 1.0–5.0 mg/day reportedly stimulate the intestinal absorption of calcium (Rutherford *et al.*, 1975).

The most recent synthetic vitamin D_3 analogue used for the treatment of vitamin D-resistant renal osteodystrophy is 1α-hydroxycholecalciferol (1α-OHD_3) (Peacock *et al.*, 1974; Catto *et al.*, 1975; Chalmers *et al.*, 1973; Tougaard *et al.*, 1976; Catto *et al.*, 1975; Pierides *et al.*, 1976, Davie *et al.*, 1976; Nielsen *et al.*, 1976; and Chan, *et al.*, 1977). This analogue has comparable biological activity on a weight basis to 1,25-$(OH)_2D_3$ in the stimulation of intestinal calcium transport and bone calcium mobilization in the normal and anephric state (Holick *et al.*, 1973b). Unlike 1,25-$(OH)_2D_3$, which is more effective when administered intravenously rather than orally (Silverberg *et al.*, 1975), 1α-OHD_3 is active orally as well as parenterally (Pechet and Hesse, 1974). The onset of the biological activity of 1α-OHD_3 is rapid with daily doses of 2.5 μg effectively reversing the skeletal defects of patients with nutritional osteomalacia by 8–10 days (Pechet and Hesse, 1974). Doses as small as 10 μg/day for 2–3 days in uremic patients have been associated with a two- to threefold increase in calcium absorption, an elevation in serum calcium, and a fall in circulating alkaline phosphatase (Chalmers *et al.*, 1973). More prolonged treatment (i.e., 9–10 weeks) with daily doses of 1.0–2.0 μg reveals progressive increments in both calcium absorption and skeletal mineral (Catto *et al.*, 1975). 1α-OHD$_3$ is biologically effective in the anephric state (Pechet and Hesse, 1974), although it appears to be rapidly metabolized to 1α-25-(OH)$_2$D$_3$, the latter considered to be the ultimate metabolically active form (Holick *et al.*, 1977; Holick *et al.*, 1976; Fukushima *et al.*, 1975). A hydroxy analogue of vitamin D$_2$, 1α-hydroxyvitamin D$_2$, has also been synthesized, which has biopotency comparable to that of the corresponding vitamin D$_3$ analogue 1α-OHD$_3$ (Lam *et al.*, 1974). The 1α-OHD$_2$ analogue appears presently to offer no advantages over the 1α-OHD$_3$ analogue, both of which exhibit an antirachitic potency 3 times that of the respective parent vitamin D compounds.

D. Parathyroidectomy

Whereas the early osteomalacic manifestations of uremic osteodystrophy may respond favorably to the judicious use of oral calcium, phosphate, and vitamin D therapy, the latter stages dominated by osteitis fibrosa are somewhat more resistant to most conservative modes of therapy. In addition, the decision to initiate long-term dialysis therapy in order to amerliorate the varied symptoms and biochemical abnormalities of chronic uremia inevitably results in a greater incidence of recognizable osteodystrophy. There is, however, convincing evidence that secondary hyperparathyroidism plays a significant, if not major, role in the progressive skeletal demineralization seen in the undialyzed patient with long-standing uremia, or in the subject on intermittent dialysis. Attempts to suppress parathroid activity by establishing a mild hypercalcemia either with combinations of vitamin D, oral antacids, and calcium salts or by increasing dialysate calcium concentrations have been moderately effective. However, the combination of an acquired disturbance in vitamin D metabolism which is not reversed by chronic dialysis, persistent hyperphosphatemia, and the inability to maintain suppressive levels of plasma calcium without accelerating metastatic calcification often leaves much to be desired in this form of treatment. In carefully selected cases, parathyroidectomy may offer a therapeutic advantage over conservative, medical attempts to suppress parathyroid activity (Fig. 5).

The exact indications and ideal time for parathyroid surgery are uncertain. One circumstance in which immediate parathyroidectomy appears mandatory is that of rapidly progressive vascular calcification either ln patients awaiting renal transplantation or in those destined to remain in long-term intermittent dialysis programs. In the former group vascular calcification tends to compromise the appropriate surgical anastomoses. whereas in the latter situation, vascular integrity essential for chronic rotating cannulation procedures may be severely compromised. Parathyroidectomy should not be injudiciously used to ameliorate the osteodystrophic syndrome without careful consideration of each individual case and the plans for the patient's subsequent management. This surgical procedure is not without risk in severely ill uremic patients and should not be undertaken except in those instances where adequate attempts at medical management have failed, and when symptoms of bone pain and pathological fractures are incapacitating. It must be emphasized that parathyroidectomy may be followed by severe hypocalcemia and tetany in a uremic patient who will then require chronic therapy with vitamin D after emergency administration of parenteral calcium solutions.

Subtotal glandular excision is indicated in chronic uremic patients (Gerdon *et al.*, 1972), including children (Geis *et al.*, 1973; Firor *et al.*, 1972) when prior medical treatment fails to improve X-ray or clinical evidence of osteodystrophy, soft tissue calcification, hypercalcemia with systemic symptoms, or severe pruritus. It should also be emphasized that osteodystrophy is likely to progress in spite of correction of abnormalities of vitamin D, calcium, and phosphate metabolism if excessive parathyroid hormone secretion goes unchecked (Katz *et al.*, 1969). Although Katz *et al.* (1969) believe parathyroid surgery may be indicated more frequently, the number of uremic patients subjected to this procedure vary from less than 2% (Hampers *et al.*, 1969; Gerdon *et al.*, 1972) to almost 20% (Geis *et al.*, 1973). It is maintained by some that total, rather than subtotal, parathyroidectomy is the operation of choice, particularly for those patients who are not candidates for transplantation (Massry *et al.*, 1969; Firor *et al.*, 1972; Gill *et al.*, 1969), since rapid growth of the remaining parathyroid tissue may occur, necessitating reoperation (Geis *et al.*, 1973). Total parathyroidectomy with both allo- and autograft transplantation of parathyroid tissue in the forearm has been advocated as an appropriate compromise by some (Wells *et al.*, 1975).

The clinical response to parathyroidectomy is often striking, particularly regarding pruritus (Gerdon *et al.*, 1972; Katz *et al.*, 1967, 1969; Massry *et al.*, 1969; Johnson *et al.*, 1971; Firor *et al.*, 1972; Ritz *et al.*, 1973). This often disabling complication of chronic uremia may disappear within 1 week of surgery (Katz *et al.*, 1968). Vascular complications may be slow to resolve (Katz *et al.*, 1969), and ischemic symptoms (Pendras, 1969), including angina pectoris (Ball *et al.*, 1973), relieved by subtotal parathyroidectomy. More importantly, however, the bones of parathyroidectomized uremic patients with soft tissue calcification heal quicker than those without extraskeletal mineralization (Stanbury et al., 1969; Stanbury, 1966). Total-body neutron activation measurements made before and following parathyroidectomy in uremic patients with extensive metastatic calcification show a decrease in total-body calcium concurrent with the reduction of metastatic calcification (Cohn et al., 1972). X-ray evidence of skeletal healing may occur within 3 months of parathyroidectomy (Potts et al., 1969; Gerdon et al., 1972; Gill et al., 1969) (Figs. 13 and 14), although it is often the last pathological parameter to demonstrate evidence of improvement (Katz et al., 1968). Some dialyzed patients, particularly those with severe osteomalacia may, however, continue to sustain fractures without evidence of improvement of their osteodystrophy (Parfitt et al., 1972). Whereas Ellis and Peart (1973) claim woven bone may not respond to parathyroidectomy and persist for long periods following surgery, in my experience this immature collagen may disappear within months of surgery.

E. Transplantation

The availability of renal homotransplanatation has dramatically altered the course of patients with renal failure (Marchioro, 1969; Hume et al., 1955; Woods et al., 1972, 1973; Bailey et al., 1972). Derangements in vitamin D (Avioli et al., 1968) and 25-OHD (Piel et al., 1973) metabolism which obtain prior to transplantation are effectively reversed, and in most instances the osteodystrophy heals (Fine et al., 1972). Continued and accelerated interest in renal transplantation as the definitive therapeutic procedure for patients with chronic renal failure has uncovered a new constellation of biochemical abnormalities characterized by hypercalcemia, hypophosphatemia, and hyperphosphatasia in those subjects who were hypocalcemic and hyperphosphatemic preoperatively (Geis et al., 1973; David et al., 1973; Moorhead et al., 1974; McPhaul et al., 1964; Hornum, 1971; Schwartz et al., 1970).

In general, the hypercalcemia and hypophosphatemia observed in the posttransplanation period are both mild and transient characteristically occurring in patients who attain good allograft function. Mild elevations in circulating alkaline phosphatase persist longer, presumably reflecting the process of bone repair, a pattern that is also seen during the postoperative course of patients with primary hyperparathyroidism (see Chapter 1). One prevailing opinion attributes the posttransplantation hypercalcemia and hypophosphatemia to the secondary hyperparathyroidism established during the preoperative uremic period. The alterations in serum calcium and phosphate observed after transplantation are considered sequellae of the persistent excessive rates of parathyroid hormone secretion by hyperplastic glands when the institution of normal renal function abruptly reverses the uremic state and the resistance to the biological effects of the hormone (Geis *et al.*, 1973; David *et al.*, 1973; Schwartz *et al.*, 1970; McPhaul *et al.*, 1969). Since in some instances secondary hyperparathyroidism with hypercalcemia has been evident for as long as 2 to 3 years after transplantation surgery (David *et al.*, 1973), parathyroidectomy has been advocated (Geis *et al.*, 1973; David *et al.*, 1973; McPhaul *et al.*, 1969). The operation of choice is subtotal parathyroidectomy, although in selected instances total parathyroidectomy has been performed and a fraction of one gland returned as a free autograft (Geis *et al.*, 1973). Hypophosphatemia (David *et al.*, 1973; Moorhead *et al.*, 1974), the resolution of soft tissue calcification (Hornum, 1971), the dose and duration of preoperative vitamin D therapy, and magnesium depletion have all been implicated as contributing factors to the persistent posttransplant hypercalcemic state (Geis *et al.*, 1973). Hypophosphatemia which persists postoperatively may, if untreated, lead to symptoms of phosphorus depletion such as weakness and intention tremors and radiologically detectable osteomalacia with pseudofractures (Moorhead *et al.*, 1974; Schwartz *et al.*, 1970). Both signs and symptoms of phosphate deficiency as well as the hypercalcemia can occasionally be reversed by oral sodium phosphate therapy alone in a dosage of 2–3 gm/day, although parathyroid hyperplasia may be severe enough to warrant subtotal parathyroidectomy (David *et al.*, 1973; Schwartz *et al.*, 1970).

Although it seems to have been repeatedly established that ultimately the most effective form of therapy for patients with severe renal disease and progressive renal osteodystrophy is successful transplantation, we are confronted with an abundant population of patients with mild but progressive renal failure who ultimately develop a specific osteodystrophy that defies all attempts at therapy with vitamin D_3. The fact that disordered vitamin D metabolism attends the uremic state cannot be denied. Moreover, the fact that structurally related vitamin D_3 and 1,25-$(OH)_2D_3$ analogues either exist or will become increasingly available must also be acknowledged.

Despite our ever increasing knowledge of vitamin D biochemistry and the defects in its biological activation acquired during the progression of renal failure, the clinician must weigh all potential avenues of therapy such as dialysis with solutions of appropriate calcium concentration, dietary discretion with emphasis on supplemental vitamins, low phosphate, high calcium diets and phosphate-binding gels, and subtotal parathyroidectomy if and when persistently high circulating calcium and phosphate values are associated with a severe degree of autonomous parathyroid overactivity and progressive bone demineralization. The incorporation of vitamin D, its biologically active metabolites, and/or structurally related analogues in any therapeutic regimen should be tempered by a complete understanding of: (1) the pathogenesis of the osteodystrophic syndrome; and (2) the complications attending vigorous attempts at therapeutic management using agents that not only increase calcium absorption but may in fact lead to progressive soft tissue and renal calcification when bone resorption and hyperphosphatemia continue unabated.

REFERENCES

Ahmed, K. Y., Wills, M. R., Skinner, R. K., Varghese, Z., Meinhard, E., Baillod, R. A., Moorhead, J. F. (1976). Lancet 2:439.

Ahmed, K. Y., Wills, M. R., Varghese, Z. Meinhard, E. A., and Moorhead, J. F. (1978). *Lancet* **1**, 629.

Agus, Z. S., and Goldberg, M. (1972). *Radiol. Clin. North Am.* **10**, 545.

Alfrey, A. C., and Smythe, W. R. (1975). *Artif. Kidney-Chronic Uremia Program, Nat. Inst. of Arthritis, Metab. and Dig. Dis., 1975*, p. 29.

Arnaud, S. B., Matthusen, M., Gilkinson, J. B., and Goldsmith, R. S. (1977). *Am. J. Clin. Nutr.* **30**, 1082.

Atkinson, P. J., Hancock, D. A., Acharya, V. N., Parsons, F. M., Proctor, E. A., and Reed, G. W. (1973). *Br. Med. J.* **4**, 519.

Avioli, L. V. (1972). *Arch. Intern. Med.* **129**, 345.

Avioli, L. V. (1975). *In* "Heparin" (R. A. Bradshaw and S. Wessler, eds.), p. 375. Plenum, New York.

Avioli, L. V., and Haddad, J. G. (1973). *Metab., Clin. Exp.* **22**, 507.

Avioli, L. V., and Prockop, D. J. (1967). *J. Clin. Invest.* **46**, 217.

Avioli, L. V., Scharp, C., and Birge, S. J. (1964). *Am. J. Physiol.* **217**, 536.

Avioli, L. V., Birge, S., Lee, S. W., and Slatopolsky, E. (1968). *J. Clin. Invest.* **47**, 2239.

Avioli, L. V., Birge, S. J., and Slatopolsky, E. (1969a). *Arch. Intern. Med.* **124**, 451.

Avioli, L. V., Scott, S., Lee, S. W., and DeLuca, H. F. (1969b). *Science* **166**, 1154.

Bacon, G. E., Kenny, F. M., Murdaugh, H. V., and Richards, C. (1973). *Johns Hopkins Med. J.* **132**, 127.

Baerg, R. D., Kimberg, C. V., and Gershon, E. (1970). *J. Clin. Invest.* **49**, 1288.

Bailey, A. J., Robins, S. P., and Balian, G. (1974). *Nature (London)* **251**, 105.

Bailey, G. L., Mocelin, A. J., Griffiths, H. J. L., Zschaeck, D., Ghantous, W. H., Hampers, C. L., Merrill, J. P., and Wilson, R. E. (1972). *J. Am. Geriat. Soc.* **20**, 421.

Baker, L. R. I., Ackrill, P., Cattell, W. R., Stamp, T. C. B., and Watson, L. (1974). *Br. Med. J.* **3**, 150.

Ball, J. H., Johnson, J. W., Hampers, C. L., and Merrill, J. P. (1973). *Arch. Intern. Med.* **131**, 746.

Bankowski, E., Galasinski, W., and Rogowski, W. (1970). *FEBS Lett.* **6**, 19.

Barzel, U., and Jowsey, J. (1969). *Clin. Sci.* **36**, 517.

Bayard, F., Bec, P., Ton That, H., and Louvet, J. P. (1973). *J. Clin. Invest.* **3**, 447.

Bell, N. H., and Bartter, F. C. (1964). *Ann. Intern. Med.* **61**, 702.

Benoit, F. L., and Watten, R. H. (1968). *Metab., Clin. Exp.* **17**, 20.

Benoit, F. L., Theil, G. B., and Watten, R. H. (1963). *Metab., Clin. Exp.* **12**, 1072.

Bergdahl, L., and Boquist, L. (1973). *Virchows Arch. A* **358**, 225.

Berlyne, G. M. (1968). *Lancet* **2**, 366.

Berlyne, G. M., Ben-Ari, J., Pest, D., Weinberger, J., Stern, M., Gilmore, G. R., and Levine, R. (1970). *Lancet* **1**, 494.

Berlyne, G. M., Danovitch, G. M., Ben-Ari, J., and Blumenthal, M. (1972a). *Lancet* **1,** 509.

Berlyne, G. M., Ben-Ari, J., Knopf, E., Yagil, R., Weinberger, G., and Danovitch, G. M. (1972b). *Lancet* **1,** 564.

Berson, S. A., and Yalow, R. S. (1966). *Science* **154,** 907.

Bikle, D. D., and Rasmussen, H. (1974). *Biochim. Biophys. Acta* **362,** 425.

Bikle, D. D., and Rasmussen, H. (1975). *J. Clin. Invest.* **55,** 292.

Bikle, D. D., Murphy, E. W., and Rasmussen, H. (1975). *J. Clin. Invest.* **55,** 299.

Bilbrey, G. L., Galoona, G. R., White, M. G., and Knochel, J. P. (1974). *J. Clin. Invest.* **53,** 841.

Binswanger, Y., Sherrard, D., Rich, C., and Curtis, F. K. (1973). *Nephron* **12,** 1.

Birge, S. J., and Alpers, D. H. (1973). *Gastroenterology* **64,** 977.

Bishop, M. C., Woods, C. G., Oliver, D. O., Ledingham, J. G. G., Smith, R., and Tibbutt, D. A. (1972). *Br. Med. J.* **3,** 664.

Bordier, P. J., Tunchot, S., Eastwood, J. B., Fournier, A., and DeWardener, H. E. (1973). *Clin. Sci.* **44,** 33.

Bordier, P. J., Maries, P. J., and Arnaud, C. D. (1975). *Kidney Int.* **7,** S102.

Bordier, P., Zingraff, J., Gueris, J., Jungers, P., Marie, P., Pechet, and Rasmussen, H. (1978). *Am. J. Med.* **64,** 101.

Bornstein, P. (1970). *Am. J. Med.* **49,** 429.

Brand, J. S., and Raisz, L. G. (1972). *Endocrinology* **90,** 479.

Bricker, N. S. (1972). *N. Engl. J. Med.* **286,** 1093.

Brickman, A. S., Coburn, J. W., and Norman, A. W. (1972). *N. Engl. J. Med.* **287,** 891.

Brickman, A. S., Sherrard, D. J., Jowsey, J., Singer, F. R., Baylink, D. J., Maloney, N., Massry, S. G., Norman, A. W., and Coburn, J. W. (1974a). *Arch. Intern. Med.* **134,** 883.

Brickman, A. S., Coburn, J. W., Massry, S. C., and Norman, A. W. (1974b). *Ann. Intern. Med.* **80,** 161.

Brickman, A. S., Coburn, J. W., Rowe, P. H., Massry, S. G., and Norman, A. W. (1974c). *J. Lab. Clin. Med.* **84,** 791.

Brickman, A. S., Hartenbower, Norman, A. W., and Coburn, J. W. (1977). *Am. J. Clin. Nutr.* **30,** 1064.

Brumbaugh, P. F., and Haussler, M. R. (1973). *Biochem. Biophys. Res. Commun.* **51,** 74.

Brumbaugh, P. F., and Haussler, M. R. (1974). *J. Biol. Chem.* **249,** 1251.

Brumbaugh, P. F., Haussler, D. H., Bressler, R., and Haussler, M. R. (1974). *Science* **183,** 1089.

Burnell, J. M. (1971). *J. Clin. Invest.* **50,** 327.

Burnell, J. M., Teubner, E., Wergedal, J. E., and Sherrard, D. J. (1974). *J. Clin. Invest.* **53,** 52.

Byers, P. D., and Smith, R. (1971). *Q. J. Med.* **40,** 471.

Cadnapaphornchai, P., Kuruvila, K. C., Holmes, J., and Schrier, R. W. (1974). *Am. J. Med.* **57,** 789.

Caldwell, J. G., Webber, B. L. and Avioli, L. V. (1971). *J. Clin. Endocrinol. Metab.* **33,** 105.

Calenoff, L., and Norfray, J. (1973). *Am. J. Roentgenol., Radium Ther. Nucl. Med.* [N. S.] **118,** 282.

Caner, J. E. Z., and Decker, J. L. (1964). *Am. J. Med.* **36,** 571.

Cangiano, J. L., Ramirez-Gonzales, R. E., and Ramirez-Muxo, O. (1972). *Am. J. Med. Sci.* **264,** 301.

Catto, G. R. D., MacDonald, A. F., McIntosh, J. A. R., and MacLeod, M. (1973). *Lancet* **1,** 1150.

Catto, G. R. D., MacLeod, M., Pelc, B., and Kodicek, E. (1975). *Br. Med. J.* **1,** 12.

Chalmers, T. M., Hunter, J. O., Davie, M. W., Szaz, K. F., Pelc, B., and Kodicek, E. (1973). *Lancet* **2,** 696.

Chan, J. C. M., Oldham, S. B. and DeLuca, H. F. (1977). *J. Pediatrics* 90:820.

Charnard, J., Assailly, J., Bader, C., and Funck-Bretano, J. L. (1974). *J. Nucl. Med.* **15**, 588.

Chen, T. C., and DeLuca, H. F. (1973). *J. Biol. Chem.* **248**, 4890.

Chen, T. C., Castillo, L., Korycka-Dahl, M., and DeLuca, H. F. (1974). *J. Nutr.* **104**, 1056.

Chertow, B. S., Williams, G. A., Kiani, R., Stewart, K. L., Hargis, G. K., and Flayter, R. L. (1974). *Proc. Soc. Exp. Biol. Med.* **147**, 16.

Chesney, R. W., and Haughton, P. B. (1974). *Am. J. Dis. Child.* **127**, 584.

Clarkson, E. M., McDonald, S. J., and DeWardener, H. E. (1966). *Clin. Sci.* **30**, 425.

Clarkson, E. M., Luck, V. A., Hynson, W. V., Bailey, R. R., Eastwood, J. B., Woodhead, J. S., Clemenets, V. R., O'Riordan, J. L. H., and DeWardener, H. E. (1972). *Clin. Sci.* **43**, 519.

Clarkson, E. M., Eastwood, J. B., Koutsaimanis, K. G., and DeWardener, H. E. (1973). *Kidney Int.* **3**, 258.

Coburn, J. W., Koppel, M. H., Brickman, A. S., and Massry, S. G. (1973). *Kidney Int.* **2**, 264.

Cochran, M., Bulusu, L., Horsman, A., Stasiak, L., and Nordin, B. E. C. (1973). *Nephron* **10**, 113.

Coe, F. L., Canterbury, J. M., Firpo, J., and Reiss, E. (1973). *J. Clin. Invest.* **52**, 134.

Cohen, M. E. L., Cohen, G. F., Ahad, V., and Kaye, M. (1970). *Clin. Radiol.* **21**, 124.

Cohn, S. H., Cinque, T. J., Dombrowski, C. S., and Letteri, J. M. (1972). *J. Lab. Clin. Med.* **79**, 978.

Contiguglia, S. R., Albrey, A. C., Miller, M. L., Runnells, D. E., and LeGeros, R. Z. (1973). *Kidney Int.* **4**, 229.

Corradino, R. A. (1974). *Endocrinology* **94**, 1607.

Counts, S. J., Baylink, D. J., Shen, F. H., Sherrard, D. J., and Hickman, R. O. (1975). *Ann. Intern. Med.* **82**, 196.

Clinical Pathological Conference. (1972). *Am. J. Med.* **52**, 254.

Crapper, D. R., Krishnan, S. S., and Dalton, A. J. (1973). *Science* **180**, 511.

David, D. S., Sakai, S., Brennar, L., Riggio, E. A., Cheigh, J., Stenzel, K. M., Rubin, A. L., and Sherwood, L. M. (1973). *N. Engl. J. Med.* **289**, 398.

Davie, M. W. J., Chalmer, T. M., Hunter, J. O., Pelc, B. and Kodicek, E. (1976). *Ann. Intern. Med.* 84:285.

DeBroe, M. E., Bosteels, V., and Wieme, R. J. (1974). *Lancet* **1**, 753.

DeFronzo, R. A., Andres, R., Edgar, P., and Walker, W. G. (1973). *Medicine (Baltimore)* **52**, 469.

DeLuca, H. F. (1973). *Kidney Int.* **4**, 80.

Denney, J. D., Sherrard, D. J., Nelp, W. B., Chestnut, C. H., and Baylink, D. J. (1973). *J. Lab. Clin. Med.* **82**, 226.

Dent, C. E., and Winter, C. S. (1974). *Br. Med. J.* **1**, 551.

Dent, C. E., Harper, C. N., and Philpot, G. R. (1961). *Q. J. Med.* **30**, 1.

Deshmukh, K., and Nimni, M. E. (1969). *J. Biol. Chem.* **244**, 1787.

Deshmukh, K., Just, M., and Nimni, M. E. (1973). *Clin. Orthop. Relat. Res.* **91**, 196

DeVeber, G. A., Oreopholus, D. G., Rabinovich, S., Lloyd, G. J., Meema, H. E., Beattie, B. L., Levy, D., Husdan, H., and Rapoport, A. (1970). *Trans., Am. Soc. Artif. Intern. Organs* **16**, 479.

Dobbelstein, H., Korner, W. F., Mempel, W., Grosse-Wilde, H., and Edel, H. H. (1974). *Kidney Int.* **5**, 233.

Doyle, F. H. (1972). *Br. Med. Bull.* **28**, 220.

Dubovsky, J., Pacovsky, V., and Cubovska, E. (1965). *Clin. Chim. Acta* **12**, 230.

Dufresne, L. R., Cooper, C. W., and Gitelman, H. J. (1972). *Endocrinology* **90**, 291.

Duursma, S. A., Visser, W. J., and Njio, L. (1972). *Calcif. Tissue Res.* **9**, 216.

Duursma, S. A., Visser, W. J., Mees, E. J. D., and Nijo, L. (1974). *Calcif. Tissue Res.* **16,** 129.
Eastwood, J. B., Bordier, P., and DeWardener, H. E. (1971). *Q. J. Med.* **40,** 569.
Eastwood, J. B., Stamp, T. C. B., Harris, E., DeWardener, H. E. (1976). *Lancet* **2,** 1209.
Editorial. (1974). *Nutr. Rev.* **32,** 247.
Efron, M. L., Bixby, E. M., and Pryles, C. V. (1965). *N. Engl. J. Med.* **272,** 1299.
Eisenberg, E., and Bartholomew, P. V. (1963), *N. Engl. J. Med.* **268,** 1216.
Eisman, J. E., Kream, B. E., Hamstra, A. J. and DeLuca, H. F. (1976). *Science* 193:1021.
Ellis, H. A., and Peart, K. M. (1973). *J. Clin. Pathol.* **26,** 83.
Eugenidis, N., Olah, A. J., and Haas, H. G. (1972). *Radiology* **105,** 265.
Feldman, S. L., and Cousins, R. J. (1973). *Nutr. Rep. Int.* **8,** 4.
Finalyson, G. R., Smith, J. G., Jr., and Moore, M. J. (1964). *J. Am. Med. Assoc.* **187,** 659.
Fine, R. N., Isaacson, A. S., Payne, V., and Grushkin, C. M. (1972). *J. Pediatr.* **80,** 243.
Fink, C. W., Ferguson, J. L., and Smiley, J. D. (1967). *J. Lab. Clin. Med.* **69,** 950.
Firor, H. V., Moore, E. S., Levitsky, L. L., and Galvez, M. (1972). *J. Pediatr. Surg.* **7,** 565.
Fischer, J. A., Oldham, S. B., Sizemore, G. W., and Arnaud, C. D. (1972). *Proc. Natl. Acad. Sci. U.S.A.* **69,** 2341.
Follis, R. H., Jr. (1950). *Bull. Johns Hopkins Hosp.* **87,** 593.
Fournier, A. E., Johnson, W. J., Taves, D. R., Beaubout, J. M., Arnaud, C. D., and Goldsmith, R. S. (1971). *J. Clin. Invest.* **50,** 592.
Fournier, A. E., Tunchot, S., Bedrossian, J., Idatte, J. M., and Bordier, P. (1972). *J. Urol. Nephrol.* **28,** 1001.
Frame, B., Jackson, C. E., Reynolds, W. A., and Umphrey, J. E. (1974). *Ann. Intern. Med.* **80,** 44.
Fraser, D. R., and Kodicek, E. (1973). *Nature (London), New Biol.* **241,** 163.
Friedman, S. A., Novak, S., and Thomson, G. E. (1969). *N. Engl. J. Med.* **280,** 1392.
Friis, T., Hahnemann, S., and Weeke, E. (1968). *Acta Med. Scand.* **183,** 497.
Frost, H. M. (1969). *Calcif. Tissue Res.* **2,** 211.
Fukushima, M., Suzuki, T., Tohira, Y., and Matsumaga, I. (1975). *Biochem. Biophys. Res. Commun.* **66,** 632.
Galante, L., Colston, K., MacAuley, S., and MacIntyre, I. (1972). *Lancet* **1,** 985.
Garabedian, M., Pavlovitch, H., Fellot, C., and Balsan, S. (1974). *Proc. Natl. Acad. Sci. U.S.A.* **71,** 554.
Garner, A., and Ball, J. (1966). *J. Pathol. Bacteriol.* **91,** 545.
Geis, W. P., Popovtzer, M. M., Corman, J. L., Halgrimson, C. G., Groth, C. G., and Starzl, T. E. (1973). *Surg., Gynecol. Obstet.* **137,** 997.
Genuth, S. M., Vertes, V., and Leonards, J. R. (1969). *Metab., Clin. Exp.* **18,** 124.
Genuth, S. M., Sherwood, L. M., Vertes, V., and Leonards, J. R. (1970). *J. Clin. Endocrinol. Metab.* **30,** 15.
Gerdon, H. E., Coburn, J. W., and Passaro, E. (1972). *Arch. Surg. (Chicago)* **104,** 520.
Ghazarian, J. G., and DeLuca, H. F. (1974). *Arch. Biochem. Biophys.* **160,** 63.
Ghazarian, J. G., Schnoes, H. K., and DeLuca, H. F. (1973). *Biochemistry* **12,** 2555.
Gill, G., Pallotta, J., Kashgarian, M., Kessner, D., and Epstein, F. H. (1969). *Am. J. Med.* **46,** 930.
Ginsburg, D. S., Kaplan, E. L., and Katz, A. I. (1973). *Lancet* **1,** 1271.
Gitelman, H. J. (1970). *Arch. Intern. Med.* **126,** 793.
Goldman, R., Bassett, S. H., and Duncan, G. B. (1954). *J. Clin. Invest.* **33,** 1623.
Goldsmith, R. S., and Johnson, W. J. (1973). *Kidney Int.* **4,** 154.
Goldsmith, R. S., Fursyfer, J., Johnson, W. J., Fournier, A. E., and Arnaud, C. D. (1971). *Am. J. Med.* **50,** 692.
Gonick, H. C., Drinkard, J. P., Hertoqhe, J., and Rubini, M. E. (1974). *Clin. Orthop. Relat. Res.* **100,** 315.

Goodhue, W. W., Davis, J. N., and Porro, R. S. (1972). *J. Am. Med. Assoc.* **221,** 911.

Goodman, A. D., Lemann, J., Jr., Lennon, E. J., and Relman, A. S. (1965). *J. Clin. Invest.* **44,** 495.

Grahame, R., Sutor, D. J., and Mitchener, M. B. (1971). *Ann. Rheum. Dis.* **30,** 597.

Gray, R., W., Boyle, I., and DeLuca, H. F. (1971). *Science* **172,** 1232.

Gray, R. W., Weber, H. P., Dominquez, J. H., and Lemann, J., Jr. (1974). *J. Clin. Endocrinol. Metab.* **39,** 1045.

Gray, R. W., Wilz, D. R., Caldas, A. E. and Lemann, J., Jr. (1977). *J. Clin. Endocr. Metab.* **45:**299.

Greenfield, G. B. (1972). *Am. J. Roentgenol., Radium Ther. Nucl. Med.* [N.S.] **116,** 749.

Greenwood, R. H., Prunty, F. T. G., and Silver, J. (1973). *Br. Med. J.* **1,** 643.

Griffiths, H. J., Zimmerman, R. E., Bailey, G., and Snider, R. (1973). *Radiology* **109,** 277.

Haddad, J. G., Jr., and Kyung, J. C. (1971). *J. Clin. Endocrinol. Metab.* **22,** 992.

Haddad, J. G., Jr. and Rojanasathit, S. (1976). *J. Clin. Endocr. Metab.* **42:**284.

Haddad, J. G., Jr., Min, C., Mendelsohn, M., Slatopolsky, E., and Hahn, T. J. (1977). *Arch. Biochem. Biophys.* **182:**390.

Hahn, T. J., and Avioli, L. V. (1970). *Arch. Intern. Med.* **126,** 882.

Hahn, T. J., Hendin, B. A., Scharp, C. R., and Haddad, J. G., Jr. (1972). *N. Engl. J. Med.* **287,** 900.

Hahn, T. J., Scharp, C. R., and Avioli, L. V. (1974). *Endocrinology* **94,** 1489.

Hahn, T. J., Hendin, B. A., Scharp, C. R., Boisseau, V. C., and Haddad, J. G., Jr. (1975). *N. Engl. J. Med.* **292,** 550.

Hallick, R. B., and DeLuca, H. F. (1971). *Biochem. Biophys. Res. Commun.* **44,** 1096.

Hallick, R. B., and DeLuca, H. F. (1972). *J. Biol. Chem.* **247,** 91.

Hampers, C. L., Katz, A., Wilson, R. E., and Merrill, J. P. (1969). *Arch. Intern. Med.* **124,** 282.

Handy, J. R., Hobbs, D. R., and Parks, N. M. (1969). *Clin Res.* **17,** 385.

Hartenbower, D. L., Stella, F. J., Norman, A. W., Friedlor, R. M., and Coburn, J. W. (1977). *J. Lab. Clin. Med.* **90,** 760.

Haussler, M. R., Baylink, D. J., Hughes, M. R., Brumbaugh, P. F. Wergedal, J. E., Shen, F. H., Neilsen, R. L., Counts, S. J., Bursac, K. M. and McCain, T. A. (1976). *Clin. Endocr.* **5:**151S.

Haust, M. D., Landing, B. H., Holmstrand, K., Currarino, C., and Smith, D. S. (1964). *Am. J. Pathol.* **44,** 141.

Heath, D. A., and Martin, D. J. (1970). Br. J. Radiol. **43,** 517.

Helmke, K., Federlin, K., Piazolo, P., Stroder, J., Jeschke, R., and Franz, H. E. (1974). *Gut* **15,** 875.

Henderson, R. G., Ledingham, J. G., Oliver, D. O., Small, D. G., Russell, R. G., Smith, R., Walton, R. J., Preston, C., and Warner, C. T. (1974a). *Lancet* **1,** 379.

Henderson, R. G., Ledingham, J. G. G., Oliver, D. O., Smith, R., and Woods, C. G. (1974b). *Proc. R. Soc. Med.* **67,** 10.

Henry, H. L., and Norman, A. W. (1974). *J. Biol. Chem.* **249,** 7529.

Heynen, G., and Franchimont, P. (1974). *Lancet* **1,** 627.

Hibberd, K. A., and Norman, A. W. (1969). *Biochem. Pharmacol.* **18,** 2347.

Hill, L. F., Van Den Berg. C. J., and Mawer, E. B. (1971). *Nature (London)* **232,** 189.

Holick, M. F., deBlanco, M. C., Clark, M. B., Henley, J. W., Neer, R. M., DeLuca, H. F., and Potts, J. T., J. *J. Clin. Endocr. Metab.* **44:**595.

Holick, M. F., Garabedian, M., and DeLuca, H. F. (1972). *Biochemistry* **11,** 2715.

Holick, M. F., Kleiner-Bossaller, A., Schnoes, J. K., Kasten, P. M., Boyle, I. T., and DeLuca, H. F. (1973a). *J. Biol. Chem.* **248,** 6691.

Holick, M. F., Semmler, E. J., Schnoes, H. K., and DeLuca, H. F. (1973b). *Science* **180,** 190.

Holick, M. F., Tavela, T. E., Holick, S. A., Schnoes, H. K., and DeLuca, H. F. (1976). *J. Biol. Chem.* **251**, 1020.
Holtrop, J. E., Raisz, L. G., and Simmons, H. A. (1974). *J. Cell Biol.* **60**, 346.
Hornum, I. (1971). *Acta Med. Scand.* **189**, 199.
Hosking, D. J., and Chamberlain, M. J. (1973). *Q. J. Med.* **42**, 467.
Hruska, K., Kopelman, R., Rutherford, W. E., Klahr, S., and Slatopolsky, E. (1973). *Am. Soc. Nephrol.* Abstract, p. 50.
Hume, D. M., Merrill, J. P., Miller, B. F., and Thorn, G. W. (1955). *J. Clin. Invest.* **34**, 327.
Hunter, D., and Turnbull, H. M. (1931). *Br. J. Surg.* **19**, 203.
Hutton, J. J., Tappel, A. L., and Udenfriend, S. (1967). *Arch. Biochem. Biophys.* **118**, 231.
Ingham, J. P., Stewart, J. H., and Posen, S. (1973). *Br. Med. J.* **2**, 745.
Ingham, J. P., Kleerekoper, M., Stewart, J. H., and Posen, S. (1974). *Med. J. Aust.* **1**, 873.
Ireland, A. W., Cameron, D. A., Stewart, J. H., and Posen, S. (1969). *Calcif. Tissue Res.* **4**, 282.
Jacobs, A. N., Neitzschman, H. R., and Nice, C. M., Jr. (1973). *Am. J. Roentgenol., Radium Ther. Nucl. Med.* [N. S.] **118**, 344.
Jaworski, Z. F. G., Lok, E., and Wellington, J. L. (1975). *Clin. Orthop. Relat. Res.* **107**, 299.
Johnson, J. W., Wachman, A., Katz, A. I., Bernstein, D. S., Hampers, C. L., Hattner, R. S., Wilson, R. E., and Merrill, J. P. (1971). *Metab. Clin. Exp.* **20**, 487.
Jowsey, J. (1972). *J. Clin. Invest.* **51**, 9.
Jowsey, J., and Riggs, B. L. (1968). *J. Clin. Endocrinol. Metab.* **28**, 1833.
Jowsey, J., Massry, S. G., Coburn, J. W., and Kleeman, C. R. (1969). *Arch. Intern. Med.* **124**, 539.
Jowsey, J., Johnson, W. J., Taves, D. R., and Kelly, P. J. (1972). *J. Lab. Clin. Med.* **79**, 204.
Joyce, J. R., Pierce, K. R., Romance, W. M., and Baker, J. M. (1971). *J. Am. Vet. Med. Assoc.* **158**, 2033.
Jubiz, W., Haussler, M. R., McCain, T. A. and Tolman, K. G. (1977). J. Clin. Endocr. Metab. 44:617.
Kaltreider, H. B., Baum, G. S., Bogarty, G., McCoy, M. D., and Tucker, M. (1969). *Am. J. Med.* **46**, 188.
Kalu, D. N., Doyle, F. H., Pennock, J., and Foster, G. V. (1970). *Lancet* **1**, 1363.
Katz, A. I., Hampers, C. L., Wilson, R. E., Bernstein, D. S., Washman, A., and Merrill, J. P. (1968). *Trans., Am. Soc. Artif. Intern. Organs* **14**, 376.
Katz, A. I., Hampers, C. L., and Merrill, J. P. (1969). *Medicine (Baltimore)* **48**, 333.
Kaye, M. (1969). *Arch. Intern. Med.* **124**, 656.
Kaye, M. (1974a). *J. Clin. Invest.* **53**, 256.
Kaye, M. (1974b). *J. Lab. Clin. Med.* **84**, 256.
Kaye, M., and Sagar, S. (1972). *Metab., Clin. Exp.* **21**, 815.
Kaye, M., and Silverman, M. (1965). *J. Lab. Clin. Med.* **66**, 535.
Kaye, M., and Thibault, T. (1964). *J. Clin. Invest.* **43**, 1367.
Kaye, M., Pritchard, J. E., Halpenny, G. W., and Light, W. (1960). *Medicine (Baltimore)* **39**, 157.
Kaye, M., Chatterjee, G., Cohen, G. F., and Sagar, S. (1970a). *Ann. Intern. Med.* **73**, 225.
Kaye, M., Frueh, A. J., and Silverman, M. (1970b). *J. Clin. Invest.* **49**, 442.
Kelly, P. J., Jowsey, J., and Riggs, B. L. (1965). *Clin. Orthop. Relat. Res.* **40**, 7.
Kerr, D. N. S., Walls, J., Ellis, D. H., Simpson, W., Uldall, P. R., and Ward, M. K. (1969). *J. Bone Joint. Surg., Br. Vol.,* **51**, 578.
Kessner, D. M., and Epstein, F. H. (1965). *Am. J. Physiol.* **209**, 141.
Kildeberg, P., Engel, K., and Winters, R. W. (1969). *Acta Paediat. Scand.* **58**, 321.
Kivirikko, K. I., Laitinen, O., and Lamberg, B. A. (1965). *J. Clin. Endocrinol. Metab.* **25**, 1347.

Kleeman, C. R., Massry, S. G., Cob, J. W., and Popovtzer, M. M. (1969). *Arch. Intern. Med.* **124**, 262.

Klein, L. (1964). *Metab., Clin. Exp.* **13**, 386.

Klein, L., and Teree, T. M. and (1966). *J. Pediat.* **69**, 266.

Klein, L., Albertsen, K., and Curtiss, P. H. (1962). *Metab., Clin. Exp.* **11**, 1023.

Kleiner-Bossaler, A., and DeLuca, H. F. (1974). *Biochim. Biophys. Acta* **288**, 489.

Klock, J. C., Williams, H. E., and Mentzer, W. C. (1974). *Arch. Intern. Med.* **134**, 360.

Knox, F. G., Schneider, E. G., Willis, L. R., Strandhoy, J. W., and Ott, C. E. (1973). *Kidney Int.* **3**, 347.

Kopple, J. D., and Coburn, J. W. (1973). *Medicine (Baltimore)* **52**, 597.

Kopple, J. D., and Swendseid, M. E. (1975). *Kidney Int.* **7**, S-79.

Korz, R. (1971). *Klin. Wochenschr.* **49**, 684.

Kowalewski, J., Tomaszewski, J., Hanzlik, J., Zawislak, H., and Zbikowska, A. (1971). *Clin. Chim. Acta* **34**, 123.

Kowarski, S., and Schachter, D. (1973). *J. Clin. Invest.* **52**, 2765.

Krempien, B., Ritz, E., Beck, U., and Keilbach, H. (1972a). *Virchows Arch. A* **357**, 257.

Krempien, B., Ritz, E., and Schmidt, G. (1972b). *Z. Orthop. Ihre Grenzeb.* **110**, 25.

Krempien, B., Geiger, G., Ritz, E., and Buttner, S. (1973). *Virchows Arch.* **360**, 1.

Krempien, B., Mehls, O., and Ritz, E. (1974). *Virchows Arch. A* **352**, 129.

Kumar, R., Harden, D. and DeLuca, H. F. (1976). Biochemistry 15:2420.

Lachman, E. (1955). *Am. J. Roentgenol.* **74**, 712.

Laitinen, O., Nikkila, E. A., and Kivirikko, I. K. (1966). *Acta Med. Scand.* **179**, 275.

Lam, H. Y. P., Schnoes, H. K., and DeLuca, H. F. (1974). *Science* **186**, 1038.

Leber, H. W., and Schutterle, G. (1972). *Kidney Int.* **2**, 152.

Lee, C. A., and Lloyd, H. M. (1964). *Med. J. Aust.* **1**, 992.

Lee, S. W. Russell, J., Avioli, L. V. (1977). *Science* **195**, 994.

LeGeros, R. Z., Contiguglia, S. R., and Alfrey, A. C. (1973). *Calcif. Tissue Res.* **13**, 173.

Lemann, J., Jr., Lennon, E. J., Goodman, A. D., Litzow, J., and Relman, A. S. (1965). *J. Clin. Invest.* **44**, 507.

Lemann, J., Jr., Litzow, J. R., and Lennon, E. J. (1966). *J. Clin. Invest.* **45**, 1608.

Lemann, J., Jr., Litzow, J. R., and Lennon, E. J. (1967). *J. Clin. Invest.* **46**, 1318.

LeRoy, E. C., and Sjoerdsma, A. (1965). *J. Clin. Invest.* **44**, 914.

Lewy, J. E., and New, M. I. (1975). *Am. J. Med.* **58**, 65.

Lim, V. S., and Fang, V. S. (1975). *Am. J. Med.* **58**, 655.

Liu, S. G., and Chu, H. I. (1943). *Medicine (Baltimore)* **22**, 103.

Lucas, R. C. (1883). *Lancet* **1**, 993.

Ludwig, G. D., Kyle, G. C., and DeBlanco, M. (1967). *Am. J. Med.* **43**, 136.

Lumb, G. A., Mawer, E. B., and Stanbury, S. W. (1971). *Am. J. Med.* **50**, 421.

McDermott, F. R., Galbraith, A. J., and Dalton, M. K. (1974). *Gastroenterology* **66**, 235.

McLachlan, M. S. F., Wallace, M., and Seneviratne, C. (1968). *Br. J. Radiol.* **41**, 99.

McPhaul, J. J., Jr., McIntosh, D. A., Hammond, W. S., and Park, O. K. (1969). *N. Engl. J. Med.* **271**, 1342.

Marchioro, T. L. (1969). *Arch. Intern. Med.* **123**, 485.

Martin, J. H., and Mathews, J. L. (1969). *Clin. Orthop. Relat. Res.* **68**, 273.

Martin, K. J., Hruska, K. A., Lewis, J., Anderson, C., and Slatopolsky, E. (1977). *J. Clin. Invest.* 60:808.

Massry, S., Coburn, J. W., Popovtzer, M. M., Shinaberger, J. H., Maxwell, M. M., and Kleeman, C. R. (1969). *Arch. Intern. Med.* **124**, 431.

Massry, S. G., Coburn, J. W., Lee, D. D. N., Jowsey, J., and Kleeman, C. R. (1973). *Ann. Intern. Med.* **78**, 357.

Massry, S. G., Arieff, A. I., Coburn, J. W., Palmieri, G., and Kleeman, C. R. (1974). *Kidney Int.* **5**, 437.

Matrajt, H., and Hioco, D. (1966). *Stain Technol.* **41,** 97.

Mawer, E. B., Taylor, C. M., Backhouse, J., Lumb, G. A., and Stanbury, S. W. (1973). *Lancet* , 626.

Mazess, R. B. (1970). *Arct. Anthropol.* **7,** 114.

Mechanic, G. (1971). *Isr. J. Med. Sci.* **7,** 458.

Mechanic, G., and Tanzer, M. L. (1970). *Biochem. Biophys. Res. Commun.* **41,** 1597.

Mechanic, G., Gallop, P. M., and Tanzer, M. L. (1971). *Biochem. Biophys. Res. Commun.* **45,** 644.

Meema, H. E., Rabinovich, S., Meema, S., Lloyd, G. J., and Oreopoulos, D. G. (1972). *Radiology* **102,** 1.

Meema, H. E., Oreopoulos, G., Rabinovich, W., Husdon, H., and Rapoport, A. (1974). *Radiology* **110,** 513.

Mehls, O., Ritz, E., Krempien, B., Willich, E., Bommer, J., and Scharer, K. (1973). *Pediatr. Radiol.* **1,** 183.

Melvin, K. E. W., Hepner, G. W., Bordier, P., Neale, G., and Joplin, G. F. (1970). *Q. J. Med.* **39,** 83.

Merz, W. A., and Schenk, R. K. (1970). *Acta Anat.* **76,** 1.

Messener, R. P., Smith, H. T., Shapiro, F. L., and Gregory, D. H. (1969). *J. Lab. Clin. Med.* **74,** 472.

Meyer, W. L., and Kunin, A. S., (1969). *Arch. Biophys.* **129,** 438.

Mills, B. G., and Bavetta, L. A. (1968). *Clin. Orthop. Relat. Res.* **57,** 267.

Mioni, G., Ossi, E., D'Angelo, A., Valvo, E., Lupo, A., and Maschio, G. (1973). *Biomedicine* **18,** 491.

Mirahmadi, K. S., Duffy, B. S., Shinaberger, J. H., Jowsey, J., Massry, S. G., and Coburn, J. W. (1971). *Trans., Am. Soc. Artif. Intern. Organs* **17,** 118.

Mirahmadi, K. S., Coburn, J. W., and Bluestone, R. (1973). *J. Am. Med. Assoc.* **223,** 548.

Mishkin, M. S., Hsu, T. H., Walker, W. G., and Gledsoe, T. (1972). *Johns Hopkins Med. J.* **131,** 160.

Moorhead, J. F., Ahmed, K. Y., Varghese, Z., Wills, M. R., Baillod, R. A., and Tatler, G. L. B. (1974). *Lancet* **1,** 694.

Moxley, M. A., Bell, N. H., Wagle, S. R., Allen, D. O., and Ashmore, H. (1974). *Am. J. Physiol.* **227,** 1058.

Muldowney, F. P., Donohoe, J. F., Freaney, R., Kempff, C., and Swan, M. (1970). *Isr. J. Med. Sci.* **3,** 221.

Muldowney, F. P., Carroll, D. V., Donohoe, J. F., and Freaney, R. (1971). *Q. J. Med.* **40,** 487.

Muldowney, F. P., Donohoe, J. F., Carroll, D. V., Powell, D., and Freaney, R. (1972). *Q. J. Med.* **41,** 321.

Nahara, H. T., and Williams, R. H. (1957). *Endocrinology* **60,** 285.

Neff, M., Yalcin, S., Gupta, S., and Berger, H. (1974). *Am. J. Med.* **56,** 103.

Nichols, G., Flanagan, B., and Van Der Sluys Veer, J. (1969). *Arch. Intern. Med.* **124,** 530.

Nichols, G., Flanagan, B., Van Der Sluys Veer, J., Johnson, J. W., Hampers, L., and Merrill, J. P. (1972). *Metab., Clin. Exp.* **21,** 317.

Nielsen, S. O., Binderup, E., Godtfredsen, W. O., Jensen, H. and Ladefoged, J. (1976). *Nephron* 16:359.

Oettinger, C. W., Merrill, R., Blanton, T., and Briggs, W. (1974). *N. Engl. J. Med.* **291,** 458.

Offermann, G., von Herrath, D., and Schaefer, K. (1974). *Nephron* **13,** 269.

Ogg, C. S. (1968). *Clin. Sci.* **34,** 467.

Olsen, N. S., and Bassett, J. W. (1951). *Am. J. Med.* **10,** 52.

Olson, E. B., and DeLuca, H. F. (1969). *Science* **165,** 405.

Olson, E. B., DeLuca, H. F., and Potts, J. T., Jr. (1972). *Endocrinology* **90,** 151.

Oreopoulos, D. G., Pitel, S., Husdan, H., DeVerber, G. A., and Rapoport, A. (1974). *Can. Med. Assoc. J.* **110,** 43.

O'Riordan, J. L. H., Page, J., Kerr, D. H. S., Walls, J., Moorhead, J., Crockett, R., Franz, H., and Ritz, E. (1970). *Q. J. Med.* **39,** 359.

Oxnard, S. C., O'Bell, J., and Grupe, W. E. (1974). *Pediatrics* **53,** 105.

Parfitt, A. M. (1969a). *Arch. Intern. Med.* **124,** 269.

Parfitt, A. M. (1969b). *Arch. Intern. Med.* **124,** 544.

Parfitt, A. M., Massry, S. G., Winfield, A. C., DePalma, J. R., and Gordon, A. (1971). *Am. J. Med.* **51,** 319.

Parfitt, A. M., Massry, S. G., and Winfield, A. C. (1972). *Clin. Orthop. Relat. Res.* **87,** 287.

Parker, R. F., Vergne-Marini, P., Hull, A. R., Pak, C. Y. C., and Fordtran, J. S. (1974). *J. Clin. Invest.* **54,** 358.

Pavlovitch, H., Garabedian, M., and Balsan, S. (1973). *J. Clin. Invest.* **52,** 2656.

Peacock, M., Gallagher, J. C., and Nordin, B. E. C. (1974). *Lancet* **1,** 385.

Pechet, M. M., and Hesse, R. H. (1974). *Am. J. Med.* **57,** 13.

Pellegrino, E. D., and Biltz, B. S. (1965). *Medicine (Baltimore)* **44,** 397.

Pendras, J. P. (1969). *Arch. Intern. Med.* **124,** 312.

Pendras, J. P., and Erickson, R. V. (1966). *Ann. Intern. Med.* **64,** 293.

Piazolo, P., Schleyer, M., and Franz, H. E. (1972). *Klin. Wochenschr.* **50,** 603.

Piel, C. F., Roof, B. S., and Avioli, L. V. (1973). *J. Clin. Endocrinol. Metab.* **37,** 944.

Pierides, A. M., Simpson, W., Ward, M. K., Ellis, H. A., Dewar, J. H., Kerr, D. N. S. (1976). *Lancet* **1**:1092.

Pinnell, S. R., and Martin, G. R. (1968). *Proc. Natl. Acad. Sci. U.S.A.* **61,** 708.

Platts, M. M., Grech, P., McManners, T., and Cochran, M. (1973). *Br. J. Radiol.* **46,** 585.

Pletka, P., Bernstein, D. S., Hampers, C. L., Merrill, J. P., and Sherwood, L. M. (1974). *Metab., Clin. Exp.* **23,** 619.

Popovtzer, M. M., and Robinette, J. B. (1974). *Proc. Soc. Exp. Biol. Med.* **145,** 222.

Popovtzer, M. M., Pinggera, W. F., Hutt, M. P., Robinette, J., Halgrimson, C. G., and Starzl, T. E. (1972). *J. Clin. Endocrinol. Metab.* **35,** 213.

Potts, J. T., Teitz, R. E., Deftos, L. J., Kaye, M. B., Richardson, J. A., Buckle, R. M., and Aurbach, G. D. (1969). *Arch. Intern. Med.* **124,** 408.

Preece, M. A., Tomlinson, S., Ribot, C. A., Pretrek, J., Korn, H. I., Davies, D. M., Ford, J. A., Dunnigan, M. G., and O'riordan, J. L. H. (1975). *Quart. J. Med.* **44**:575.

Prockop, D. J., and Kivirikko, K. E. (1967). *Ann. Intern. Med.* **66,** 1243.

Raisz, L. G. (1965). *Proc. Soc. Exp. Biol. Med.* **119,** 614.

Raisz, L. G., Trummel, C. L., Holick, M. F., and DeLuca, H. F. (1972a). *Science* **175,** 768.

Raisz, L., Trummel, C. L., and Simmons, H. (1972b). *Endocrinology* **90,** 744.

Read, V. H., McCaa, C. S., Bower, J. D., and McCaa, R. E. (1973). *J. Clin. Endocrinol. Metab.* **36,** 773.

Recker, R. R., and Saville, P. D. (1971). *J. Lab. Clin. Med.* **78,** 380.

Reidenberg, M. M., Haag, B. T., Channick, B. J., Shuman, C. R., and Wilson, T. G. G. (1966). *Metab. Clin. Exp.* **15,** 236.

Reiss, E. and Canterbury, J. M. (1970). Proc. Int. Congr. Nephrol. 4th, 1969, Vol. 2, p. 166.

Reiss, E., Canterbury, J. M., and Kanter, A. (1969). *Arch. Intern. Med.* **124,** 417.

Reiss, E., Canterbury, J. M., Bercovitz, M. A., and Kaplan, E. L. (1970). *J. Clin. Invest.* **49,** 2146.

Reynolds, J. J. (1973). *Hard Tissue Growth, Repair Remineralization, Ciba Found. Symp. 1972* No. 11 (new series).

Richardson, J. A., Harron, G., Reitz, R., and Layzer, R. (1969). *Ann. Intern. Med.* **71,** 129.

Ritz, E. (1970). *Z. Gesarnte Exp. Med.* **152,** 313.

Ritz, E., and Jantzen, R. (1969). *Klin. Wochenschr.* **47,** 1112.

Ritz, E., Franz, H. E., and Jajns, E. (1968). *Trans., Am. Soc. Artif. Intern. Organs* **14**, 385.
Ritz, E., Krempien, B., Riedasch, G., Kuhn, H., Hackeng, W., and Heuck, F. (1971). *Dial. Renal Transplant., Proc. Cen. Eur. Dial. Transplant Assoc., 7th, 1970* p. 131.
Ritz, E., Malluche, H. H., Roher, H. D., Krempien, B., Koch, K. M., and Andrassy, K. (1973). *Dtsch. Med. Wochenschr.* **98**, 484.
Rodgers, C. M., Fisher, J. W., and George, W. J. (1974). *Clin. Res.* **22**, 67a.
Rojkind, M., and Gutierrez, A. M. (1969). *Arch. Biochem. Biophys.* **131**, 116.
Rolle, G. K. (1969). *Calcif. Tissue Res.* **3**, 142.
Roof, B. S., Piel, C. F., Rames, L., Potter, D., and Gordan, G. S. (1974). *Pediatrics* **53**:404.
Roth, S. I., and Marshall, R. B. (1969). *Arch. Intern. Med.* **124**, 397.
Rubenstein, A. H., and Spitz, I. (1968). *Diabetes* **17**, 161.
Rucker, R. B., Parker, H. E., and Rogler, J. C. (1969). *Biochem. Biophys. Res. Commun.* **34**, 28.
Russell, J. E., and Avioli, L. V. (1972). *J. Clin. Invest.* **51**, 3072.
Russell, J. E., and Avioli, L. V. (1974). *J. Lab. Clin. Med.* **84**, 317.
Russell, J. E., and Avioli, L. V. (1975). *Kidney Int.* **7**, S-333.
Russell, J. E., Termine, J. D., and Avioli, L. V. (1973). *J. Clin. Invest.* **52**, 2848.
Russell, J. E., Avioli, L. V., and Mechanic, G. (1975). *Biochem. J.* **145**, 119.
Rutherford, W. E., Hruska, K., Blondin, J., Holick, M., DeLuca, H. F., Klahr, S., and Slatopolsky, E. (1975). *J. Clin. Endocrinol. Metab.* **40**, 13.
Sagar, S., Borra, S., and Kaye, M. (1971). *Nephron* **8**, 270.
Samaan, N. A., and Freeman, R. M. (1970). *Metab., Clin. Exp.* **19**, 102.
Sarnsethsiri, P., Jaworski, F., Shimizu, A. G., and Frost, H. M. (1969). *Arch. Pathol.* **88**, 49.
Schachter, D. (1963). *In* "The Transfer of Calcium and Strontium Across Biological Membranes" (T. J. Wasserman, ed.), p. 197. Academic Press, New York.
Schaefer, K., Schaefer, P., Poeppe, P., Opitz, A., and Hoffler, D. (1968). *Ger. Med. Mon.* **13**, 575.
Schreiner, G. E. (1975). *Kidney Int.* **7**, S-270.
Schwalbe, S. L., Betts, P. R., Rayner, P. H. and Rudd, B. T. (1977). *Brit. Med. J.* 1:679.
Schwartz, G. H., David, D. S., Riggio, R. R., Saville, P. F., Whitsell, J. C., Stenzel, K. H., and Rubin, A. L. (1970). *Am. J. Med.* **49**, 42.
Scribner, B. H., and Babb, A. L. (1975). *Kidney Int.* **7**, S-349.
Shain, S. A. (1972). *J. Biol. Chem.* **247**, 4404.
Shear, L. (1969). *J. Clin. Invest.* **48**, 1252.
Shelton, E., Yonemasu, K., and Stroud, R. M. (1972). *Proc. Natl. Acad. Sci. U.S.A.* **69**, 65.
Sherman, H. C., Gillett, L. H., and Pope, H. M. (1918). *J. Biol. Chem.* **34**, 373.
Sherrard, D. J., Baylink, D. J., Wergedal, J. E., and Maloney, N. A. (1974). *J. Clin. Endocrinol. Metab.* **39**, 119.
Siddiqui, J., and Kerr, D. H. S. (1971). *Br. Med. Bull.* **27**, 153.
Siegel, R. C., and Martin, G. R. (1970). *J. Biol. Chem.* **245**, 1653.
Siersbaek-Nielsen, K., Skovsted, L., Hansen, J. M., Kristensen, M., and Christensen, L. K. (1971). *Acta Med. Scand.* **189**, 485.
Silverberg, D. S., Ulan, R. A., Fawcett, D. M., Dossetor, J. B., Grace, M., and Bettcher, D. (1973). *Can. Med. Assoc.* **109**, 282.
Silverberg, D. S., Bettcher, K. B., Dossetor, J. B., Overton, T. R., Holick, M. F., and DeLuca, H. F. (1975). *Can. Med. Assoc.* **112**, 190.
Slatopolsky, E., Caglar, S., Pennell, J. P., Taggart, D. D., Canterbury, J. M., Reiss, E., and Bricker, N. S. (1971). *J. Clin. Invest.* **50**, 492.
Slatopolsky, E., Caglar, S., Gradowska, L., Canterbury, J., Reiss, E., and Bricker, N. S. (1972). *Kidney Int.* **2**, 147.
Smith, F. R. and Goodman, D. S. (1971). *J. Clin. Invest.* **50**, 2426.
Spanos, E., Colston, K. W., Evans, M. S., Galante, L. S., Macauley, S. J. and MacIntyre, I. (1976). *Mole. Cell. Endocrinol.* **5**:163.

Sreepada Rao, R. K., and Friedman, E. A. (1975). *Kidney Int.* **7**, 125.

Stamp, T. C. B., Round, J. M., Towe, D. J. F., and Haddad, J. G. (1972). *Br. Med. J.* **4**, 9.

Stanbury, S. W. (1966). *Ann. Intern. Med.* **65**, 1133.

Stanbury, S. W. (1967). *In* "Renal Disease" (D. A. K. Black, ed.), 2nd ed., p. 665. Davis, Philadelphia, Pennsylvania.

Stanbury, S. W., and Lumb, G. A. (1962). *Medicine (Baltimore)*, **41**, 1.

Stanbury, S. W., and Lumb, G. A. (1966). *Q. J. Med.* **35**, 1.

Stanbury, S. W., Lumb, G. A., and Nicholson, W. F. (1960). *Lancet* **1**, 793.

Stanbury, S. W., Lumb, G. A., and Mawer, E. B. (1969). *Arch. Intern. Med.* **124**, 274.

Stewart, W. K., Fleming, L. W., and Hutchinson, F. (1973). *Scott. Med. J.* **114**, 114.

Sullivan, J. F., and Eisenstein, A. B. (1970). *Am. J. Clin. Nutr.* **23**, 1339.

Swenson, R. S., Weisinger, J. R., Ruggeri, J. L., and Reaven, G. M. (1975). *Metab., Clin. Exp.* **24**, 199.

Tanaka, Y., and DeLuca, H. F. (1974a). *Science* **183**, 1198.

Tanaka, Y., and DeLuca, H. F. (1974b). *Proc. Natl. Acad. Sci. U.S.A.* **71**, 1040.

Tanaka, Y., Frank, H., and DeLuca, H. F. (1973). *Science* **181**, 564.

Tanzer, F. S., and Navia, J. M. (1973). *Nature (London), New Biol.* **242**, 221.

Tanzer, M. L., Monroe, D., and Gross, H. (1966). *Biochemistry* **5**, 1919.

Tatler, G. L. V., Baillod, R. A., Varghese, Z., Yound, W. B., Farrow, S., Wills, M. R., and Moorhead, J. F. (1973). *Br. Med. J.* **4**, 315.

Teitelbaum, S. L., Bone, J. M., Stein, P. M., Gilden, J. J., Bates, M., Boisseau, V. C., and Avioli, L. V. (1976). *J. Am. Med. Assoc.* **235**, 164.

Terman, D. S., Alfrey, A. C., Hammond, W. S., Donndelinger, T., Ogden, D. A., and Holmes, J. H. (1971). *Am. J. Med.* **50**, 744.

Termine, J. D. (1972). *Clin. Orthop. Relat. Res.* **85**, 207.

Thiele, J., Georgii, A., and Reale, E. (1974). *Klin. Wochenschr.* **52**, 444.

Tougaard, L., Sorensen, E., Brochner-Mortensen, J., Rodbro, P. and Sorensen, A. W. S. (1976). *Lancet* 1:1044.

Tsai, H. C., and Norman, A. W. (1973). *J. Biol. Chem.* **248**, 5967.

Tsai, H. C., Midgett, R. J., and Norman, A. W. (1973). *Arch. Biochem. Biophys.* **157**, 339.

Uitto, J., and Laitinen, O. (1968). *Acta Chem. Scand.* **22**, 1039.

Van Stone, J. C., Frank, D. E., and Bradford, W. R. (1977). J. Lab. Clin. Med. 89:1168.

Verberckmoes, R., Boullon, R., and Krempien, B. (1975). *Ann. Intern. Med.* **82**, 529.

Villanueva, A. R., Jaworski, Z. F., Hitt, O., Sarnsethsiri, P., and Frost, H. M. (1970). *Calcif. Tissue Res.* **20**, 288.

Wachman, A., and Bernstein, D. S. (1970). *Clin. Orthop. Relat. Res.* **69**, 252.

Walker, W. G., and Cooke, C. R. (1973). *Kidney Int.* **3**, 1.

Walter, R., and Bowman, R. H. (1973). *Endocrinology* **92**, 189.

Wells, S. A., Jr., Gunnells, J. C., Shelburne, J. D., Schneider, A. B., and Sherwood, L. M. (1975). *Surgery* **78**, 34.

Wilde, C. D., Jaworski, Z. F., Villanueva, A. R., and Frost, H. M. (1973). *Calcif. Tissue Res.* **12**, 137.

Wills, M. R., Fairney, A., Varghese, Z., Tatler, G. L. V., Baillod, R. A., and Moorhead, J. F. (1974). *Clin. Chim. Acta* **57**, 83.

Woods, J. E., Johnson, W. J., Anderson, C. F., Leary, F. J., Palumbo, P. J., Frohnert, P. P., Donadio, J. V., Jr., and DeWeerd, J. H. (1972). *Lancet* **2**, 795.

Woods, J. E., Anderson, C. F., Johnson, W. J., Donadio, J. V., Jr., Frohnert, P. P., Leary, F. J., DeWeerd, J. H., and Tashwell, H. F. (1973). *Surg., Gynecol. Obstet.* **137**, 393.

Wray, J. B., Sugarman, E. D., and Schneider, A. J. (1963). *J. Am. Med. Assoc.* **182**, 118.

Wright, A. D., Lowry, C., Russell-Fraser, T., Spitz, I. M., Rubenstein, A. H., and Bersohn, I. (1968). *Lancet* **2**, 789.

3

Hypoparathyroidism

CHARLES NAGANT DE DEUXCHAISNES AND
STEPHEN M. KRANE

I. Postoperative Hypoparathyroidism	218
A. Parathyroid Function after Operations for Hyperparathyroidism	220
B. Parathyroid Function after Thyroid Surgery	224
II. Nonsurgical Damage to the Parathyroid Glands	245
A. Radioactive Iodine Therapy	245
B. L-Asparaginase	247
C. Hemochromatosis	247
D. Metastatic Involvement of the Parathyroid Glands	248
E. Infarction of a Parathyroid Adenoma	249
F. Trauma to the Parathyroid Glands	249
G. Other Nonsurgical Damage to the Parathyroid Glands	250
III. Functional Hypoparathyroidism of Diverse Etiology in the Newborn	251
A. Early Neonatal Hypocalcemia	251
B. Late Neonatal Hypocalcemia	254
C. Primary Hypomagnesemia with Secondary Hypocalcemia	255
IV. Secondary Hypoparathyroidism Due to Hypercalcemia, with Special Reference to the Newborn Infant of a Hyperparathyroid Mother	257
V. Secondary Hypoparathyroidism Due to Hypermagnesemia	258
VI. Acquired Metabolic Resistance to Parathyroid Hormone	259
A. Hypomagnesemia	261
VII. Hypoparathyroidism Due to the Secretion of Ineffective Parathyroid Hormone	268
VIII. Idiopathic Hypoparathyroidism	269
A. Incidence	270
B. Genetic Classification of Idiopathic Hypoparathyroidism and Physiopathological Considerations	271
C. Idiopathic Hypoparathyroidism and Steatorrhea	283
D. Spasmophilia	290

217

Copyright © 1978 by Academic Press, Inc.
All rights of reproduction in any form reserved
ISBN 0-12-068702-X

IX. Pseudohypoparathyroidism and Related Disorders 296
    A. Blood Chemistries 298
    B. Incidence 303
    C. Genetics 304
    D. End-Organ Resistance to PTH 308
    E. The Adenyl Cyclase–Cyclic AMP System................. 325
    F. Special Studies in Pseudohypoparathyroidism 331
    G. Pathogenesis of Pseudohypoparathyroidism 355
    H. Special Forms of Pseudohypoparathyroidism and Related
       Conditions 367
    I. Associated Endocrinopathies 382
    J. Typical Signs of Pseudohypoparathyroidism 385
X. Signs and Symptoms of Hypocalcemia 395
    A. Neurologic Features 395
    B. Ectodermal Changes 399
    C. Dental Abnormalities 399
    D. Ocular Findings 400
    E. Cardiac Disease 401
XI. Biological Findings 402
XII. Treatment.. 405
XIII. Concluding Remarks 415
    References 415

Hypoparathyroidism is not common, yet much of our knowledge, concerning mineral ion homeostasis and skeletal metabolism in man has stemmed from studies of patients with deficient function of the parathyroid glands. The most frequent cause of hypoparathyroidism is the removal of or damage to parathyroid tissue during thyroidectomy or other neck operations. Hypoparathyroidism also occurs spontaneously in two major forms. In the first, idiopathic hypoparathyroidism, the parathyroid glands are either atrophied, absent or replaced by fat. In the second major form, pseudohypoparathyroidism, the parathyroid glands are not only present but are hyperplastic and even hyperfunctioning. Since the hormone in the latter situation is ineffective in maintaining serum calcium levels, a state mimicking hypoparathyroidism results.

In this chapter we will review in detail the clinical features, differential diagnosis and pathophysiology of the forms of hypoparathyroidism and their variants, illustrating many of the problems with our own studies. Finally, an approach to therapy will be presented.

I. POSTOPERATIVE HYPOPARATHYROIDISM

A well known hazard of neck surgery is loss of parathyroid function, either complete or partial. In the mildest degree only latent hypoparathyroidism may ensue, i.e., a condition in which parathyroid reserve is

diminished and hypoparathyroidism becomes manifest only under conditions of stress.

Loss of parathyroid function may be permanent or transient. Transient
hypoparathyroidism is probably much less frequent than is assumed. Too
often, especially in the early literature, postoperative tetany has been
equated with postoperative hypoparathyroidism. Tetany may occur postoperatively at any level of serum calcium, however, especially if there has
been a rapid fall in the serum calcium level (for example, from 10.2 to 8.7
mg/dl) or as a consequence of hyperventilation. Harrold and Wright (1966)
reported normal serum calcium values in 20% of the patients who were
symptomatic after thyroid removal, whereas in the experience of Heaton
et al. (1962), 31% of the patients symptomatic after parathyroid surgery
had an average serum calcium value of 9.7 mg/dl, with an average drop of
3.6 mg/dl. In the series of Evans et al. (1968) the incidence of normocalcemia was 71% in the patients who presented "clinical signs of calcium
deficiency" after operations for hypoparathyroidism.

In thyrotoxicosis the preoperative calcium value is on the average 0.5
mg/dl higher than in normal subjects (Adams et al., 1967) and as many as
20% of hyperthyroid patients may have abnormally elevated values (Baxter and Bondy, 1966) (Chapter 4) which sometimes require attention
(Twycross and Marks, 1970). Elevated serum calcium levels may also be
present in any malignant disease, usually as a consequence of the presence of osteolytic metastases (Chapter 6) which are characteristic of
carcinoma of the thyroid (McCormack, 1966). The incidence of bone
metastases on roentgenologic examination was 11.7% in carcinoma in
general in the series studied by Clain (1965) and 12.7% as reported by
McCormack (1966). The autopsy findings of Abrams et al. (1950)
suggested that the true incidence of bone involvement in carcinoma of the
thyroid is 3.5 times higher than the figures quoted from the examination of
roentgenograms, and indeed Silverberg et al. (1970) found skeletal metastases in 40.7% of 54 cases of thyroid carcinoma with a higher incidence in
those with medullary and follicular carcinoma. Although it does occur,
hypercalcemia associated with carcinoma of the thyroid is not seen in
more than 2% of the cases of hypercalcemia associated with malignant
diseases (Myers, 1960; Warwick et al., 1961). In these cases, serum
calcium levels may eventually diminish after operation as a consequence
of low oral calcium intake, parenteral fluid administration, parathyroid
damage, and ^{131}I therapy directed toward the eventual metastases. The
patient who had adapted to a higher level, sometimes for a long period of
time, may react to a lower (albeit normal or subnormal) serum level
postoperatively with the characteristic neuromuscular symptoms. This is
postoperative tetany but does not necessarily represent postoperative
hypoparathyroidism.

The same condition may occur in diseases in which the turnover of bone is very high. After the stimulus for elevated bone turnover is removed, high rates of bone formation may persist for long periods during the process of bone repair when excessive bone resorption and the pathological picture of osteitis fibrosa, characteristic of both hyperparathyroidism and bone involvement in hyperthyroidism (Krane *et al.*, 1956; Adams and Jowsey, 1967) has been present. The result of this may be postoperative tetany ("recalcification tetany") and although relative functional hypoparathyroidism may be present, the levels of circulating parathyroid hormone are increased rather than decreased and secondary hyperparathyroidism exists instead of postoperative hypoparathyroidism.

Conversely, the disappearance of postoperative tetany may be taken as a sign that the bone disease is healed and the hypoparathyroidism is considered "transient" when it is really "asymptomatic" or "slightly symptomatic." The vague symptoms of ill health, cramps, anxiety, depression, headaches, and mental dullness may give way at any time to tetany or hypocalcemic seizures, sometimes presenting as overt epilepsy. Ectodermal manifestations including cataracts may also occur. Seldom does this situation cause death although it may do so indirectly through cardiac abnormalities and severe mental depression which may lead to suicide (Painter, 1960; Hellström and Ivemark, 1962; Watkins *et al.*, 1962; Alveryd, 1968; Nicholson, 1969).

A. Parathyroid Function after Operations for Hyperparathyroidism

Postoperative tetany, overt or latent, is extremely frequent after operations for hyperparathyroidism. Chvostek's sign is rarely absent, although in one series full-blown tetany developed in only 3 patients out of 68 (Pyrah *et al.*, 1966), one of whom suffered laryngeal spasm. Tetany usually appears on the second to fifth postoperative day, occasionally later. Analysis of the postoperative data provided by Heaton *et al.* (1962) shows that in the cases without tetany (5 out of 18) the average serum calcium drop was 2.9 mg/dl and the lowest average serum calcium value reached was 9.6 mg/dl. The average values were 3.0 and 9.3 mg/dl respectively in the cases of transient paresthesias only, 3.3 and 8.7 mg/dl in the cases of transient minimal tetany, 3.7 and 8.2 mg/dl in the cases of transient mild tetany, and 5.3 and 8.0 mg/dl in the case of transient frank tetany. From these data one gains the impression that as a greater negative correlation develops between the drop in serum calcium and the value of the lowest serum calcium reached, there is a systematic progression in the severity of the symptoms.

The incidence and severity of the symptoms will depend essentially on the degree of preoperative bone involvement, which is present roentgenologically in one third (Dent, 1962; Hellström and Ivemark, 1962; Borowy, 1969) to one fourth (Riddick and Reiss, 1962; Coffey *et al.*, 1965; Purnell *et al.*, 1971) of the cases. Tetany developed in all the patients with bone involvement in the series of McGeown (1965), and in the series of Hellström and Ivemark (1962) the serum calcium fell below 8.0 mg/dl in the two weeks following operation in 52% of the cases with bone involvement (as shown radiographically) versus 5% in cases without skeletal disease. The incidence remained 24% versus 6% respectively after a period of at least one year. The striking difference between the two groups is related to three factors. The first involves the "hungry bones" or repair syndrome which develops only in patients with bone involvement and may last from several weeks to several months up to two years (see Chapter 1).

The second factor accounting for the difference in postoperative serum calcium values is the much greater incidence of renal glomerular failure in the group with bone involvement as compared with the group without this feature: 71% versus 17%, respectively, according to Hellström and Ivemark (1962) and 56% versus 7% according to Dent (1962). This complication may be responsible *per se* for persistent hypocalcemia. In the experience of Hellström and Ivemark (1962) about half of the patients with bone involvement and persistent low serum calcium values after more than a year suffered from renal failure.

The third factor contributing to hypocalcemia in patients with bone involvement is postoperative development of hypomagnesemia concurrently with hypocalcemia, which aggravates the neuromuscular irritability. In one series postoperative hypomagnesemia occurred in 18 of the 28 patients with adequate data for analysis (Pratley *et al.*, 1973). In some cases postoperative hypocalcemia can only be corrected by magnesium administration (Davies and Friedman, 1966), although in the absence of magnesium supplements the serum calcium may return to normal before the serum magnesium changes, especially if hypomagnesemia is not too severe.

In patients with bone disease and postoperative hypomagnesemia and hypocalcemia, convulsions have been described resulting in femoral neck and/or pelvic fractures (Davies and Friedman, 1966). To prevent these complications some recommend preoperative calciferol or dihydrotachysterol therapy (Jackson and Dancaster, 1962; Davies and Friedman, 1966). In other instances personality disturbances have been described with hallucinations, behavioral disturbances, or serious depression (Vincent *et al.*, 1962; Newton and Sumick, 1968). When corrective surgery was delayed (not an unusual decision years ago), patients died because of "complete exhaustion" on the twentieth (Beck, 1928) or the seventy-fifth

(Mandl, 1933) postoperative day. In a more recent report, death on the fifth postoperative day was ascribed to unrecognized hypomagnesemia (Nicholson, 1969).

The incidence of permanent true postoperative hypoparathyroidism in patients with primary hyperparathyroidism can be fully appreciated only in those cases without renal insufficiency in which sufficient time has elapsed for skeletal remineralization. In the series of Hellström and Ivemark (1962), about 6% of patients without bone involvement presented with serum calcium levels lower than 8.0 mg/dl after more than one year postoperatively. In most series insufficient data are available to ascertain the true incidence of permanent hypoparathyroidism. Some authors apparently did not encounter this complication (Blalock, 1971), whereas others report figures of 2% (Pratley *et al.*, 1973), 4% (Evans *et al.*, 1968), 5% (Thorén and Werner, 1969), 7% (Borowy, 1969), 8% (Paloyan *et al.*, 1969), 11% (Heaton *et al.*, 1962), and 12.5% (Preisman and Mehnert, 1971). In McGeown's experience (1965), 6.7% of the patients with preoperative bone involvement remained hypoparathyroid. The paucity of data concerning permanent postoperative hypoparathyroidism in patients with primary hyperparathyroidism is surprising in view of the abundant literature on the medical and surgical aspects of this disease. Although changes in circulating calcium in the immediate postoperative period have been well described, relatively little information exists concerning the later course in these patients except in those cases where recurrence of the disease has attracted attention.

Clearly several factors influence the development of postoperative hypoparathyroidism. The difficulty and duration of surgical procedure and the routine biopsy of normal glands is obviously contributory in this regard. The more extensive the operation, the less chance there is to leave residual parathyroid tissue intact. Moreover with primary parathyroid hyperplasia most of the parathyroid tissue will have to be removed, leaving, for example, only 30 to 50 mg of tissue (Paloyan *et al.*, 1969) for continuing parathyroid function (Chapter 1).

One must also consider changing trends in the surgical approach to primary hyperparathyroidism. In the past this was often conservative, as described by Cope (1960), who removed an amount of abnormal parathyroid tissue roughly proportional to the severity of the disease. If an adenoma of sufficient size was found, the operation was terminated. If hyperplasia was identified during the operation and one gland was small, it might have been left behind with only a small fragment removed for identification (Cope, 1960). This policy usually minimized the complications of permanent hypoparathyroidism but resulted in a certain number of reoperations, as was the case for four of Cope's patients (1966). The first step toward a more aggressive attitude was complete exploration of all the parathyroid glands, both normal and abnormal, in the search for possible multiple adenomas, a practice performed by many surgeons (Adams and Murphy, 1963; Coffey et al., 1965; Judd et al., 1966; Haff et al., 1970). Subsequently, because of continued problems in those patients with recurrent or persistent disease after a simple operation (accounting in some series for 3% (Bruining, 1971), 4% (Purnell et al., 1971), and 15% (Paloyan et al., 1969)) "near-total" parathyroidectomy was systematically performed (Paloyan et al., 1969), i.e., excision or biopsy of all parathyroid glands, leaving behind as little as 30 to 50 mg of tissue. Although this policy was successful in drastically reducing recurrence or persistence of the disease, the incidence of permanent hypoparathyroidism was, of course, greater (Paloyan et al., 1969; Bruining, 1971; Johansson and Segerström, 1972) than that observed with more conservative surgical procedures.

The number of cases of permanent postoperative hypoparathyroidism has been increased by the performance of total parathyroidectomy in cases of secondary or "tertiary" hyperparathyroidism related to azotemic renal osteodystrophy (Felts et al., 1965; Davies and Friedman, 1966; Ogg, 1967; Fine et al., 1970; Esselstyn and Popowniak, 1971; Gordon et al., 1972), as recommended by Berson and Yalow (1967); subtotal parathyroidectomy is performed with increasing frequency in these situations unless long-term dialysis is anticipated (Pendras, 1969; Buck and Robertson, 1971; Esselstyn and Popowniak, 1971) (see Chapter 2). The same policy of total parathyroidectomy has been advocated in cases of primary chief cell hyperplasia as well (Adams et al., 1965; Block et al., 1967). However, all do not agree with the radical approach (Chapter 1). Finally, one must always consider the operative skill and experience of the surgeon, his ability to recognize (with as little delay as possible) abnormal parathyroid tissue and to avoid disturbing the vascular supply of residual parathyroid tissue.

The incidence of transient hypoparathyroidism cannot be defined exactly in the absence of sensitive and specific determinations of circulating, biologically active parathyroid hormone levels. In the series of Borowy (1969) 3 of 28 patients developed "hypoparathyroidism with tetany, the symptoms being mild, requiring no treatment." This does not indicate that 11% of these patients had transient hypoparathyroidism. It only reflects the highest possible figure for this complication in this series. From the data of Hellström and Ivemark (1962) where 5% of the operated cases without bone involvement had hypocalcemia during the two weeks after operation versus 6% of the same group on follow-up after more than one year, it would appear that true transient hypoparathyroidism is relatively uncommon. The reason why detailed and long-term postoperative observations are so rare is that immediate and often inappropriate therapy for hypocalcemia makes it difficult to follow the natural history of postoperative biological events.

That transient hypoparathyroidism may occur after removal of hyperfunctioning parathyroid tissue has been shown in cases in which the level of immuno reactive hormone has dropped to undetectable levels after a few hours or days (Berson and Yalow, 1967 and 1968; Buckle, 1969). Residual parathyroid tissue is more likely to be atrophic if the preoperative serum calcium has been high for a long period of time. That this actually occurs was shown by the studies performed by Black (1969) on the remaining glands which were biopsied during an operation in which a parathyroid adenoma was removed. On light microscopy the glands showed abundant fat with widely separated trabeculae of small chief cells. The ultrastructure on electron microscopy confirmed the impression of atrophic or inactive tissue. The cells contained large quantities of lipid, the Golgi apparatus was poorly developed, and rough surfaced endoplasmic reticulum was reduced to a few scattered dilated profiles; secretory granules were not present in most cells. These observations confirm those made by Roth and Munger (1962) in their studies on the rim or remnant of normal parenchyma around functional adenomas. Although these observations represent indirect evidence of glandular hypofunction, there is good correlation between morphological structure and parathyroid function in animals under experimental or pathological conditions characterized by chronic hypocalcemia or hypercalcemia (Capen et al., 1968). How long it takes for these hypoactive glands to resume their normal function after months and (more often) years of inhibition is not known.

B. Parathyroid Function after Thyroid Surgery

The problem of hypoparathyroidism complicating thyroid surgery, especially as manifested by tetany, has attracted attention ever since Wölfler (1879) and Weiss (1881 and 1883) reported the first cases in Billroth's Clinic in Vienna. It has been the subject of numerous reports, in contrast to the lack of papers devoted solely to this complication following operations for hyperparathyroidism. Excellent historical accounts of the early literature have been compiled by Welsh (1898a), Delore and Alamartine (1910), Jeandelize (1902), and Morel (1912). Although the parathyroid glands had been well described and identified by Sandström in 1880, their role in the etiology of postoperative tetany was not understood until the experimental work of Gley (1891), who showed that thyroparathyroidectomy and not thyroidectomy alone was necessary for tetany to occur. Uncertainty about the number of parathyroid glands and their function was finally resolved by the work of Kohn (1895), Vassale and Generali (1896a and 1896b) and Erdheim (1906). The biochemical hallmarks of hypoparathyroidism were identified when MacCallum and Voegtlin (1909) showed that hypocalcemia was the underlying basis of postoperative tetany and again when Greenwald (1913) reported hyperphosphatemia associated with hypocalcemia.

It is reasonable to use the term postoperative hypoparathyroidism in the cases where hypocalcemia with or without varying characteristic symptoms (among which tetany is the most common) follows thyroid surgery. Such simplification is unjustified, however, when the hypocalcemia is transient (lasting for days, weeks, or months) and the underlying disorder has been thyrotoxicosis. Many authors report that tetany is more frequent after thyroid surgery for hyperthyroidism than for other thyroid maladies (Delore and Alamartine, 1910; Lachmann, 1941; Cattell, 1949; Bartels, 1952; Wijnbladh, 1952; Beahrs *et al.*, 1956; Painter, 1960; Wade, 1960; Krane, 1961; Murley and Peters, 1961; Michie *et al.*, 1965; Wade *et al.*, 1965a; Blondeau *et al.*, 1973). There is also evidence that hyperthyroidism may be associated with high bone turnover, as shown by kinetic studies after the administration of ^{45}Ca (Krane *et al.*, 1956), by the determination of total hydroxyproline output in the urine (Dull and Henneman, 1963; Kivirikko *et al.*, 1965; Uitto *et al.*, 1967), histomorphometric studies on bone specimens (Adams *et al.*, 1967; Bordier *et al.*, 1967; Bianchi *et al.*, 1972), as well as by the existence of slightly elevated serum alkaline phosphatase levels (Nielsen, 1952; Cook *et al.*, 1959; Cassar and Joseph, 1969; Michie *et al.*, 1971; Siersbaek-Nielsen *et al.*, 1971; Bianchi *et al.*, 1972). Therefore when thyrotoxic patients are subjected to subtotal thyroidectomy, hypocalcemia may ensue. As noted for patients subjected to parathyroid surgery, the hypocalcemia results from rapid bone repair where the rate of bone formation exceeds that of bone resorption. Hypocalcemia following thyroid surgery which results from rapid bone repair is not unusual since the usual period of preoperative antithyroid drug treatment which renders the patient euthyroid is insufficient to restore bone turnover to normal for periods which may last for 6 months (Siersbaek-Nielsen *et al.*, 1971) up to 2 years (Fraser *et al.*, 1960).

The following observation by one of us (C.N.) is pertinent to these considerations. A 60-year-old woman developed sudden hyperthyroidism in June, 1970. The diagnosis was established at the end of July, and the patient was treated with methimazole in high doses. On July 28, her serum protein-bound iodine level was 12.0 μg/dl and on August 18, it had dropped to 4.4 μg/dl (T_3 resin uptake at that time: 27.3%). Because of a high serum calcium (11.1 mg/dl) and alkaline phosphatase (95 U/liter) discovered on August 18, she was studied further in September. At that time she had been treated for 6 weeks and had been clinically and chemically euthyroid for 1 month. The serum calcium had not yet normalized (10.4 mg/dl) and despite low values for thyroid function (serum P.B.I. : 2.0 μg/dl; T_3 resin uptake : 23.8%; serum T_4 : 0.7 μg/dl), the serum alkaline phosphatase (90 U/liter) and urinary excretion of total hydroxyproline (88 mg/24 h) were still elevated. She was treated further with decreasing doses of methimazole. In November, after 3 months of correction of hyperthyroidism, her serum calcium was still 10.5 mg/dl. The patient was restudied in January 1971. At that time she had been euthyroid and eventually hypothyroid for 5 months. While she was clinically hypothyroid the serum calcium level had finally normalized (9.9 mg/dl), but the alkaline phosphatase level was still elevated (79 U/liter), as was the urinary excretion of total hydroxyproline (52 mg/24 h). Thus, bone turnover had not yet normalized. The immunoreactive parathyroid hormone level in this patient was normal (185 pg bovine parathyroid hormone equivalent per ml) as determined according to the method of Lequin *et al.* (1970).

With this in mind it should be recognized that when thyroid function in thyrotoxicosis is suppressed radically as is the case after subtotal thyroidectomy, "recalcification tetany" associated with bone repair may occur and the accompanying hypocalcemia may not reflect hypoparathyroidism. On the contrary, such a state should be accompanied by secondary *hyper*parathyroidism if the parathyroid glands are responsive.

What the exact frequency may be of postoperative hypocalcemia ascribable to bone repair is unknown. Cases which exemplify this condition may be found in reports of Dent and Harper (1958), Krane (1961), and Michie *et al.* (1971). The latter authors stress the very early appearance of hypocalcemia and tetany in their 28 affected patients; two had tetany within 24 hours of operation and a further 10 required supplementary calcium within the first postoperative day, as compared with a later onset of symptoms and hypocalcemia (a few days) when parathyroid glands are removed in diseases associated with normal bone turnover. It is Kurth's opinion (1972) that tetany occurring within 10 hours after surgery characterizes the "hungry bone" phenomenon as compared with a time lag of usually 24 to 48 hours for tetany arising from lack of parathyroid hormone. Cattell (1953) felt that if tetanic and related symptoms developed before the third postoperative day, they were not due to parathyroid insufficiency. In the cases described above, hypocalcemia would be expected to be transient. These may be examples of cases of so-called "delayed recovery" or "late reversion" of postoperative "hypoparathyroidism," which have intrigued several workers (Lachmann, 1941; Watkins *et al.*, 1962; McNeill and Thomson, 1968; Parfitt, 1972a).

Children and adolescents comprise another group of patients in whom bone turnover is increased prior to surgery. If thyrotoxicosis supervenes, antithyroid drugs will at most correct the fraction of the increase in turnover rate owing to this disease (unless myxedema develops). Thus these patients have two reasons for high calcium "avidity" of the skeleton. Hypocalcemia (6.0–8.2 mg/dl) and tetany occurred in 17% of such young patients, the condition being noticed "most frequently on the second day" after surgery in a report by Saxena *et al.* (1964). These results were not confirmed by Reeve *et al.* (1969). In the series described by Michie *et al.* (1971) the highest incidence of hypocalcemia was found in the youngest patients, those in their third decade (37% versus an overall incidence of 18%). The same incidence at that age group has been noted by Parfitt (1971). There is still some growth continuing in the beginning of the third decade and the daily output of total urinary hydroxyproline is on the average higher in this decade as compared with values obtained in older subjects (Jones *et al.*, 1964; Anderson *et al.*, 1965; Eisinger *et al.*, 1969).

Theoretically one should be able to distinguish postoperative bone repair from hypoparathyroidism by serum phosphate levels which are low in the former condition and elevated in the latter. Unfortunately, serum phosphate levels are seldom given in the series in which postoperative hypoparathyroidism has been reviewed. Difficulty arises when the serum phosphate level is normal, a condition compatible with a certain degree of parathyroid deficiency (serum calcium in the range of 7.5–8.5 mg/dl, Parfitt, 1972a) as well as with a certain amount of bone healing. Furthermore, the two conditions may be associated and produce a state in which the serum calcium shows a late tendency to rise though normal levels are never reached.

Whatever the reason for thyroid surgery, transient tetany may appear postoperatively in about two-thirds of patients, or there may be vague symptoms of neuromuscular irritability (tingling, muscle cramps, or numbness) in as many as 90% of the cases (Buckwalter *et al.*, 1955). Unless the condition is severe, the symptoms will disappear so that the great majority of patients—some authors say almost all (Painter, 1960)—are practically symptomless three months after operation. The appearance of these symptoms does not necessarily mean that hypocalcemia is present, although a slight fall in the serum calcium is the rule postoperatively; conversely if hypocalcemia does exist, the disappearance of symptoms does not necessarily mean that the situation has corrected itself. The incidence of tetany is highly variable according to the series and depends on the definition of the condition. The lowest incidence (0.2%) is that reported in a series of 13,000 patients (Swinton, 1937) and probably relies on postoperative tetany as reported in the patients' records. In several series serum calcium levels were determined only when patients presented typical symptoms related to postoperative tetany; under such conditions hypocalcemia appeared in 3.7% of the patients described by Michie *et al.* (1965). In the same center, when serial postoperative serum calcium determinations were made routinely and "hypoparathyroidism" was diagnosed on biochemical and/or clinical suspicion "stringently sought" (for example, paresthesias only), the incidence rose from 3.7 to 13% (Michie *et al.*, 1965). If the cases displaying simple paresthesias without abnormal calcium values are omitted, the incidence of the latter falls to 8.4%. All these figures are open to question since the definition of "low serum calcium level" itself varies widely. In the series just quoted the lower limit was 8.0 mg/dl and in the tables from that report 6 of 13 patients with "paresthesias only" had recorded serum calcium levels between 8.0 and 8.4 mg/dl, values which most authors would consider "low" by any method used. If these patients are included, the incidence of postoperative hypocalcemia becomes 10.4%. Therefore one obtains, according to the definition adopted, incidences of 3.7, 8.4, 10.4 and 13% in the same center. In contrast, Jones and Fourman (1963b) consider serum calcium levels below 8.9 mg/dl as abnormally low. For these reasons no attempt will be made to establish the exact incidence of hypocalcemia and/or related symptoms after thyroid surgery in this review. However, it must be emphasized that thyroid surgery may alter parathyroid function, permanently or transiently, and at times severely. Definite, permanent hypoparathyroidism may be assumed to exist either if hypocalcemia (with or, more often, without symptoms) persists or if normocalcemia can be maintained only with therapy (consisting of calcium supplements and/or vitamin D or analogs) after a sufficient time postoperatively to assume that the situation will not revert itself or that the hypocalcemia is not the result of skeletal remineralization. This time period has usually been considered one year (Buckwalter *et al.*, 1955; Wade, 1960; Freeman, 1970) or longer (Wade *et al.*, 1965a; Dimich *et al.*, 1967). As cited earlier it may take 2–3 years for bone turnover to return to normal in thyrotoxic patients after corrective surgery.

Using the above criteria and if one excludes the series devoted solely to surgery for malignant diseases, the incidence of this complication varies from zero (Rose, 1963) with an average interval of 10 years between operation and follow-up, to 22% (Jones and Fourman, 1963b), based on systematic retrospective serum calcium determinations performed more than three years after operation. In Lachmann's follow-up series (1941) performed on 213 patients more than three years after surgery for toxic goiter, hypoparathyroidism was detected in 5, an incidence of 2.3%. In two of these patients hypocalcemia was extremely severe (5.5–6.5 mg/dl). In the series reported by Iversen *et al.* (1957), 1.1% of the 442 patients operated on for thyrotoxicosis and reviewed after an average period of 9.2 years (4–14 years) remained under treatment for hypocalcemia or related symptoms, whereas 3.6% of the remaining patients had a serum calcium level between 8.0 and 8.9 mg/dl. Davis *et al.* (1961) reviewed 80 patients who had undergone thyroidectomy on the average 10 years previously: 2.5% were found to be hypocalcemic. John and Wills (1964) found hypocalcemia (<8.5 mg/dl) in 1.9% of the patients who underwent sub-total thyroidectomy for thyrotoxicosis or nodular goiter more than three years prior to their study. It should be noticed that in the latter two surveys the low serum calcium values never fell below 8.0 mg/dl. The review by Painter (1960) of 172 patients operated on for toxic goiter after an average interval of 4.3 years does not quite match the criteria set for an optimum review, since some cases were restudied less than 18 months after surgery, and the interval since operation is not given individually for the patients who presented with hypocalcemia. There are very few retro-spective systematic studies that offer sufficient follow-up periods (without overlap with a postoperative period) of at least two or three years.

1. Causes and determining factors of postoperative hypoparathyroidism

All degrees of parathyroid insufficiency may develop as a consequence of thyroid surgery, from complete absence of parathyroid secretion to latent hypoparathyroidism, a condition in which parathyroid function is clearly insufficient only under conditions of hypocalcemic stress. The outcome depends on the degree of damage to the blood supply of the parathyroid glands which may function more or less as autogenous grafts. This view has been reemphasized by Parfitt (1972a) who showed that unlike the situation in idiopathic (congenital) hypoparathyroidism, there is a continuous spectrum of serum calcium values among the postoperative cases from the very lowest levels, such as are found in idiopathic cases, up to the lower limit of normal and within the normal range as well.

Although explicitly mentioned as a cause of postoperative hypopara-thyroidism by some authors (Cattell, 1953; Kyle *et al.*, 1954) almost all agree that inadvertent partial parathyroidectomy is not an important fac-tor in the pathogenesis of this complication (Lachmann, 1941; Watkins *et al.*, 1962; Girling and Murley, 1963; Turunen and Saxén, 1963; Michie *et al.*, 1965; Wade *et al.*, 1965b). The early work of Welsh (1898b) showed that removal of 3 out of 4 parathyroid glands in the cat never led to hypoparathyroidism, and in the previous section it was pointed out that even subtotal parathyroidectomy does not necessarily lead to permanent hypoparathyroidism. Inadvertent parathyroidectomy has been reported in 4% (Wade, 1965b) and 8.7% (Michie et al., 1965) of the cases. These are clearly minimal figures, the exact incidence depending upon the zeal of the pathologist in looking carefully for parathyroid tissue within the material removed at operation, as shown by Murley and Peters (1961).

There has been more emphasis on the importance of sparing the blood supply to the parathyroid glands during thyroid operations. Halsted and Evans (1907) stated: "It is in the control of hemorrhage that we sacrifice the parathyroid glandules" and demonstrated that the parathyroids were each supplied by one single parathyroid artery entering at the hilus and arising from the inferior thyroid artery or from the anastomosing channel between the inferior and superior thyroid vessels. These observations have been confirmed by the more recent anatomical study of Mauro (1950).

Routine ligation of the inferior thyroid arteries has been blamed both in the early literature (Halsted and Evans, 1907; Pool, 1907; Delore and Alamartine, 1910; de Quervain, 1923) and more recently (Keynes, 1963; Chamberlin et al., 1964; Blondeau et al., 1973). Careful studies have completely discarded this factor as an aggravating event (Cattell, 1953; Kalliomäki et al., 1961b; Lange, 1963; Michie et al., 1965), owing to the numerous anastomoses existing between the branches of these arteries and the esophageal and tracheal arteries. On the contrary, Wade et al. (1965b) have advocated this procedure in order to reduce the bleeding in the operative field and therefore the number of sutures that have to be used. It is part of the surgical routine in the most recent descriptions of the operative technique (Freeman, 1970).

Hypocalcemia may result from two types of interference with the blood supply of the parathyroid glands (Michie et al., 1965). The first type is due to "congestion" of the thyroid remnant and is transient by definition. This would account for the frequent transitory fall (albeit seldom to very abnormal values) in serum calcium levels postoperatively with restoration after a period of 7–14 days. The second type would result from definite damage to the end-artery of the parathyroid glands, their sole source of blood supply. In this case hypocalcemia would be more or less severe but, as a rule, permanent. The parathyroid glands would function as autogenous implants with little chance of compensatory hypertrophy since adequate vascularization seems necessary for this to occur. A third theoretically possible mechanism is damage to the nerve supply of the parathyroid vessels. Adrenergic fibers, which have been studied by

Yeghiayan *et al.* (1972) may play a crucial role not only in the control of parathyroid gland blood flow but also possibly in the physiological regulation of parathyroid hormone secretion itself (Fischer *et al.*, 1973). If the vascularity of the parathyroid glands is particularly vulnerable to trauma resulting in ischemia of the glands, it is important to determine those factors which are likely to increase this possibility.

It seems that the most important factors in sparing the blood supply of the parathyroid glands are the surgical technique itself, the skill and the experience of the surgeon, the difficulties encountered at the operation, the extent of the operation to be performed, and the number of operations sustained by any one gland, all elements that may be critical in the final outcome of parathyroid function.

The importance of the surgical technique is illustrated by the results of modifying the operative procedure to protect the parathyroid glands during surgery as a result of a high rate of postoperative hypoparathyroidism in Cardiff. There was a dramatic diminution of this complication: 4% (Wade *et al.*, 1965b) versus at least 28% (Jones and Fourman, 1963b), a sevenfold reduction defined on the basis of EDTA tests (cf. infra). The most important single factor that these authors were able to pinpoint which correlated closely to the development of postoperative (latent) hypoparathyroidism was the number of ligatures and sutures close to the parathyroid glands that were needed to achieve hemostasis during the operation.

Second, it is obvious that experienced surgeons, as pointed out by Parfitt (1971) and Blondeau *et al.* (1973), do have fewer complications than their inexperienced colleagues. Parfitt (1971) showed that there were more surgeons performing fewer thyroid operations so that the number of operations performed each year by each surgeon had been steadily decreasing from an average of 18 to an average of 5 over the two decades of his survey. Paralleling this trend, the overall incidence of postoperative tetany had increased by a factor of almost five, from 0.8% (1944–1964) to 3.8% (1964–1969). He also demonstrated that for any single surgeon, the critical number of operations seemed to be about 100–125; a seven-fold decrease in postoperative tetany was noticed when approximately this number of operations had been performed.

Third, the extent of the operation and the underlying disorder play a very important role as well. If the operation is performed for thyrotoxicosis, not only are transient tetany and hypocalcemia more frequent, but also the incidence of permanent hypoparathyroidism increases by a factor or two (Wijnbladh, 1952) to nine (Beahrs *et al.*, 1956). One reason why permanent hypoparathyroidism is more frequent after operations for toxic goiter is the higher vascularity of the goitrous tissue as compared with nontoxic goiters. This requires the use of more hemostatic ligatures and sutures which may compromise the blood supply to the parathyroid glands. Several authors have noticed an increase in post-operative tetany when preoperative treatment with antithyroid medications was introduced, and suggested that the medications rendered the thyroid gland even more vascular and friable (Cattell, 1949; Michie *et al.*, 1965).

Besides the quality and vascularity of the thyroid tissue the amount to be removed is also a factor of paramount importance. Painter (1960) did not record a single case of permanent hypoparathyroidism after "partial" thyroidectomy (removal of ⅞ of the gland), versus an incidence of 13% when "subtotal" thyroidectomy (leaving a thin button of thyroid tissue on each side) was performed. Parfitt (1971) also was unable to find any case of postoperative tetany after hemithyroidectomy, versus an incidence of 0.7% after partial thyroidectomy and of 2.4% after radical subtotal thyroidectomy. Block *et al.* (1966) recorded no permanent hypoparathyroidism after subtotal thyroidectomy, whereas total thyroidectomy for thyroid carcinoma resulted in a 9% incidence of permanent hypoparathyroidism. These authors point out that this incidence essentially depends on the extent of dissection and the care taken in dissections in both tracheoesophageal groove regions. When bilateral removal of the lymph nodes involved in the metastatic process was performed, the incidence of permanent hypoparathyroidism was 44%. Similarly, Beahrs and Pasternak (1969) record permanent tetany in 0.3% of their cases after conservative surgical procedures, 4% after "total" thyroidectomy, and "40% or more" after extensive radical thyroidectomy.

Surgery for carcinoma of the thyroid represents a particular challenge to the parathyroid glands. The incidence of permanent hypoparathyroidism following "total" thyroidectomy is alarmingly high in all series: 12.8% (Clark *et al.*, 1966), 26.7% (Hardin and Hardy, 1971), 27% (McKenzie, 1971). Hardin and Hardy (1971) observed that since the adoption of a conservative policy of total lobectomy on the involved side and radical subtotal lobectomy on the contralateral side, the incidence of hypoparathyroidism has fallen from 26.7% (total thyroidectomy with or without various degrees of associated radical neck dissection) to zero. If even more extensive neck surgery accompanied by mediastinal dissection is performed, with removal of the "total thyroid and parathyroid complex" (as well as any eventual accessory parathyroid tissue) for such diseases as recurrent stomal carcinoma, post-cricoid and cervical esophagus carcinoma, as well as advanced thyroid carcinoma, permanent hypoparathyroidism may ensue in as many as 74% of the cases (Sisson and Vander Aarde, 1971). It is therefore not surprising that the incidence of hypoparathyroidism is correlated with the incidence of vocal cord paralysis (Ranke and Holinger, 1955; Iversen *et al.*, 1957; Shearman *et al.*, 1965; McNeill and Thomson, 1968). It seems obvious that a safe *in vivo* staining procedure for the parathyroid glands is needed for parathyroid gland identification. Experiments with toluidene blue (Klopper and Moe, 1966; Hurvitz *et al.*, 1968; Singleton and Allums, 1970; Skjoldborg and Nielsen, 1971; Tardy and Tenta, 1971) have been less than satisfactory in this regard. Finally, the risk of permanent hypoparathyroidism is also considerably higher after recurrent ("secondary") operations (Boothby *et al.*, 1931; Lachmann, 1941; Cattell, 1953; Wade, 1960; Jones and Fourman, 1963a), with the incidence of tetany increasing by a factor of four (Bell and Bartels, 1951). Bartels (1952) points out that 25% of his patients with permanent tetany and 33% of those with transient tetany had previous thyroidectomy for toxic goiters. In Swinton's huge series (1937), 38% of the cases of both transient and permanent tetany followed recurrent operations which constituted some 20% of all operations performed. The same is true for other complications including vocal cord paralysis (Shearman *et al.*, 1965).

In addition to those factors discussed above, there are a few others of importance. One of the most quoted is sex distribution, with females far outranking males with regard to the incidence of postoperative complications (Boothby *et al.*, 1931; Swinton, 1937; Lachmann, 1941; Bertelsen and Bruun, 1947; Ranke and Holinger, 1955; Turunen and Saxén, 1963; Shearman *et al.*, 1965; and Parfitt, 1967a and 1971). Only the series of Buckwalter *et al.* (1955) and O'Malley and Kohler (1968) contain any number of affected males (7 versus 43 females and 4 versus 39 females, respectively). However, in most series the proportion of females to males undergoing thyroidectomy [9:1, Lachmann (1941); 5:1, Bertelsen and Bruun (1947); 7:1 Parfitt (1971); 9:1, Painter (1960); 12:1, Rose (1963); and 13:1, McNeill and Thomson (1968)], and therefore at risk, is such that the sex ratio of postoperative complications cannot be considered of significance. In the past when lower sex ratios were reported [3:1, Boothby *et al.* (1931) and 4:1, Swinton (1937)], too much emphasis was placed on postoperative symptoms rather than on long term systemic postoperative serum calcium determinations. It is possible that females present more symptoms than males after this type of operation. So-called "idiopathic tetany" or "spasmophilia" often of psychoneurotic origin is a disease affecting females almost exclusively. When more males are liable to be at risk than females, such as in extensive neck surgery for all kinds of carcinomatous processes, the reverse proportion may actually be observed. In the series studied by Sisson and Vander Aarde (1971) 9 males versus 1 female suffered permanent hypoparathyroidism.

The last factor that has been blamed by some authors as either causative (Watkins *et al.*, 1962) or contributory (Wade *et al.*, 1965a) to postoperative hypoparathyroidism is aggressive, postoperative medical treatment "artificially" correcting the serum calcium level and therefore not allowing the remaining parathyroid tissue to hypertrophy since the stimulus for its function has been suppressed. Whereas withholding calcium replacement therapy temporarily so that compensatory hypertrophy of the parathyroid glands appears reasonable (Wade *et al.*, 1965a), measures designed to elevate the serum calcium postoperatively do not necessarily result in permanent hypoparathyroidism as contended by Watkins *et al.* (1962). In hyperparathyroid patients, prolonged inhibition of parathyroid function in the non-adenomatous glands does not prevent the latter from resuming their activity once an adenoma has been removed.

2. Natural History of Postoperative Hypoparathyroidism

As a general rule, the serum calcium falls after an operation on the thyroid gland. Lachmann (1941) recorded an average fall of 1.2 mg/dl after surgery for *toxic goiters* in 140 out of 144 patients with a nadir usually observed after one to two days. In 14% of the cases the serum calcium value fell below 9.0 mg/dl (which Lachmann considered abnormal) and in half of these cases the values had returned above this level prior to discharge from the hospital. The fall in serum calcium averaged 0.5 mg/dl in patients with *non-toxic goiters* and in only 4.5% of 44 cases did the value drop to abnormal levels.

With the exception of Lange (1963), most authors confirm this systemic fall although not of the magnitude indicated by Lachmann (1941). From the tables of Wade *et al.* (1965b), it can be computed that in 50 consecutive patients who underwent subtotal thyroidectomy for simple or toxic goiter (in a ratio of 3 to 1), the serum calcium, measured on the fifth postoperative day, fell on the average by 0.6 mg/dl although it returned to preoperative levels 3 months later. In 30% of the patients the serum level fell below 8.9 mg/dl; only 4% remained below this value after 3 months. John *et al.* (1966), studying 34 patients prior to and after subtotal thyroidectomy for toxic and non-toxic goiter (in a ratio of one to one), found an average fall of 0.5 mg/dl on the first postoperative day (18% of values lower than 8.5 mg/dl), the same average value on the seventh postoperative day, and a complete restoration to initial values after 6 weeks (yet still 12% of the values were lower than 8.5 mg/dl). Two of the patients who were hypocalcemic after this period of time were restudied after one year: one remained hypocalcemic (7.9 mg/dl), the other had apparently recovered (from 8.0 to 8.7 mg/dl). Simultaneously, these authors studied serum calcium levels after operations not involving the thyroid gland. The slight fall (0.3 mg/dl) detected on the first postoperative day did not reach statistical significance and had completely disappeared on the seventh postoperative day. Michie *et al.* (1965) also followed a group of patients with nonthyroid operations who had no change in serum calcium value at any time postoperatively. Suzuki *et al.* (1968) ascribed the significant fall of serum calcium during thyroid operations, which reached its lowest level within one hour after the beginning of the manipulation of the gland, to release of calcitonin during the operation. That calcitonin may play a role during surgery on the thyroid glands has been shown experimentally by Adie (1973) in the rat. To what extent the same factor may operate in man is still unkown (Chapter 4).

Further changes in calcium and phosphate levels depend on parathyroid function and bone "avidity" for these mineral ions. Krane (1957) pointed out that hypocalcemia is the primary event after thyroid surgery and that at the time this is first noticed, the serum phosphate level is not necessarily elevated. The rise in serum phosphate level frequently takes several days to manifest itself (Krane, 1961); in milder cases, it will not occur at all (Parfitt, 1972a). It should be emphasized that less parathyroid hormone is necessary to maintain normal renal handling of phosphate than to mobilize calcium from bone (Chapter 1).

Whereas overt permanent hypoparathyroidism may present with dramatic symptoms of neuromuscular irritability, it may also be completely asymptomatic. For this reason it is important to monitor the serum calcium systematically and repeatedly postoperatively. In Lachmann's retrospective study (1941) seven patients with pronounced hypoparathyroidism were detected out of the 113 investigated three months to three years after surgery; only two of them had presented tetany during hospitalization. In another group, five cases with permanent hypoparathyroidism were detected out of 213 patients reviewed more than three years after operation. One of these had been asymptomatic during her hospital stay and in three cases the symptoms had been considered to be transient since they had subsided prior to hospital discharge. Lachmann (1941) quotes a sixth patient in this series who was not examined because of his demise during a bout of tetany one year postoperatively. In Krane's series (1961), five of 18 patients had transient symptoms but persistent hypocalcemia. In three patients, the diagnosis was delayed for 4 to 16 years. Another patient developed permanent asymptomatic hypoparathyroidism five years postoperatively. In Parfitt's analysis (1967a) of cases with a delayed diagnosis (5–20 years postoperatively) of chronic hypoparathyroidism, 6 out of 15 patients had not suffered from postoperative tetany or related symptoms, a condition termed by Wade (1960) "masked hypoparathyroidism," and by Osborn and Jones (1968) "non-tetanic hypoparathyroid state."

Whether "hypoparathyroidism of delayed onset" exists is a matter of dispute. Lachmann (1941) reported one case, with "quite normal" levels of serum calcium after 6–8 weeks, in which hypocalcemia (7.9 mg/dl) was detected 3–4 months postoperatively, with appearance of symptoms which had required therapy for one year at the time of his writing. Several authors, including Bertelsen and Bruun (1947), have searched specifically for cases like this, but were unable to detect any. Parfitt (1967a) concluded that one of his cases belonged in this category and advanced several hypotheses to explain late failure of parathyroid glands: ischemic atrophy or infarction of the remaining parathyroid tissue, fibrosis of the remaining glands as a result of the operation or of the underlying thyroid disease; or some autoimmune process initiated during the surgical act. Whatever the cause, these cases must be rare indeed and it is more probable that in instances of slight postoperative hypocalcemia the level of serum calcium may depend on dietary intake of calcium and phosphorus as well as calcium requirements. Another possibility is that the remaining parathyroid tissue may function for a certain period as an autogenous graft which eventually ceases to function. If such were the case, however, more instances should have been documented unless they are simply overlooked on the ground that on early follow-up the serum calcium was normal and therefore was not checked again.

3. Provocative Tests to Stress Parathyroid Function

There are two tests which are used to evaluate parathyroid function indirectly and to uncover latent hypoparathyroidism, both based on the role of the parathyroid glands in maintaining normal serum calcium levels when the organism is deliberately deprived of calcium (Chapter 1).

The first consists of the administration of sodium phytate (sodium inositol hexaphosphate), a substance which complexes calcium in the intestine (Mellanby, 1949; Bronner et al., 1954). In subjects with a normal serum calcium, normal vitamin D intake or endogenous synthesis and normal parathyroid function, sodium phytate (9 g daily in divided doses), administered for short periods of time (3 to 7 days) to patients on low calcium diets (140–170 mg/24 hr), will not decrease the level of serum calcium (Smith et al., 1960; Friis and Hahnemann, 1964), whereas it will do so in cases of diminished parathyroid responsiveness (Smith et al., 1960; Rose, 1963; Osborn and Jones, 1968; John and Wills, 1964).

The use of phytate in this manner raises an important theoretical point. Not only is calcium chelated in the gut, but one half to two thirds of the phytate phosphorus is hydrolyzed (Henneman et al., 1956) and a considerable fraction of this is absorbed (Fig. 1) in amounts which may affect the level of serum calcium, especially if bone turnover is rapid and excess

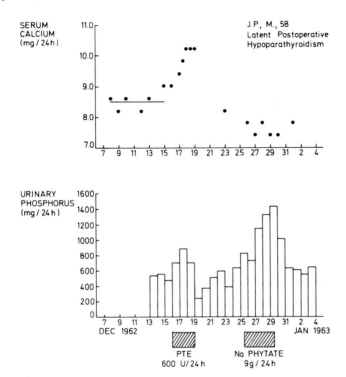

Fig. 1. Effects of the administration of PTE and sodium phytate in a patient with latent postoperative hypoparathyroidism following subtotal parathyroidectomy for hyperparathyroidism. See text for details of interpretation.

osteoid tissue is present (Nagant de Deuxchaisnes and Krane, 1967). Such is the case after some (if not most) operations for thyrotoxicosis. Phosphate infusions are associated with a drop in serum calcium, which in hypoparathyroid individuals may lead to tetany (Thompson and Hiatt, 1957).

Another point of interest is that phytate is also hydrolyzed into various polyphosphate esters of inositol. The latter (at least the di- and triphosphoesters) are potent inhibitors of mineralization *in vitro* (Thomas and Tilden, 1972; Van Den Berg *et al.*, 1972) and *in vivo* in the rat (Van Den Berg *et al.*, 1972). However, little of these polyphosphate esters is absorbed by the intestinal mucosa, so that the practical impact of this is probably negligible.

In Fig. 1 the results are illustrated of a "positive" response to sodium phytate in a 58-year-old man who had been operated on 26 months earlier for chief cell hyperplasia of the parathyroids. On the 8th postoperative day, the serum calcium fell from 14.4 (the preoperative value) to 6.4

mg/dl, a value still maintained on the twelfth postoperative day. The patient had been discharged on vitamin D_2 (100,000 U/24 h) and calcium supplements (4.8 g of elemental calcium given as calcium lactate). He was able to discontinue therapy and was readmitted without treatment for evaluation on long-term follow up. Serum calcium value was 8.5 mg/dl, serum phosphorus 4.0 mg/dl. Blood urea nitrogen and serum creatinine values had remained normal. It can be seen in Fig. 1 that the intramuscular administration of parathyroid extract (600 U/24 h) for 3 days raised the serum calcium from 8.5 to 10.2 mg/dl, while the urinary phosphorus excretion increased from an average of 525 mg/24 h to a maximum of 949 mg/24 h, followed by a characteristic decrease to 240 mg/24 h. The subsequent administration of sodium phytate orally during 4 days produced a drop in the serum calcium to 7.4 mg/dl, while the urinary phosphorus rose to a maximum of 1433 mg/24 h, a 0.9 g/24 h increase over the baseline value. Since 9 g sodium phytate contains approximately 1.5 g elemental phosphorus, these figures would indicate a very high degree of intestinal hydrolysis and absorption in this patient. The response, as far as serum calcium is concerned, is characteristic of that in latent hypoparathyroidism, but the exact significance of the calcium decrease is hard to evaluate in view of the fact that the alkaline phosphatase level was still elevated (8.2 Bodansky U). Furthermore kinetic studies performed with [47]Ca showed a rather high calcium deposition rate in bone (see Table IX, patient J.P.) whereas a lower than normal value would have been anticipated if pure latent hypoparathyroidism had existed. It is probable that the bone turnover was still slightly elevated and that part of the fall in serum calcium was phosphate-mediated. The entire study was performed on a low calcium-low phosphate diet.

A second procedure used to evaluate the function of the parathyroid glands consists of inducing sudden hypocalcemia by the intravenous administration of a sodium (disodium or trisodium) salt of EDTA (ethylene diamine tetraacetic acid), which chelates calcium into a stable, soluble, and physiologically inert complex, which is rapidly excreted in the urine. The fall in the ionized, physiologically active fraction of serum calcium is the stimulus for parathyroid hormone secretion. Under these circumstances, immunoreactive parathyroid hormone levels can indeed be shown to increase in humans (Berson and Yalow, 1966) as they do in the cow and goat (Sherwood et al., 1966). Parathyroid responsiveness is evaluated by studying the rate at which unchelated serum calcium, as measured by the usual titration methods, returns to the initial pre-infusion level.

Kaiser and Ponsold (1959) first described a standardized test using EDTA. Modifications have been made by Kalliomäki et al. (1961a), Jones and Fourman (1963a), Klotz *et al.* (1963), Estep *et al.* (1965), King *et al.* (1965), Rosenbaum (1965 and 1966), and Parfitt (1969).

In normal subjects, the preinfusion levels should be restored within 12 hours after the initiation of the test. Parathyroid insufficiency would be marked if after 24 hours the serum level is still lower than 8.5 mg/dl, a criterion adopted by Jones and Fourman (1963a) as representing latent hypoparathyroidism "of clinical importance." The same patients had a positive phytate test as defined by Smith *et al.* (1960).

The main criticism in the evaluation of these results is that little attention is given to the shape of the restoration curve after the maximum decrease in serum calcium level has been reached. If one patient does not reach or barely reaches the arbitrary serum calcium level of 8.5 mg/dl after 24 hours because his basal serum calcium value was 8.9 mg/dl whereas another patient reaches a value of 9.0 mg/dl because his basal calcium level was 9.5 mg/dl, both patients have an identical 95% restoration potential. Yet the former is usually considered abnormal or borderline whereas the latter is not. An analysis which considers several points of the curve or the entire shape of the restoration curve toward the preinfusion value with results expressed as percentages of basal levels is much more representative of parathyroid reserve, especially when the results are submitted to statistical evaluation (Klotz *et al.*, 1963; King *et al.*, 1965; Parfitt, 1969). The studies of King *et al.* (1965) and of Parfitt (1969) on carefully selected groups of patients revealed that two degrees of parathyroid insufficiency can be distinguished on the basis of the results of the "EDTA test." The "first degree" is characterized by a normal or near-normal serum calcium value after 24 hours whereas the 12-hour value remains low by about 1.0 mg/dl. This corresponds closely to the criteria set by Klotz *et al.* (1963), and has been designated as an insignificant "sluggish parathyroid response" by Jones and Fourman (1963a). The "second degree" of parathyroid insufficiency is characterized by a serum calcium value (after 24 hours) that remains low by about 0.8 mg/dl which usually corresponds to the limit set by Jones and Fourman (1963a).

It should be noted that administration of parathyroid hormone restores a normal curve of recovery in hypoparathyroid patients (Jones and Fourman, 1963a; Klotz *et al.*, 1963; Fujita *et al.*, 1966), as does the administration of calcium or dihydrotachysterol, the latter only when given in sufficient amounts to raise the basal serum calcium value to the upper limit of normal, or higher. All hypoparathyroid subjects with a normal curve have had initial serum calcium values higher than 10.0 mg/dl (Kaiser *et al.*, 1960; King *et al.*, 1965; Rosenbaum, 1966; Parfitt, 1969). If calciferol is given and the serum calcium level brought from 8.6 to 9.4 mg/dl, for example, the response to the EDTA test will be better after therapy than before (Stowers *et al.*, 1967), although it will be subnormal. It should be noted that as a group, the basal serum calcium level is lower in patients with latent parathyroid insufficiency than in normal subjects (Kaiser *et al.*, 1960) by about 0.4 mg/dl in grade I and 0.8 mg/dl in grade II insufficiency (Parfitt, 1969), although by definition the values are within normal limits. If not, the hypoparathyroidism is considered "definite." Therefore, this initial value is of limited interest in an individual patient.

The experience of one of us (C.N.) with this test is illustrated in Fig. 2. Patient M.C. had a parathyroid adenoma removed 18 months prior to test. Patient C.D. had thyroid surgery performed 23 years prior to the investigation. Patients A.L., M.V., and G.L. suffered from proven hyperparathyroidism, cured by surgery. Patient A.B. suffered from "heparin osteoporosis." The six other patients were so-called "spasmophiliacs," i.e., patients presenting with typical attacks of tetany, normal serum calcium and magnesium levels and positive electromyographic findings of repetitive discharge of doublets, triplets and/or multiplets.

It can be seen that according to Fourman's definition, only the patient operated on for parathyroid adenoma (M.C.) had parathyroid insufficiency

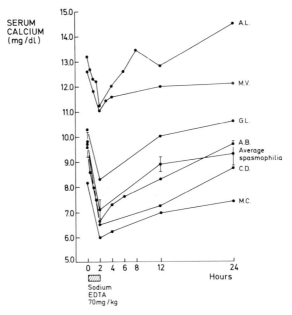

Fig. 2. Results of the EDTA test to evaluate parathyroid gland responsiveness in patients with a variety of disorders. See text for details.

"of clinical importance." This is not surprising since her basal serum calcium was low.

The response in the group of patients with hyperparathyroidism was strikingly different from all others; not only was the restoration of the serum calcium extremely vigorous, but the decrease induced in the serum calcium was of lesser magnitude despite the use of an identical technique. For 3 patients, calcium level 2 hours after infusion was on the average only 85% of zero time, whereas for the other 9 patients it fell to an average of 72%. The amount of parathyroid hormone produced during an EDTA perfusion is higher when hyperparathyroidism is present than under normal circumstances (Lockefeer *et al.*, 1973 and 1974), or in parathyroid insufficiency. The increased circulating parathyroid hormone probably maintains bone resorption at an increased rate, preventing the serum calcium from falling as steeply as it usually does under other circumstances.

Subtle distinctions between grades of parathyroid insufficiency may be demonstrable when measurements of immunoreactive PTH (iPTH) are made during EDTA-induced hypocalcemia. When 5 patients with primary hyperparathyroidism and excessive immunoreactive parathyroid hormone release in the circulation under the influence of EDTA were restudied postoperatively by Lockefeer *et al.* (1974), normal responses were observed in all. In contrast, in a case of primary parathyroid hyperplasia, studied by Murray *et al.* (1972), where 4.9 g of an estimated 5 g of hyperplastic parathyroid tissue were removed, no increase in circulating iPTH could be detected during the hypocalcemic challenge, in contrast to the striking increase during the same test preoperatively.

When EDTA is infused, not only does the unchelated serum calcium fall, but the serum phosphorus does as well (Mazzuoli and Naccarato, 1959; Kalliomäki *et al.,* 1961; Rosenbaum, 1965; Estep *et al.,* 1965; Parfitt, 1969) owing to a shift of phosphate into cells and an increase in parathyroid hormone secretion. The latter probably accounts for the delayed increase in phosphate clearance by the kidney, which in one study was maximal 3 to 6 hours after the end of the infusion (Rosenbaum, 1965). No such increase in phosphate clearance was noticed in any of the 4 hypoparathyroid patients studied (Rosenbaum, 1966). These changes have been confirmed by Estep *et al.* (1965) who demonstrated a progressive decrease in tubular reabsorption of phosphate for 3 to 4 hours after the end of the infusion, whereas patients with hypoparathyroidism showed a slight increase in tubular reabsorption of phosphate, a phenomenon that the authors attributed to an effect of decreased amounts of circulating calcium on the kidney tubule. It has been speculated that studies on phosphate excretion might be useful in distinguishing between the two levels of parathyroid insufficiency; increased phosphate clearance might persist in grade I parathyroid insufficiency, whereas this might be absent in grade II if Parfitt's assumptions are correct (1969).

Sudden hypocalcemia after EDTA may induce symptoms of paresthesias, cramps, anxiety and depression (Jones and Fourman, 1963b; Wade *et al.*, 1965a; Stowers *et al.*, 1967). The highest incidence of hypocalcemic symptoms during the procedures occurred in patients who had had a thyroidectomy within the previous two years (Michie *et al.*, 1965). More side effects will be encountered if the rate of infusion is twice as rapid (King *et al.*, 1965). Despite the fact that less EDTA was infused and less profound hypocalcemia observed, 65% of the patients tested experienced paresthesias of the face and extremities; 7% had a Chvostek or Trousseau sign. When EDTA was even more rapidly infused (35–45 minutes), 20% of the patients had a Chvostek sign and more experienced paresthesias of the face and extremities, as well as tightness in the chest. This illustrates that symptoms produced by hypocalcemia correlate better with the rate at which the serum calcium falls rather than with the absolute value reached. Tetany in itself has been seldom observed (Kaiser and Ponsold, 1959; Stowers *et al.*, 1967; Klotz *et al.*, 1963). The test should not be performed in patients whose serum calcium is below the lower limit of normal (Jones and Fourman, 1963b). More serious toxicity has been seen in patients given repeated EDTA infusions at much higher dosages (440 mg/kg body weight) for treatment of hypercalcemia and death with excessive bleeding and renal insufficiency has been reported (Dudley *et al.*, 1955). No severely ill patients or individuals with such disorders as renal failure or a bleeding tendency should be subjected to the procedure.

In order to minimize all side effects, Fujita *et al.* (1966) modified the standard EDTA test by substituting infusions of calcium disodium EDTA. When this is done, the total serum calcium usually increases strikingly owing to the addition of chelated calcium to the ordinary calcium fractions, but the unchelated calcium remains unchanged (Rosenbaum, 1965; Parfitt, 1969) and side effects are nil (Rosenbaum, 1965). More experience is needed with this test before its usefulness can be delineated.

4. Latent Hypoparathyroidism

Using the phylate test, Smith *et al.* (1960) induced clinical tetany and very low serum calcium levels (< 7.0 mg/dl) in 3 patients with postoperative hypoparathyroidism whose treatment with oral calcium supplements had been interrupted one month prior to the test. In two patients who had suffered overt transient hypoparathyroidism, phytate administration did not produce tetany, but in both the serum calcium level fell to about 8.0

mg/dl or lower. These differences show the evolution from transient definite hypoparathyroidism to permanent latent hypoparathyroidism.

The high incidence of latent hypoparathyroidism (24%) in patients after thyroidectomy, as reported by Davis *et al.* 1961) and determined by the phytate test, was later shown to be due to the surgical technique then in use. Once the surgical procedure had been modified, EDTA tests performed one year postoperatively yielded only two abnormal responses out of 50 patients tested, an incidence of 4% (Wade *et al.*, 1965b).

John and Wills (1964) studied 21 patients whose serum calcium level (8.5–9.5 mg/dl) was below the midpoint of their normal range (8.5–10.5 mg/dl) and obtained intermediate results: 3 patients out of 21 (14%) had an abnormal response several years post-thyroidectomy. One of them developed clinical tetany when the serum calcium level reached 6.5 mg/dl. This patient too had suffered from overt transient hypoparathyroidism, but had been free of symptoms for 18 months with a basal level of serum calcium at 8.6 mg/dl. Rose (1973) was unable to detect a single case of latent hypoparathyroidism with the phytate test among 15 patients post-thyroidectomy.

As a group, however, patients who undergo thyroidectomy undoubtedly have less parathyroid reserve than normals. This is shown by the study of Friis and Hahnemann (1964) who compared 10 normal subjects and 10 patients who had undergone subtotal thyroidectomy for toxic and non-toxic goiter (in a ratio of one to one). The basal serum calcium level was identical in both groups (9.8 mg/dl), but the lowest value in the normal subjects while on phytate reached, on an average, 9.5 mg/dl (no single value below 9.0 mg/dl), whereas the average value in the operated individuals was 8.9 mg/dl, a statistically significant difference. Five patients out of ten had a serum calcium which fell below 9.0 mg/dl; one was lower than 8.5 mg/dl.

Wade *et al.* (1965b) using the EDTA test estimated parathyroid reserve after thyroid surgery in 50 patients studied preoperatively, and 5 days, 3 months, and 1 year postoperatively; latent hypoparathyroidism was revealed after the operations in 22, 6, and 4% at the respective time periods. They concluded that latent hypoparathyroidism is more likely to be transient than permanent as contrasted with definite hypoparathyroidism, which is more likely to be permanent. When overt hypoparathyroidism was transient, permanent latent hypoparathyroidism developed in 7 out of 10 such patients studied, as demonstrated by the response to EDTA evaluated 2–11 years after surgery (Wade *et al.*, 1965a). Two of these 7 cases could have also been considered as suffering from asymptomatic permanent definite hypoparathyroidism, although of a mild degree. They did indeed eventually develop fluctuating basal serum calcium levels, at times below the normal limits. Such patients do not show any later tendency to raise their serum calcium levels (Fourman *et al.*, 1963). Thus latent hypoparathyroidism may be a permanent condition unless episodes of transient definite hypoparathyroidism supervene. On the other hand, if definite transient hypoparathyroidism has existed, latent permanent hypoparathyroidism will usually ensue.

As with the phytate test, the data collected with the EDTA test on patients who have undergone thyroidectomy show that these patients have a definitely diminished parathyroid reserve (Jones and Fourman, 1963a; King *et al.*, 1965; Parfitt, 1969). Patients who present with postoperative evidence of transient hypoparathyroidism are more likely to suffer from the more severe, grade II level of parathyroid insufficiency, whereas patients who do not present with evidence of prior parathyroid insufficiency are more likely to fall into the category of grade I latent hypoparathyroidism.

Pertinent to this subject is the work conducted by Reeve (1967) with EDTA administration in the rat, an animal which has only two parathyroid glands. When the animals were used as their own controls, the most highly abnormal responses to EDTA other than in totally parathyroidectomized animals were found in those rats where the vasculature of the parathyroid gland had been disturbed by clamping for only five seconds. This disturbed the response to EDTA more than the removal of one and one-half parathyroid glands, adding additional weight to the vascular theory of latent hypoparathyroidism (the basal serum calcium values remained unaffected).

The subject of the clinical significance of latent hypoparathyroidism is a highly controversial one. Davis (1961) and Davis *et al.* (1961) described a series of vague, ill-defined symptoms such as mental depression, lassitude, loss of interest, paresthesias, headaches, cramps, abdominal pain, and ectodermal lesions. Most subjective symptoms were more prominent at the premenstrual period and raised the problem of differential diagnosis with the syndrome of premenstrual tension. Fourman *et al.* (1963) found that such symptoms in 122 thyroidectomized patients were more frequent with serum calcium levels which were decreased, although still within normal range. This was especially conspicuous as far as headaches, lassitude, and mental depression were concerned. Treatment of these patients with large oral doses of calcium supplements (3 to 4 g daily), and eventually vitamin D as well, produced a disappearance of all symptoms in 19 patients, an improvement in another 20, and no change in the complaints of only 3. The most striking subjective improvement was a change in the patients' sense of well-being (Davis *et al.*, 1961; Fourman *et al.*, 1963), as shown most often in their personal appearance.

These data have been criticized on the basis that no double-blind trial was performed and that the alleged symptoms were nonspecific and common in middle-aged women. Rose (1963) was unable to induce any significant improvement with oral calcium supplements administered in a double-blind trial as were Stowers *et al.* (1967). However, the latter authors gave only minimal amounts of oral calcium supplements (0.7 g/24 h), whereas in the series of the former author neither definite nor latent hypoparathyroidism was identified. These trials therefore remain inconclusive. Fourman *et al.* (1967) later conducted a double-blind crossover trial using 3 g of oral calcium supplements daily administered to thyroidectomized patients with and without latent hypoparathyroidism and performed a psychiatric assessment of their symptoms. Only the patients with diminished parathyroid reserve improved significantly as far as their mental symptoms were concerned. The increase in serum calcium values amounted to only 0.3 mg/dl on the average and did not reach statistical significance, perhaps owing to the small number of patients tested.

It is difficult to accept that a striking improvement in symptoms could be ascribed to such a trivial increase in serum calcium. Fourman *et al.* (1963) have advanced the hypothesis that intracellular rather than extracellular calcium concentrations might be changed by this therapy, if not the gradient from cell to extracellular fluid. Some support for this concept is found in the publications of Borle (1968), DeLuca *et al.* (1968), and Park and Talmage (1968). Another possibility is that calcium therapy in such high pharmacological doses might affect neuromuscular irritability and mood nonspecifically.

II. NONSURGICAL DAMAGE TO THE PARATHYROID GLANDS

A. Radioactive Iodine Therapy

The parathyroid glands are relatively resistant to radiation damage so that definite hypoparathyroidism, permanent or transient, is a rare event following ^{131}I treatment for thyroid disease. Only massive doses of external radiation will destroy parathyroid tissue in several animal species (Berdjis, 1972).

Doses of ^{131}I which are nearly lethal for thyroid tissue (>4 mCi/g of thyroid tissue) caused irreversible destruction of the parathyroid glands in certain strains of mice (Gorbman, 1950). Parrott *et al.* (1960), using 5 mCi/kg body weight in the rat, found that none of the parathyroid glands removed from the ^{131}I-irradiated animals was undamaged. The most severe alterations consisted of fibrous invasion and diminished cellularity with small clusters of cells separated from each other by large septa of connective tissue. These authors found a rough correlation between the microscopic appearance of the parathyroid tissue and the ensuing hypocalcemia of the animal at parturition. The determining factor in the severity of the parathyroid alteration was the topographic location of the glands, those deeply embedded within the thyroid tissue showing much more severe damage than those located at the surface. In addition to direct effects, radiation may also induce local changes which through fibrosis can alter blood supply or neural function of the parathyroid glands.

Although the dose used in these rats is higher than that which is commonly utilized in humans for treatment of thyrotoxicosis, in the treatment of metastatic thyroid carcinoma as much as 100–500 mCi may be administered, a dose which may correspond to the 5 mCi/kg body weight used by Parrott et al. (1960).

Some of the largest (Blumgart et al., 1955), as well as the most recent series (Bhatia et al., 1968; Sagel et al., 1972) reviewing the subject of ^{131}I therapy specifically note the absence of "symptomatic" hypoparathyroidism among the patients treated. An analysis of the literature discloses only 7 cases of overt hypoparathyroidism. All had been treated for thyrotoxicosis; in 4 cases the hypoparathyroidism was permanent (Gilbert-Dreyfus et al., 1958; Townsend, 1961; Hélou et al., 1964; Eipe et al., 1968). The duration of hypoparathyroidism in one case is not stated (Orme and Conolly, 1971). Only in two cases were serum calcium levels recorded prior to ^{131}I therapy. In the first case, serum calcium fell from 10.2 to 6.8 mg/dl after 2.5 months (Hélou et al., 1964) and in the second from 9.0 to 4.5 mg/dl after 16 months (Eipe et al., 1968). The average serum calcium on appearance of symptoms was 5.8 mg/dl (range: 4.5–6.8 mg/dl) and the average concomitant serum phosphate level was 6.4 mg/dl (range: 5.0–8.2 mg/dl). Typical hypocalcemic symptoms were described including tetany, spasms, cramps, paresthesias, confusion with seizure-like movements, and grand mal seizures. In one case, typical bilateral cataracts developed after 20 months (Gilbert-Dreyfus et al., 1958).

Two cases suffered transient overt hypoparathyroidism. In one (Tighe, 1952), tetany, hypocalcemia and hyperphosphatemia appeared 2.5 months after the administration of a single dose of 4 mCi of ^{131}I to a 14-year-old boy. Healing occurred after 6 weeks and no further treatment was necessary. In another (Freeman et al., 1969), hypocalcemia developed 5 days after the administration of 3.5 mCi of ^{131}I and coincided with the appearance of thyroiditis and a thyroid crisis. The hypocalcemia, which was readily corrected, was probably due more to local trauma and edema resulting from the abnormal response of the thyroid gland than to radiation damage as such.

A greater number of patients may be affected by latent than by overt hypoparathyroidism after radiation treatment. Adams and Chalmers (1965) studied a group of 60 patients who had received ^{131}I for thyrotoxicosis. They measured the response to EDTA infusions in 12 of these subjects and found that 58% of the patients tested, and therefore at least 11% of the entire group, demonstrated diminished parathyroid reserve. Goldsmith et al. (1968) performed an identical study on 74 patients post-radiation and found a significant difference between the serum calcium values of the patients after 12 hours as compared with those of a control group of 19 normal subjects. Better et al. (1969) and Harden et al. (1963), measuring responses to intravenous and oral phosphate, obtained results similar to those with EDTA. As a whole the probable incidence of documented permanent hypoparathyroidism post-radiation is only 6 cases out of an estimated 300,000 patients so treated, an incidence of 0.002%, whereas postoperatively this value probably lies between 0.2–2.0%.

The radionuclide ^{125}I, recently introduced as a therapeutic agent, is also able to destroy the thyroid gland and to induce hypothyroidism (Bremner et al., 1973). However, since it emits no β-irradiation, it should be harmless to the parathyroid glands. [125]I has a very low penetrating potential in tissue, travelling less than 30 μm (McDougall et al., 1971), as compared to 2000 μm for the β-rays of [131]I.

B. L-Asparaginase

Administration of L-asparaginase, an antileukemic agent derived from *Escherichia coli,* has been shown to lead to necrosis of chief cells (and the appearance of numerous oxyphil cells) in rabbit parathyroid glands with ensuing hypoparathyroidism and eventual death if the serum calcium is not corrected. These findings, made by Tettenborn et al. (1970), have been amply confirmed by two other groups (Chisari et al., 1972; Young et al., 1973) on biochemical and histological grounds but do not apply in species other than the rabbit. To date, no case of hypoparathyroidism due to L-asparaginase has been documented in humans, but thorough studies on this subject have not been carried out.

C. Hemochromatosis

Excessive iron storage, either primary or secondary, results in iron deposition in many organs, especially the liver, the pancreas, and the parathyroid glands. It is therefore not surprising that in some instances of hemochromatosis hypoparathyroidism develops as reviewed by de Sèze *et al.* (1972b). Vachon *et al.* (1970) reported two cases of hypoparathyroidism, de Sèze *et al.* (1972a) and Pawlotsky *et al.* (1972) one case each associated with primary hemochromatosis. Sherman *et al.* (1970) have reported one instance of hypoparathyroidism ascribed to secondary hemochromatosis in a patient who had received 541 pints of blood over a period of six years for temporary aplastic anemia. Other similar cases have been described by Newns (1973) and Oberklaid and Seshadri (1975).

In none of these cases is there definite proof that hemochromatosis is the cause of the hypoparathyroidism, especially since no biochemical findings are available in the period before the onset of the iron storage disease. Coincidental idiopathic hypoparathyroidism and hemochromatosis cannot be ruled out. A link between the two disorders seems possible, however, in view of what is known about the predilection of iron for deposition in the parathyroid glands. Hypoparathyroidism is not frequent in hemochromatosis; Pawlotsky *et al.* (1972), reviewing 44 cases, were unable to find another instance of hypocalcemia other than in the one case they had described. Lack of interference with parathyroid function may be explainable by the relative absence of fibrosis accompanying iron deposition in the parathyroid glands (Sheldon, 1935).

D. Metastatic Involvement of the Parathyroid Glands

Although Thiele *et al.* (1975) in a necropsy study of 589 unselected cases found metastatic involvement of the parathyroid glands in only three instances in which generalized metastases occurred, the glands are often affected when cases of malignancy are considered [12% of the cases in a prospective study including all malignant conditions (Horwitz *et al.*, 1972)]. Most of the tissue of all the glands has to be invaded in order for hypoparathyroidism to occur. Horwitz *et al.* (1972) provided evidence of this in two instances of breast carcinoma where hypocalcemia as well as hyperphosphatemia developed in the absence of renal failure. At autopsy at least 70% of all parathyroid tissue was replaced by metastatic tumor, possibly sufficient to impair parathyroid hormone secretion. It remains to be proven by immunoreactive parathyroid hormone determination since these cases were complicated by extensive metastases of the mixed type (osteoblastic and osteolytic), which are known to produce hypocalcemia. In one case hypomagnesemia was also present and, although correction of this abnormality was attempted during a period of 5 days, normomagnesemia was not achieved. In the second case, serum magnesium levels were apparently not determined. The implications of low serum magnesium values in the plasma will be discussed later.

King and Goldsmith (1964) also reported one case of breast carcinoma with clinical and biological manifestations of hypoparathyroidism (serum calcium, 5.8 mg/dl; serum phosphorus, 5.4 mg/dl). At autopsy only remnants of parathyroid glands could be identified, the rest of the parathyroid tissue being invaded by metastatic tissue. Whatever reservations might be made about particular cases, the possibility of metastasis-induced hypoparathyroidism should be kept in mind, especially when the primary tumor is breast carcinoma. This malignancy has even been shown to metastasize to a parathyroid adenoma (Margolis and Goldenberg, 1969).

E. Infarction of a Parathyroid Adenoma

Bleeding into a parathyroid adenoma may result either in aggravation of the hypercalcemia, eventually resulting in so-called parathyroid crisis (Lemann and Donatelli, 1964; Chodack et al., 1965; DeGroote, 1969) or a state of more or less severe hypocalcemia following the disappearance of all functioning adenomatous tissue (Norris, 1946; Howard et al., 1953a; Johnston and Schnute, 1961; Northcutt et al., 1969). The latter may represent either hypoparathyroidism, if the other glands do not resume their normal function, or recalcification hypocalcemia (and eventual tetany) as described in the section on hypoparathyroidism following parathyroid surgery. A mixture of both conditions is a third possibility. The sequence of events has seldom been documented by details of blood chemistries. Most of the evidence, except in one case (Howard et al., 1953b), rests on the patient's past history or on typical roentgenological changes which healed after the infarction. The latter event is usually heralded by an episode of pain in the neck, sometimes accompanied by a palpable and tender mass. Pain and tenderness are presumably produced by the sudden increase of the gland size with stretching of the capsule. Deliberate injury to the parathyroid glands has been used as an experimental technique in the therapy of hyperparathyroidism (Marx et al., 1974; Doppman et al., 1975).

F. Trauma to the Parathyroid Glands

Whether nonsurgical trauma to the cervical area may result in parathyroid failure has not been proved. Friedlaender (1930) reported the death of a 3-month-old child who had suffered convulsions during the previous month. At autopsy, three parathyroids showed hemorrhage and the fourth hyperemia. These changes are not specific, however, since hemorrhage into the parathyroid glands is common in infants coming to autopsy (Grosser and Betke, 1911). The case described by Mosonyi and Szilagyi (1964) of a hematoma in the cervical area is not convincing as a cause of parathyroid failure since no evidence was provided for preexisting normal parathyroid function. It seems unlikely that enlargement of the thyroid gland, such as occurs in Graves' disease, exerts sufficient pressure on the parathyroid glands or their blood supply to result in permanent hypoparathyroidism, as claimed by Dahl *et al.* (1962).

G. Other Nonsurgical Damage to the Parathyroid Glands

Drake *et al.* (1939) have reviewed the literature on this subject from 1899 through 1935 and reported their pathological findings, ascribed to various focal lesions such as those from bacterial emboli, tuberculosis and syphilis, rheumatic and suppurative parathyroiditis, primary or secondary fibrosis, old hemorrhagic cysts, amyloidosis, chronic passive congestion, hydrops with mild inflammation. It is difficult to evaluate these findings, since the connection between pathological and clinical manifestations is not always apparent. Not all cases necessarily represent true hypoparathyroidism. Blood chemistries were seldom available and the precise criteria for diagnosis of hypoparathyroidism which were set by Drake *et al.* (1939) led them to include only 8 cases in which this diagnosis was justified. In 1958 Bronsky *et al.* accepted only 5 of these 8 cases as hypoparathyroidism, and added one more case; none of these nine cases came to autopsy.

Recent pathological findings show that some lymphocytic infiltration of the parathyroids may be seen in a number of "normal" parathyroid glands (Reiner *et al.,* 1962; Seemann, 1967; Van de Casseye and Gepts, 1973), as well as intrafollicular amyloid deposits in one or more glands (Lieberman and DeLellis, 1973; Anderson and Ewen, 1974; Thiele *et al.,* 1975), when the parathyroids are systematically analyzed on autopsy. This is not necessarily a sign of parathyroid disease, but may have been interpreted as such in the past, owing to a lack of control series. More definite signs of inflammatory, so-called autoimmune, atrophic parathyroiditis may be more significant, as have been found in a number of well-established cases of "idiopathic" hypoparathyroidism (cf. infra!). In systemic amyloidosis, all four parathyroid glands have shown extensive amyloid deposits (Fanconi, 1969; Lieberman and DeLellis, 1973; Anderson and Ewen, 1974; Thiele *et al.,* 1975); the interstitium and perivascular spaces were heavily infiltrated with an entirely different distribution than in normal parathyroid glands. Apparently hypoparathyroidism does not ensue (Fanconi, 1969), although this cannot be stated with certainty in the absence of estimations of iPTH, since these patients usually die in renal failure with hypocalcemia and hyperphosphatemia (Fanconi, 1969). Whether cytomegalovirus may invade parathyroid tissue and cause hypoparathyroidism has not been proven. The association of hypoparathyroidism with cytomegalic inclusion disease led Curtis *et al.* (1962) to suggest an etiologic relationship, although this remains only an hypothesis.

III. FUNCTIONAL HYPOPARATHYROIDISM OF DIVERSE ETIOLOGY IN THE NEWBORN

Two types of hypocalcemia in newborns have been distinguished, according to the age of the infant at onset (see Chapter 7). If hypocalcemia occurs within the first three days after birth, it is called "early." Symptoms were observed in only 18% of such cases in the series of Rösli and Fanconi (1973) and the course is generally benign. When occurring later after birth (between the fifth and eighth days) the hypocalcemic symptoms are much more severe; most cases present with convulsions which are of the clonic type. The prognosis is usually good (Bakwin, 1937; Brown *et al.*, 1972b).

A. Early Neonatal Hypocalcemia

As described in Chapter 7, "early" hypocalcemia occurs within the first 2 or 3 days of life and thereafter corrects itself spontaneously before the end of the first week (usually on the fifth day of life). Its peak incidence is found between the 24th and 30th hours (Rösli and Fanconi, 1973) or between 30 and 40 hours of age (Radde *et al.*, 1972). Rösli and Fanconi (1973) consider the average serum calcium level in the healthy full-term newborn at the time to be 8.5 ± 0.5 mg/dl (range: 7.0–9.6 mg/dl); the values of Snodgrass *et al.* (1973) are slightly higher [8.9 ± 0.8 mg/dl (range: 6.2–11.3)]. Both figures reflect some "physiological" transient hypocalcemia. Pathological hypocalcemia has been variously defined by Brown *et al.* (1972a), Rossier *et al.* (1973), Keen and Lee (1973) and Rosen *et al.* (1974), all of whom consider values less than 7.5 mg/dl as definitely abnormal. The influence of gestational age, however, is such that several authors (Tsang *et al.*, 1972; Rösli and Fanconi, 1973) have arbitrarily defined serum calcium values as pathological if lower than 8.0 mg/dl in full-term infants, and lower than 7.0 mg/dl in preterm infants.

Prematurity is one of the most frequent causes of early neonatal hypocalcemia; 57% of the preterm infants had serum calcium values below 7.0 mg/dl in the series of Rösli and Fanconi (1973), versus none of the full-term healthy infants. The incidence varied from 35% in those born after 37 weeks (8½ months of gestation) to 85% in those born after 24–29 weeks (about 6 months of gestation). Other factors involve maternal diabetes (Tsang *et al.*, 1972), perinatal complications (including abnormal or difficult delivery), and especially birth asphyxia (Tsang *et al.*, 1974). The course is considered benign by some (Rösli and Fanconi, 1973) but others have stated that early neonatal hypocalcemia is associated with only a 50% chance for normal development (Volpe, 1973), owing to the various conditions associated with such hypocalcemia.

Early hypocalcemic tetany may reflect transient functional hypoparathyroidism, as suggested by Bakwin (1937), since the parathyroid glands do not respond to a decreased serum calcium with the expected increase in secretion. In normal full-term infants, the serum calcium level in the placental umbilical vein is unusually high: 10.4 ± 0.6 mg/dl and the decrease during the first day amounts on the average to 1.5 mg/dl (Snodgrass *et al.*, 1973), whereas the serum phosphate level rises from an average cord value of 5.7 ± 0.9 mg/dl to an average of 6.3 ± 1.0 mg/dl. The same pattern is observed in the sick neonate where the serum calcium level falls from 10.4 mg/dl (cord blood) to an average of 7.3 mg/dl within 24 hours, a 30% decrease (Radde *et al.*, 1972). Brown *et al.* (1972a) demonstrated the existence of a linear correlation between ionized and total calcium in the plasma of infants under 72 hours of age.

The fall in serum calcium may result from a cessation of active transport through the placenta, sequestration by the newborn's skeleton, vitamin D deficiency (Rosen *et al.*, 1974)—there exists a positive correlation between maternal and cord serum concentrations of $25(OH)D_3$ (Hillman and Haddad, 1974)—or excess secretion of calcitonin (Bergman *et al.*, 1974), either as a reaction to the elevated serum ionized calcium level at birth or as a response to glucagon secretion in response to hypoglycemia. While the serum levels of calcitonin increase manyfold from normal values in the cord blood to elevated levels after 24 hours and may affect the serum calcium levels in infants whose bone turnover is elevated, the serum levels of immunoreactive parathyroid hormone (iPTH) do not increase over 48 hours (Bergman *et al.*, 1974). David and Anast (1973) demonstrated transient relative hypoparathyroidism in the majority of newborns with early hypocalcemia who presented with low or nondetectable blood iPTH, compared with older hypocalcemic infants. When the parathyroids of infants were stressed by sudden hypocalcemia resulting from exchange transfusions, significant increments in iPTH were noted only in infants older than 48 hours. Tsang *et al.* (1973b) confirmed these findings, and furthermore observed a more sluggish rise in blood iPTH in premature infants in response to either spontaneous early hypocalcemia or artificially induced hypocalcemia through exchange transfusions than their full-term counterparts. Since measurements of iPTH may not reflect biologically active PTH, these results must be interpreted with caution.

Thus, it appears that there may be some degree of parathyroid unresponsiveness to hypocalcemia during the first two days of life which, when normalized, probably contributes to the increase in and stabilization of serum calcium, usually achieved by the fifth day. The cause of this transient functional hypoparathyroidism is unclear. It does not appear to be due to immaturity of the parathyroid glands since they are able to function in a hyperactive manner *in utero* (vide infra). It is also possible, however, that both kidney and bone are relatively resistant to PTH. Tsang *et al.* (1972; 1973a; 1974) repeatedly demonstrated that bone did respond to exogenous parathyroid hormone, but data concerning the renal response are equivocal. Connelly *et al.* (1962) and Linarelli *et al.* (1972) were unable to produce a phosphaturic response on the first day of life with intravenously administered parathyroid hormone. The fact that there was a spontaneous rise between the first and third day in the cyclic AMP/creatinine ratio without any stimulation (Linarelli *et al.*, 1972) may be evidence of increased levels of circulating parathyroid hormone. The finding of increasing renal responsiveness to PTH between days 1 and 3 may reflect maturation of the adenyl cyclase system within the renal cortex. Recent data from Marks *et al.* (1973) support the hypothesis that peripheral resistance to PTH (as measured by the urinary cyclic AMP secretion and response to treatment) may play a role in the pathogenesis of neonatal tetany.

It is more likely that transient functional hypoparathyroidism is a mild expression of secondary hypoparathyroidism, owing to physiological maternal hyperparathyroidism, as pointed out by Bakwin (1937). Ionized serum calcium falls significantly from an average 4.4 mg/dl to an average 4.2 mg/dl between the second and third trimester of pregnancy (Tan *et al.*, 1972). Similarly, the level of iPTH increases progressively from the 24th week (5.5 months) to achieve maximum values at 36–40 weeks (9 months) and decreases quickly thereafter (Lequin *et al.*, 1970; Cushard *et al.*, 1972). Bouillon and De Moor (1973) have found a highly significant increase in iPTH levels only during the last week of pregnancy. The levels declined slowly after delivery and at the end of the first postpartum week were still elevated. The urinary excretion of cyclic AMP also increases during pregnancy and is ascribable to the nephrogenous fraction of cyclic AMP, presumably dependent on PTH (Babka *et al.*, 1974). Possibly this hyperparathyroidism contributes to the high cord blood calcium levels which are assumed to suppress, at least transiently, parathyroid hormone secretion.

B. Late Neonatal Hypocalcemia

The late onset variety of neonatal hypocalcemia occurs with a peak incidence on the sixth to eighth day after birth, and always within the first two weeks of life. Because it is not related to any of the factors operating in the early onset variety and since brain damage is less frequent, the prognosis is better (Brown *et al.*, 1972b). Volpe (1973) states that this variety of hypocalcemia is associated with an 80–100% chance of normal development. The disturbances of mineral metabolism associated with late neonatal hypocalcemia are so prominent that Brown *et al.* (1972b) have termed them "metabolic convulsions," whereas Rösli and Fanconi (1973) speak of "transient idiopathic hypoparathyroidism" (Fanconi and Prader, 1967). Two abnormalities distinguish this hypocalcemia from the early onset type: definite hyperphosphatemia (average value: 9.1 ± 1.6 mg/dl) and hypomagnesemia (average value: 1.4 ± 0.3 mg/dl). If hypocalcemia (average: 6.3 ± 0.9 mg/dl) is the common denominator, it represents the sole biochemical abnormality in less than 20% of the cases (Cockburn *et al.*, 1973).

Definite hyperphosphatemia (i.e., >8.5 mg/dl) is present in 64% of these cases with "metabolic convulsions." They occur in hyperalert (Brown *et al.*, 1972b), large, full-term infants, voraciously consuming non-human milk of high phosphate content (Cockburn *et al.*, 1973; Snodgrass *et al.*, 1973). Bone turnover is high in these infants; therefore high phosphate intake decreases serum calcium presumably by increasing the rate of calcium deposition in bone. In addition, renal function is immature and there is decreased clearance of phosphate loads compared with adults. McCrory *et al.* (1952) have shown that adult-like responses in phosphate excretion to parathyroid hormone occur only after 7 to 12 days of age, and the increased renal response to parathyroid hormone between days 1 and 3 after birth shown by the ratio of cyclic AMP/creatinine excretion (Linarelli *et al.*, 1973) is short of what is observed in the adult. Furthermore, a high serum phosphate level might inhibit the renal hydroxylation of vitamin D (Tanaka and DeLuca, 1973) and thus diminish the response to parathyroid hormone.

Finally, high phosphate intake interferes with intestinal absorption of magnesium and may lead to hypomagnesemia. Definite hypomagnesemia (i.e., <1.5 mg/dl) is the second biochemical abnormality of late neonatal hypocalcemia, characterizing 53% of the cases described by Cockburn *et al.* (1973). These authors demonstrated the existence of a significant positive correlation between serum calcium and magnesium levels in this condition, confirming the earlier findings of Gittleman *et al.* (1964). That low magnesium levels, especially in infants and children, actually cause serum calcium levels to fall is a well recognized fact. Under those circumstances, the administration of supplemental calcium, vitamin D, or parathyroid extract is not effective; only the administration of magnesium supplements will correct to both the hypomagnesemia and the hypocalcemia (Paunier et al., 1968; Seelig, 1971). The cause of hypomagnesemia in the absence of diarrhea is not entirely clear, although excessive intake of non-human milk with its ratio of P/Mg of 7.5/1 versus 1.9/1 in human milk is probably the single most important factor, as suggested by Anast (1964). An excessive phosphate load would lead to hypomagnesemia (Seelig, 1971), as it does to hypocalcemia, and the hypomagnesemia might in turn enhance the hypocalcemia.

In a series of normal infants, the concentration of iPTH rose from an average level of 97 pg/ml in cord blood to 217 pg/ml at 6 days of age, with no further increase during the next 9 months of life (Fairney et al., 1973). Levels of iPTH have not been systematically studied in infants with "metabolic convulsions" as they have been in those with early hypocalcemia. Low magnesium levels per se increase parathyroid hormone secretion, whereas more severe magnesium depletion has opposite effects; in some clinical situations if serum magnesium is low, the levels of iPTH may be lower than would be expected from the serum calcium values (Chase and Slatopolsky, 1974). In addition, parathyroid hormone effectiveness may be reduced in the presence of magnesium depletion. The situation may be best characterized as inadequate and/or inefficient parathyroid hormone secretion. The hypothesis of transient congenital idiopathic hypoparathyroidism, as advanced by Fanconi and Prader (1967), is open to question; one would not expect administration of vitamin D_3 (20,000 IU per day) or AT 10 to cause the initially normal serum alkaline phosphatase to rise while normal serum calcium levels were attained, as in their study, if idiopathic hypoparathyroidism were present. The evidence of Fairney et al. (1973) that iPTH levels in infants with late hypocalcemia were significantly lower than normal is of interest. However, the group of 13 infants studied was extremely heterogeneous, many severe complicating factors were present, and neither serum phosphate nor serum magnesium levels were reported. Therefore this study does not allow conclusions to be drawn about what happens in "ordinary" cases of metabolic convulsions.

C. Primary Hypomagnesemia with Secondary Hypocalcemia

This disorder of "congenital and/or primary hypomagnesemia with magnesium-dependent secondary hypocalcemia" apparently results from a permanent and specific disorder in absorption of the Mg ion from the small intestine (Friedman *et al.*, 1967; Skyberg *et al.*, 1968) which affects only male infants with a single exception (Haljamäe and MacDowall, 1972), usually at 3 weeks to 4 months after birth. It may be familial (Stromme *et al.*, 1969; Vainsel *et al.*, 1970). Only magnesium supplements are able to correct both biochemical abnormalities in the serum.

Unlike the less severe hypomagnesemia so frequently encountered in late neonatal hypocalcemia, infants with primary hypomagnesemia have serum levels of Mg lower than 1.0 mg/dl, at times as low as 0.1 mg/dl* (Woodard *et al.*, 1972). In most cases only subnormal levels were established, even with massive Mg supplementation, and treatment with Mg supplements must be prolonged for an indefinite period (Salet *et al.*, 1966: Friedman *et al.*, 1967; Paunier *et al.*, 1968; Skyberg *et al.*, 1968; Nordio *et al.*, 1971; Haljamäe and MacDowall, 1972). In one case, the disorder seems to have been transient (Keipert, 1969), but the case described by Paunier *et al.* (1968) still required magnesium supplements after 8 years (Suh *et al.*, 1973). The effects of magnesium withdrawal (Haljamäe and MacDowall, 1972) (i.e., decreased serum Mg and Ca with increased P while phosphate clearance falls) are identical with regard to Ca and P metabolism to those which result from decreased parathyroid hormone secretion. No information is available on the morphological state of the parathyroid glands in children with this disorder who came to autopsy (Stromme *et al.*, 1969; Vainsel *et al.*, 1970).

Administration of high doses of parathyroid extract to children with primary Mg defect usually results in the normalization of serum calcium (Salet *et al.*, 1966; Paunier *et al.*, 1968; Skyberg *et al.*, 1968; Stromme *et al.*, 1969) and serum phosphate levels (Salet *et al.*, 1966; Skyberg *et al.*, 1968). Only the serum magnesium level remains unchanged. This is indirect evidence that lack of parathyroid hormone is not responsible for the hypomagnesemia, nor is severe end-organ unresponsiveness to parathyroid extract the main cause of hypocalcemia. Although there has been considerable confusion between primary hypomagnesemia and "idiopathic hypoparathyroidism with hypomagnesemia," several distinctions can be made. Therapy with high magnesium supplements can "cure" the former but not the latter. In addition, the serum phosphate level in primary hypomagnesemia is not generally as high as that observed in idiopathic hypoparathyroidism. Finally, if levels of iPTH are measured, it may be anticipated that they will be detectable in primary hypomagnesemia, and so it was in one case (Smales, 1974) whereas in idiopathic hypoparathyroidism they should not. The pathophysiology of this condi-

---

* In this chapter levels of serum Mg are variously reported in mg/dl and mEq/l. Since the equivalent weight of Mg is 12, the units are approximately interchangeable.

tion pertains to the problem of hypomagnesemia which has been alluded to and will be discussed in detail (cf. infra).

IV. SECONDARY HYPOPARATHYROIDISM DUE TO HYPERCALCEMIA, WITH SPECIAL REFERENCE TO THE NEWBORN INFANT OF A HYPERPARATHYROID MOTHER

In secondary hypoparathyroidism the parathyroid glands are inhibited by the negative feedback action of hypercalcemia. The source of the hypercalcemia is unimportant and by definition the state of secondary hypoparathyroidism is always transient, provided the suppressed parathyroid glands have not been harmed.

A similar situation may exist in the newborn, whenever functional or pathological hyperparathyroidism is present in the mother; delivery may be compared to sudden surgical removal of the source of excess parathyroid secretion and transient hypoparathyroidism may ensue.

It has been well known that pathological maternal hyperparathyroidism may be the cause of neonatal tetany since the first case reported by Friderichsen (1938, 1939), a follow-up of which has been published 30 years later (Friderichsen and Rosendal, 1968). Since then, 23 children of 14 hyperparathyroid mothers have been reported to have suffered from neonatal tetany (Ludwig, 1962; Johnstone et al., 1972; Willi and Baumann, 1966; Ertel et al., 1969; Bronsky et al., 1970; Bocquentin et al., 1973, and Joly, 1973). Undoubtedly, maternal hyperparathyroidism results in high fetal mortality and morbidity. Prematurity is frequent and its effect on the incidence of early neonatal hypocalcemia has been stressed in a previous section. Neonatal tetany occurred in 62% of the living children of hyperparathyroid mothers versus 1% in a control population where maternal pathological hyperparathyroidism accounts for less than 1 case out of 1000 (Boonstra and Jackson, 1971).

In these cases of secondary hypoparathyroidism, the assumption is made that the fetal parathyroid glands have been suppressed by the high serum ionized calcium concentrations that cross the placenta and bathe the parathyroid glands of the fetus. PTH as such does not cross the placenta. In animal experimentation it has been shown that the size of the fetal parathyroid glands varies inversely with maternal serum calcium concentration (Sinclair, 1942). In the offspring of hypercalcemic rats, the serum calcium level was significantly lower on the first day of life than in control offspring of normocalcemic rats (Fairney and Weir, 1970).

Secondary hypoparathyroidism due to maternal hyperparathyroidism has two features which distinguish it from the common types of neonatal hypocalcemia. First, the hypocalcemia is persistent, and treatment is frequently required for longer periods of time. Normal serum calcium levels were attained after 26 and 40 days, respectively, in cases described by Bocquentin *et al.* (1973), 29 days in the case described by Ertel *et al.* (1969), and 2 months in the cases reported by Friderichsen (1939) and by Wagner *et al.* (1964). McGeown and Field (1960) were able to diminish the dose of calcium supplements after 33 days, but calcium withdrawal could only be achieved after 3 months for symptoms present from the 4th day after birth. It would therefore seem that suppression of function of the parathyroid glands *in utero* may have long lasting effects; whether this may lead to suppression of parathyroid maturation or development remains to be proven. One infant born to a hyperparathyroid mother had permanent hypoparathyroidism (Bruce and Strong, 1955) and in another who died after 5 days no parathyroid tissue at all could be identified at autopsy (Johnstone *et al.*, 1972).

A second difference between these cases and those of neonatal tetany is the time of onset of symptoms. In most cases of the latter they become manifest within the first two weeks of life, whereas in the former condition some cases have been described of later onset, usually at the time nonhuman milk is used to replace breast feeding. In the case of Willi and Baumann (1966), symptoms appeared 18 days after birth, in Friderichsen's case (1938), 5 months after birth, and in the case described by Bruce and Strong (1955), at age one year. This situation is analogous to that of transient neonatal adrenal insufficiency which may occur in the offspring of mothers suffering from Cushing's syndrome (Kreines and DeVaux, 1971). The mirror image of this situation is that which is represented by infants born with transient hyperparathyroidism to mothers suffering from untreated hypoparathyroidism during pregnancy (Gerloczy and Farkas, 1953; Aceto *et al.*, 1966; Bronsky *et al.*, 1968; Schlack, 1969; Landing and Kamoshita, 1970; Orr and Graham, 1972). There is one striking difference, however, between the two situations. The fetus of the hyperparathyroid mother does not have hypoparathyroidism *in utero* but only after delivery. The fetus of an untreated hypoparathyroid mother does have hyperparathyroidism *in utero*. At birth, he may show histological evidence of osteitis fibrosa.

V. SECONDARY HYPOPARATHYROIDISM DUE TO HYPERMAGNESEMIA

Although the level of ionized serum calcium is known to be the primary stimulus for parathyroid secretion (Sherwood *et al.*, 1968), serum levels of magnesium ion exert a similar negative feedback control on the parathyroid glands (MacIntyre *et al.*, 1963; Buckle *et al.*, 1968; Sherwood *et al.*, 1970). Any significant increase in the magnesium ion concentration of the extracellular fluid will suppress parathyroid hormone secretion, as has been shown experimentally in the nephrectomized rat by Gitelman *et al.* (1968) and in the dog by Massry *et al.* (1970). These physiological studies have been confirmed by Altenähr and Leonhardt (1972) in a morphometric ultrastructural study of the parathyroid glands in the rat, which provided evidence that both hormone secretion and synthesis were inhibited. The authors concluded from their studies that Ca and Mg were interchangeable in their ability to suppress the parathyroid glands. There is little chance for clinical hypoparathyroidism to occur in humans as a result of hypermagnesemia, although diminished parathyroid secretion is possible in cases of excessive use of Mg-containing antacids, for example. In renal failure, the most common single cause of hypermagnesemia, hypocalcemia is seldom absent and is the more powerful stimulus acting on the parathyroid glands (Massry *et al.*, 1970). Finally, if excessive magnesium intake resulted in elevated levels of serum Mg, the pharmacologic effects of this ion might overshadow the symptoms of hypoparathyroidism; instead of neuromuscular hyperexcitability, the clinical picture would be that of neuromuscular depression.

VI. ACQUIRED METABOLIC RESISTANCE TO PARATHYROID HORMONE

When metabolic abnormalities interfere with the peripheral action of parathyroid hormone (PTH) in such a fashion that it can no longer maintain the calcium concentration in the plasma and extracellular fluid within normal limits, functional hypoparathyroidism may be said to exist; it may be termed metabolic (relative) hypoparathyroidism.

Several hormones (estrogens, calcitonin, glucocorticoids) are antagonistic to PTH but their administration does not lead to frank hypocalcemia. Although estrogens lower the serum calcium level significantly (Parfitt, 1965; Young *et al.*, 1968) and have therefore been given to postmenopausal women with primary hyperparathyroidism (Gallagher and Nordin, 1972; Gallagher and Wilkinson, 1973) and to a man with parathyroid carcinoma (Sigurdsson *et al.*, 1973), never, to our knowledge, has this led to *hypocalcemia*. Similarly, even if acute calcitonin administration produces hypocalcemia, the latter biochemical abnormality is not a feature of medullary carcinoma of the thyroid, a calcitonin-producing tumor.

The effect of glucocorticoids had been appreciated from observations that adrenal cortical failure alleviates (Leonard, 1946; Leifer and Hollander, 1953; Morse *et al.*, 1961; Kenny and Holliday, 1964), whereas the administration of adrenal glucocorticoids aggravates the manifestations of hypoparathyroidism (Moehlig and Steinbach, 1954; Myers and Lawrence, 1958; Morse *et al.*, 1961; Kahn *et al.*, 1964; Eliel *et al.*, 1965 and 1971), whether treated or untreated, and regardless of the mode of therapy: parathyroid extract, vitamin D, or dihydrotachysterol. Whether this adverse activity exerts itself entirely or partially through its antagonism to vitamin D, as suggested by Eliel *et al.* (1965), or by some other mechanism, is unknown. Only the antagonistic action to vitamin D has been well documented recently (Favus *et al.*, 1973a and 1973b). It is well established that glucocorticoids do not interfere adversely with the intermediary metabolism of vitamin D, but probably induce biochemical alterations in the intestinal mucosal cells involved in calcium absorption (Favus *et al.*, 1973a). Prednisolone has even been shown to increase the concentration of $1,25\text{-}(OH)_2D_3$ in rat serum, yet intestinal transport of calcium is inhibited in these animals (Lukert *et al.*, 1973). This question, however, remains unresolved since recent data have shown that large doses of prednisolone (20 mg/kg/day for 5 days) stimulate further metabolism of $1,25\text{-}(OH)_2D_3$ to more polar, biologically inactive intestinal metabolites (Carré *et al.*, 1974), as had been shown previously by Avioli *et al.* (1968).

Other substances interfere with the PTH-induced bone resorption, although they do not produce overt hypocalcemia, at least not by this mechanism. This is especially true of inorganic pyrophosphate (DeLong *et al.*, 1971), imidazole (Avery *et al.*, 1971), corticosteroids (Raisz *et al.*, 1972b), phenytoin (Harris *et al.*, 1974; Jenkins *et al.*, 1974), chlorpropamide (Numann and Moses, 1974), and sodium fluoride (Phang *et al.*, 1968; Messer *et al.*, 1973), although the effect of fluorides in one study could not be reproduced (Kraintz, 1969). The same has been shown recently as far as aspirin is concerned (Powles *et al.*, 1973). Although this widely used drug is not known to induce hypocalcemia, the authors are aware of one case in whom aspirin administration repeatedly produced profound hypocalcemia. The action of ethanol (Peng and Gitelman, 1974) is more striking, since hypocalcemia develops upon acute exposure, but it is self-limited. Chronic alcoholism is not associated with chronic hypocalcemia unless the liver is severely involved. Mithramycin is another agent which causes acute hypocalcemia and interferes with PTH-induced bone resorption, both *in vivo* (Robins and Jowsey, 1973) and *in vitro* (Minkin, 1973). Bone resorbing effects of PTH are also suppressed by colchicine *in vitro* (Heath *et al.*, 1972; Raisz *et al.*, 1973). In exceptional cases of self-poisoning, hypocalcemia may result (Ellwood and Robb, 1971), as regularly occurs in rats given 0.05-0.2 mg/g intraperitoneally (Heath *et al.*, 1972). One of us (C.N.) is aware of an individual who consumed 40 mg of colchicine, enough to produce complete medullary aplasia, yet hypocalcemia did not develop. In the case reported by Ellwood and Robb (1971), 25-30 mg of colchicine was ingested and a low serum calcium level (7.0 mg/dl) was detected 2 days later and persisted for two weeks. The authors postulated depressed PTH production but produced no evidence in support of this idea.

Other disorders are associated with significant, chronic, and eventually symptomatic hypocalcemia. They are hypomagnesemia, vitamin D deficiency, renal failure, and other disorders of vitamin D metabolism. Interactions of vitamin D and PTH and abnormalities of vitamin D metabolism are discussed elsewhere in this volume and will not be considered further here.

A. Hypomagnesemia

Hypomagnesemia, either primary or secondary (Wacker and Parisi, 1968) may produce hypocalcemia which can be corrected only by magnesium supplementation (Heaton and Fourman, 1965). The means whereby this hypocalcemia occurs is a controversial matter. One possible mechanism which has been postulated is end-organ unresponsiveness to parathyroid hormone. One has to take into account at least two factors in the interpretation of the findings. First, the degree of magnesium depletion and its duration and, second, the amount of parathyroid hormone administered. If subtle differences are to be shown, physiological rather than pharmacological amounts of parathyroid extracts must be administered. In dogs, the amount necessary to maintain serum calcium within normal limits in the acutely parathyroidectomized animal has been estimated from 0.1 U/kg/h (Copp *et al.*, 1961) to 0.4 U/kg/h (Suh *et al.*, 1971) when using crude parathyroid extract. If highly purified bovine parathyroid hormone is infused at a constant rate, the dosage necessary to obtain the same effect is 0.05 U/kg/h (i.e., 25 ng/kg/h), whereas 0.2 U/kg/h (i.e., 100 ng/kg/h) produces marked hypercalcemia in all dogs (Parsons and Reit, 1974). If those data may be extrapolated to other species or to humans, it must be realized that very often much higher dosages have been given. Experiments in which parathyroid extract has been given to Mg-deficient animals have not shown evidence of end-organ resistance to the hormone (Hahn *et al.*, 1972b), but these doses were greater than physiological. Rayssiguier and Larvor (1974) found no difference in the hypercalcemic effect in rats when injecting large doses of PTE (500 U/kg) into normal or Mg-depleted animals. Similarly, in cases of primary hypomagnesemia in infants in which "normal responses" to PTE are claimed, the doses commonly employed were often as large as those used in adults, despite the differences in body weights (Salet *et al.*, 1966; Paunier *et al.*, 1968; Suh *et al.*, 1973). In contrast, Woodard *et al.* (1972), using 80 U/day for 2 days, did not see any rise in the serum calcium level in an infant whose serum Mg level was 0.3 mg/dl. Another infant tested with very low serum Mg values and no response to PTE (dose not given), has been reported by Aziz (1972). It therefore seems that if "physiological" doses of parathyroid extract are given to severely Mg-depleted infants, end-organ responsiveness is defective. Furthermore, when retested after magnesium supplementation, the infant of Salet *et al.* (1966) showed a brisk response on the very first day of administration with a serum calcium of 16.3 mg/dl and clinical signs of calcium intoxication despite the use of only 100 U of PTE. Serum Mg level at that time was 1.3 mg/dl, evidence for only mild magnesium deficiency. Similarly, the second administration of PTE by Paunier *et al.* (1968) was followed by a much brisker response. Even if Mg supplements had been withdrawn before the test, Mg depletion was much less pronounced at that time, as witnessed by a definitely higher serum Mg level (about 0.9 mg/dl, versus 0.5 mg/dl during the first test).

Further evidence that low levels of Mg in the plasma may be associated with functional hypoparathyroidism was provided by Estep *et al.* (1969), who administered PTE to 13 hypocalcemic alcoholic patients. Five had a normal response to PTE and eight showed resistance at both end-organs: bone (as measured by serum calcium and urinary hydroxyproline) and kidney (as measured by tubular reabsorption of phosphorus). The average serum Mg level in the PTE-resistant group was 0.8 ± 0.3 mg/dl versus 1.8 ± 0.2 mg/dl in the PTE-sensitive group; there was no overlap between the values in these two groups. When the Mg-depleted state was corrected, the peripheral resistance to PTE disappeared. Muldowney *et al.* (1970) found end-organ (bone) resistance to PTE in their severely Mg-depleted (0.6 mEq/l) patiets with steatorrhea, versus a normal response in normomagnesemic patients. After magnesium replenishment, a normal hypercalcemic response was observed in the previously PTE-resistant patients (Muldowney *et al.*, 1970; Connor *et al.*, 1972). It should be realized that comparing Mg-depleted with Mg-repleted patients—even if each subject serves as his own control—may be misleading since one may also be comparing hypocalcemic with normocalcemic patients in the process and there is some evidence that normocalcemic patients respond better to PTE (Au and Raisz, 1967). Intracellular calcium may function as a second messenger for PTE, and an alternative to cyclic AMP (Parsons and Robinson, 1971; Robinson *et al.*, 1972), in the process of initiating bone resorption. On the other hand, comparing Mg-depleted patients with hypoparathyroid patients may be valid only if there is not excess PTH secretion in the hypocalcemic hypomagnesemic patients.

In cases of hypomagnesemia, a sluggish response to PTE has been demonstrated in bone (Coenegracht and Houben, 1974) or kidney (Medalle and Waterhouse, 1973). On the other hand, Chase and Slatopolsky (1974) found a normal renal response to PTE as judged by cyclic AMP excretion, although they did not compare the response before and after Mg supplementation. Serum calcium increased from 7.2 to 9.2 mg/dl after 3 days of parathyroid extract administration (800 U/day) in one patient whose serum Mg level was 0.8 mEq/l and from 4.8 to 6.2 mg/dl after 4 days of an equal dose of PTE in another with serum Mg of 0.5 mEq/l. In conclusion, it seems that if the serum Mg level is very low and provided physiological rather than pharmacological doses of PTH are used, some degree of end-organ unresponsiveness towards PTH exists in Mg-depleted infants and adults.

The exact pathophysiology of end-organ unresponsiveness is not clear. It is true that Mg is an essential cofactor for adenyl cyclase and thus influences the conversion of ATP to cyclic AMP. However, if this were the mechanism whereby magnesium deficiency achieved end-organ unresponsiveness, it would have to affect simultaneously most of the reactions that are cyclic AMP-mediated, which is obviously not the case. *In vitro* studies showed that PTE had less effect on bone from Mg-deficient rats than on bones from control rats as far as release of calcium, inorganic phosphate, and hydroxyproline into the incubation medium was concerned (MacManus *et al.*, 1971). Furthermore, Raisz and Neimann (1969) found less calcium release from cultures of embryonic bone when PTE was delivered in the presence of a low Mg concentration. Several authors have suggested that there might exist in this situation an alteration in the exchange of calcium between extracellular fluid and bone which favors net movement of calcium into the skeleton. In chicks, endosteal bone resorption is markedly reduced when Mg depletion is produced (Reddy *et al.*, 1973), and in man radiocalcium kinetic studies have actually shown the bone resorption rate (v_{o-}) to be nil in a single instance (Vesin *et al.*, 1974).

Besides end-organ unresponsiveness another possible cause of magnesium-dependent hypocalcemia is failure of the parathyroid glands to respond to hypocalcemia or hypomagnesemia. Reports in the literature are contradictory. Some authors have found elevated PTH levels (Connor *et al.*, 1972; Coenegracht and Houben, 1974), others inappropriately normal levels (Suh *et al.*, 1973; Medalle and Waterhouse, 1973; Chase and Slatopolsky, 1974) and some undetectable levels (Anast *et al.*, 1972). Magnesium supplementation is followed by a temporary rise in iPTH levels above normal values (Anast *et al.*, 1972; Chase and Slatopolsky, 1974) before a return to the normal range, an example of the "parathormone-like effect" of magnesium replenishment described by Muldowney *et al.* (1970) and Rude *et al.* (1975). The rise in serum calcium is accompanied by an increase in phosphate clearance by the kidney and an increase in alkaline phosphatase levels in the serum (Muldowney *et al.*, 1970), a pattern of response which could result either from an increase in PTH secretion, or a restoration of end-organ responsiveness, or both (as is probable).

"Inadequate" levels of iPTH were found in two Mg-depleted dogs by Levi *et al.* (1974), and they did not increase while hypocalcemia was developing. There seems to be little doubt that during Mg depletion, failure of parathyroid hormone secretion (or synthesis) occurs. Under these circumstances, a phosphate load which lowers the serum ionized calcium fraction does not result in an increase of iPTH levels in man (Anast *et al.*, 1972), as expected. In the Mg-deficient rat the serum calcium falls to abnormal levels only under the influence of a phosphate load (Rayssiguier and Larvor, 1974). It would seem that there exists some critical level of serum Mg concentration that is necessary for PTH secretion (or synthesis?) to occur. Targovnik *et al.* 1971) showed *in vitro* that the PTH secretion diminishes strikingly when the concentration of Mg in the incubation medium falls below 0.7 mg/dl.

Since data in the literature are scarce and often fragmentary, dealing, for example, either with iPTH levels or with end-organ resistance, and since little or no histologic information is available on the underlying bone disorder, it is of interest to review briefly our own experience in this field (Rombouts-Lindemans *et al.*, unpublished).

Several patients were studied. Basic data are given in Table I. Four patients had steatorrhea: J.P. in association with idiopathic hypoparathyroidism, C.R. and F.G. owing to large ileal resections due to regional enteritis, A.L. as a result of celiac sprue. M.C. had primary hyperparathyroidism with bone involvement. End-organ responsiveness to exogenous PTH was evaluated by measuring urinary excretion of cyclic AMP and by analyzing bone biopsies with quantitative histomorphometric techniques; in some instances levels of iPTH were determined in addition to routine pertinent biochemical analyses on serum and urine. Four out of five patients were hypomagnesemic, but only two (C.R. and M.C.) were severely depleted. Upon Mg replenishment, serum calcium of C.R. became normal (cf. Fig. 3A), that of F.G. remained normal, and that of J.P., the hypoparathyroid patient, remained low. However, in the latter instance, complete refractoriness to treatment with crystalline dihydrotachysterol (DHT) disappeared and only when the serum Mg had

Basic Data on Five Hypomagnesemic Patients, including iPTH Levels and the Results of Histomorphometric Measurements, as Applied to Trabecular Bone Obtained Through Transiliac Bone Biopsy. (cf. Figs. 3A and 3B)

Parameters	Normal values[a]	J.P.	C.R.	F.G.	M.C.	A.L.
Age		16	59	57	43	71
Sex		M	F	F	F	F
Weight (kg)		51	46	39	65	43
Serum magnesium (mEq/l)[b]	1.4– 1.9	1.17	0.49	1.28	0.85	1.38
Serum calcium (mg/dl)	8.5–10.5	5.3	7.9	8.8	14.1	8.4
Serum phosphorus (mg/dl)	2.8– 4.0	5.9	3.5	3.3	2.0	2.0
Urinary calcium (mg/24 h)	80–250	24	35	40	405	29
Urinary total hydroxyproline (mg/24 h)	15–35	106	21	19	262	75
Serum carotene (µg/dl)	>100	54	8	18	(—)	28
Relative resorption surface (%)[b]	<4	1.9	2.5	1.0	8.5	3.3
Mean surface periosteocytic lacunae (µm²)	50.6 ± 5.2	53.1	45.4	43.1	67.2	55.8
Relative osteoid volume (%)	<4	1.0	1.3	1.2	4.0	13.5
Relative osteoid surface (%)	<25	8.3	9.0	4.7	18.4	(—)
Mean thickness osteoid seams (µm)	<12	6.6	7.1	8.9	10.4	23.0
Calcification fronts	++	++	++	++	++	None
Cortical bone (g/cm²)	0.60	0.48	0.68	0.53	0.59	(—)
Trabecular bone (g/cm²)	0.35	0.29	0.40	0.28	0.46	0.30
iPTH (pg bPTH Eq/ml)[c]	214 ± 95	N.D.	300	230	1510	550

[a] Many values are age- and sex-dependent, especially those concerning bone histomorphometry and photon absorptiometry. The "normal values" represent an oversimplification but do indicate some limit beyond which numbers may be considered definitely abnormal. N.D. means "not detectable" and (—) means that either the measurement was not performed or that for technical reasons it could not be determined.

[b] See Meersseman (1973).

[c] Performed by Dr. R. Bouillon, Rega Institute, Leuven University, using antiserum A VI-2 (Bouillon et al., 1974) and expressed in terms of bovine PTH equivalent (bPTH Eq) (Bouillon et al., 1974).

been normal for some time could the serum calcium be brought to normal as well with reduced doses of DHT. The effects of Mg administration in patient M.C. were difficult to evaluate owing to the changes occurring in the postoperative period.

Relative renal resistance to PTE was demonstrated in C.R., as shown by increased cyclic AMP excretion after 3 days of Mg supplementation (Fig. 3A). No difference could be seen in J.P. (Fig. 3A) and in F.G. (not shown), possibly since Mg depletion was less severe. Four successive studies were performed on patient M.C. (Fig. 3B). Prior to her operation, 9/16/1971, when an excess quantity of iPTH was circulating, or afterwards, when presumably a normal amount was present, her response to exogenous PTE was very poor as long as the Mg level was low (respectively 0.85 for "M.C.I." and 1.00 mEq/1 for "M.C.II.") When this level was corrected, a normal response was obtained on two different occasions ("M.C.III" and "M.C.IV").

It should be noted that in no patient studied, except A.L., was any excess osteoid tissue present, shown by histomorphometric measurements. This is probably due to the high serum phosphate levels in J.P., C.R. and F.G. There were no signs of hyperparathyroidism in C.R.,

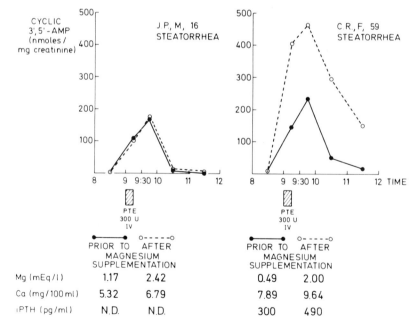

Fig. 3A. Response of urinary cAMP to exogenous PTE before and after Mg supplementation in two patients with steatorrhea.

despite chronic low serum calcium and magnesium levels, or in F.G., despite chronic low magnesium levels. It is known that excessive osteo-clastic resorption surfaces in trabecular bone and/or an increase in the mean surface of periosteocytic lacunae characterize patients with hyper-parathyroidism. In the series studied by Meunier *et al.* (1972), both these parameters were abnormal in 85% of the cases, and in all cases one was present. This is especially conspicuous in patient M.C., while patient A.L. is somewhat intermediate between C.R. and F.G. on the one hand, and M.C. on the other. These measurements provide different informa-tion than the radioimmunoassays for circulating PTH, since they show the effects of biologically active PTH over the entire period the bone has been exposed to the hormone. In addition, urinary excretion of total hy-droxyproline in both C.R. and F.G. was low, in contrast to the elevated values in M.C. and A.L. In J.P., the high value reflects the growth spurt of an adolescent boy.

Levels of iPTH were normal in both C.R. and F.G. In contrast, the

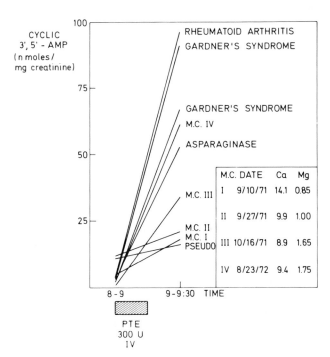

Fig. 3B. Response of urinary cAMP to exogenous PTE in various subjects. In patient M.C. with primary hyperparathyroidism, the response was measured on 4 separate occa-sions: MC I: prior to parathyroidectomy (high iPTH, low serum Mg, 0.85 mEq/liter). MC II: after parathyroidectomy (normal iPTH, how serum Mg, 1.00 mEq/liter). MC III and MC IV: after parathyroidectomy and Mg supplementation (normal iPTH, normal serum Mg).

level of iPTH, determined on three occasions in A.L., the normomagnesemic patient, was elevated for a serum calcium level intermediate between that of C.R. and F.G. On Mg replenishment, iPTH increased in C.R. to abnormally high levels (Fig. 3A), confirming the results obtained by Anast *et al.* (1972) and Chase and Slatopolsky (1974). Simultaneously, urinary hydroxyproline hardly changed (21 to 28 mg/24 h). It is even possible that severe chronic hypomagnesemia might have prevented osteopenia in C.R. by inhibiting the development of secondary hyperparathyroidism.

It is apparent that different individuals with magnesium depletion show different responses when tested, but these data also show that (1) severe Mg depletion (serum Mg levels ≤1.0 mEq/l, i.e., ≤1.2 mg/dl) may interfere with but not abolish renal responsiveness to PTH as expressed by cyclic AMP excretion; (2) secondary hyperparathyroidism does not occur, as judged by morphometric analysis of bone biopsies and radioimmunoassay of circulating PTH; (3) upon Mg replenishment, the iPTH level increases; and (4) no excess osteroid tissue was present in the hypomagnesemic patients studied.

VII. HYPOPARATHYROIDISM DUE TO THE SECRETION OF INEFFECTIVE PARATHYROID HORMONE

In section VI failure to respond to normal parathyroid hormone was considered as a cause of disordered calcium and magnesium metabolism. Here we turn to the theoretical possibility of the secretion of an ineffective, abnormal parathyroid hormone. If this occurred, one would expect to see the clinical and biochemical hallmarks of hypoparathyroidism, excess amounts of abnormal parathyroid hormone in the circulation, and a normal response to the administration of exogenous parathyroid hormone, assuming no competition between endogenous and exogenous hormones at the end-organs.

Nusynowitz and Klein (1973) hypothesized a defect in the conversion of secreted proparathyroid hormone to an active form and coined the term of "pseudoidiopathic" hypoparathyroidism for this syndrome. A troublesome finding in this case is the severe hypomagnesemia (0.7 mg/dl) which is not a classical biochemical finding in IHP. Lerner and Lukert (1974) recently described another case. Since these cases are based on radioimmunoassay of endogenous, circulating parathyroid hormone, more precise information will depend on refinement of the assay procedure. Some authors report that patients with idiopathic hypoparathyroidism do not always have undetectable levels of PTH as measured by immunoassay (Roof *et al.*, 1973; Carson *et al.*, 1973; Bouillon *et al.*, 1974; Hawker, 1975; Burckhardt *et al.*, 1975; Werder *et al.*, 1975). Some of them at least are due to lack of specificity of the radioimmunoassay. Hawker (1975) found measurable levels of iPTH in all 40 patients with hypoparathyroidism (22 with IHP, 18 postoperatively), and admits that all or much of the iPTH detected in these patients must have been due to background or blank in the assay. Others found undetectable levels in all patients with hypoparathyroidism (Reiss and Canterbury, 1968; Arnaud *et al.*, 1971; Deftos *et al.*, 1972; Fujita *et al.*, 1972; Conaway and Anast, 1974; Woo and Singer, 1974). In the authors' experience, however, some patients with idiopathic hypoparathyroidism and some with longstanding severe postoperative hypoparathyroidism have had levels of iPTH that were undetectable, normal, or even elevated. If some cases of idiopathic hypoparathyroidism are to be classified as "pseudoidiopathic" hypoparathyroidism by this assay, one should at least demonstrate that EDTA infusion produces a significant increase and calcium infusion a decrease of iPTH levels; both secondary and primary hyperparathyroidism respond appropriately to such stimuli (Murray *et al.*, 1972). EDTA infusion can be performed after hypocalcemia has been corrected with vitamin D or one of its metabolites or analogs. This procedure has only been applied by Burckhardt *et al.* (1975). Possibly one single patient studied by these authors qualifies for the entry under discussion, since upon EDTA infusion iPTH, as measured with an antiserum predominantly directed against the amino terminal end of the molecule, did not change whereas it rose when determined with an antiserum predominantly directed against the carboxyterminal end. This is compatible with the existence of biologically inert material and the absence of active hormone, but whether such is really the case remains to be confirmed.

VIII. IDIOPATHIC HYPOPARATHYROIDISM

Idiopathic hypoparathyroidism (IHP) is an infrequent condition, of unknown etiology, in which no parathyroid hormone is secreted. It was probably first described by Beumer and Falkenheim (1926). Drake *et al.* (1939) proposed criteria which remain generally useful for diagnosis of "chronic idiopathic hypoparathyroidism": biochemical findings (hypocalcemia and hyperphosphatemia, in the absence of renal insufficiency), clinical findings (signs and symptoms of tetany, in the absence of alkalosis), and negative radiological findings (excluding rickets and osteomalacia although the two diseases may coexist). Signs of tetany may be slow to appear or be mild enough to be overlooked and very different presenting symptoms have been recorded.

The idiopathic variety of hypoparathyroidism can be diagnosed only by excluding all other possible etiologies. It is necessary to establish the existence of end-organ responsiveness by evaluating the renal response to PTH via measurement of cyclic AMP. iPTH levels should be undetectable in the blood, and should not increase upon EDTA perfusion, which can be performed after correction of hypocalcemia.

Hypocalcemia is always present and often severe; in the review of Bronsky *et al.* (1958) of 50 cases, serum calcium values averaged 5.4 mg/dl (range 3.0–7.4 mg/dl). Hyperphosphatemia is almost always present but must be interpreted with respect to age in children. Serum phosphate values averaged 8.2 mg/dl in the above series (range 4.0–13.4 mg/dl).

The serum calcium level was lower than 7.4 mg/dl and the serum phosphate level higher than 4.0 mg/dl in all of the reported cases. The data of Dimich *et al.* (1967) are more recent and deal with a more homogeneous group of 10 patients, collected over 10 years. Here the average serum calcium level was 5.3 ± 0.6 (S.D.)/mg/dl and the average serum phosphate level was 7.2 ± 2.0 mg/dl. The highest serum calcium value was 6.3 mg/dl and the lowest phosphate level 4.5 mg/dl.

A. Incidence

Idiopathic hypoparathyroidism (IHP) is a rare disorder. Robins (1963) found only 151 cases in the English and American literature. Only 28 cases were reported from five teaching hospitals in the United States (Buckwalter *et al.*, 1955; Krane, 1961; Dimich *et al.*, 1967; Fonseca and Calverly, 1967; O'Malley and Kohler, 1968), where cases had been carefully recorded during one to three decades, versus 168 cases of postoperative origin, a ratio of 1 to 6. In reviewing 213,025 admissions at the Queens General Hospital between 1935 and 1950, Steinberg and Waldron (1952) were able to pinpoint only one single case of IHP, Bronsky *et al.* (1958) also recorded only one case among 434,768 admissions to the Cook County Hospital over a period of 5 years (1953–1957), while Wise and Hart (1952) detected two cases from about 620,000 admissions in Kings County Hospital in a 10-year period. The disease is being recognized with increasing frequency. While screening records in the Department of Medicine at St-Pierre University Hospital in Louvain, one of us (C. N.) found four cases out of 10,599 admissions over a period extending from 1970 through 1973. Since two-thirds of all cases manifest themselves before the age of 15 (Robins, 1963), many others were diagnosed in the

Department of Pediatrics. A greater incidence has been found by Hsien-Yi *et al.* (1964) who detected 12 cases of IHP among 25,311 admissions to Tientsin Medical College Hospital between 1947 and 1963, 7 of which were diagnosed within the last 3 years of search, an overall incidence of 1:2,100.

The true frequency is difficult to assess. When systematically screening serum calcium values in all patients at a general medical clinic, Boonstra and Jackson (1965) found the incidence of hypoparathyroidism to be 6 out of 26,000 determinations, i.e., 1:4333 patients with an equal distribution between idiopathic and postoperative cases, an incidence of IHP of 0.01%. This is probably an underestimation of the frequency of the disease since in the study all individuals were excluded "on whom serum calcium determinations had been requested specifically." In a systematic study of serum phosphate levels, the incidence of hyperphosphatemia due to hypoparathyroidism was 1:6684 (Betro and Pain, 1972) or 0.01%.

The average interval between onset of symptoms and diagnosis of IHP was 6.3 years in the study by Robins (1963). The sex distribution seems about equal (Bronsky *et al.*, 1958), except when IHP is associated with moniliasis and/or an endocrinopathy, where female preponderance is 2:1. If one analyzes the data from 74 patients collected by Blizzard *et al.* (1966) one finds that isolated IHP predominates in women (2:1), whereas sex distribution is equal when IHP occurs in association with Addison's disease (Spinner *et al.*, 1968). All in all, it seems that females with IHP probably outnumber males.

B. Genetic Classification of Idiopathic Hypoparathyroidism and Physiopathophysiological Considerations

Peden (1960) was the first to make a clear distinction between cases of IHP with early onset (within the first year of life) and those of late-onset, with familial and sporadic cases in both categories. She suggested a sex-linked genetic transmission for the familial cases of early-onset, whereas the familial cases of late-onset were probably autosomally transmitted. Several other classifications have also been offered (Taitz *et al.*, 1966; Hallström, 1967; and Barr *et al.*, 1971).

1. Sporadic Cases

Most cases of IHP are sporadic, whether of early- or late-onset.

a. Early-onset. Among the sporadic cases of early onset, at least three different varieties can be distinguished:

1. The cases called by Fanconi (1969) "persistent congenital idiopathic hypoparathyroidism," whose onset occurs within the first 3 weeks of life. Fanconi lists 14 of these cases which show a male predominance (10 M, 4 F). Additional cases have been reported by Orme (1971). It is believed that these children are born without parathyroid glands or with aplastic or hypoplastic glands, which do not become functional.

2. Those cases of infantile IHP (the "acquired" form) which manifest themselves within the first year of life.

3. All cases of the so-called III/IV pharyngeal pouch syndrome (Di-George syndrome), a disease characterized by absence, hypoplasia, or ectopy of (nonfunctional) parathyroid glands and congenital malformations of the other main structures derived from the third and fourth pharyngeal pouches, which may involve a variety of serious abnormalities, especially aplasia or hypoplasia of the thymus, leading eventually to the impairment of immunological defense mechanisms.

The association of severe multiple congenital abnormalities with congenital IHP has been recognized since the first cases were reported by Rössle (1932, 1938); others have been described by Lobdell (1959) and Huber et al. (1967). The importance of the congenital absence of the thymus and its immunological consequences have been emphasized by DiGeorge (1965, 1968), Lischner et al. (1967) and Taitz et al. (1966). The latter authors coined the term "III/IV pharyngeal pouch syndrome," because of the common embryological origin of parathyroids and thymus. Miller et al. (1972) insisted that association with congenital defects in tissues from all branchial pouches and arches could be observed, and suggested the broader term of "branchial dysembryogenesis." This syndrome, which is not familial, may occur as a result of some injury during the fourth or fifth week of fetal life. One case of IHP with abnormalities of structures arising from the first and second branchial arches was found to have the rare ring chromosome 16 (Pergament et al., 1970). The frequency of the DiGeorge syndrome is relatively high. Miller et al. (1972), reviewing their 13 cases of IHP, judged 4 to have associated congenital abnormalities of branchial origin. Reviewing 143 cases in the literature, together with their own 13 cases, they found that 33 (21%) had signs of dysembryogenesis, with 99 separate instances of 40 different types of branchial anomalies associated with IHP. The syndrome carries a poor prognosis in the most typical and severely affected cases (Taitz et al., 1966; Nézelof et al., 1975), owing to the severity of the associated abnormalities (33% mortality in the first year of life), but the prognosis is much better when the manifestations of branchial dysembryogenesis are mild, such as hypernasal speech owing to cleft palate or functional and anatomic abnormalities of the velo-pharyngeal musculature (Miller *et al.*, 1972). It has also been pointed out that congenital absence of the parathyroid glands may coexist with various malformations of derivatives of the pharyngeal pouches but without absence of the thymus (Vesterhus *et al.*, 1975).

Comments are appropriate concerning the sudden infant death syndrome (SIDS) occurring in infants aged 2 to 4 months (the so-called "crib deaths" or "cot deaths"), which has been considered by some as a disease of "congenital subvalidity" of the parathyroids (Geertinger, 1967). This author pointed out a high frequency of morphological abnormalities of the parathyroid glands, which were absent on necropsy in 34% of the cases he examined, versus 3% in a control series of infants who died from unknown conditions. Furthermore, complete fusion of thymus and parathyroids was present in 31% of the cases where parathyroids were identified, and in none of the 37 cases of the control group. Valdés-Dapena and Weinstein (1971) were unable to detect any difference in their series of autopsies between 88 infants dead from the SIDS versus a control group of 49 infants, as far as the number of parathyroid glands were concerned. The fusion of parathyroids and thymus, more frequent in the SIDS series than in controls, was considered to be a variant of normal in the infant. It seems unlikely that inadequate parathyroid gland function contributes to this syndrome since SIDS usually supervenes in full health, without any past history of tetany or convulsions. Recent investigations implicate different etiologic factors (Ferris, 1973; Ferris *et al.*, 1973; Naeye, 1974; Anderson and Ewen, 1974; Guilleminault *et al.*, 1975).

b. Late-onset. Most cases of *isolated idiopathic hypoparathyroidism* represent an acquired form of the disease and are sporadic and of late-onset. The average age at which symptoms first appear is 20 years (Bronsky *et al.*, 1958) when all cases with moniliasis and/or associated endocrinopathy are excluded, although undoubtedly, and as often demonstrated by careful dental analysis, the disease may begin earlier and remain unnoticed. The sequence of events has seldom been adequately documented, but in at least 3 cases, a normal serum calcium level has been documented from 1 to 3 years prior to the onset of symptoms of IHP and the discovery of hypocalcemia (Berezin and Stein, 1948; Axelrod, 1959; and Robins, 1963). Furthermore, despite the fact that average serum calcium values are definitely lower in IHP than in pseudohypoparathyroidism, symptoms of the latter, which is a congenital condition, occur much earlier, at the average age of 8.5 years (Bronsky *et al.*, 1958).

Cases of this acquired form of idiopathic hypoparathyroidism which have come to autopsy invariably show the parathyroids to be absent, rudimentary, atrophic, or replaced by fat (Drake *et al.*, 1939; Cantarow *et al.*, 1939; Kopin and Rosenberg, 1960; Treusch and Cohen, 1962; Hsien-Yi *et al.*, 1964). In several cases, some parathyroid tissue has been found at autopsy. Treuch and Cohen (1962), in a case of onset in adulthood at age 46, described the single parathyroid they could find as atrophic. Its greatest diameter was 1 mm, versus an average of 6.4 mm for a normal parathyroid gland (Gilmour, 1938). Microscopically, they found increased fibrosis, cellular atrophy and nuclear pyknosis. Kopin and Rosenberg (1960) also described a case with symptomatic onset at age 65 who came to autopsy at age 79. A single parathyroid gland was found and considered normal histologically. The gland was not weighed but its greatest diameter was "1 to 2 mm." Some cellular atrophy may have been present (Treusch and Cohen. 1962).

2. *IHP in association with moniliasis and various endocrinopathies*

In sporadic cases of IHP associated with diverse endocrinopathies, as well as with superficial moniliasis, the average age of onset of symptoms is 8 years. *Candida albicans* infection of skin, mucosa (mouth: Figure 4, and vaginal area), and nails (Figure 5) is present in about 14% of all cases with IHP. It always occurs in cases of the juvenile-onset form of the disease (less than 15 years), which comprise two thirds of all cases.

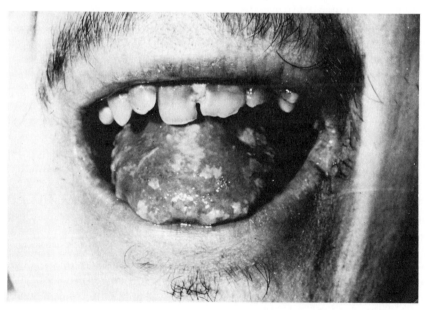

Fig. 4. Moniliasis affecting the tongue in a case of IHP in a 24 year old male. Infection had been present since age 2. Hypocalcemia (6.3 mg/dl) and hyperphosphatemia (6.5 mg/dl) were discovered on routine examination.

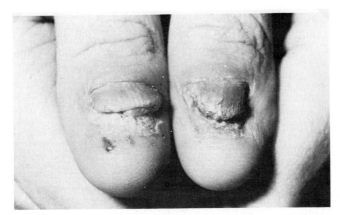

Fig. 5. Moniliasis of the fingernails as seen in the patient described in Figure 4.

Usually moniliasis precedes the onset of symptoms of IHP, and even that of hypocalcemia as has been documented in one single instance (Case Records of the Massachusetts General Hospital, 1954). It has been hypothesized that it could be the cause of hypoparathyroidism, an assumption still held by Bronsky *et al.* (1958). However, the results of autopsy have never shown involvement by *Candida albicans* of the viscera or of the parathyroid glands (Whitaker *et al.*, 1956; McMahon *et al.*, 1959; Drury *et al.*, 1970). Whitaker *et al.* (1956) favored the view that moniliasis actually resulted from dystrophic lesions of the skin, mucosa, and nails due to hypoparathyroidism, lesions which may precede chemical changes in the serum by a long interval. This hypothesis seems unlikely since moniliasis precedes the onset of IHP by an average of 5 years and dystrophic ectodermal changes improve when IHP is treated, while moniliasis usually remains intractable as shown by Sutphin *et al.* (1943). Sjöberg (1966), and Windorfer (1970) argue that moniliasis produces a toxic effect on the other glands, but it has never been possible to demonstrate this. If a causal relationship between this cutaneous disorder and the ensuing endocrinopathies could be established, Jellinek (1971) felt there would be a case for amputation of the ends of the fingers because of the high mortality of unrecognized disease. Certainly it is important to be aware of the association between the two conditions, although their exact relationship is unknown. It is possible that there may be a genetic predisposition toward developing moniliasis and IHP in association.

In order to understand this association, studies have been made on the pathogenesis of chronic moniliasis. In normal serum, there may be an inhibitory factor that prevents the growth of *Candida albicans* (Roth *et al.*, 1959; Louria and Brayton, 1964) and that might be deficient in sera of patients with intractable moniliasis. Only 4 out of 16 patients (25%) with moniliasis and IHP exhibited this antimonilial factor versus 3 out of 66 children (5%) aged 3 months to 15 years with trivial skin disease (superficial bacterial pyoderma). This difference may be significant, but the study of Esterly *et al.* (1967) showed that the presence or absence of this inhibitor is not a determining factor for the disease. Various abnormalities in cell-mediated immunity are summarized by Kirkpatrick *et al.* (1971) and by Block *et al.* (1971), who described a case of IHP and moniliasis (as well as Addison's disease and primary ovarian failure) in which the patient was unable to develop a delayed hypersensitivity response to *Candida albicans in vivo*, despite evidence of immune cellular activity *in vitro* (lymphocyte stimulation and release of a migratory inhibition factor). There is evidence for a significant role for impaired cellular immunity in the report of Levy *et al.* (1971) in which oral moniliasis cleared in a 17-year-old male with chronic mucocutaneous moniliasis, Addison's disease, pernicious anemia, and malabsorption following transplantation of fetal thymus tissue on two occasions. High titres (1/120–1/480) of antibodies against *Candida albicans* were found in all three cases of the two associated diseases described by Sjöberg (1966).

The first endocrinopathy to have been reported in association with IHP is Addison's disease (Leonard, 1946), which occurs in about 10% of all cases. Since in one-third of these cases moniliasis is present as well, this triad has been termed the HAM (hypoparathyroidism–Addison's disease–moniliasis) syndrome by Taitz *et al.* (1966). Addison's disease usually follows IHP, and moniliasis usually precedes IHP, but there are exceptions. Addison's disease may occasionally precede the onset of IHP, but it never appears before moniliasis in the HAM syndrome. If unrecognized, Addison's disease may lead to death. On the other hand, the symptoms of hypoparathyroidism are considerably relieved when hypoadrenalism supervenes and return upon glucocorticoid replacement therapy. Case 2 of Morse *et al.* (1961) exemplifies the sequence of events in a spectacular manner. IHP was diagnosed at age 11 (serum calcium level: 5.5 mg/dl). Treatment was instituted, but discontinued by the patient after 2 months. One year later he was readmitted and had developed Addison's disease; his serum calcium level had risen spontaneously to 10.3 mg/dl. On glucocorticoid replacement therapy (without additional vitamin D therapy), the serum calcium fell to 4.7 mg/dl. Similar cases have been reported by Leonard (1946), Leifer and Hollander (1953), Papadatos and Klein (1954), and Quichaud *et al.* (1969). Conversely, in a case described by Kenny and Holliday (1964), the occurrence of Addison's disease in a patient treated for IHP coincided with an elevation of the serum calcium to 14.5 mg/dl, which required intravenous infusions of sodium sulfate. Whether the destruction of the adrenal cortex may be limited to the adrenal zona glomerulosa and produce isolated hypoaldosteronism, as in the case of a 12-year-old girl with IHP and superficial moniliasis reported by Marieb *et al.* (1974), remains to be shown.

Other endocrinopathies which may be associated with IHP or with the complete or incomplete HAM syndrome include hypothyroidism (Himsworth and Maizels, 1940; Perlmutter *et al.*, 1956; Carter *et al.*, 1959; Presley and Paul, 1960), Hashimoto's thyroiditis (Kenny and Holliday, 1964; Drury *et al.*, 1970), and ovarian failure (Sjöberg, 1966; Irvine *et al.*, 1968; Golonka and Goodman, 1968; Hermans *et al.*, 1969; Block *et al.*, 1971; Vazquez and Kenny, 1973; Jehanne and Guivarch, 1974; Kleerekoper *et al.*, 1974; Lorenz and Burr, 1974). Several patients developed severe, multiple endocrine insufficiency, involving in one case the parathyroids, the adrenals, the thyroid, and the ovaries in that order (Vazquez and Kenny, 1973). Moniliasis was the first manifestation of the disease. The pituitary gland has not been found to be directly involved, although associated hypopituitarism owing to a pituitary tumor has been described (Thew and Goulston, 1962).

Other diseases may be associated with IHP as well; pernicious anemia is the most common (Reisner and Ellsworth, 1955; Hurwitz, 1956; McMahon *et al.*, 1959; Morse *et al.*, 1961; Hung *et al.*, 1963; Visakorpi and Gerber, 1963; Ikkala *et al.*, 1964; Sjöberg, 1966; Siurala *et al.*, 1968; Comin *et al.*, 1969; Drury *et al.*, 1970; Olin and Poindexter, 1972). Pernicious anemia usually follows IHP by 5 to 10 years, with the exception of an adult case of Comin *et al.* (1969). Circulating gastric antibodies are usually demonstrable. Early acquired atrophy of the gastric mucosa is probably the etiological factor, as in the "adult-form" of pernicious anemia. However, a distinction should be made between these cases of true pernicious anemia, in which a lack of intrinsic factor can be demonstrated, and those in which there is impaired vitamin B_{12} absorption, owing either to steatorrhea or to nonspecific changes in the gastric mucosa, such as gastritis or achlorhydria secondary to chronic hypocalcemia. Ikkala *et al.* (1964) showed that these latter changes may also occur in cases of postoperative hypoparathyroidism. In similar cases of IHP, correction of the hypocalcemia has occasionally been followed by disappearance of impaired vitamin B_{12} absorption (Halmos *et al.*, 1962; Gay and Grimes, 1972).

Other less frequent conditions associated with IHP include phlyctenular kerato-conjunctivitis, as described by Emerson *et al.* (1941), Sutphin *et al.* (1943), and Leonard (1946). In a review of the subject Gass (1962) reported 12 cases, all with associated moniliasis and/or endocrinopathies. Alopecia totalis is another frequently mentioned complication (Leonard,

1946; Blizzard et al., 1966; Blizzard and Gibbs, 1968; Irvine et al., 1968; Fields et al., 1971; Jehanne and Guivarch, 1974; Kleerekoper et al., 1974) or alopecia areata (Kleerekoper et al., 1974), as are "juvenile cirrhosis" (Blizzard et al., 1966 and 1968), posthepatitic cirrhosis (Whitaker et al., 1956; Williams and Wood, 1959; Gass, 1962; Kunin et al., 1963), vitiligo (Perlmutter et al., 1956; McMahon et al., 1959; Fisher and Fitzpatrick, 1970; Fields et al., 1971), cystic fibrosis or muco-viscidosis (McMahon et al., 1959; Morse et al., 1961), and steatorrhea, which will be dealt with separately in the following section.

In a large series reviewed by Fanconi (1969) moniliasis occurred in 72% (at the mean age of 3), Addison's disease in 58% (mean age of 11), steatorrhea in 26% (mean age of 8) and pernicious anemia in 9% (mean age of 16.5). The full HAM syndrome occurred in 32% whereas moniliasis alone with IHP occurred in 40% and Addison's disease alone with IHP in 28%. One third of the patients died from Addison's disease.

In the 74 patients whose sera were analyzed by Blizzard et al. (1966) 42 had isolated IHP, while 32 had one or more associated diseases: moniliasis (66%); Addison's disease (56%); pernicious anemia (22%); thyroid disease (19%); alopecia totalis (13%); premature menopause, before the age of 25 (6%); and juvenile cirrhosis (6%). Steatorrhea was not mentioned in this series.

3. Familial cases

a. Early-onset. Several familial cases of IHP have been reported with an early-onset (Peden, 1960; Lelong et al., 1962, 1968; Benson and Parsons, 1964; Gorodischer et al., 1970; Barr et al., 1971). The small number of well documented cases, both sporadic and familial, precludes definite conclusions as to their genetic transmission. Because a significant proportion of male patients, but none of the females, have affected male siblings and from the study of a single kindred, it was concluded that one form of early-onset IHP probably results from a sex-linked mendelian recessive trait (Peden, 1960; Taitz et al., 1966). In several other families studied (Lelong et al., 1962 and 1968; Benson and Parsons, 1964; Gorodischer et al., 1970; Barr et al., 1971), an autosomal dominant mode of transmission seemed more likely. The question of an autosomal recessive type of transmission, as suggested by Niklasson (1970), will have to wait further clarification, since the diagnosis in these cases (congenital hypoparathyroidism or primary hypomagnesemia with Mg-dependent secondary hypocalcemia) is open to question.

b. Late-Onset. Most cases of the isolated form of IHP are sporadic, but some familial cases do occur. Not surprisingly, some of these may be seen in families where cases of early-onset IHP are present as well. This is not true for the sex-linked recessive type of transmission, but does occur in those families with an autosomal dominant form of inheritance, as mentioned above. Except for these few instances, most of the familial cases of isolated IHP do not exhibit any mendelian distribution (Spinner *et al.*, 1968 and 1969).

IHP in association with an endocrinopathy (chiefly Addison's disease) and/or various other above mentioned diseases, and especially the HAM syndrome, has a familial incidence in about half of the cases. Whitaker *et al.* (1956) termed the syndrome "familial juvenile hypoadrenocorticism, hypoparathyroidism and superficial moniliasis." The distribution is compatible with an autosomal recessive pattern (Spinner *et al.*, 1968 and 1969).

One mechanism which could account for the occurrence of IHP and associated disorders could be immunologically mediated tissue damage. The evidence on which such a hypothetical mechanism is based is circumstantial and immunologically mediated damage has not been proven. It is, however, useful to review the data which form the basis for this thinking.

The frequent familial occurrence of IHP syndrome is compatible with a genetic tendency to disordered immune mechanisms. In the family described by Drury *et al.* (1970), it is possible that both (consanguinous) parents carried a recessive trait with incomplete penetrance, since clinical pernicious anemia was present in the father and his sister, and parietal cell antibodies were detected in the serum of both father and mother. The manifestations of apparent autoimmunity in their children were pronounced and occurred early. The daughter had moniliasis (age 7), hypothyroidism (age 15), Addison's disease (age 15), hypoparathyroidism (age 16), pernicious anemia (age 22) and ovarian failure (no menarche and no secondary sex characteristics). At autopsy (age 24), no adrenal tissue could be identified macroscopically or histologically. Rudimentary ovaries and uterus were identified; no follicles were present in the ovaries, no endometrium could be detected in the uterus. Only one small focus of probable parathyroid tissue could be identified after careful search. The thyroid gland was almost totally replaced by acellular fibrotic tissue, in which small foci of surviving thyroid tissue remained, histologically consistent with Hashimoto's thyroiditis. Her brother had moniliasis and steatorrhea (age 7), probable undiagnosed Addison's disease (age 11) which led to death, and probable IHP, masked by Addison's disease. At autopsy, both adrenals were extremely thin and atrophic. Parathyroid glands could not be identified. Another sibling had died in childhood "from gastroenteritis" and the fourth child could not be examined, but was reportedly in good health. There are numerous similar case reports.

Olin and Poindexter (1972) described two sisters, one of whom developed the full HAM syndrome as well as pernicious anemia, the other IHP and moniliasis. Both sisters carried adrenal antibodies. Since the older girl did not develop Addison's disease until age 19 (1970), it is still possible that her younger sister, born in 1953, will develop the same endocrinopathy. The proband with pernicious anemia had a gastric biopsy which showed a normal mucosa, except for the absence of parietal cells. She carried antibodies against parietal cells, as did her mother and another healthy sibling born in 1954.

Kunin et al. (1963) reviewed the autopsies of 9 patients with IHP and Addison's disease. Parathyroid tissue was found in only 3 instances. The cortical tissue of the adrenal glands was uniformly atrophic. Cystic fibrosis of the pancreas was present in one case with lung involvement, consistent with that disorder, whereas in two other cases bronchiectasis was found. Thyroid abnormalities were detected in 3 cases. Hepatic abnormalities were found in 8 cases and were consistent with posthepatitic cirrhosis. A viral etiology was proposed to account for the syndrome but not proven. It thus seems advisable to screen all patients with hepatitis and IHP for the presence of hepatitis antigens. In several instances, hepatitis has followed, rather than preceded, the onset of IHP (Williams and Wood, 1959; Chaptal et al., 1960). A few cases might also have had chronic active hepatitis. Another possible explanation for hepatic involvement is the increased vulnerability of the liver in the absence of parathyroid glands. Parathyroidectomy in dogs has led to necrosis of liver cells (Larson and Elkourie, 1928). Rixon and Whitfield (1972) showed that in the rat PTH may initiate liver regeneration after partial hepatectomy. Following this procedure, DNA synthesis and cell proliferation are reduced 50% and delayed 12–14 hours in the absence of PTH. It was later shown that PTH was necessary to maintain the ability of liver parenchymal cells to proliferate after partial hepatectomy rather than to initiate this process itself (Rixon and Whitfield, 1974). The liver is known to be one of the target organs of PTH (Neuman et al., 1975a, 1975b, and 1975c). Canterbury et al. (1974) showed that PTH stimulates liver adenyl cyclase maximally at concentrations equivalent to those reported for bone and kidney. How these data pertain to possible liver regeneration and/or protection is not known.

The role of hypocalcemia per se should also be considered. One of us (C.N.) and his co-workers (Rombouts-Lindemans et al., unpublished) observed an adolescent with IHP (patient J. P. in Table I) and steatorrhea (age 13), who subsequently developed Addison's disease (age 16) and pernicious anemia (age 16.5), with antibodies against intrinsic factor as well as parietal cell antibodies, although the latter were found in low titer (courtesy of Professor D. Doniach). His brother (two years older) also suffered from IHP. On each of three occasions when the proband presented with a severe hypocalcemia, increases were observed in serum transaminases and leucine aminopeptidase, and bromsulphalein retention was 17%. When the serum calcium was normal, these abnormalities disappeared. Australia antigen was absent from the serum. Liver biopsy showed necrosis of some hepatocytes. There were no fatty infiltration, periportal fibrosis, or abnormal inflammatory cells. Liver disease in IHP may sometimes be merely "functional." The authors have never observed signs of impaired liver function with hypocalcemia where parathyroid glands are functional. Whether steatorrhea contributed to these transient episodes of liver damage could not be determined. Mild derangement of liver function tests has been noticed in a similar situation by Sjöberg (1966) and Lorenz and Burr (1974).

Williams and Wood (1959) and Kenny and Holliday (1964) raised the possibility of hypersensitivity or "autoimmune disorder" as the etiologic mechanism for the syndrome. Kenny and Holliday (1964) described two sisters, the first suffering from moniliasis (age 6), hypoparathyroidism (age 6.5), Addison's disease (age 8) and Hashimoto's thyroiditis (age 16.5). Circulating antibodies to adrenal and thyroid tissue were detected in her serum. She later developed pernicious anemia (age 18) and was found to suffer from ovarian failure (Vazquez and Kenny, 1973). Her only sibling developed moniliasis (age 5), hypoparathyroidism (age 5), Hashimoto's thyroiditis (age 15.6) and ovarian failure. In both girls circulating antibodies to thyroid, adrenal, and ovarian tissues could be detected. The mother had Hashimoto's thyroiditis and the father antithyroid antibodies. Golonka and Goodman (1968) also postulated an autoimmune process as the cause of the coexistence in a patient of IHP (age 3), primary ovarian failure (age 15) and idiopathic Addison's disease (age 17). Antibodies to the adrenal cortex, to thyroid antigens, and to parietal cells of the gastric mucosa were detected in the patient's plasma.

Blizzard et al. (1966) found circulating parathyroid antibodies, as detected by the indirect immunofluorescent technique, in 41% of IHP with associated conditions, in 33% of isolated "acquired" IHP, in 26% of isolated Addison's disease, in 12% of isolated Hashimoto's disease, and in 6% of a control population. In none of the 4 patients with congenital hypoparathyroidism could parathyroid antibodies be shown. The specificity of these antibodies was not established. Adrenal antibodies were found in 11% of patients with IHP without symptoms or signs of Addison's disease, versus 53% in patients with idiopathic Addison's disease, and none in patients with Hashimoto's thyroiditis, virilizing adrenal hyperplasia, adrenal tumors, or Cushing's syndrome. In four patients with

IHP in whom the authors had previously found adrenal antibodies, Addison's disease subsequently developed. The incidence of gastric antibodies directed towards parietal cells was 71% in IHP associated with pernicious anemia, 22% in IHP associated with any of the other conditions, 13% in isolated IHP, 4% in Hashimoto's thyroiditis, and 2% in a control population. Finally, the incidence of cytoplasmic thyroid antibodies was 13% in IHP without associated thyroid disease, versus 1% in normal control children. Whether some of the patients with circulating adrenal, gastric, or thyroid antibodies have subclinical disease or are likely to develop Addison's disease, pernicious anemia, or Hashimoto's thyroiditis is not known.

Irvine and Scarth (1969) described the unequivocal presence of IgG antibody to parathyroid oxyphil cells in the serum of one out of 9 patients with IHP. This serum also reacted with parathyroid chief cells. They could not exclude the possibility that the other patients' sera contained antibody to chief cells in low titer. The positive serum also contained antibodies against parietal cells, steroid-producing cells of the gonads, and all three layers of human adrenal cortex. Only against human thyroid cytoplasm could no antibodies be shown. In the family described by Lorenz and Burr (1974), the proband with moniliasis, IHP, and steatorrhea also had antibodies to parathyroid tissue. Her brother had died at age 6 from the full HAM syndrome. Several members of the immediate family had antibodies to thyroid, parathyroid, or gastric mucosa. Consanguinity was revealed three generations previously. Bottazzo et al. (1975) found that 3 of 17 patients with IHP had evidence of antibodies to human parathyroid gland tissue; there was a high incidence (53%) of prolactin-cell antibodies in these patients, the significance of which is not established. The presence of adrenal antibodies in the serum of patients with IHP has been confirmed by Spinner et al. (1969), Irvine and Barnes (1972), and Bottazzo et al. (1975). IHP is the only condition, besides idiopathic Addison's disease, in which adrenal antibodies occur (Nerup, 1974). These antibodies are absent even in tuberculous Addison's disease. These various circulating antibodies should not be considered responsible per se for the atrophic disease process but at the present time are useful markers for some abnormalities.

Evidence for disordered cellular immunity in IHP was presented by Moulias et al. (1971) who measured inhibition of leukocyte migration in vitro against parathyroid tissue. Rao et al. (1974) recently showed that some patients with IHP, but none with postoperative hypoparathyroidism and none with pseudohypoparathyroidism, have impaired cell-mediated immunity. Rameis et al. (1972) performed skin tests with phytohemagglutinin and streptokinase and found defects in delayed hypersensitivity in their patients with IHP as compared to the healthy members of their families. A patient with the HAM syndrome (Fields *et al.*, 1971) was reported to have cutaneous anergy to various antigens (Fragola, 1971).

All these data indicate that immune mechanisms may be abnormal in at least some of the patients with IHP. The occurrence of lymphocytic parathyroiditis in a few cases is also consistent with such a possibility (Craig *et al.*, 1955; Kössling and Emmrich, 1971; Mitschke *et al.*, 1973; Van de Casseye and Gepts, 1973). The case described by Williams and Wood (1959) includes autopsy findings of parenchymatous atrophy and lymphocytic infiltration in the parathyroid and adrenal glands. Confirmation of possible immunologically mediated tissue damage necessitates production of similar lesions in animals. Lupulescu *et al.* (1965, 1968) succeeded in producing experimental parathyroiditis with isoimmune hypoparathyroidism by active immunization (repeated inocculation with homologous parathyroid tissue plus Freund's adjuvant) of dogs and rats. Altenähr and Jenke (1974) were able to produce immune parathyroiditis by passive immunization in 3 out of 15 rats, without overt signs of hypoparathyroidism, however.

The existence of a possible autoimmune etiology for IHP is suggested by comparing it to idiopathic Addison's disease. The latter is found in association with moniliasis, lymphocytic thyroiditis, pernicious anemia, and ovarian failure, with or without IHP. The presence of these associated diseases, none of which is ever present in postoperative hypoparathyroidism nor in pseudohypoparathyroidism, suggests a common pathogenetic mechanism whether the parathyroid gland participates or not.

In this regard the report of Hooper *et al.* (1973) is of interest. Two siblings were described, one of whom developed IHP at age 13 and the other, isolated Addison's disease at age 12.5. The latter became clinically apparent 6 months after adrenal antibodies were detected which rose in titer from 1:4 to 1:64 after the disease became manifest. The patient with IHP never had measurable adrenal antibodies.

That the predisposition to develop isolated or, more often, associated atrophic polyendocrine disorders can be genetically inherited is shown by the unique case described by Rameis *et al.* (1972). In this kindred the full HAM syndrome developed in 2 siblings (aged 16 and 18) and in the 3-year-old daughter of a third, healthy 26-year-old female sibling. This is, to our knowledge, the first reported instance of this syndrome in two successive generations.

C. Idiopathic Hypoparathyroidism with Steatorrhea

The association of IHP and steatorrhea represents a puzzling problem for both diagnosis and pathogenesis. Whatever their relationship may be, their association is too frequent to be fortuitous (Jackson, 1957) and steatorrhea should be removed from the diagnostic criteria proposed by Drake *et al.* (1939) which exclude IHP. From a practical point of view, fat absorption should be assessed in all patients with IHP at least by measurement of serum carotene levels. Conversely, all patients with steatorrhea should have, at least, determinations of their serum phosphate level, as recommended by McMahon *et al.* (1959). It is not always easy to determine which patients with steatorrhea have hypoparathyroidism. Not all cases with steatorrhea and hypocalcemia have hypophosphatemia owing to secondary hyperparathyroidism (Bennett *et al.*, 1932; Salvesen and Böe, 1953).

Intestinal malabsorption of a "substance of lipid nature" necessary for normal parathyroid activity, as postulated by Salvesen and Böe (1953) and Cochrane *et al.* (1960), has not been substantiated. "Exhaustion hypoparathyroidism," as hypothesized by Bennett *et al.* (1932) and Williams and Wood (1959), does not seem to occur, although one recent abstract has suggested that this situation could exist (Relkin, 1974). In this case the underlying disorder, however, was chondrosarcoma and the evidence rested entirely on finding undetectable iPTH levels each time the serum calcium fell, as well as high serum phosphate levels. It is unlikely that parathyroid gland function would decrease with stimulation of hypocalcemia unless severe hypomagnesemia is present. Hypomagnesemia of some degree is bound to accompany a number of cases of severe steatorrhea. Peripheral resistance to the action of PTH, as well as diminished PTH secretion and/or synthesis, has been postulated in these cases.

Another classical biochemical abnormality which may accompany steatorrhea is vitamin D deficiency. In rare instances of vitamin D deficiency the blood chemical findings can mimic those of hypoparathyroidism, as in the group of male adolescents alluded to by Lumb and Stanbury (1974), and the children described by Taitz and de Lacy (1962), and represent "acquired (secondary) pseudohypoparathyroidism." Lowe *et al.* (1950) postulated in a case initially reported to be pseudohypoparathyroidism that continued excessive PTH production caused constant stimulation of the renal tubules until these eventually became refractory to further hormonal effects. This case has since been shown to be IHP with steatorrhea and several other abnormalities (Gomez *et al.*, 1972); iPTH was undetectable in the serum. Measurement of serum 25-OHD$_3$ levels, iPTH, and bone histomorphometry could help clarify abnormalities of calcium and phosphorus levels in steatorrhea.

There are several hypotheses to explain the relationship of IHP to steatorrhea. It has been claimed that parathyroid hypofunction either disturbs intraluminal fat digestion or damages the small bowel mucosa so that absorption of fat is impaired. Peroral suction biopsy of the proximal small bowel should provide the most useful information as to the underlying mechanisms but, unfortunately, the findings have been varied. A flat jejunal mucosa has occasionally been found (Russell, 1967) in patients in whom "secondary coeliac syndrome" was the diagnosis. Usually, however, a normal jejunal mucosa is found (Williams and Wood, 1959; Taybi and Keele, 1962; Siurala et al., 1968; Miettinen and Perheentupa, 1971; Lorenz and Burr, 1974). Defective intraluminal fat digestion should then be considered the cause of steatorrhea. Sometimes, jejunal biopsy has yielded equivocal results (Clarkson et al., 1960).

There are several ways in which a lack of PTH might affect the function of the small bowel. One of these mechanisms, as studied in three children (9–14 years of age) and one adult with IHP by Miettinen and Perheentupa (1971), may be to bring about bile salt deficiency, causing impairment of micellar solubilization of fat. In IHP bile flow is diminished, as seen on cholecystography where the gall bladder normally fills but fails to contract, even after the administration of cholecystokinin. That PTH in some way affects gall bladder function can be implied by the high incidence of cholelithiasis in primary hyperparathyroidism, as recently documented by Selle et al. (1972) and confirmed by others (Brünner and Rothmund, 1973a and 1973b; Funk et al., 1974). If bile flow is diminished in hypoparathyroidism with severe hypocalcemia, cholelithiasis may also be a complication as was observed in the case of Lowe et al. (1950). At age 28 months, this hypoparathyroid child suffered from jaundice and malnutrition. A cholecystectomy was performed and multiple pigment-containing stones were found (Gomez et al., 1972). It should be noted that in parathyroidectomized rats the bile flow is increased rather than decreased (Heidbreder et al., 1975).

Another mechanism to explain the relationship between IHP and steatorrhea is the decreased motility of the gastrointestinal tract which results from lack of PTH. Experimental findings have been unconvincing or conflicting concerning the action of PTH on the propulsive motility of the small bowel in the animal (Scaletta and Consolo, 1960; Johansson and Segerström, 1972; Segerström, 1973; Nilsson and Segerström, 1973). In humans decreased motility with IHP has occasionally been shown, with (Leifer and Hollander, 1953; Jackson et al., 1956; Clarkson et al., 1960; Taybi and Keele, 1962). Correction of hypocalcemia in the other cases was followed by normalization of intestinal motility (Clarkson et al., 1960; Snodgrass and Mellinkoff (1962). There is some evidence, reviewed by Snodgrass and Mellinkoff (1962), that intestinal hypomotility may promote steatorrhea. It may even, on theoretical grounds, favor overgrowth of intestinal bacteria which may alter the bile salts and produce fat maldigestion. Abnormal D-xylose absorption (Clarkson *et al.*, 1960; Sjöberg, 1966; Siurala *et al.*, 1968) or an abnormal Schilling test (Clarkson *et al.*, 1960; Morse *et al.*, 1961; Kunin *et al.*, 1963) has been found in more cases of IHP and steatorrhea than would be expected from the usually normal histological appearance of the jejunal wall. Occasionally, however, the xylose test (Vesakorpi and Gerber, 1963) and the Schilling test (Lorenz and Burr, 1974) have been normal.

Finally, adequate calcium ion concentrations in the pancreatic juice are necessary for maintaining the molecular configuration of lipase (Benzonana, 1968), and high concentrations of calcium ion are required for the activity of lipase (Sarda *et al.*, 1957). On theoretical grounds, severe hypocalcemia may thus indirectly interfere with fat digestion by impairing the intraluminal hydrolysis of triglycerides to fatty acids and monoglycerides which can be readily incorporated into the bile salt micelles.

Whatever the pathogenesis, treatment of the underlying condition, i.e., correction of the hypocalcemia, usually brings relief of the symptoms related to steatorrhea (DiGeorge and Paschkis, 1957; Clarkson *et al.*, 1960; Morse *et al.*, 1961; Kunin *et al.*, 1963; Visakorpi and Gerber, 1963; Sjöberg, 1966; Russell, 1967; Siurala *et al.*, 1968). Butler (1957) even declared that "some older patients can make a pretty good appraisal of their vitamin D therapy from the frequency of the bowel movements!" In contrast, gluten-free diets have usually been unsuccessful in alleviating this condition (Williams and Wood, 1959; Clarkson *et al.*, 1960; Siurala *et al.*, 1968), with a single exception where some improvement was noted (McMahon *et al.*, 1959). The hypothesis is therefore unlikely that these patients suffer from sprue, a diagnosis sometimes suggested from the roentgenological appearance of the small bowel after a barium meal (Jackson *et al.*, 1956; McMahon *et al.*, 1959; Clarkson *et al.*, 1960; Snodgrass and Mellinkoff, 1962). When improvement has been obtained, not only does the frequency of the bowel movements diminish, but in one case xylose absorption improved (Siurala *et al.*, 1968). and repeated jejunal biopsies in the only cases where the mucosa was strikingly abnormal showed improvement (Clarkson *et al.*, 1960; Russell, 1967).

If correction of the underlying biochemical abnormalities is a prerequisite for improvement of the malabsorption syndrome, steatorrhea as a rule recurs when treatment is abandoned, and in several cases it may persist throughout and the cases are then declared "difficult to manage" (Lorenz and Burr, 1974). Medium-chain triglyceride (MCT) diet may be of help under those circumstances (Carson *et al.*, 1973; Lorenz and Burr, 1974). Fat given as MCT does not require intraluminal digestion to be absorbed so that this measure can achieve control of the steatorrhea when the use of vitamin D (with oral calcium supplements) or its equivalents has not. This is further indirect evidence that the underlying disorder in the pathogenesis of IHP-associated steatorrhea is one of fat maldigestion rather than fat malabsorption.

Occasionally, steatorrhea in IHP may be induced by pancreatic disease, which results in insufficient lipase reaching the intestine to hydrolyze triglycerides. This may happen when cystic fibrosis occurs, and was probably the case in the steatorrhea reported by McMahon *et al.* (1959). Although cystic fibrosis was also diagnosed in case 2 reported by Morst *et al.* (1961), it is not likely that this played a determining role in the pathogenesis of steatorrhea in this case, since the latter completely disappeared on vitamin D therapy. In cases without cystic fibrosis, studies of the exocrine pancreatic function have often been cursory. Normal (McMahon *et al.*, 1959; Clarkson *et al.*, 1960) or abnormal (Sjöberg, 1966) secretin responses have been reported. In the instance when the secretin response was abnormal, restoration of the serum calcium level was accompanied by an improved response (Sjöberg, 1966). Administration of pancreatic extracts has not as a rule brought improvement in the amount of excreted stool fats (Visakorpi and Gerber, 1963; Lorenz and Burr, 1974). Salvesen and Böe (1953) ascribed their case to monilial involvement of the intestine, since *Candida albicans* was cultured from the stools as it was in the case described by Lorenz and Burr (1974). This possibility cannot be ruled out, but is unlikely, since *Candida* is a commensal of the digestive tract.

The question remains whether steatorrhea results from the hypoparathyroid state so that the relationship between the two is functional (Clarkson *et al.*, 1960; Siurala *et al.*, 1968, or whether the intestinal disease represents another of the "associated diseases" enumerated in the previous section which complicate the course of IHP. Three points argue in favor of the latter view. First, steatorrhea is not a complication of postoperative hypoparathyroidism or pseudohypoparathyroidism. Cases in which it was claimed to coexist with the latter disease by Lowe *et al.* (1950) have not been accepted (Gomez *et al.*, 1972) and those of MacGregor and Whitehead (1954) and Jackson *et al.* (1956) had none of the morphological characteristics of pseudohypoparathyroidism. Their diagnoses rested on failure of the renal tubule to respond to parathyroid extract; whether lack of vitamin D played a role is not known. It may be difficult to evaluate the phosphaturic response of the kidney to a single arbitrary injection of PTE or the dose given may have been too small (MacGregor and Whitehead, 1954). The only instance of intestinal malabsorption in association with pseudohypoparathyroidism is that reported by Mautalen *et al.* (1967). Lactase deficiency was conclusively demonstrated. The only cases of which the authors are aware where steatorrhea was associated with postoperative hypoparathyroidism are those reported by Siurala *et al.* (1968), one of which had hypothyroidism with high titers of thyroid antibodies and the other Waldenström's macroglobulinemia, both diseases known to be associated with alterations of gastrointestinal function. The only other instance is that reported as case No. 1 by Dent and Friedman (1964). This case, however, was not investigated preoperatively, and subtotal villous atrophy was found on the jejunal biopsy specimen. The frequency of severe cases of postoperative hypoparathyriodism and the absence of any reference to associated intestinal disease contrasts with the relative scarcity of cases of IHP and the emphasis on major manifestations of steatorrhea in these instances. At least 20 cases of this association have been formally described, to which the four cases of Miettinen and Perheentupa (1971) should be added. In addition, the discussion which followed the case presentation by DiGeorge and Paschkis (1957) showed that in the audience, Klein, Wilkins, Ulstrom, Butler, and Parrott, probably among others, followed one or several similar cases. If this can be confirmed, steatorrhea, like moniliasis, might serve as a useful clinical guide in the differential diagnosis between IHP and pseudo-hypoparathyroidism.

Second, it is suggested that steatorrhea does not result from hypoparathyroidism since in a few cases its onset may have preceded that of IHP. The "onset" of IHP is difficult to ascertain, however, and claims that steatorrhea occurred before the first manifestations of IHP by Collins-Williams (1950), Leifer and Hollander (1953), and Jackson *et al.* (1956) do not constitute proof that IHP was not present earlier. In only one case, that reported by DiGeorge and Paschkis (1957), was this sequence of events documented. All associated diseases and/or endocrinopathies accompanying IHP usually follow the onset of IHP, with the exception of moniliasis, but all of them may occasionally occur first with the exception of pernicious anemia. Steatorrhea usually manifests itself almost simultaneously with the onset of symptoms of IHP. It is probable that the onset of steatorrhea, which impairs calcium absorption, aggravates preexisting, inapparent IHP. In the case of Russell (1967), the diagnosis of steatorrhea and IHP was made at the age of 58, but the patient had been operated on for a cataract at the age of 23! The same mechanism has been evoked to explain the "onset" of IHP following gastric surgery (Vlietstra, 1973) when the latter would unmask the underlying condition.

A third argument for the existence of IHP and steatorrhea as associated diseases may be found in the fact that the great majority of cases occur together with other typical associated conditions or in cases where siblings also have IHP and associated diseases (Colling-Williams, 1950; Leifer and Hollander, 1953; Salvesen and Böe, 1953; Case Records, 1954;

Jackson *et al.*, 1956; DiGeorge and Paschkis, 1957; McMahon *et al.*, 1959; Williams and Wood, 1959; Morse *et al.*, 1961; Taybi and Keele, 1962; Kunin *et al.*, 1963; Visakorpi and Gerber, 1963; Sjöberg, 1966; Siurala *et al.*, 1968; Lorenz and Burr, 1974). Only four cases (20%) were without known associated diseases or known familial involvement (Lowe *et al.*, 1950; MacGregor and Whitehead, 1954; Russell, 1967; Carson *et al.*, 1973).

A final argument in favor of the hypothesis that steatorrhea is indeed to be considered as an "associated disease" is that it is found in combination with other well-known associated conditions, such as moniliasis, Addison's disease, thyroid insufficiency, severe persistent bilateral keratitis, and chronic active hepatitis (Wuepper and Fudenberg, 1967), or with moniliasis, Addison's disease, and pernicious anemia (Levy *et al.*, 1971), or with moniliasis and Addison's, disease (Hermans *et al.*, 1969), without coexisting IHP. Hypoparathyroidism cannot be blamed for the occurrence of steatorrhea in these cases. Similarly, unexplained steatorrhea occurs in association with other typical conditions but not IHP in siblings of cases with IHP and associated conditions (Collins-Williams, 1950; Craig *et al.*, 1955). "Associated diseases" without IHP are known to occur in the families of patients with IHP (Hooper *et al.*, 1973).

The case of J. P., whose basic data are given in Table I exemplifies the association of steatorrhea and hypoparathyroidism. Both conditions were discovered at the same time, followed by Addison's disease and true, "adult-type" pernicious anemia. One of his siblings has, to date, isolated IHP. Steatorrhea has been difficult to manage in this patient. In 1971, oral calcium supplements (3g/24 h as elemental calcium) and AT 10 (2 mg/24 h), as well as a gluten-free diet, restored the serum calcium to only 6.8 mg/dl from 3.8 mg/dl. Only when PTE was given (100 Units USP/day) intramuscularly did this value reach normal levels. Whenever the serum calcium fell, the steatorrhea increased and vice versa. In 1973, he was hypocalcemic (3.9 mg/dl) on admission, and for the first time hypomagnesemic as well (0.94 mEq/l). Serum phosphate level was high (8.2 mg/dl) and serum carotene low (35 μg/dl). Hypomotility of the small bowel was striking and the barium meal reached the cecum in 7.5 hours, instead of 2 hours. D-xylose absorption was normal, with 5.0 of 25 g administered recovered in the urine and a 2 hour serum peak of 64 mg/dl. Secretin test was normal as well. Jejunal mucosa biopsy showed only a slight unevenness of the villi. Steatorrhea was striking (15 g/24 h). Serum calcium could not be raised to above 7.0 mg/dl, despite the administration of oral supplements of calcium (3 g daily of elemental calcium), and oral administration of crystalline dihydrotachysterol (1.2 mg/24 h), as well as calcium infusions (0.5–1.5 g/24 h of elemental calcium). Magnesium infusions (0.6

g/24 h of elemental magnesium) readily corrected the hypomagnesemia without any change in the hypocalcemia, probably because normal parathyroid function was not restored. Magnesium repletion seemed to restore peripheral skeletal responsiveness, since after its administration infusions of calcium (0.75 g/24 h) were able to restore the serum calcium in 48 hours, without any further decrease. As shown in Fig. 3A, Mg replenishment did not alter the renal response to PTH as measured by cyclic AMP production. Bile flow was normal in this patient and the gallbladder vigorously responded to the administration of cholecystokinin, but bile salt deficiency developed during hypocalcemic episodes, disappearing when serum calcium was normalized (Rombouts-Lindemans et al., unpublished). This therefore was a contributing, but not a causative factor.

Treatment of these patients may be difficult. Some steatorrhea persisted even when calcium was maintained at normal levels, although malabsorption was less severe. However, when for unknown reasons hypocalcemia recurred, malabsorption was striking and hypocalcemia refractory to treatment, especially if Mg depletion coexisted. Administration of PTH was usually effective in restoring the serum calcium level to normal which could then be maintained within normal limits. Lorenz and Burr (1974) encountered similar difficulties in treatment of their case and stated that "low concentration of serum calcium predispose to further steatorrhea, which in turn aggravates the hypocalcemia." In another case, correction of hypocalcemia did not improve the steatorrhea (Carson et al., 1973). MCT are currently being administered in order to assure more prolonged control of the steatorrhea in the hope of maintaining normal serum calcium levels.

D. Spasmophilia

Some adult patients present with a number of symptoms which in the aggregate resemble those of hypoparathyroidism. They include mental depression (with crying spells), lassitude, headache, abdominal pain, muscle cramps, paresthesias, and ectodermal lesions. Occasionally typical attacks of tetany are present. Hypocalcemia is not a feature, however (Kramer, 1936a and 1936b).

The majority of such patients are women. It has not been established whether these patients have a "latent" form of idiopathic hypoparathyroidism or have another unrelated disorder. Several terms have been used to describe this clinical "syndrome," including "chronic constitutional tetany" (Klotz et al., 1962), "cryptotetany" (Rosselle and De Doncker, 1959), or "idopathic tetany" (Fanconi and Rose, 1958; Jesserer, 1958; and Lamberg et al., 1960). We prefer the term "spasmophilia" introduced by

Klotz in 1958, with the understanding that this is a vague entity usually considered only in the Old World although a single case has recently been described in New York City (Seelig *et al.*, 1975). Not only is the serum ionized calcium normal (Zuyderhoudt *et al.*, 1974) as predicted by Klotz and Jungers (1959) and shown earlier by Fanconi and Rose (1958), but the magnesium level is also normal (Durlach *et al.*, 1967; Gounelle *et al.*, 1970; Durlach *et al.*, 1971; Hioco, 1974; Puissant *et al.*, 1975) despite earlier reports to the contrary (Rosselle and De Doncker, 1959; Durlach and Lebrun, 1959).

It has usually been assumed that such normocalcemic tetany is due to hyperventilation with consequent alkalosis and decrease in level of ionized calcium (Collip and Backus, 1920; Greenwald, 1922; O'Donovan, 1948; George *et al.*, 1963; Saltzman *et al.*, 1963). The decrease in serum ionized calcium induced by respiratory alkalosis has only recently been documented *in vivo* using calcium specific electrodes in animals (Höffken *et al.*, 1971) and in man (Lindgärde, 1972). In man the changes induced by forced hyperventilation were small (a mean change in [Ca^{2+}] of -7%) but were accompanied by the appearance of Chvostek and Trousseau signs.

The commonest cause of normocalcemic tetany is due to hyperventilation alkalosis. In patients with hyperventilation tetany, respirations tend to be deep rather than rapid and symptoms may be relieved by holding the breath or by rebreathing into a paper bag (Albright, 1941). The question remains whether all cases of normocalcemic tetany are due to hyperventilation, and if so whether hyperventilation always occurs on an emotional basis. In the English-speaking countries, it is commonly assumed that cases of nonhypocalcemic tetany are due to "hysterical hyperventilation" (Talbott *et al.*, 1938).

There is some doubt, however, whether anxiety hyperventilation is causative, rather than a manifestation of the attack of tetany itself, as suggested by Alajouanine *et al.* (1954). Jesserer (1958) and Klotz *et al.* (1962) distinguished idiopathic tetany from hyperventilation tetany, and separated cases of "pseudotetany," a truly hysterical manifestation. Why certain individuals are more sensitive to hyperventilation or to other factors, such as stress, while others may undergo the same events and yet not suffer from any symptoms, remains unexplained. It has been hypothesized that these patients have a lowered threshold to stimulation of their motornerve fibers (Layzer and Rowland, 1971). A pertinent question is whether normocalcemic tetany bears any relationship to partial hypoparathyroidism (F. Kramer, 1936). Before discarding any role played in certain cases by the latter factor, three points should be given consideration.

First of all, perhaps 10% of patients with spasmophilia may have cataracts "of the endocrine type" or subcapsular lenticular opacities (Klotz and Fiks, 1962). On the other hand, in the presence of idiopathic subcapsular opacities, manifestations of spasmophilia occur in approximately 50% (Klotz and Fiks, 1962). If this can be confirmed, the presence of these lenticular opacities provides an objective physical finding within a framework of predominantly psychosomatic symptoms. They have been observed in normocalcemic tetany by Leriche and Jung (1936), Hoesch (1937), Lachmann (1941) and one of us (C.N.) in a recent case.

Secondly, two cases have been described by Levin et al. (1961) of intracranial calcifications and *normal* serum calcium values. Pneumoencephalographic studies, and in one case a biopsy of the right frontal cortex and adjacent white matter, showed them to be basal ganglia, convolutional, or dentate nuclear calcifications. The description of the second case is consistent with that of spasmophilia, whereas in the first case the proof of normocalcemic seizures is lacking. Intracranial calcifications have not often been reported in normocalcemic tetany, but it is doubtful that they have been systematically looked for. Furthermore, many patients are too young for these calcifications to have developed sufficiently to be demonstrated on standard roentgenograms.

Thirdly, if the parathyroid reserve of these patients is not normal, provocative tests to stress parathyroid function might unmask the glandular failure. Klotz and Witchitz (1963) measured the response to disodium EDTA infusion in 34 patients with spasmophilia, 7 patients with spasmophilia and in addition "endocrine" cataract, as compared to 15 controls. The percentage of abnormal responses 12 hours after the initiation of the perfusion was, respectively, 68%, 86%, and nil in the three groups. After 24 hours, it was, respectively, 53%, 71%, and 13%. Similarly, Hartemann et al. (1971) found 15% of definite abnormalities in 45 tests performed using disodium EDTA infusions in patients with spasmophilia. In the small group of six patients (Fig. 2) tested by one of us (C. N.) with EDTA, at least two patients out of six had an abnormal serum calcium value after 12 hours. Evidence of abnormalities from kinetic studies performed with radiocalcium are not convincing, (Milhaud et al., 1959 and 1962). The point made by Milhaud et al. (1959), that upon treatment of 8 patients with normocalcemic tetany with vitamin D_2 (or DHT), with average dosages of 1.75 mg/24 h (70,000 IU/24 h), the calcium pool (P) increased from an average of $4,736 \pm 1.180$ to an average of $6,085 \pm 2.388$ mg and the v_{0+} from an average of 610 ± 253 to an average of $1,027 \pm 616$, is well taken. However, these changes are not specific and did not reach statistical significance.

Klotz et al. (1962) have provided an extensive description of the syndrome of "chronic constitutional tetany," emphasizing the hereditary character of the condition. In their experience, 68% of the 125 children examined from a total of 85 affected mothers and 7 affected fathers had signs of spasmophilia. Among 25 pairs of identical twins, the concordance rate was 100% (Klotz *et al.*, 1962). Diagnostic criteria for the syndrome are as follows: (1) Serum calcium level is normal, although it may occasionally fluctuate with borderline low values. (2) Presence of Chvostek's sign as defined by Albright and Reifenstein (1948). The incidence of this sign found in the literature varies in the control population from 5% (Bell and Bartels, 1951) to 24% (Hoffman, 1958), with a higher incidence in older children (Graham and Anderson, 1924; Hoffman, 1958). (3) Trousseau's sign [blood pressure cuff kept inflated 20 mmHg above the systolic blood pressure for 3 min with appearance of "main d'accoucheur" (flexion of the wrist and metacarpal-phalangeal joints, extension of both proximal and distal interphalangeal joints, tonic adduction of the thumb and fingers)]. Normocalcemic tetany cannot be distinguished from true, severe, well established IHP on the basis of this sign. (4) Von Bonsdorf's sign, a combined test which couples the mechanical pressure of Trousseau's sign (3 min) overlapping for 2 min with a 3-min period of hyperpnea. (5) Electromyographic findings of typical repetitive electrical discharges, displaying double spikes of identical appearance (doublets) (Turpin *et al.*, 1943), repeating themselves at a frequency of 6 to 10/sec, or multiple spikes (triplets, multiplets) at a frequency of 0.5 to 10/sec, (Lefebvre and Lerique, 1962). Multiplets is a term suggested by Alajouanine *et al.*, (1954) to characterize the multiple spikes typical of repetitive activity. An example is shown in Fig. 6.

In latent tetany, spontaneous iterative motor-unit action potentials do not occur. They only manifest themselves when so-called "facilitating" procedures are utilized, i.e., local ischemia (Magladery *et al.*, 1950; Kugelberg and Cobb, 1951) or hyperventilation (Turpin and Lefebvre, 1943). The sequence of the procedures is usually performed as suggested by Alajouanine *et al.* (1954). Activation of human nerves by hypocalcemia, ischemia, or hyperventilation results in the same electrical response with respect to the order of activation of spikes of various sizes and the frequency of discharge as demonstrated by Kugelberg (1948) in a detailed study of these phenomena.

In the electromyographic investigations of subjects suspected of having spasmophilia on the basis of the evocative symptoms mentioned earlier, only 56% had typical electrical repetitive activity (Rosselle and De Doncker, 1959). All patients with Trousseau's sign were in this group, as were patients with a past history of tetany. Chvostek's sign was present in 7% of the EMG-negative patients and in 30% of the EMG-positive patients. In a recent study of patients with spasmophilia by Puissant *et al.* (1975),

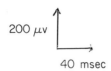

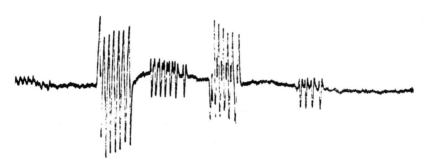

Fig. 6. Electromyogram showing multiple spikes of repetitive activity (multiplets). These electrical discharges correspond to individual motor units excited by single or multiple discharges of an individual nerve fiber. With increasing tetany new motor units join the discharge. The spikes themselves have a high internal frequency of ~ 80 cps for doublets (interval of ~ 12 msec and of ~ 80 to 250 cps for multiplets (interval of ~ 12 to 4 msec). The test is performed by inserting a needle in the first dorsal osseous muscle of the hand. In the example given, interval frequency is 180 cps.

Chvostek's sign was present in 21% of the EMG-negative and in 51% of the EMG-positive patients, whereas ectodermal lesions could be found in 15% of the EMG-negative and in 42% of the EMG-positive patients. Incidentally, no significant difference between the EMG-negative and the EMG-positive groups could be found with respect to serum or erythrocyte magnesium concentrations (Puissant *et al.*, 1975).

Cathala and Contamin (1957) also found it exceptional to have "false-positive" results with this technique. Others have considered as positive responses only those in which repetitive activity was displayed during more that 10 minutes in the postischemic period (Giudicelli *et al.*, 1967; Monod *et al.*, 1970). Indeed, most of their control subjects showed repetitive activity only during 2 to 5 minutes. Our own studies, conducted with the help of Dr. Knoops (Department of Physical Medicine and Rehabilitation, Louvain University), using the classical tourniquet test at adequate blood pressure and a concentric needle electrode, showed a very high incidence of positive results in controls, as did Puissant *et al.* (1975). Positive electromyographic responses in control populations have increased strikingly over the years, from a few percent in the 1950's (Cathala and Contamin, 1957; Rosselle and De Doncker, 1959), and some 15% in young males in the late 1960's (Giudicelli *et al.*, 1967; Giraud *et al.*, 1967; Monod *et al.*, 1970) to even higher percentages in the mid 1970's (Puissant *et al.*, 1975 and ourselves). Whether or not these differences are ascribable to changes in instrumentation, new criteria will have to be developed to consider repetitive activity significant (Monrod *et al.*, 1970).

It is clear that all the diagnostic criteria for spasmophilia are nonspecific. They may be present in as much as 8% of the population with a predominant female distribution (82%). In one series of 187 cases (Klotz *et al.*, 1962) Chvostek's sign was present in 76%; the combined test (Von Bonsdorf's sign) was positive in 97%; Trousseau's sign was present in 19%; and typical electromyographic findings were present in 65%. As far as symptoms are concerned (Klotz *et al.*, 1962), they are exactly those described earlier in the cases of postoperative latent hypoparathyroidism, as well as occasional episodes of loss of consciousness and sensations of thoracic oppression, if not of precordial pain.

In collecting our (C. N.) series of 29 cases, we have insisted that patients have true normocalcemic tetany, as observed by a practitioner, as well as typical abnormal electromyographic findings, and Chvostek, Trousseau, or von Bonsdorf's sign. These more rigid criteria would eliminate about 90% of the patient material studied by Rosselle and De Doncker (1959). The acute response to EDTA infusion in 8 such patients is shown in Table II. Although more profound hypocalcemia was produced

TABLE II

Effect of a 2-Hour (T0-T2) Disodium-EDTA Infusion (50 mg/kg Body Weight) on the Serum Calcium Levels and iPTH Values of 8 Patients (2 Males, 6 Females) with Repeated Episodes of Normocalcemic Tetany, as Compared with 15 Controls[a]

	Serum calcium (mg/dl)					iPTH (pg bPTH Eq/ml)				
	T0	T1	T2	T3	T4	T0	T1	T2	T3	T4
Controls (n = 15)										
Av.	9.62	8.82	8.04	8.31	8.47	264	430	503	454	434
S.D.	0.46	0.57	0.56	0.57	0.66	69	80	133	90	105
Normocalcemic tetany (n = 8)										
Av.	9.18	7.99	7.19	7.32	7.42	202	325	385	340	332
S.D.	0.51	0.40	0.45	0.38	0.34	73	71	93	61	64
p	<0.05	<0.005	<0.005	<0.025	<0.001	N.S.	<0.01	<0.05	<0.005	<0.025

[a] iPTH was measured by Dr. R. Bouillon (Dept. of Experimental Medicine, University of Leuven) with antiserum A VI-2 (Bouillon et al., 1974). Controls were those of Dr. Bouillon as well.

than in controls during (T1), at the end (T2) and, respectively, one hour (T3) and two hours (T4) after discontinuing the EDTA infusion, the response of the parathyroid glands to the hypocalcemic stimulus was less, as shown by the iPTH levels.

It is not easy to interpret these findings. Either these patients have a diminished parathyroid reserve and should therefore be considered as suffering from idiopathic latent hypoparathyroidism, or their release of PTH is defective owing to a derangement of their autonomic nervous control system, which plays a role in the feedback control of calcium regulation, as emphasized earlier. Basal serum calcium levels show more variation than controls and occasionally low levels of serum calcium have been described (Levin et al., 1961; Klotz et al., 1962). In the experience of Klotz et al. (1962), symptoms of "chronic constitutional tetany" are more frequent during periods of increased calcium requirements (pregnancy, lactation, starvation, increased intestinal loss), as well as at the end of the winter, when less endogenous vitamin D is produced. It is conceivable that some of these patients in the heterogeneous group may suffer from idiopathic latent hypoparathyroidism. This would be consistent with the data of Hioco (1974) showing low serum alkaline phosphatase levels and decreased urinary excretion of total hydroxyproline in spasmophilia. Hyperventilation, if it occurs in these patients, might then produce a sudden decrease in the ionized serum calcium level, precipitating an attack of tetany.

IX. PSEUDOHYPOPARATHYROIDISM AND RELATED DISORDERS

Pseudohypoparathyroidism (PHP) is a condition first described by Albright et al. (1942) in which the serum chemistries (and ensuing clinical symptoms and complications) are those of IHP, although lack of endogenous PTH is not the cause of the disorder and administration of exogenous PTH does not correct it. They attributed the condition to a failure in end-organ responsiveness to the hormone. Resistance to exogenous PTH was demonstrated. It was proposed that circulating endogenous PTH was normal or excessive, since normal (Albright et al., 1942) or hyperplastic (Elrick et al., 1950) parathyroid glands were found upon cervical exploration. Patients with this disorder display a variety of somatic alterations, among which are characteristic osteochondrodystrophic lesions (especially brachydactyly), short stature, a round face, obesity, some degree of mental retardation, and subcutaneous bone formation. All these abnormalities, somatic and biological, are of congenital origin. PHP has been reviewed extensively by MacGregor and Whitehead (1954), Bronsky *et al.* (1958), Nagant de Deuxchaisnes *et al.* (1960b), Forbes (1962), Mann *et al.*, (1962), Schwartz (1964), Bartter (1966), Potts (1972), and Potts and Deftos (1974).

Pseudo-pseudohypoparathyroidism (PPHP) is the (controversial) term applied by Albright *et al.* (1952) to a variant of PHP in which the blood chemistries and end-organ responsiveness to PTH are normal but somatic alterations, mental dullness, and ectopic bone formation remain. This disorder has no connection with abnormalities of parathyroid hormone secretion or effectiveness, although it may be detected in families in which members have PHP, and has a similar sex distribution. The two conditions are, therefore, genetically linked.

A common error has been to equate normal (or so-called normal) blood chemistries within this framework with the diagnosis of PPHP. In some instances, end-organ resistance to PTH may only be partial, with serum calcium levels approaching normal during certain periods, and be abnormal only at times of greater calcium demands by the organism such as adolescence, pregnancy, or restricted calcium intake. These cases have been described as progressing from PHP to PPHP, or vice versa. These instances of "normocalcemic PHP" are more accurately described as PHP characterized by intermittent normocalcemia.

Another error leading to overdiagnosis of PPHP is to include subjects based upon inadequate criteria. Subcutaneous bone formation may be absent and if the osteochondrodystrophy is not highly characteristic, or if it is representative of another congenital disease, cases may be mistaken for PPHP, especially since Albright *et al.* (1952) recognized the existence of incomplete cases of the syndrome. Isolated features of PPHP will be found in familial brachydactylia or hereditary peripheral dysostosis (Brailsford, 1945; Newcombe and Keats, 1969; Riccardi and Holmes, 1974), hereditary multiple exostoses (Jaffe, 1943), multiple epiphyseal dysplasia (Jackson *et al.*, 1954), hereditary deforming chondrodysplasia (Bartter, 1966), myositis ossificans progressiva (Albright *et al.*, 1952; Bland *et al.*, 1973), familial calcification of the basal ganglia (Matthews, 1957; Moskowitz *et al.*, 1971), the Holt-Oram syndrome (Holt and Oram, 1960; Kaufman *et al.*, 1974), the Ellis-van Creveld syndrome or chrondro-ectodermal dysplasia (Caffey, 1952), pleonosteosis (Léri, 1926), dyschondrosteosis (Léri and Weill, 1929) with Madelung's deformity (Madelung, 1878; Felman and Kirkpatrick, 1969), acrodysostosis (Maroteaux and Malamut, 1968), diastrophic dwarfism (Lamy and Maroteaux, 1960), acromesomelic dwarfism (Maroteaux *et al.*, 1971), cryptodontic brachymetacarpalia (Gorlin and Sedano, 1971), and the Marchesani (or Weill-Marchesani) syndrome (brachydactyly, short stature, and spherophakia), Laurence-Moon-Biedl syndrome, and Dudley Morton's syndrome (short first metatarsals), among many others.

The difficulties in classifying individual patients have been best described by Hortling *et al.* (1960), Todd *et al.* (1961), Gorman *et al.* (1962), and Arkless and Graham (1967). The differential diagnosis has been discussed by these authors and others (Nagant de Deuxchaisnes *et al.*, 1960b; Gibson, 1961; Mann *et al.*, 1962; Goeminne, 1965; Steinbach and Young, 1966; Hertzog, 1968).

A. Blood Chemistries

Serum calcium and phosphorus levels in PHP are similar to those of IHP. However, since the refractoriness to PTH may be only partial, both hypocalcemia and hyperphosphatemia are less pronounced (Table III). Some confusion has arisen in this field from the tables published by Bronsky *et al.*, (1958) and their interpretation by Parfitt (1972a). Bronsky *et al.* recorded not the average pre-treatment values, but the extreme ones, i.e. the very lowest serum calcium and the very highest serum phosphorus levels measured. We have, therefore, analyzed his 40 case reports of PHP and 50 case reports of IHP to determine mean pre-treatment values. The numbers reported in Tables III, IV, and V are based on these values.

We have also correlated the values with the age at which the blood specimen was drawn, since Bronsky *et al.* (1958) give only the (pre-

TABLE III

Mean Pretreatment Values of Serum Calcium and Phosphorus in Patients with PHP and IHP[a]

	Serum calcium (mg/dl)		Serum phosphorus (mg/dl)		Age (years)[b]	
	PHP	IHP	PHP	IHP	PHP	IHP
Number	40	50	39	50	40	50
Mean	6.41	5.45[c]	7.30	8.23[d]	20.25	23.25[e]
S.E.	0.18	0.14	0.35	0.32	1.94	2.67

[a] The *p* values have to be considered horizontally and within the same broad column.
[b] Age refers to age at time of analysis.
[c] *p* < 0.001.
[d] *p* = 0.05.
[e] *p* = N.S.

sumed) age of onset of symptoms, which may differ from the age at which the quoted serum chemistries were determined by as many as 4 decades. Parfitt (1972a) did not consider the distinction between "age at onset" of the disease and age at which the serum was actually analyzed. For example, he compared the findings of 9 infants (0–4 years) with PHP, 24 children (5–16 years), and 4 adults (age 17+), whereas the chemistries actually relate to 4 infants, 12 children, and 24 adults with PHP. His conclusions, which have been generally accepted, that "the plasma P level falls with increasing age in IHP but not in PHP," that "the plasma P levels in adults are higher in PHP that in IHP for the same degree of hypocalcemia," that "the mean plasma Ca is significantly lower in IHP than in PHP both in infants and in children, but not in adults," and that "the mean plasma P levels in IHP and PHP do not differ significantly in any age group" are therefore not suggested by the data. In addition, it cannot be concluded that "the higher plasma P in PHP than in IHP suggests that in most cases of PHP the resistance to PTH of the renal tubular reabsorption of phosphate is relatively greater than the resistance to PTH of calcium release from bone."

Table III shows that the average serum calcium level is 1.0 mg/dl higher in PHP than in IHP, this difference being statistically highly significant ($p < 0.001$). The serum level of inorganic phosphorus is 0.9 mg/dl lower in PHP than in IHP, a difference that is statistically valid at the 5% level. The ages at which the quoted serum values were determined are comparable in both groups. If the mean serum calcium in PHP is 6.4 mg/dl with a standard deviation of 1.1 mg/dl (C.V.: 17%), the range is 4.1–8.9 mg/dl and therefore overlaps accepted normal values. As pointed out by Parfitt (1972a), this is in contrast to the reported cases of IHP where the range of serum calcium is 3.0–7.4 mg/dl. Some cases which were not frankly hypocalcemic and hyperphosphatemic may not in the past have been considered as cases of IHP, although such cases have occasionally been reported (Levin *et al.*, 1961). Cases of "borderline" PHP are more likely to be reported as PHP or PPHP because of the associated somatic abnormalities and eventual ectopic bone formation, which attract attention

Hyperphosphatemia is striking in PHP: 7.3 mg/dl with a standard deviation of 2.2 mg/dl (C.V.: 30%) (Fig. 7). The fact that the range of serum P levels is almost identical in PHP (4.2–13.3 mg/dl) and IHP (4.0–13.4 mg/dl) whereas serum calcium values are so different suggests that the abnormalities relating to calcium metabolism may be less striking indeed than those related to phosphate metabolism. There is an inverse correlation between serum Ca and serum P both in PHP and IHP (Parfitt, 1972a). In PHP, the regression line is P = 11.46 − 0.65 Ca (SE = 2.05) with a regression coefficient of −0.34 (p = 0.031). In IHP, the regression line is P

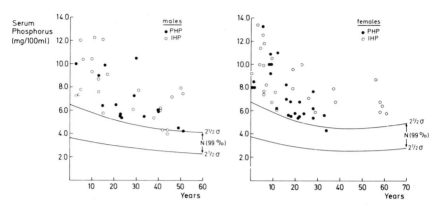

Fig. 7. Serum phosphorus values in males and females with PHP (●) or IHP (○) compared to those for normal individuals as a function of age. There is little or no overlap between normal values and those for either PHP or IHP.

$= 11.80 - 0.66$ Ca (SE $= 2.22$), with a regression coefficient of -0.28 (p $= 0.045$).

The serum chemistries in Table IV have been divided into three groups according to age: infants (0–4 years), "children" (5–16 years), and "adults" (> 17 years). As can be seen, the serum calcium level is lower by 0.9–1.0 mg/dl in IHP than in PHP in all age groups; it reaches maximal statistical significance in the adults (p < 0.001), probably owing to the greater number of patients. Longitudinally, the serum Ca level increases by 0.5 mg/dl in both diseases when comparing infants to adults, but there is little difference between "children" and "adults" (0.16 mg/dl in PHP; 0.11 mg/dl in IHP). The serum phosphorus level in PHP is lower in both infants and adults than in IHP, but, owing to the small number of affected infants, this reaches statistical significance only in adults at the 5% level. In "children," the serum P value is equal in both groups of patients. Longitudinally, the serum P level falls dramatically when comparing children and adults, especially in PHP. The difference amounts to 3.25 mg/dl in PHP and is highly significant (p < 0.001). The regression coefficient between the serum P level and age is -0.66 (p < 0.01) in PHP and -0.50 in IHP (p < 0.01). When considering the period of "childhood," it is -0.69 (p < 0.02) in PHP, versus -0.26 (p N.S.) in IHP. This means that whatever mechanism accounts for the elevated serum P level during adolescence is fully operational in both PHP and IHP. Growth hormone probably plays the most significant role in maintaining the relatively high P level in children and adolescents, predominantly through a direct action on the renal tubule (Corvilain and Abramow, 1962) opposite to that of PTH. When PTH is absent, the tubular reabsorption of P is

TABLE IV

Serum Calcium and Phosphorus Values in Patients with PHP and IHP Arranged According to Age at Time of Analysis[a]

Age	Serum calcium (mg/dl)		Serum phosphorus (mg/dl)	
	PHP	IHP	PHP	IHP
0–4				
Number	4	6	4	6
Mean	6.03	5.08[e]	8.63	9.60[e]
S.E.	0.38	0.48	0.47	1.06
Av. Age	1.9	3.1	1.9	3.1
5–16				
Number	12	20	12	20
Mean	6.35	5.42[d]	9.28	9.24[e]
S.E.	0.44	0.23	0.59	0.49
Av. Age	11.8	9.3	11.8	9.3
17+				
Number	24	24	23	24
Mean	6.51	5.53[c]	6.03	7.05[d]
S.E.	0.20	0.19	0.27	0.36
Av. age	28.4	39.8	28.8	39.6

[a] The p values apply to the paired comparisons of PHP and IHP within each age group and with respect to serum calcium and serum phosphorus.
[b] The figures represent mean pretreatment values.
[c] $p < 0.001$.
[d] $p = 0.05$.
[e] $p = $ N.S.

increased, thus increasing the serum P level. Growth hormone enhances this action, and therefore maximal serum P levels are to be expected in hypoparathyroid growing children (Table IV). The fact that this is the case in PHP as well as in IHP, whereas the serum calcium is significantly higher in the former, shows that although the renal tubule is resistant to the action of PTH in PHP, it is highly sensitive to the action of growth hormone. From the data in Table V it can be concluded for the same degree of hypocalcemia, the plasma P levels in adults, or in children and adults combined, are not higher in PHP than in IHP. On the contrary, the serum P levels remain 0.7–0.8 mg/dl lower, although this does not reach statistical significance.

In Table VI we have considered serum values of aklaline phosphatase in PHP and IHP. Only those values were included which were expressed in terms of either, Bodansky Units or King-Armstrong Units, the latter

TABLE V

Comparison of Serum Phosphorus Levels in Children (Age 5+) and Adults (Age 17+) with Severe Degrees of Hypocalcemia (Serum Ca < 6.5 mg/dl) due to Either PHP or IHP

| | Severity Grade 5 (serum Ca < 6.5 mg/dl) | | | |
| | Serum calcium (mg/dl) | | Serum phosphorus (mg/dl) | |
Age	PHP	IHP	PHP	IHP
5+				
Number	16	34	16	34
Mean	5.51	5.09^a	7.76	8.43^a
S.E.	0.19	0.12	0.58	0.37
Av. age	23.1	26.6	23.1	26.6
17+				
Number	11	20	11	20
Mean	5.80	5.28^a	6.61	7.44^a
S.E.	0.19	0.17	0.45	0.36
Av. age	28.9	39.0	28.9	39.0

^{a} p = N.S., considered as in Table IV.

TABLE VI

Serum Values of Alkaline Phosphatase in Males and Females with IHP or PHP

| | Males[a] | | Females[a] | |
	PHP	IHP	PHP	IHP
Age				
Number	8	17	17	11
Av.	23.8	25.1	13.1	27.4
S.E.	4.6	4.5	1.8	7.6
Alkaline phosphatase (Bodansky units)				
Number	8	17	17	11
Av.	7.5	5.9	6.0	5.7
S.E.	3.1	0.9	0.8	1.3

[a] There is no statistical difference of the means for the age between male patients with PHP (pseudohypoparathyroidism) or IHP (idiopathic hypoparathyroidism), nor for the alkaline phosphatase for male and for female patients with either PHP or IHP. The mean age of female patients with IHP is significantly higher ($p < 0.05$) than that of female patients with PHP.

being converted into Bodansky Units by applying the conversion factor of 0.32, the mean of the conversion factors of 0.30 and 0.34, respectively, determined by Schwartz *et al.* (1960) and Deren *et al.* (1964). In 53 case reports pretreatment values were available. Dent and Harper (1962) observed that normal adult females had a lower alkaline phosphatase level (mean 5.6; S.D. 1.8 K.A. units) than normal adult males (mean 7.6; S.D. 1.9). We therefore analyzed males and females separately; no significant sex-related difference between the values was seen. There is no difference either between the values in PHP and in IHP. However, whereas in males the ages for both PHP and IHP are comparable, this was not the case in females. Since growth and adolescence have greater influences on alkaline phosphatase levels than sex (Clark and Beck, 1950; Salz *et al.*, 1973) we chose to pool the sexes and to compare the age groups in which the alkaline phosphatase values are relatively stable. According to Clark and Beck (1950), there exists a plateau in alkaline phosphatase values in both sexes between the ages of 2.1 and 10.0 years, following which the values increase in males and decrease in females. We have computed from their data that for the 191 children examined between age 2.1 and 10.0, the mean alkaline phosphatase level is 6.3 Bodansky Units for an average age of 7.0 years. The sex difference is very small in this group: 6.49 B.U. for the girls ($n = 83$) and 6.17 B.U. for the boys ($n = 108$).

From Table VII it is seen that there is no difference in the alkaline phosphatase values between PHP and IHP in both age groups considered. Taking into account the difference which may exist between the sexes in adults, males were considered separately. The average values are, respectively, 3.8 B.U. in PHP and 3.6 B.U. in IHP. In general, PHP is not a disease characterized by elevated alkaline phosphatase values which are commonly encountered in cases of secondary hyperparathyroidism.

B. Incidence

Although there are insufficient data regarding the incidence of PHP; this disorder appears to occur less frequently than IHP. The temptation to report a case of PHP is greater than to report a case of IHP, because of the multiple fascinating and complex aspects of the former. This undoubtedly represents a bias. Most authors encountered only a few cases (Lachmann, 1941; Buckwalter *et al.*, 1955; Bronsky *et al.*, 1958; Dimich *et al.*, 1967; Fonseca and Calverly, 1967; O'Malley and Kohler, 1968). One of us (C.N.) recorded 4 cases of IHP over a 4 year period but no cases of PHP screening with the aid of a computer 10,599 admissions in the Department of Medicine in St. Pierre University Hospital in Louvain. The 12 cases

TABLE VII

Age and Alkaline Phosphatase Values in Patients with PHP or IHP Considered according to Two Age Groups in Which Alkaline Phosphatase Values are Known to Be Relatively Stable[a]

	Age 2.1–10.0		Age 21–61	
	PHP	IHP	PHP	IHP
Patients				
Number	7	8	9	11
	(1M, 6F)	(4M, 4F)	(6M, 3F)	(7M, 4F)
Average Age	6.8	5.7	27.6	50.4
S.E.	0.8	0.8	2.8	2.3
Alk. P′se[b]				
Av.	7.2	8.6	3.9	3.0
S.E.	1.3	1.5	0.6	0.5

[a] There is no statistical difference between the means for the age of the young patients (age 2.1–10.0) between subjects with PHP (pseudohypoparathyroidism) or with IHP (idiopathic hypoparathyroidism), nor for the alkaline phosphatase for both age groups with either PHP or IHP. The mean age of the patients in the older age group (age 21–61) is significantly higher ($p < 0.001$) for IHP than for PHP.

[b] Alkaline phosphatase.

followed at the MGH by Forbes (1962) include all the original cases and constitute, to our knowledge, the largest single series in the literature. Two years later, she reported on the dermatoglyphics and palmar-flexion creases of 19 patients with "PHP or PPHP" (Forbes, 1964). Okano et al. (1969) recorded all cases reported in Japan and were able to collect only 10. When Beaudoing et al. (1970) reviewed the literature, they found 146 cases of PHP and 123 cases of PPHP, although the criteria for establishing the diagnoses were not detailed. The sex ratio in these 269 cases was 2.1:1 in favor of the females (183 F, 86 M). Spech and Olah (1974) reviewed 186 cases of PHP and found 61% affecting females.

C. Genetics

Elrick et al. (1950) proposed that PHP is a genetic disorder involving three genes, one causing end-organ resistance to PTH, one leading to dyschondroplasia, and one inducing ectopic bone formation. Albright et al. (1952) hypothesized the existence of a mutation in one gene controlling the different traits. Whether polymeric or pleiotropic, the disease does not seem to involve chromosomal aberrations, as had been suggested by various observations (Forbes, 1962; Jancar, 1965; Zisman et al., 1969) including common somatic features in PPHP and Turner's syndrome (Engel *et al.*, 1956; Nagant de Deuxchaisnes, 1959; van der Werff ten Bosch, 1959; Hortling *et al.*, 1960; Forbes, 1964; Minozzi *et al.*, 1964; Miller *et al.*, 1965; Nedok *et al.*, 1968; Lieschke and Witkowski, 1968; Gardner, 1970). The hypothesis of Nagant de Deuxchaisnes *et al.* (1960b), which ascribed the phenotypic abnormalities common to PPHP and Turner's syndrome to unfavorable intrauterine conditions at about the sixth to ninth week of gestation, was conceived at a time before abnormalities of the sex chromosomes were known to be responsible for Turner's syndrome (Ford *et al.*, 1959).

PHP and PPHP have a high familial incidence. If reported cases of both are pooled (Beaudong *et al.*, 1970), 105 cases (43 PHP, 62 PPHP) are familial, versus 164 cases (103 PHP, 61 PPHP) apparently sporadic although not all members of the families have been thoroughly investigated in all cases. The genetic mechanism of inheritance is a matter of dispute. Most authors have accepted the conclusions of Mann *et al.* (1962) that both syndromes are transmitted as a sex-linked dominant trait, based on the following evidence: lack of well-documented male-to-male transmission, presence of a consistent pattern when two or more generations were affected, and a female to male ratio of approximately 2:1. Union of two recessive gene carriers was considered statistically unlikely and there was no record of consanguinity in the affected families. Aurbach (1970, 1971) explained why some of the female patients in the same family had PHP and others PPHP according to the Lyon hypothesis (Lyon, 1961, 1962, and 1963): inactivation of one of the X chromosomes or a part of it (the "abnormal chromosome," carrying the "PTH resistance" trait) about 16 days after conception, could lead to PPHP. If the normal X chromosome (or a part of it) was inactivated, PHP would result. As Potts (1972) has observed, this explanation could not account for the occurrence of PPHP in males.

Male-to-male transmission of the disorder rules out the hypothesis of an X-linked inheritance. These cases are of special interest and several may be quoted from the literature up to the review of Mann *et al.* (1962). The paternal grandmother and two paternal uncles (or aunts) of a male case with PHP were described by Mackler *et al.* (1952) as having thickened skulls and a tendency to short and thick metacarpal bones. The father of a male with PHP reported by Buchs (1954) had short first metacarpals and first metatarsals which were short and stumpy with a tendency to exostoses formation. Royer *et al.* (1959) described a male with PHP who had a paternal uncle who was short, mentally retarded, and round faced. The father of a male patient with PPHP was reported to have short thumbs (Wallach *et al.*, 1956). In a family of PPHP, where the male propositus had brachydactyly, a round face, and mental retardation, the father had brachydactyly as well, and the paternal grandfather a round face and brachydactyly (Klotz *et al.*, 1962).

Since then, many other cases have been reported, including those of Minozzi *et al.* (1963), Hermans *et al.* (1964), Goeminne (1965), and Spranger and Rohwedder (1965), but all these cases are characterized essentially by brachydactyly. Whether these represent true PPHP rather than familial brachydactyly, type E (i.e., hereditary peripheral dysostosis), cannot be settled; there are no cases of true PHP in these families, which would confer more significance to the presence of brachydactyly, especially since short stature and a round face are also features of familial brachydactyly (Hertzog, 1968). Bartter (1966) concluded that the "true" PHP–PPHP syndromes are indeed X-linked conditions, while the other cases do not represent PPHP and are inherited according to an autosomal dominant pattern. It should be noted, however, that such features as exostoses (Minozzi *et al.*, 1963; Spranger and Rohwedder, 1965), radius curvus (Goeminne, 1965), and subcutaneous bone formation (Goeminne, 1965) have been seen in some members of the above-quoted families, in addition to short stature and round face, adding some presumptive evidence that PPHP might have been the correct diagnosis. Only mental retardation has been conspicuously absent. Our own feeling is that these cases should not be discounted entirely.

When PHP occurs in a kindred, the characteristic abnormalities of "physiognomy," a term used by Albright *et al.* (1942, 1952), are most likely to represent PPHP in other members of the same kindred. This was the case in the above mentioned pedigrees in only three instances (Mackler *et al.*, 1952; Buchs, 1954; Royer *et al.*, 1959), and not all three cases were convincing. Similar cases have been reported since. Weinberg and Stone (1971) described a family where PPHP was present in one son and one daughter of a man with PHP who also had a sister with PHP. The only abnormalities in the proband were short stature and multiple subcutaneous ossifications, also present in the three other affected members of the family, but he was only 31 months old when examined and other features of the disease may appear later. Reinhart *et al.* (1973) studied a kindred with three affected females and five affected males in three generations. The conclusion in both reports was that autosomal dominant inheritance characterizes the transmission of PHP and PPHP, as had been postulated earlier by Minozzi *et al.* (1963), Hermans *et al.* (1964), Goeminne (1965), Spranger and Rohwedder (1965), and McKusick (1966). The available pedigrees from the literature may be examined in the reports of Mann *et al.* (1962), Schwarz and Bahner (1963), Spranger and Rohwedder (1965), and Spranger (1969).

However, if these syndromes are not X-linked dominant disorders, one must account for the fact that the sex ratio is 2.1:1 and not equal, as in an autosomal dominant mode of inheritance. Spranger and Rohwedder (1965) felt this ratio was biased in favor of females. They reviewed the literature, excluding all cases they felt to be doubtful, including all cases of Turner's syndrome, and came to a ratio of 1.79:1 in PHP ($n = 109$), and 1.76:1 in PPHP ($n = 89$). Studying all available cases in the pedigrees, they obtained, when excluding the probands, a female to male ratio of 1.1:1, very close to an equal distribution indeed. According to these authors, selection bias in favor of females may be accounted for by the fact that females for esthetic reasons more readily seek medical attention, or that the disease is more severe in females than in males, with a tendency for more complete expression, so that the affected males are more easily overlooked in the population at large and are detected at their true incidence only as siblings of affected probands, when systematically and carefully investigated. If sex-linked dominant inheritance were the mode of transmission, one might expect that the disease would be more severe in males as a consequence of Lyon's hypothesis, since in females one of the X chromosomes is randomly inactivated. In the males, no such inactivation is possible. Mann *et al.* (1962) recognized that males were not more severely involved, a finding that is generally consistent with the descriptions in the literature.

Whether hereditary transmission occurs only through one mechanism, or whether there is heterogeneity in the mode of inheritance is not known. Cederbaum and Lippe (1973) suggested an autosomal recessive mechanism of transmission, based on a well-studied family in which two siblings suffered from classic PHP (a brother and a sister), while the parents and maternal grandparents were normal, as were (supposedly) the paternal grandparents. A similar situation has been described by Fanconi *et al.* (1964), where one son and two daughters of normal parents (and grandparents) suffered from PHP. A dominant mode of transmission with a wide difference in penetrance and expressivity remains a theoretical possibility. When more pedigrees become available and can be studied with modern techniques involving cyclic AMP response to PTH administration, there will be a more useful approach to understanding the inheritance of these syndromes.

Another approach involves study of the histocompatibility antigens. Farriaux *et al.* (1975) reported on a family described earlier on two occasions (Maillard *et al.*, 1966; Christiaens *et al.*, 1967), in which four of the five siblings suffered from PHP and the mother from PPHP. Of the four affected siblings (three females and one male), three had brachydactyly (two females, one male), which they apparently inherited as a separate trait from their father. In all four members with brachydactyly (three siblings and their father), and in no other member of the family, segregation occurred between brachydactyly and the haplotype HLA A3 and HLA BW5. If this did not occur by chance, the gene governing brachydactyly (as it may in hereditary peripheral dysostosis) could be located on chromosome 6. In this family PHP seemed to be inherited from the mother, but brachydactyly from the father, a most unusual pattern of inheritance.

D. End-organ Resistance to PTH

Albright *et al.* (1942) demonstrated that PHP was characterized by a failure of PTH to effect its normal response on phosphate excretion and on serum calcium and phosphorus values in contrast to results obtained in IHP. They proposed their hypothesis of target-organ resistance. Albright used the expression "Seabright-Bantam syndrome" to characterize this type of resistance, since in this species of cockerel the males develop, under the influence of endogenous androgens, tailfeathers of the female type. This is a misnomer, as pointed out by Alexander and Tucker (1949), since castration of this type of fowl is followed by the development of a male type of tail plumage. It therefore represents a "perversion" of response, rather than a true end-organ refractoriness. Albright was quick in abandoning this term (Elrick *et al.*, 1950), but it still has been used for many years, among others by Prentice (1954) and Laymon and Zelickson (1959). Not only is this term a misnomer, but it also has been misspelled, as it applies to an old British breed of bantam fowls designated after Sir John S. Sebright, an English agriculturist (*Webster's Third New International Dictionary*, unabridged, 1971). The Sebright-Bantam appellation should be dropped, and only remain as an example of the many colorful and imaginative digressions of Albright's universal mind.

The protocol of Ellsworth and Howard (1934) has generally been followed to test the response of the kidney tubule to PTE. PTE (200 Units USP or 40 Units BPC) is administered intravenously over a 10 to 15-minute period and phosphate excretion is measured in hourly urine collections. Phosphate or the P to creatinine ratio is measured in the urine and compared prior to (usually three hourly urine collections) and after (usually three to four hourly urine collections) the injection of PTE. In normal subjects, the phosphate excretion increases by a factor of 2 to 4 and in hypoparathyroid patients (other than PHP) this increase is even more striking, occasionally reaching 4 to 10 times control values (Ellsworth and Howard, 1934; Albright *et al.*, 1942; Elrick *et al.*, 1950). Sometimes phosphate clearance has been measured hourly, or the phosphate-creatinine clearance ratio, providing the percent tubular reabsorption of phosphorus (T.R.P.), as advocated by Kleeman and Cooke (1951). T.R.P. in normal individuals falls 8 to 29% (mean 15%) (Purnell *et al.*, 1968) or 12 to 30% (Birtwell *et al.*, 1970) after PTE injection. In contrast to patients with hypoparathyroidism, hyperparathyroid patients tested in this manner demonstrate a blunted response (Becker *et al.*, 1964; Gershberg *et al.*, 1966; Purnell *et al.*, 1968), a point of paramount importance.

There are good reasons for measuring the T.R.P. or performing the Ellsworth–Howard test on a control subject with hypoparathyroidism other than PHP. Commercially available parathyroid extracts may produce a rise in the filtered P in normal subjects as a result of an increase in glomerular filtration rate (action of the extract on renal hemodynamics), whereas in patients with hypoparathyroidism there is in addition a diminution in the tubular reabsorption of P (Hiatt and Thompson, 1957). According to Lowe and Calcagno (1955), this increase in glomerular filtration rate does not occur if PTE is injected intramuscularly in normal subjects, or in patients with PHP, whether by the intramuscular or the intravenous route. This is not so in all cases with PHP. Schwarz (1960) demonstrated a normal phosphaturic response in a patient with PHP, which was entirely accounted for by an increase in the glomerular filtration rate.

Another means to measure the response of the kidney tubule to PTE is to study the maximal tubular reabsorptive capacity for phosphate (Tm_P) prior to and after the administration of PTE. The ratio Tm_P/GFR or "theoretical renal phosphate threshold" is the most useful means to study renal tubular phosphate handling (Bijvoet, 1969), but it is a tedious procedure unless computed from the nomogram of Bijvoet and Morgan (1971). Aperia *et al.* (1967) studied the theoretical renal phosphate threshold in two patients with IHP, as compared with two patients with PHP, prior to and 60 minutes after the administration of PTE. This value in IHP, initially very high, decreased after the administration of PTE to values well within the normal range, whereas in two patients with PHP, the value was initially high but did not change after PTE administration.

The classic Ellsworth–Howard test has been criticized by Dent (1953), MacGregor and Whitehead (1954), Royer *et al.* (1959), Mann *et al.* (1962), and Surks and Levenson (1962). The main objection has been that often little or no phosphaturic action has been demonstrable in normal or hypoparathyroid subjects, and therefore differential diagnosis between IHP and PHP could not be made on the basis of a "less-than-none-response." It has been argued that commercially available PTE is assayed based upon its calcium-raising power and not on its phosphaturic action, and that the latter may therefore not be present in the extract (Dent, 1953). There is evidence that both actions are linked in the hormonal polypeptide, although the response of both target organs may not be the same. To complicate the issue further, it should be noted that the end-organ resistance in PHP is only partial and strikingly different only when compared to cases of IHP (Elrick *et al.*, 1950).

Finally, consideration should be given to the spontaneous diurnal variation in phosphate excretion which is characterized by a rise during the morning hours from 9 AM till noon (Ollayos and Winkler, 1943; Mills and Stanbury, 1952; Lubell, 1957), apparently under the influence of the diurnal variation of cortisol secretion (Goldsmith *et al.*, 1965) and interaction of this hormone with PTH, thyroid hormone, and growth hormone. Patients with IHP do not have any appreciable spontaneous increase of P excretion during the morning hours (Goldsmith *et al.*, 1965). Therefore certain authors recommend the Ellsworth–Howard test be performed in the midafternoon (injection at 3 PM) in a patient kept fasting since breakfast. Spontaneous variation of P excretion between 1 PM and 7 PM seems to be minimal indeed (Lubell, 1957; Bethune *et al.*, 1964). In the series of these authors, there was no overlap between the PTH-induced maximal increase post-injection, compared with the pre-injection urinary P excretion, when considering normal subjects (average increase by a factor of 2.4, range 2.0–2.8), patients with IHP (average increase: 3.8, range: 3.1–5.1) and a single patient with PHP (increase: 1.4). The discrimination was even better when a low phosphate diet (200 mg/m²/day) was given for five days (including the control day and test day) and aluminum hydroxide gel administered (30 ml with each meal and at bedtime) to prevent phosphate absorption in the intestine.

The Ellsworth-Howard test is still useful if careful conditions prevail: the patient should be in the fasting state, supine except for voiding, under standard hydration conditions (200 ml of distilled water every hour), under a low dietary phosphate intake at least three days before the test. Control studies should be carried out to evaluate the spontaneous variation of phosphodiuresis under the same conditions in the same subject, as well as identical study (spontaneous variation and test) in a control subject, normal or preferably hypoparathyroid, using the same batch of PTE. If the latter has biological potency, and has been stored under proper conditions, there will be little difficulty in evaluating the difference between responses of patients with PHP and IHP. If the test can be performed with purified PTH, the difference will be even more striking as shown in Fig. 8 and 9.

Examples of carefully controlled studies in which the PTE-induced increases in urinary P/creatinine ratio were measured are shown in Table VIII. In all five controls the ratio of PTH-induced spontaneous rise in P excretion was equal to or higher than 2.1 (range: 2.1–13.7), whereas the

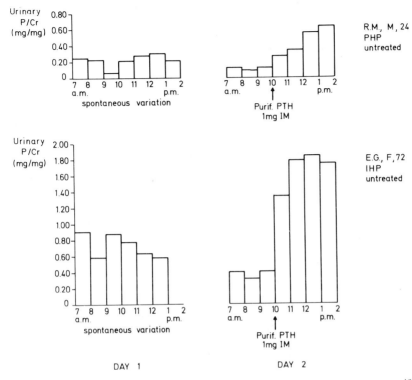

Fig. 8. Differences in acute response of urinary phosphorus (urinary P/Cr) to purified PTH as seen in PHP and IHP. Spontaneous diurnal variations in excretion are included.

rise in the four untreated patients with PHP was equal to or less than 2.1 (range: 1.2–2.1). If the ratio of PTH-induced to spontaneous variation is considered with respect to PTE administration, the data for two controls and one patient have to be discarded. It remains that in both controls this ratio was equal to or greater than 1.6 (range: 1.6–5.5), whereas all three untreated patients with PHP had a ratio equal to or less than 1.6 (range: 1.1–1.6). In both modes of expression, there was no overlap between the results of untreated patients with PHP and controls. The obvious exception in the baseline tests was patient M.B. with treated PHP whose response was more consistent with the normal pattern. This will be elaborated on later.

Another way of examining the data is to express the results as the difference between the mean control output and the peak postinjection response, as advocated by Bronsky *et al.* (1958). Recalculating our data in this manner does not substantially alter our conclusions. Bronsky *et al.* reviewed the tests in the literature and computed that on the average

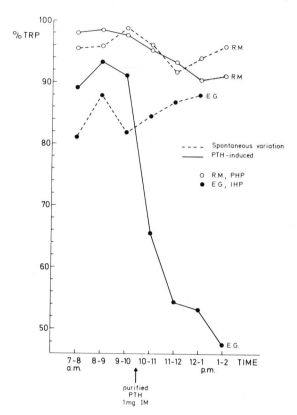

Fig. 9. Differences in acute response of % TRP to purified PTH in patients with PHP and IHP. Resistance to the effects of PTH at the level of kidney tubule is seen in PHP and serves to distinguish it from IHP.

patients with PHP (n = 19) barely double their P output, while patients with hypoparathyroidism (n = 26) had on the average a 4.5 fold increase, and the normoparathyroid controls (n = 19), a 2.5-fold increase. The latest comparative study (Coulson and Moses, 1975) indicated an average 1.7-fold increase in PHP (n = 2), a 2.5-fold increase in normal subjects (n = 6), and a 3.7-fold increase in hypoparathyroidism (n = 5). There was no overlap between the results in the latter group and those in PHP. This corresponds generally with the data in Table VIII. Most tests in the literature unfortunately lack either control data or the study of the spontaneous variation, or both. If the latter had not been examined in patient R.M., who consistently had a spontaneous increase of 1.4 to 1.9 (on four occasions preoperatively), he might have been considered to have responded to PTH (Fig. 10). This may be the cause of the so-called positive

TABLE VIII

Data on Spontaneous and PTH-Induced Rises in Urinary Phosphorous Excretion in Treated and Untreated Hypoparathyroid and Pseudohypoparathyroid Patients and Controls with Other Disorders

Patient	Sex	Age	Diagnosis	Treatment	Serum (mg/dl) Ca	P	Rise in P output[d] (mg/mg creatinine) Spontaneous	PTH-induced	Ratios Spontaneous	PTH-induced	PTH/spontaneous	PTH used
E.G.	F	72	Hypoparathyroidism	Untreated	6.5	4.2	0.79–0.66	0.36–1.67	0.8	4.6	5.8	purified
A.L.	M	52	Paget's disease	$Al(OH)_3$	9.0	3.2	N.D.	0.03–0.41	N.D.	13.7	N.D.	Batch A
J.T.	M	64	Liver cirrhosis	None	8.3	2.9	0.44–0.60	0.38–0.85	1.4	2.3	1.6	Batch B
G.K.	M	73	Paget's disease	None	9.0	3.2	0.61–0.70	0.33–0.73	1.2	2.2	1.8	Batch D
							N.D.	0.23–0.49	N.D.	2.1	N.D.	Batch C
M.L.	F	57	Hypoparathyroidism	D_2 100,000/day[a]	8.6	3.3	0.92–0.74	0.51–2.27	0.8	4.4	5.5	Batch E
		59		D_2 50,000/day	7.5	4.2	0.34–0.34	0.35–1.05	1.0	3.0	3.0	
					8.3	4.2	0.44–0.48	0.49–1.28	1.1	2.6	2.4	
M.A.	F	46	Pseudohypoparathyroidism	Untreated	6.7	3.8	0.21–0.21	0.31–0.51	1.0	1.6	1.6	Batch A
				D_2 50,000/day	9.4	2.4	0.14–0.10	0.38–0.70	0.7	1.8	2.6	Batch C
		47		AT 10 1mg/day	9.2	3.8	0.49–0.25	0.28–0.93	0.5	3.3	6.6	
M.B.	F	47	Pseudohypoparathyroidism	Untreated	8.8	5.6	N.D.	0.48–0.59	N.D.	1.2	N.D.	Batch B
K.D.	M	13	Pseudohypoparathyroidism	Untreated	4.6	5.6	0.49–0.50	0.47–0.70	1.0	1.5	1.5	Batch D
O.M.	M	47	Pseudohypoparathyroidism	Untreated	9.5	4.0	0.46–0.48	0.12–0.55	1.0	4.6	4.6	
				D_3 100,000/day	6.6	5.0	0.18–0.26	0.12–0.46	1.4	3.8	2.7	
R.M.	M	24	Pseudohypoparathyroidism	Untreated	7.4	4.5	0.26–0.49	0.40–0.84	1.9	2.1	1.1	purified
		25		D_2 100,000/day	9.4	3.6	0.42–0.73	0.43–0.66	1.7	1.5	0.9	Batch B
				D_2 50,000/day	9.0	4.2	0.36–0.52	0.32–0.54	1.5	1.7	1.1	
		27		D_2 100,000/day[b]	9.4	4.6	0.26–0.20	0.28–0.42	0.8	1.5	1.9	Batch E
		28		Untreated[c]	7.7	5.0	0.28–0.36	0.31–0.72	1.3	2.3	1.8	

[a] plus 1 ml AT 10 daily.

[b] plus 2 ml AT 10 daily, 2 weeks after PTX.

[c] 9 months after PTX.

[d] P output has been determined during fasting. The 1st value represents the average of three consecutive hourly collections prior to 10 A.M., the 2nd value is an average of four consecutive hourly collections after 10 A.M. PTH, when given, was always administered at 10 A.M.

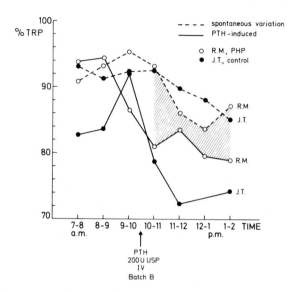

Fig. 10. The acute response of the kidney tubule to PTH (expressed as % TRP) in a patient with PHP. Control studies include spontaneous variation in phosphodiuresis for the same patient under identical conditions as well as an identical test in a control subject, using the same batch of PTH.

responses observed exceptionally in patients with PHP, such as seen in one patient of Elrick *et al.* (1950).

The Ellsworth–Howard test is a useful approach to the problem of renal tubular resistance to PTE, and in a cooperative patient can be performed on an ambulatory basis. It therefore is applicable to studies of members of affected kindreds. A much better measure of resistance, however, is obtained by prolonged administration of PTE and comparison, on a constant diet low in P, of the daily urinary excretion of phosphate prior to, during, and especially the day after PTE administration. In contrast to the action of the acute (single) injection of PTE, prolonged administration of PTE does not produce changes in renal hemodynamics, but leads to a decrease in maximal tubular reabsorption of phosphate (Hiatt and Thompson, 1957) in both normal and hypoparathyroid subjects. This procedure also enables one to evaluate the calcium-mobilizing action of PTE on bone.

Albright *et al.* (1942) performed Ellsworth–Howard tests in two of their initial cases and also administered PTE for several days (17 days in case 1, 5 days in case 3) in increasing amounts (from 300 U/day to 1500 U/day) in a 28-year-old adult, and from 100 U/day to 500 U/day in a 3-year-old infant. Only the blood chemistries were recorded. Urinary phosphate, as well as calcium and total hydroxyproline excretion should be followed prior to, during, and after PTE administration. The prolonged test has been standardized by Dancaster *et al.* (1960) who injected 200 to 800 U/day of PTE over three to seven consecutive days.

The changes produced by the prolonged administration of PTE are exemplified by the study of patient J.T. (Fig. 11). The serum Ca increased from an average 8.3 mg/dl to a maximum of 10.6 mg/dl while the serum P fell from an average of 2.9 mg/dl to a low of 2.3 mg/dl. The urinary P output rose immediately and fell the day after withdrawal of PTE to 384 mg/24 h, half the control value. We have regularly observed this "re-

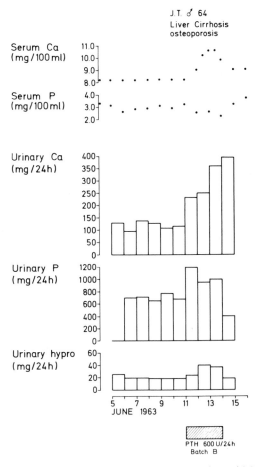

Fig. 11. Effects of prolonged administration of PTH in a patient with hepatic cirrhosis and osteoporosis.

bound" phosphate retention and consider it characteristic of the phosphaturic response to administration of PTE. The urinary calcium output rose progressively, and continued for a few days after withdrawal of PTE. Urinary output of total hydroxyproline also increased from an average of 19.2 mg/24 h to a high of 39.9 mg/24 h.

PTE can be given for longer periods of time and at higher doses. The impression gained from the study of Dancaster et al. (1960) that PTE ceases to exert an effect in the normal adult beyond the second or third day of administration may not be correct. Keiser et al. (1964) administered 600 U/day for 10 to 12 days to one control and three patients with postoperative hypoparathyroidism. The serum calcium continued to increase, albeit slightly, as did both urinary calcium and total hydroxyproline output. However, little change occurred after the sixth day of administration. No further information is gained by prolonging this procedure. The changes in serum P levels also occur in the first period of administration, and owing to the fall of serum P the increase of P output in the urine is maximal on the first or second day of the test period. Quantification of the changes in hydroxyprolinuria by Keiser et al. (1964) are also of interest. They ranged from 127 to 187% of control values on the first day of the treatment period, to reach peak levels of 142 to 228% of control values. Average increase in the three patients with hypoparathyroidism was from 23.7 to 40.3 mg/24 h (170% of control values). We have opted to administer 600 U daily for a period of three days, adequate for diagnostic purposes and for comparisons of the same patient under different conditions.

Surks and Levenson (1962) gave 2000 U/day of PTE for 3 days and reviewed the nine tests of protracted PTE administration performed in the 1950's in patients with PHP for variable periods and with varying dosages. In none did the serum Ca level increase by more than 0.6 mg/dl. Since then, more tests have been performed with dosages ranging from 800 to 4000 U/day, administered for periods of time up to 14 days (Bell et al., 1963; Hagen et al., 1964; Arnstein et al., 1966; Mautalen et al., 1967; Felitti and McAfee, 1968; Suh et al., 1969). Average serum Ca increase was 0.8 mg/dl (range: 0.0–1.5), as compared to a 2.6 mg/dl and a 2.1 mg/dl average increase respectively observed in normal subjects by Hiatt and Thompson (1957) and by Dancaster et al. (1960), both using lower dosages and shorter periods of administration. Purified bovine PTH was given by Mautalen et al. (1967) and Suh et al. (1969).

The first to use purified PTH to study PHP were Pechet et al. (1961). They demonstrated a sluggish phosphaturic response, which ceased after the second to fourth day of administration; the changes in the urinary calcium excretion were negligible. Some effect on serum Ca and serum P was noted, although below the range observed in normal and hypoparathyroid subjects. These studies demonstrated the resistance of PHP to PTE, crude or purified, both at the bone and kidney level. Since PHP is characterized by partial resistance to PTH, however, some response can be observed in all cases so treated.

A detailed account follows of more recent cases which are often quoted as having shown a better response to the administration of PTE. Zisman et al. (1969) administered PTE, 210 U/days for 4 days, 450 U/day for 8 days, and 900 U/day for another eight days to a patient with PHP with characteristic phenotypic abnormalities and subcutaneous ossifications. Not much change occurred before 900 U/day were given, but at the end of this 20 day period, the serum Ca had risen from an average of 6.3 to a high of 11.3 mg/dl, the serum P had dropped from an average of 5.7 to a low of 3.9 mg/dl, while the urinary P rose from an average of 655 to a high of 1000 mg/24 h, and urinary total hydroxyproline from an average of 19 to a high of 40 mg/24 h. This is almost a normal response, although the urinary calcium remained undetectable throughout. Lower doses (100–200 U/day) would have been sufficient in a hypoparathyroid subject to obtain this response (Hiatt and Thompson, 1957; Dancaster et al., 1960). Of interest is the fact that in this case iPTH was undetectable. Although the radioimmunoassay was not sensitive enough to measure normal amounts of circulating PTH, the existence of elevated levels was seemingly excluded. Since radioimmunoassay does not measure biologically active PTH (see Chapter 1), too much weight should not be given to the levels of iPTH. This case could therefore represent the first example of IHP which has developed in a patient with PPHP, as was later described by Moses et al. (1974). Another possibility is that the two measurements of serum calcium, which led to the conclusion that normalization was attained, were erroneous. Undetectable urinary calcium in the presence of a serum calcium of 11.3 mg/dl has never been observed in a patient with normal glomerular function. This would not explain the effect of PTE on serum and urinary P, however.

The second case of Zisman et al. (1969) also responded, but in an abnormal way, 450 U/day of PTE was given reportedly for eight days (twelve days according to the published graph) without any response, and at a dosage of 900 U/day for another twelve days. The serum Ca increased from an average of 8.0 mg/dl to a high of 10.0 mg/dl, while once more the urinary calcium remained undetectable, possibly reflecting action upon the tubular reabsorption of calcium. Serum and urinary P remained unchanged, whereas the urinary output of total hydroxyproline decreased. This case is a better example of resistance to PTE, except for its effect on the (distal) tubular reabsorption of calcium. The crucial role of the kidney as a target organ in serum Ca homeostasis has been stressed by Peacock *et al.* (1969) and reassessed by Nordin and Peacock (1969). Renal tubular reabsorption of calcium may be an important regulator, in particular when bone turnover is low (Kalu *et al.*, 1974).

The three cases of Bell *et al.* (1972) showed increases in serum calcium, concomitant with increases in urinary calcium. PTE was given for three days, 12 U/kg body weight/day, which amounted to a dose of 600 U/day in two patients and 900 U/day in the third. This increase was unimpressive in patient J.C., and amounted to slightly more than 1.0 mg/dl in patient F.N. Only in patient J.B. did the serum calcium normalize (+2.0 mg/dl). Total hydroxyproline excretion was not measured, however, so that the total effect on bone cannot be appreciated. A modest phosphaturic response was observed without any change in the serum P levels, perhaps a nonspecific effect secondary to the increase in serum calcium. Comparison of two patients suffering from postoperative hypoparathyroidism shows a striking difference. Phosphate clearance changed from an average of 7.1 to an average of 21.9 ml/min in hypoparathyroidism in response to PTE, while changes were from an average of 5.9 to an average of 9.4 ml/min in PHP.

Birkenhäger *et al.* (1973) observed normalization of serum Ca level (from 7.0 to 9.6 mg/dl) in a patient given 300 U PTE/day for 3 days (no changes) followed by 900 U/d for another 3 days. There was no change in the total hydroxyproline excretion or in the urinary components of calcium balance. Probably PTE acted to increase distal tubular reabsorption of calcium, as was suggested in case 2 of Zisman *et al.* (1969). The serum P level fell from 5.4–5.7 to 4.9 mg/dl while urinary P increased from an average of 507 to a maximum of 760 mg/24 h. These changes are modest and distinct from those in patients with IHP. All in all, with the single possible exception of case 1 of Zisman *et al.* (1969), cases of PHP have been shown to be refractory even to prolonged exogenous PTE administration.

The dose of 600 U/day for three days may only affect the serum Ca level when it is not too low to start with, as in case J.B. of Bell *et al.* (1972), where it was 8.6 mg/dl. All cases of Bell *et al.* (1972) were treated with vitamin D throughout the study period. In general, it seems that two consecutive 3-day periods, one with 600 U/day, the following with 900–1200 U/day, would be perfectly adequate. The first period, using physiological dosages of PTE, would serve diagnostic purposes and ascertain that hypercalcemia does not develop, as might occur in a patient with IHP. The second period would serve to evaluate all parameters of calcium metabolism, including the urinary excretion of total hydroxyproline, under the effect of pharmacological dosages of PTE. 600 U/day is probably a physiological dosage. It is equivalent in an adult of 70 kg to 0.36 U/kg/h, very close to the dose needed to maintain normal serum Ca in parathyroidectomized dogs (0.1–0.4 U/kg/h) and rats (0.5–0.6 U/kg/h) and consistent with the normal secretion rate for PTH in humans calculated by Froeling and Bijvoet (1974).

Children are prone to intoxication with PTE if they are not resistant and doses must be adapted to their weight or body surface. We would suggest no more than 10 U/kg/day. The recommended doses for children in the literature have ranged from 300 U/m^2/day (Hermier *et al.*, 1972) to 500 U/m^2/day (Fanconi, 1969) for the test of prolonged PTE administration, whereas for the Ellsworth–Howard procedure doses of 50 U/m^2– (Nakajima *et al.*, 1966) to 150 U/m^2 (Royer *et al.*, 1959) have been injected. In infants, the intramuscular route has been used (Royer *et al.*, 1959), with some theoretical advantage in the normal subject (Lowe and Calcagno, 1955).

Another way of examining skeletal and kidney resistance to PTH is to investigate the response to endogenous PTH by inducing acute hypocalcemia with the administration of sodium EDTA. This test may be dangerous if the basal serum Ca is lower than 8.0–8.5 mg/dl. Estep *et al.* (1965) applied this test to two patients with PHP, whose basal Ca levels were 7.8 and 8.3 mg/dl, and compared them with three patients with hypoparathyroidism and eight normal subjects. Recovery from acute hypocalcemia was 93% 7 hours after initiation of the test in the normal subjects, versus 81% in patients with hypoparathyroidism and 83% in patients with PHP. Despite profound hypocalcemia, the expected decrease in T.R.P., measured in four consecutive two-hour urine collections with blood drawn at the midpoint of each, did not occur. On the contrary, it rose progressively and consistently from 94 to 97 in hypoparathyroidism and from 88 to 93% in PHP. Serum P remained unchanged in PHP throughout. In contrast, the serum P in normal subjects dropped from 3.4 to 3.0 mg/dl and % T.R.P. decreased progressively from 92% to 82%. Bone and kidney responses are thus very similar in hypoparathyroidism and PHP. Whatever additional endogenous PTH is secreted during this procedure in PHP is incapable of affecting calcium mobilization of phosphaturia as can be observed in normal persons.

Parfitt (1969) infused sodium EDTA in four patients with PHP, whose serum Ca levels ranged from 8.6 to 9.5 mg/dl, and who (apparently) were receiving vitamin D. Average recovery after 12 hours was 83% and after 24 hours, 92%, compared with values of 90% and 95%, respectively, established by Klotz *et al.* (1963) as a normal response. The results might have been more striking if vitamin D had been withheld.

The fact that the kidney in PHP does not respond normally to PTE does not mean that it cannot respond to other stimuli. The infusion of calcium in patients with hypoparathyroidism results in a significant increase in phosphate clearance and a lowering of the serum P levels (Eisenberg, 1965). Thus the serum Ca concentration directly affects the ability of the kidney tubule to excrete phosphate and this ability is restored to normal when hypocalcemia is corrected. This was observed in a patient with PHP as well (Mautalen et al., 1967). Oral P loading barely alters the P clearance in the hypocalcemic hypoparathyroid individual, whereas an oral P load given during Ca infusion produces the expected increase in phosphate clearance. This should be taken into account in the interpretation of any phosphaturia which accompanies a PTE-induced rise in serum Ca level whenever the prolonged test of PTE administration is used. No such interference accompanies acute (single) injections of PTE, since the serum Ca value remains unaffected. If the mechanism for tubular excretion of phosphate were congenitally impaired in PHP, such a response would not be observed. Schwartz (1960) demonstrated a definite phosphaturic response when Ca was infused (15 mg/kg body weight for four hours). Moore and Smith (1963), Hagen et al. (1964), Zampa and Zucchelli (1965) and Arnstein et al. (1966) also observed an increase of urinary P on the day of Ca infusion in patients with PHP. This is in contrast with the results obtained in two cases of PHP by Bell et al. (1963) and one case by Birkenhäger et al. (1973). These divergent results may be explained by the existence of gross radiological and histological signs of secondary hyperparathyroidism in one case of Bell et al. (1963), and by the existence of florid histological osteomalacia (anticonvulsant-induced) in the case of Birkenhäger et al. (1973).

PTH affects renal tubular handling of many electrolytes, as well as amino acids and hexoses (Aurbach and Heath, 1974; Froeling and Bijvoet, 1974; Diaz-Buxo and Knox, 1975), but there has been no thorough study of these effects in cases of PHP. Circumstantial evidence suggests a normal response to PTH in distal tubular reabsorption of calcium. Thus, hypercalciuric hypocalcemia is not unusual after correction of hypoparathyroidism with vitamin D and is ascribed to the lack of PTH, the calcium-sparing principle at the kidney level (Kleeman et al., 1961). It may even be seen in the absence of vitamin D and has been ascribed to sun exposure (Granström and Hed, 1965). It does not occur as a rule in PHP when vitamin D is administered, as demonstrated by Litvak et al. (1958) and reemphasized by Forbes (1962). Hypocalcemic hypercalciuria developed in 10 out of 15 treated patients with hypoparathyroidism but in none of 6 treated patients with PHP.

The mechanism of glucose reabsorption was not impaired in PHP in the single case studied by Halver (1966). He found a high Tm_g/gFR ratio, well within the range of the values obtained in primary hyperparathyroidism, whereas patients with hypoparathyroidism have a low ratio (Halver, 1967). Accurate determination of maximal tubular reabsorption of glucose is difficult, and no other patients with PHP have, to our knowledge, been tested.

New insight into the nature of end-organ resistance to PTH was provided by the demonstration of Chase *et al.* (1969) that patients with PHP did not appreciably increase cyclic AMP excretion in the urine upon PTH administration. Purified PTH (300 U) was given intravenously between 9:00 and 9:15 AM and cAMP in the urine (expressed either as nmoles/min or nmoles/mg of creatinine) was compared in normal subjects, and in patients with PHP, PPHP, and both idiopathic and postoperative hypoparathyroidism. The procedure was performed fasting and 250 ml water consumed hourly from 6 AM till noon. This forced hydration not only ensured adequate urine flow, but also suppressed endogenous secretion of vasopressin, another hormone which influences cAMP production in the kidney, although at a different site (Chase and Aurbach, 1968).

Following PTH infusion, there was a sharp rise in urinary cAMP, usually maximal during the first half hour, with a rapid return towards normal values. The ratio of peak postinjection excretion over basal excretion was 20.6 in normal subjects, 2.4 in PHP, 15.3 in PPHP, and 25.9 in other forms of hypoparathyroidism. Chase *et al.* (1969) concluded that cAMP determination in the urine after PTH is a much better discriminant than P excretion between PHP and IHP and between PHP and PPHP. Why the cAMP response to PTE administration does not discriminate between PHP and PPHP as well as between PHP and normal subjects is due to an unexplained higher than normal basal output of cAMP in PPHP and not to a less striking increase after PTE infusion. In Fig. 12 is shown our experience with the response of urinary cAMP to PTH in four patients with PHP compared with a patient with multiple basal-cell nevi syndrome and a patient with postoperative hypoparathyroidism. An increase in patients with PHP was barely detectable, except in M.A. Results in two other subjects were shown in Fig. 13.

Measurement of cAMP excretion after PTE administration has several advantages over the study of P excretion alone. The order of magnitude of the response is 20 times over the basal output for cAMP versus 2.5 times for P (Chase *et al.*, 1969). Excretion of cAMP is little affected by impurities in the parathyroid gland extracts as contrasted with phosphorus excretion although cAMP excretion is influenced by glomerular filtration rate (Broadus *et al.*, 1970). There is also no appreciable circadian variation of cAMP excretion (Chase *et al.*, 1969; Kopp *et al.*, 1972; Murad and Pak, 1972; Sagel *et al.*, 1973) and while dietary phosphate intake will

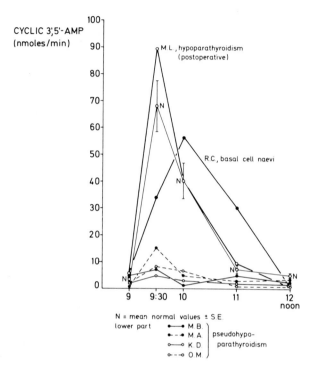

Fig. 12. Measurement of cAMP in the urine after administration of PTH to 4 patients with PHP compared with results in a patient with basal cell naevi (nevi) syndrome and another with postoperative hypoparathyroidism. N = normal subjects studied by Chase *et al.* (1969).

significantly affect urinary P response to PTE administration (Bethune *et al.*, 1964), dietary variations do not affect the response of cAMP excretion. In contrast to the Ellsworth–Howard test, response of cAMP excretion can be measured at any time of day, parathyroid extract is as useful as purified PTH, and there is little need to test the biologic potency of the extract.

However, there are limitations. One of the subjects with PHP described by Chase *et al.* (1969) demonstrated a normal response. This may be an instance of the entity later reported by Drezner *et al.* (1973) and Rodriguez *et al.* (1974) under the term "pseudohypoparathyroidism type II." Severe magnesium depletion may interfere with the response to PTE, as may severe vitamin D deficiency. However, in the latter instance it may be the secondary hyperparathyroidism which interferes with the cAMP response (response of the kidney tubule is already maximal). Aida *et al.* (1975) showed that in primary hyperparathyroidism the response of cAMP to

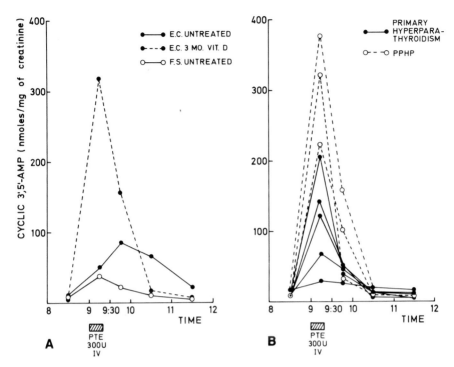

Fig. 13. Response of urinary cAMP in patients with various disorders. (A) Patients E.C. and F.S. had osteomalacia secondary to steatorrhea. The underlying disease was regional enteritis in E.C. and pancreatic insufficiency in F.S. Patient E.C. was studied before and after 3 months of oral vitamin D_2 which decreased serum iPTH from 560 to 230 pg bPTH Eq/ml (normal 214 ± 95). (B) Comparison of response in 5 patients with primary hyperparathyroidism and 3 with PPHP.

PTE administration was not different from that in PHP. Chase *et al.* (1969) inhibited endogenous PTH secretion by calcium infusion and showed that exogenous PTH did not normally stimulate urinary cAMP excretion in PHP. Finally patients with nephrogenic diabetes insipidus also have a moderately blunted cAMP response to PTE administration (Fichman and Brooker, 1972). Some of the abnormal responses are illustrated in Figure 13.

The cAMP response to PTH is dose-dependent (Kaminsky *et al.*, 1970; Tze *et al.*, 1975; Coulson and Moses, 1975), whereas smaller doses are sufficient to obtain a substantial phosphaturic response. Coulson and Moses (1975) administered 15 U of PTE to normal subjects and obtained a 1.5 ratio in the phosphaturic response, while the cAMP barely increased to less than 5 nmoles/mg creatinine. This is similar to the response of patients with PHP, given larger doses of PTE, where ratios of phosphaturic response seldom exceeded 1.5 and where the average peak response of cAMP to PTH reached 6.1 nmoles/mg creatinine (Chase *et al.*, 1969). To obtain a normal (2.5) ratio of phosphaturic response, 250 U of PTH were needed at which point urinary cAMP reached 260 nmoles/mg creatinine (Coulson and Moses, 1975). In PHP, neither the 2.5 ratio of phosphaturic response was reached, nor was the urinary output of cAMP greater than 20 nmoles/mg creatinine.

The mechanism of the blunted response in urinary cAMP excretion in PHP remains unexplained. Bell *et al.* (1972), who injected dibutyryl cyclic AMP (DB-cAMP) to patients with PHP and reproduced all the actions of PTH, indicated that the cellular response mechanism to cAMP was intact. The possibility still existed of an absence or an abnormality of adenyl cyclase in the cellular membrane, or an absence or abnormality of the receptor for PTH, or both. Marcus *et al.* (1971) showed that the adenyl cyclase in a membrane suspension from the renal cortex of a patient with PHP responded normally to PTH *in vitro*, with a log-linear dose response to the hormone. Until proven otherwise, one would have to conclude that in PHP, adenyl cyclase is normal (at least in the one patient examined) and responsive to PTH (Marcus *et al.*, 1971) and that cAMP reproduces all characteristic actions of PTH (Bell *et al.*, 1972). Another possibility is that once cAMP is formed within the cell, it is metabolized at an increased rate, presumably by a phosphodiesterase. The physiological significance of the findings of Marcus *et al.* (1971) remains to be shown.

Several authors have accepted the hypothesis that since PTH does not produce any appreciable cAMP excretion in the urine, PHP is a "disease of the second messenger." One should recall Albright's extraordinary intuition when he wrote that there might be "a deficiency in or interference with some hypothetical substance with which the parathyroid hormone reacts" (Albright *et al.*, 1942). The situation in PHP is analogous to that of nephrogenic diabetes insipidus in which, unlike primary (hypothalamic) diabetes insipidus, urinary cAMP does not increase upon the administration of vasopressin (Fichman and Brooker, 1972).

There are alternatives to the hypotheses that PTH-induced cAMP production is impaired in PHP, or that cAMP destruction is promoted. The possibility of defective transport of cAMP across the kidney tubules was considered by Marcus *et al.* (1971), but rejected, because this would result in an accumulation of cAMP within the cell of the kidney tubule, a situation deemed unlikely on the ground that this would not be compatible with the functional state of hypoparathyroidism which characterizes PHP. It remains to be proved that all PTH-induced phosphate excretion is mediated by cAMP formation.

Whether PHP is a disease of cAMP production, cAMP destruction, or cAMP release, the role of the adenyl cyclase-cAMP system in the pathogenesis of the disease is of paramount importance. Although aspects of cAMP metabolism are covered elsewhere in this volume, certain features will be analyzed here with respect to the role cAMP plays in the phosphaturic, as well as hypercalcemic response to PTH. In any event the impaired response of cAMP output to PTE serves as an important tool in the diagnosis of classic PHP (type 1). Conversely, the absence of an impaired response is a prerequisite for the diagnosis of PPHP. Caution should be exercised that the test is performed in the absence of profound hypomagnesemia, severe vitamin D deficiency, and/or striking secondary hyperparathyroidism. The patients are therefore best tested when their serum calcium level has been corrected and iPTH levels are normalized.

E. The Adenyl Cyclase–Cyclic AMP System

PTH, the first messenger, increases the permeability of the target cell membrane to calcium ions and thereby increases cellular uptake of calcium which acts as a second messenger. Simultaneously, PTH stimulates adenyl cyclase in the cell membrane which catalyzes the conversion of adenosine triphosphate (ATP) to adenosine $3',5'$-monophosphate (cAMP) within the cytoplasm. cAMP, acting as another second messenger, then promotes the function unique to that cell, presumably stimulating specific protein kinases which control the moment-to-moment activity of several other enzyme systems by phosphorylation of specific proteins (see Chapter 1). Other enzymatic reactions are also stimulated which are not calcium dependent, just as calcium ion stimulates enzymatic reactions which are not cAMP-dependent (Kurokawa and Rasmussen, 1973).

cAMP is destroyed by phosphodiesterases and maintained by agents which inhibit phosphodiesterase, particularly methylxanthines. Dibutyryl cyclic AMP is an analogue of cAMP used in many experiments because it penetrates tissues more readily and is not as easily converted to other compounds. It also inhibits phosphodiesterase. On the other hand, cAMP degradation is enhanced by agents which stimulate phosphodiesterase activity, such as imidazole. In the parathyroidectomized rat, theophylline produces an increase in serum calcium, as well as a decrease in serum P (Wells and Lloyd, 1967), demonstrating a PTH-like action; conversely imidazole causes hypocalcemia or blocks the action of PTH (Wells and Lloyd, 1968).

PTH stimulates the formation of cAMP in its two main target organs, the kidney cortex (Chase and Aurbach, 1967; Rasmussen and Tenenhouse, 1968; Dousa and Rychlik, 1968; Streeto, 1969; Melson *et al.*,

1970) and bone (Chase et al., 1969; Aurbach and Chase, 1970; Chase and Aurbach, 1970; Herrmann–Erlee and Konijn, 1970; Murad et al., 1970). A PTH-sensitive adenyl cyclase has been detected in the liver (Canterbury et al., 1974), as well as in isolated renal glomeruli (Sraer et al., 1974; Imbert et al., 1974) and in cells cultured from human giant cell tumors of bone (Goldring et al., 1978). As far as the intestine is concerned, no acute changes in cAMP are detected within a 60 min period following PTH administration to dogs (Gray and Gitelman, 1973). This would lend indirect support to the hypothesis that the action of PTH on the intestine is an indirect one, through stimulation of the biosynthesis of $1,25\text{-}(OH)_2D_3$.

As previously noted, PTH when administered to humans (Chase and Aurbach, 1967) rapidly increases urinary output of cAMP. cAMP also increases in the plasma, particularly in draining renal veins compared to peripheral veins (Tomlinson et al., 1974), indicating that the kidney makes the major contribution to the PTH-induced changes in plasma cAMP concentration. Under basal conditions in man, the kidneys contribute about 20–50% of the total cAMP in the urine. After administration of PTE, this contribution increases to more than 90% (Kaminsky et al., 1970). Anephric subjects fail to show any significant increase in plasma concentration of cAMP (Kaminsky et al., 1970; Tomlinson et al., 1974). Among the subjects studied by Chase et al. (1969), only one patient with hypoparathyroidism failed to respond to PTH administration with increased cAMP output in the urine. This patient also had renal insufficiency. cAMP output in the urine is high in hyperparathyroidism, low in hypoparathyroidism, and even lower in renal insufficiency. Average values in one study were for these groups, respectively, 5719 ± 1200 ($\pm$ SEM), 1943 ± 312, and 596 ± 208 nmoles/24 h (Taylor et al., 1970). This value has since been used by some in the differential diagnosis of hypercalcemia (Dohan et al., 1972; Murad and Pak, 1972; Neelon et al., 1973; Schmidt-Gayk and Röher, 1973; Shaw et al., 1974; Debacker et al., 1974; Bartley et al., 1975a and 1975b).

Substances other than PTH activate adenyl cyclase in the renal tubule and bone. This has been shown for calcitonin (Murad et al., 1970; Marx et al., 1972; Rodan and Rodan, 1974; Kurokawa et al., 1974), adenosine (Peck et al., 1974a); acetazolamide (Rodriguez et al., 1974); prostaglandins E_1 and E_2 (Chase and Aurbach, 1970), and catecholamines such as epinephrine, norepinephrine, and isoproterenol. The effect of the latter is associated with β-adrenergic stimulation and is abolished by propranolol, a β-adrenergic blocker, but not by phentolamine, an α-adrenergic blocker (Kurokawa and Massry, 1973). On the other hand, puromycin specifically inhibits the renal adenyl cyclase system responsive to PTH independently of its effects on protein synthesis (Fratkin et al., 1972).

When high doses of this substance are used, the hypercalcemic action of PTH is abolished as well (Kunin and Krane, 1965). Other factors also seem to inhibit PTH-dependent cyclic AMP production in the kidney tubule. These include calcium ion concentration (Beck *et al.,* 1974b), metabolic acidosis (Beck *et al.,* 1974a), and potassium depletion (Beck and Davis, 1975). Chlorpropamide also affects this system (Numann and Moses, 1974; Coulson and Moses, 1975).

Substances which inhibit phosphodiesterase include not only theophylline (Wells and Lloyd, 1967) and dibutyryl-cyclic AMP (Heersche *et al.,* 1971; Klein and Raisz, 1971), but also L-thyroxine (Marcus, 1975). Some consider propranolol another inhibitor of phosphodiesterase (Weitzman and Murad, 1973a).

Not only does PTH activate cAMP in the kidney tubule and bone, but there is also evidence that some of the PTH-induced actions are mediated by this system. In the kidney, cAMP and its dibutyryl derivative mimic the renal action of PTH (Chase and Aurbach, 1967; Rasmussen *et al.,* 1968; Kaminsky *et al.,* 1970), whether given systemically or into the renal artery (Agus *et al.,* 1971), particularly the phosphaturic action, probably through an inhibition of proximal tubular reabsorption of phosphate. The latter originates from the kidney tubule, the extracellular fluid (and thus from bone), and the soft tissues such as muscle and liver (Meyer and Meyer, 1974).

Crucial to this discussion is the fact that cAMP excretion precedes (Chase and Aurbach, 1967; Potts *et al.,* 1971; Tomlinson *et al.,* 1974; Kurokawa *et al.,* 1974; Czekalski *et al.,* 1974) rather than follows phosphate excretion, as had been suggested by Sallis (1970). The latter concluded that PTH-stimulated phosphaturia is not mediated by cAMP, but his experiments have not been confirmed. Stop-flow studies in dogs have shown that the PTH-induced urinary cAMP enters the tubular fluid in the same proximal area of the tubule in which PTH is known to affect phosphate reabsorption (Scurry and Pauk, 1974), other indirect evidence that cAMP may be the intracellular mediator of the action of PTH on the kidney cortex. The action of PTH on other ions may also be cAMP-mediated in the proximal tubule, especially sodium (Gill and Casper, 1971; Agus *et al.,* 1971; Puschett *et al.,* 1974) and potassium (Pushett *et al.,* 1974), but apparently not calcium (Puschett *et al.,* 1974). cAMP and its dibutyryl derivative also influence the permeability of the proximal convoluted tubule (Lorentz, 1974).

Pertinent to the adenyl cyclase–cAMP system is the fact that among the three distinct immunoreactive species of PTH present in human serum, only two with estimated molecular weights of respectively 9,500 (probably the glandular hormone) and 4,500–5,000 were able to activate kidney cortical adenyl cyclase, whereas the 7,000–7,500 Mol Wt fraction proved inactive in this respect (Canterbury *et al.*, 1973). Also of importance is the fact that the plasma membranes of renal cortex in the rat demonstrate a considerable proteolytic activity towards PTH, resulting in degradation of the hormone (active or inactive, i.e., the H_2O_2-oxidized form) to a host of fragments (Chu *et al.*, 1975). Enhancement of this proteolytic activity could, on a theoretical basis, account for more rapid degradation of the hormone into inactive fragments. Recent experimental evidence *in vitro* showed, however, that there is no correlation between the rate of inactivation of PTH at the level of kidney membranes and the effectiveness of PTH in stimulating adenyl cyclase activity in kidney (Moseley *et al.*, 1975).

So far as bone is concerned, Vaes (1968) showed that the addition of DB-cAMP to the medium bathing embryonic mouse calvariae in culture caused an increased rate of bone resorption similar to that seen when PTH was added. This was confirmed by Raisz and Klein (1969). Using DB-cAMP, Wells and Lloyd (1969) produced hypercalcemia and hypophosphatemia in parathyroidectomized rats. Phang and Downing (1973) showed that cAMP, DB-cAMP, as well as PTH, stimulated the uptake of proline and hydroxyproline by fetal rat calvariae. Peck *et al.* (1974b) showed that the same substances all stimulated uridine incorporation by isolated bone cells. By separating the latter into four different types of cell populations, it could be shown that the adenyl cyclase responsive to PTH is present in osteoblasts and osteoclasts, but not in the periosteum, nor in the marrow cells, supposed to contain the osteoprogenitor cells (Smith and Johnston, 1974). Cells from mouse bone in culture can be separated by their different adherence properties into those that respond predominantly to PTH or to calcitonin (Wong and Cohn, 1975).

A point of particular importance is the concentration of PTH required to achieve these actions. According to Peck *et al.* (1974a), physiological concentrations (1 ng/ml) of PTH are active in isolated bone cells, provided adenosine is present. In its absence, higher doses of PTH are necessary (of the order of 100 ng/ml). Using preparations of freshly isolated bone cells, Rodan and Rodan (1974) were able to obtain cAMP production with doses of PTH as low as 0.01 pg/ml.

In addition, cAMP also acts through the other main second messenger of PTH, i.e., the cytoplasmic calcium ion concentration, by an instantaneous release of calcium from the mitochondria (in less than 3 seconds). Only low concentrations of cAMP are necessary for this action and the cytoplasmic (extramitochondrial) calcium concentrations achieved are proportional to the cAMP concentrations within the range 0.1–3 μM (Borle, 1974). This reaction is self-limited, because of the negative feedback action of the calcium ion concentration on adenyl cyclase activity. The second product of the adenyl cyclase reaction, inorganic pyrophosphate, formed at the cell surface, also increases calcium influx into the cell and the exchangeable calcium pool (Borle, 1970; Reik et al., 1970). Pyrophosphate acts within minutes and its effect on calcium influx is proportional to its concentration (Borle, 1970).

Not only does cAMP mediate PTH action on kidney and bone, but it may also affect release of PTH by the parathyroid glands upon stimulation by decreased calcium and Mg ion concentrations (Matsuzaki and Dumont, 1972; Dufresne and Gitelman, 1972; Sherwood et al., 1972; Williams et al., 1973). DB-cAMP, as well as theophylline and epinephrine, caused increased PTH release equal to that induced by low calcium concentrations in vitro (Williams et al., 1973). Epinephrine also leads to an increase of PTH release in vivo in cows (Fischer et al., 1973) which is abolished by propranolol, suggesting a possible role of the autonomic nervous system in the physiological regulation of PTH secretion. The same effect is produced by the administration of aminophylline in the rat (Bowser et al., 1975). Williams et al. (1974) showed that the β-adrenergic agent isoproterenol, at the usual therapeutic dosage in man, stimulated PTH secretion, preceded by an increase in plasma cyclic AMP. Epinephrine, another β-adrenergic agent, also induces hypersecretion of PTH, whereas the α-adrenergic agent phenylephrine does not (Kukreja et al., 1975). The β-blocker propranolol significantly inhibited PTH secretion emphasizing the important role played by the β-adrenergic stimuli in the physiological control of PTH secretion in man (Williams et al., 1974; Kukreja et al., 1975). Propranolol may even produce hypocalcemia in rats, but the pathogenesis of this action is more complex (Lund et al., 1975).

Clearly the adenyl cyclase–cAMP system plays a central role both for PTH action and PTH release. The question remains whether appreciable PTH action can occur in the absence of an intact, responsive adenyl cyclase-cAMP system. Unpublished data gathered by the authors ten years ago in man indicate that this is so. The evidence will be produced later. Sallis (1970) was the first to question the critical mediating role of cAMP in PTH-induced phosphaturia. His experiments have largely been ignored and although the graphs produced by Potts et al. (1971), Tomlinson et al. (1974), Kurokawa et al. (1974), and Czekalski et al. (1974) indicate that cAMP is excreted at a more rapid rate than phosphate, reaching peak concentrations between 2 and 7 min after injection (Tomlinson et al., 1974), Sallis (1970) was the only one to make observations in vivo after injecting [32]P. In the rat, Sallis et al. (1967) observed an increased excretion of phosphate 60 sec after PTH administration. Rasmussen and

Tenenhouse (1968), however, showed that within one minute of infusing PTH, there was a dramatic rise in cAMP in the renal tissue of the rat. It should also be noted that the dog does not respond to PTH administration with an increase in the urinary excretion of cAMP (Blonde et al., 1974).

In rats chlorpropamide inhibits cAMP production, yet the phosphaturic response to PTH is increased (Numann and Moses, 1974). Similarly, Herrmann-Erlee and v.d. Meer (1974), working on embryonic mouse calvaria in tissue culture, found that propranolol stimulated lactate production. High doses of DB-cAMP caused significant uptake (rather than release) of calcium, and the interaction of DB-cAMP and aminophylline with PTE resulted in decreased, rather than increased, Ca, P_i, and lactate release. The authors concluded that cAMP is not the exclusive mediator of the action of PTH on bone, but that one or more other PTH-dependent processes are involved. Further work from this laboratory (Herrmann-Erlee et al., 1975), using isoptin, a potent calcium ion antagonist, led to the hypothesis that the lactate response to PTH in embryonic bone in vitro is indeed cAMP mediated, but that the citrate response as well as the osteolytic action are mediated through the calcium ion concentration. Recent data from Dziak and Stern (1975) also support the idea that calcium ion concentration is the intracellular mediator of PTH action on bone, as measured by ^{45}Ca transport in isolated bone cells. In this system, neither cAMP nor DB-cAMP caused any change in calcium transport. Agents which increased cAMP concentration, such as methylisobutylxanthine, were equally ineffective. Finally, Nagata et al. (1975) were able to produce significant elevation of plasma calcium in the rat by administering small doses of PTH without stimulating the accumulation of cAMP in calvaria or in plasma.

In humans, similar discrepancies may occasionally be observed. Estep et al. (1969) observed hypocalcemia in a patient operated on for hyperthyroidism by thyroparathyroidectomy which proved resistant to high doses of calcium supplements and vitamin D (400,000 U/day). Under those conditions, the administration of PTH produced a striking increase in the serum calcium level (from 6.5 to 11.0 mg/dl), phosphodiuresis, and a marked decrease in the serum phosphate level. Each time PTH was given the urinary phosphate rose significantly, but the urinary cAMP remained unchanged. Here also, other mediators must have been operative and the renal effects of PTH were not paralleled by changes in the urinary excretion of cAMP. Clearly more data are needed to pinpoint the exact role played by cAMP in the response to PTH by the kidney and bone. That it does play a facilitating role, amplifying the response, is indisputable. Whether this is indispensable for PTH action seems unlikely.

F. Special Studies in Pseudohypoparathyroidism

The authors have performed studies relating to the pathogenesis of PHP which also pertain to the concept of adenyl cyclase-cAMP action. Although portions of these studies have been alluded to by Tashjian *et al.* (1966), Potts (1972), and Potts and Deftos (1974), and analyses performed on tissues (Aliapoulios *et al.*, 1966) or peripheral blood (Gudmundsson *et al.*, 1970) have been reported, and while the cAMP studies have been included among other patients with PHP (Chase *et al.*, 1969), the studies performed by the authors have never been formally described, although they have been presented (Nagant de Deuxchaisnes and Krane, 1971).

All patients reported here as having PHP have had tests of response of cAMP excretion to administration of 300 U PTE intravenously. None demonstrated an appreciable response. Four responses are depicted in Fig. 12. Furthermore, in all patients the serum Mg level was normal. None had signs of kidney failure, nor of intestinal malabsorption.

1. Studies in Twin Sisters Presenting PHP

The twin sisters, M.B. and M.A., were studied on a metabolic ward under identical dietary conditions, simultaneously, and using the same batch of PTE.

Patient M.B. is case III reported by Elrick *et al.* (1950). She is the identical twin sister of patient M.A., by all criteria, including histocompatibility blood typing, although homologous skin grafting was not performed. These are the only two identical twins presenting with PHP who are known to us and therefore are of considerable interest. Both had had tetany off and on "all their lives" beginning at age of three. They presented with a single attack of convulsion at the age of five while suffering from measles. Menstrual periods aggravated the symptomatology, as did any trivial illness, emotional upsets and hyperventilation. The latter was most obvious and traditional in these Catholic nuns on Christmas evening, when singing Christmas carols in the church choir.

Figure 14 shows the sisters when they were infants and later when they were admitted for study in the metabolic ward. Typical is the aspect of fat babies with a fat, rounded head, so well illustrated by Alexander and Tucker (1949) and by Forbes (1962). This, however, did not persist, perhaps owing to the rigors imposed by their religious life. Their height was 1.57 m for M.A. and 1.60 m for M.B. at age 47. Mental function was normal.

The sisters were neither tall, nor dwarfed. To see whether they were short as compared to other members of the family, written information was obtained concerning all siblings. M.B. answered she was 1.56 and M.A. 1.59 m, a good approximation indeed, while three male siblings

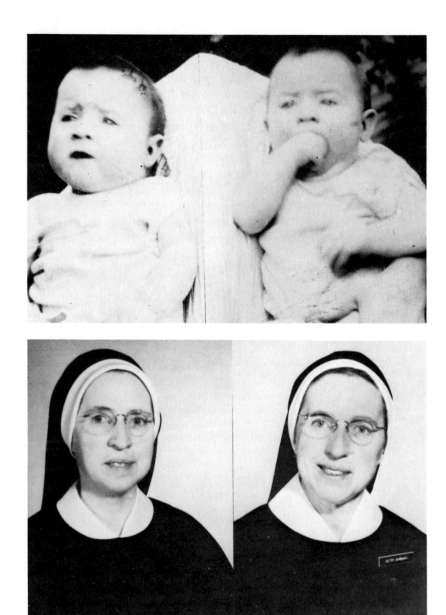

Fig. 14. Twin sisters M.A. and M.B. with PHP shown as infants and at time of study described.

reported heights of respectively 1.85, 1.83 and 1.88 m and two female siblings heights of respectively 1.75 and 1.72 m. Within this kindred, they were definitely short.

The sisters were born at term (birth weight: 3.8 kg each) from healthy parents (except for hypertension), when the mother was 40 and the father 47. There is no history of either deranged calcium metabolism, or of PPHP-like features either in the parents or the other five siblings. A sixth sibling died in youth from tuberculosis. The mother had one miscarriage. She had a goiter removed in 1925, 6 years after delivery of M.A. and M.B. The maternal grandfather had suffered from diabetes mellitus.

Both sisters have had essential hypertension, as has also been present in both parents. M.A. was told so at the age of 20, M.B. at the age of 32. Teaching in different schools, they lived hundreds of miles apart for the last 15 years. Despite this, they claim to have had attacks of tetany at the same time, even when they were engaged at different tasks, but they also have their menstrual periods simultaneously and suffer from the same illnesses (for example a common cold) at the same time. Tetany may also appear, without any known reason, in both twins simultaneously. This has allegedly been checked for years by the sisters and common witnesses. The twins seem to suffer from simultaneous disease. They began to have hay fever the same day, suffered from headaches, nose bleeding or gastric discomfort at the same time, presented with sore throats simultaneously. An infection of the right big toe followed by nail extraction occurred simultaneously in two different states. Both sisters underwent hysterectomy for metropathia hemorrhagica, M.B. in 1963 and M.A. in 1964. These details are given because they contribute somewhat to the probability that these sisters are indeed identical twins.

Both sisters have apparently normal teeth, but both have developed calcifications of the basal ganglia (with a similar amount and distribution), visible at age 34, while lenticular opacities in both patients were noticed at age 46. They did not show ectopic ossifications. Brachymetatarsia IV is present unilaterally in M.A., but not in M.B., in whom the abnormalities in length and configuration of the fingers and toes are mild. Despite reports of "minimal shortening of the fourth and fifth metacarpals," these changes seemed most unimpressive to the present observers. Both sisters have sacralization of L5, the same degree of mild scoliosis with the top at L3–L4 and the same degree of degenerative changes in the dorsal spine.

Evidence for the existence of PHP in M.B. rested on the existence of (1) life-long symptoms of hypoparathyroidism, having produced lenticular opacities and calcifications of the basal ganglia, (2) typical blood chemistries with a serum calcium level in the 7.4–7.8 mg/dl range and a serum P in the 4.3–4.8 mg/dl range at age 34, in the absence of abnormal serum Mg level, kidney failure, and signs of malabsorption, (3) the existence of short stature and a round face, (4) the resistance of the kidney tubule as ascertained by an Ellsworth–Howard test (Cfr. "S.M.B." in Fig. 13 of the paper published by Elrick *et al.*, 1950), (5) the existence of a hyperplastic (left lower) parathyroid gland, as demonstrated by a biopsy performed on February 25, 1950, by Dr. Oliver Cope (Elrick *et al.*, 1950).

Dr. Albright's file discloses that during the Ellsworth–Howard test, performed on December 6, 1949, the urinary P output increased from an average 7.9 mg/h pre-injection, to an average 16.0 mg/h post-injection value (ratio: 2.0; percentile increase: 106%). The spontaneous variation of P excretion in the urine was not studied. This is consistent with the average 90% percentile increase in cases of PHP as found in the literature by Bronsky *et al.* (1958). The response of urinary cAMP to PTE is shown in Fig. 12, and is pathognomonic for PHP, as it is for M.A. as well. Fig. 15 shows the effects of prolonged PTE administration (72 hours) of 200 U every 8 hours performed simultaneously in patient M.A. and patient M.B. with batch A of parathyroid extract. Patient M.A. showed essentially no response to PTE. Serum calcium prior to the test period averaged 6.7 (range 6.2–7.0) mg/dl. Highest serum calcium level the last day of PTE administration reached 7.8 mg/dl. Urinary calcium did not appreciably change. Similarly, urinary P output changed from an average 404 mg/24 hours to a high of 580 mg/24 hours, with some negative rebound excretion at the end of the test. In contrast, patient M.B. increased her serum calcium level from an average 9.4 (range 8.6–9.8) mg/dl to a high 13.0 at the end of the test, while urinary calcium rose from a mean 80 mg/24 hours to a high 214 mg/24 hours. Urinary P output increased from a mean 337 mg/24 hours to a high 833 mg/24 hours, with a negative rebound excretion as low as 91 mg/24 hours.

The results were surprising indeed, and possible explanations on the differences between the twin sisters were analyzed. Three factors could be considered. First, M.A. had brachymetatarsia and M.B. not. It was suggested that the PTH resistance-gene was located closely to the gene responsible for brachydactyly. M.A. would have more severe disease than M.B., as also witnessed by her basal serum calcium level of 6.7 mg/dl, versus 7.6 mg/dl for M.B. This was not so for serum P, however, since it was 3.9 mg/dl for M.A. and 4.4 mg/dl for M.B. However, even if M.B. had been a less severe case to start with, she had been as ill as her sister all her life, enough so to end up her fourth decade with lenticular opacities and calcifications of the basal ganglia. With no response of cAMP to PTH, she was as certain a case of PHP as her twin sister, yet demonstrated a normal response of calcium and P to exogenous PTE.

The second difference between M.A. and M.B. was that, when tested, M.B. had been treated since February 1958 continuously with adequate

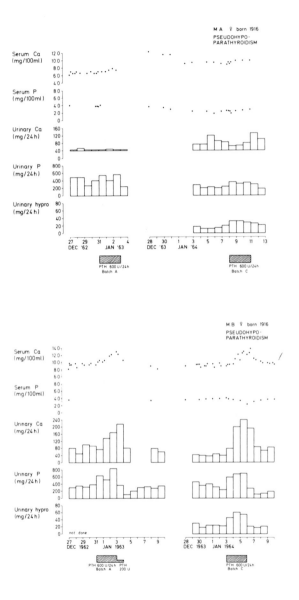

Fig. 15. Response to prolonged administration of parathyroid hormone (PTH) in twin sisters with PHP. See text for details.

335

dosages of either AT 10, or vitamin D_2, or both, with an episode of intoxication in May, 1961. When tested, she was taking 1 ml/day of AT 10 and had normal serum calcium and serum P levels. The possibility was raised that endogenous secretion of a defective PTH had been suppressed, making the receptor sites available for exogenous PTE at the target organs. The possibility of the existence of an abnormal hormone which combines with sites at the end-organs, exerting a diminished hormonal effect but competing successfully with exogenous normal hormone for the receptor sites, had been considered specifically by one of us (Krane, 1961).

The third difference between the sisters that was considered is that M.B. had undergone a cervical exploration in 1950 with search for parathyroid glands. Only one gland was found and biopsied, and although all glands were not meticulously searched for, due consideration was given to the possibility that biopsy of one gland and exploration of the area might possibly have interfered with the blood supply of other parathyroid glands such that this patient with PHP would have become a case of postoperative hypoparathyroidism. This did seem highly unlikely, since only one side of the neck had been thoroughly explored, and because, although tetany had occurred on several occasions in the immediate postoperative period, the serum calcium had not changed, a factor whose significance became more apparent to us a few years later. Finally, the absence of hypocalcemic hypercalciuria also argued against the existence of frank postoperative hypoparathyroidism, although it does not exclude it (Litvak et al., 1958).

Rejecting as decisive factors the first and third differences between M.B. and M.A., we decided to check on the second difference, the only one which was easy to verify. Therefore, patient M.A. was treated vigorously, while patient M.B. was continued on vitamin D, and both sisters were retested in December 1963. M.B. was taking vitamin D_2 150,000 U/day and M.A. 100,000 U/day with an episode of intoxication in July 1963 (serum calcium: 11.4 mg/dl), and one at the end of December 1963. When she entered the hospital on December 28, the serum calcium was 12.2 mg/dl and the serum P was 3.9 mg/dl (see Fig. 15). Blood urea nitrogen was 46 mg/dl. Vitamin D was discontinued and in 3 days the serum calcium dropped to 9.0 mg/dl and remained there, while it took 5 days for the BUN to normalize at 25 mg/dl. The serum alkaline phosphatase remained unchanged in M.A. (3.1 versus 3.3 Bodansky Units prior to the onset of therapy). In M.B., this value was 2.8 on first testing and 3.7 Bodansky Units on second testing.

Table IX shows basal chemistries, as well as the results of kinetic studies performed with ^{47}Ca, according to methodology described elsewhere (Nagant de Deuxchaisnes and Krane, 1964 and 1967). It can be seen that the calcium deposition rate in bone (v_{0+}) of M.B. was low. In M.A., it did not increase upon normalization of the serum calcium level, whereas the calcium pool (P) normalized reflecting the normalization of the serum calcium level.

The studies were then undertaken both on M.A. and M.B., M.A. not taking vitamin D while tested but with perfectly normal blood chemistries, M.B. under vitamin D therapy. The results were unchanged as compared with those obtained one year previously. As seen in Fig. 15, the serum calcium was normalized, as was the serum P. However no noticeable increase in serum Ca was produced with Batch C PTE 200 U every 8 h × 3 days (highest value 9.8 mg/dl from a base-line value of 9.2 mg/dl), nor any noticeable decrease in serum P which had fallen quite low after the episode of intoxication (2.4 mg/dl).

Whether this was a direct effect of vitamin D intoxication cannot be proven, but has occasionally been described (Lordon *et al.*, 1966). Urinary calcium did not increase, while urinary P increased from an average 227 mg/24 hours to a high 348 mg/24 hours without subsequent negative rebound excretion. Only the urinary excretion of total hydroxyproline seemed to respond, increasing from an average 15.3 mg/24 hours to a maximum of 32.3 mg/24 hours.

In contrast, patient M.B. responded normally by all criteria. Serum calcium increased from an average 9.2 to a high 13.8 mg/dl, while the urinary calcium output increased from an average 51 mg/24 hours to a high 244 mg/24 hours, and the total hydroxyproline in the urine rose from an average 23.1 mg/24 hours to a maximum of 60.8 mg/24 hours. The serum P level dropped from an average 3.8 mg/24 hours to a low 2.2 mg/24 hours at the end of the test, while the urinary P increased from an average 353 mg/24 hours to a high 713 mg/24 hours with a subsequent negative rebound excretion of 122 mg/24 hours.

At the beginning of the prolonged period of PTE administration, an Ellsworth–Howard test was performed, the results of which are shown in Table VIII. A 1.8-fold increase in P/creatinine excretion is seen in M.A., versus a 1.6-fold increase one year previously, and versus a 3.3-fold increase in patient M.B. The data on M.B. can be compared with those obtained in 1949, if urinary P is considered. Average pre-injection P output in the urine was 7.6 mg/hour, and increased to an average 25.0 mg/hour post-injection value (ratio: 3.3; percentile increase: 229%). Spontaneous increase of P output is absent in this patient: 13.2 mg/hour pre-injection time, versus 4.8 mg/hour post-injection time. The PTE-induced increase in P excretion is very close to the average 230% percentile increase recorded by Bronsky *et al.* (1958) in normal subjects. These

values may be compared with those found in Dr. Albright's file on patient
M.B. and recorded above. The present response is more striking. Thus,
the treatment in M.A. had not substantially altered her pattern of response, despite a normalization of the blood chemistries. Whatever the
cause, it was clear that cAMP output could be impaired, and indeed when
we found out later that it was even more impaired upon PTE administration in M.B. than in M.A., it was felt that cAMP response to PTE, even if
pathognomonic of PHP, was not necessarily related to effectiveness of
response to PTH. We investigated further the influence of correcting
serum calcium with vitamin D in other patients to see whether PTE-
resistance could not be overcome. Some of these studies are as follows.

2. Studies of the Effect of the Normalization of Serum Calcium with Vitamin D

The first patient (O.M.) was diagnosed in the course of an observation
preceding cataract extraction. He was short (1.62 m) and had a round
face, although no definite brachydactyly could be demonstrated
roentgenographically. Roentgenograms of the pelvis disclosed opacities
adjacent to the lower rami of the pubis. Tendon attachments of the lesser
trochanter were calcified. Mental function was normal. The patient was
the heaviest in his family at birth, weighing 4.2 kg. At age of 5 months, his
weight was 12.0 kg and he won the "largest baby" award in his commu-
nity. He was the second child of a mother with mild diabetes mellitus who
had 9 children and two miscarriages. The father also had mild diabetes
mellitus. Two paternal aunts of the propositus were diabetic and one
sister of the propositus had "hyperglycemia" after a course of glucocorticoids.

When he was admitted to the metabolic ward, the patient was 47. He
had frank cataracts, the onset of which was unknown, although the
patient complained of increasing difficulty in seeing for the last 22 years.
Symptoms of tetany occurred for the last 15 years. At age 31, he had
sudden rapid balding which stabilized after about one year, leaving the
patient with marked thinning of hair on the top of the scalp. Trousseau's
sign and Chvostek's sign were prominent. There was no hypertension.
Episodes of carpal spasm occurred 2 to 4 times weekly. He also had
benign episodes of laryngospasm, accompanied by stridor and hoarse-
ness. Dental examination (Dr. N. Treager) showed that there was no
evidence that he had suffered from severe metabolic disease before the
age of 8 to 9 years. Noneruption of the upper left wisdom tooth, despite its
nonimpacted-nonobstructed position, may indicate a problem in relation
to metabolic disease around age 17 to 20.

Fig. 16 shows a prolonged test of PTE administration (200 U every 8

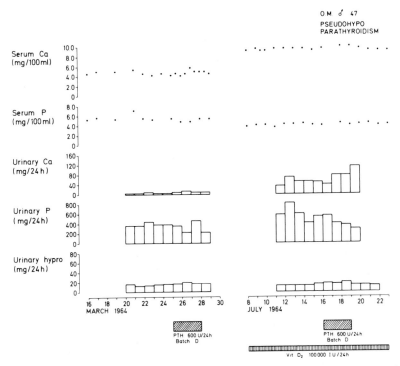

Fig. 16. Response to prolonged administration of parathyroid hormone (PTH) in a patient with PHP before and after treatment with vitamin D₂.

hours for 72 hours). There was essentially no response to Batch D PTE. Highest serum calcium was 5.8 mg/dl from an average 4.6 (range: 4.2–5.0) mg/dl pretreatment value, while the urinary calcium was unaltered and total urinary hydroxyproline excretion increased slightly from a mean 14.4 to a maximum 20.2 mg/24 hours. Lowest serum P level during the treatment period was 4.8 versus an average 5.6 (range: 5.1–70) mg/dl pretreatment value. Urinary P output increased slightly from an average 344 mg/24 hours pretreatment value to a high 423 mg/24 hours. Treatment with vitamin D₂ (Deltalin) orally was conducted, with a poor response (Fig. 17). Whereas the serum Ca had been normalized in three days with AT 10 prior to cataract extraction, vitamin D₂ had to be increased to 200,000 U/day to normalize the serum calcium, which was achieved after two months.

Upon retesting three months later (Fig. 16), the serum calcium had normalized from 4.6 to 9.5 mg/dl, while the serum P had dropped from 5.6

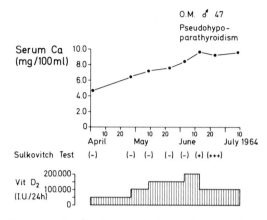

Fig. 17.   Response of serum Ca to oral vitamin D₂ in a patient with PHP.

to 4.0 mg/dl. As shown in Table IX, no substantial change occurred in the alkaline phosphatase level which actually fell slightly from 3.4 (range: 3.3–3.7) to 2.1 (range: 1.9–2.4) Bodansky Units. The urinary excretion of total hydroxyproline remained unchanged: 13.3 versus 12.7 mg/24 hours. The calcium pool normalized and the calcium deposition rate in bone increased, without reaching normal values. Whether this represents a true increase in "bone formation rate" or reflects the increase of the calcium pool cannot be settled. The slope of disappearance of the isotope from plasma was not significantly different (-0.00227 versus$-$ 0.00205).

The same batch of PTE was used at the same dosage during the same period of time, and vitamin D₂ therapy was continued (100,000 U/day) throughout the study period. Highest serum calcium achieved was 10.0 mg/dl from the base-line 9.5 (range: 9.2–9.6) mg/dl value, while the urinary calcium increased from an average 68 to a high 128 mg/24 hours, and the urinary total hydroxyproline excretion from an average 13.3 to a high 20.3 mg/24 hours. Serum P did not decrease, while urinary P output increased from an average 500 to a high 786 mg/24 hours without subsequent negative rebound excretion.

To make sure batch "D" of PTE was active, it was given to a patient (A.L.) with severe Paget's disease of bone. It can be seen (Fig. 18) that the serum calcium promptly rose from an average 9.2 to a high 11.8 mg/dl while the urinary calcium increased from an average 180 to a high of 720 mg/24 hours, and total urinary hydroxyproline from an average 730 to a high 1050 mg/24 hours. These responses, especially the unusual calciuric response, might be due to the very nature and activity of the underlying condition (Paget's disease). Serum P dropped from an average 4.0 to a low 3.0 mg/dl, while urinary P increased from an average 620 to a high 1850

TABLE IX

Serum Chemistries and Calcium Kinetics in Treated and Untreated Hypoparathyroid and Pseudohypoparathyroid Patients

Subject	Disease	Sex	Age	Weight (kg)	Height (cm)	Serum Ca (mg/dl)	Serum P (mg/dl)	Serum alkaline phosphatase (BU)	Urinary hydroxyproline (mg/24 h)	Hydroxyproline/creatinine (mg/gm)	^{47}Ca Specific Activity at 24 hours (% dose/g Ca)	v_l (mg/24 h)	v_u (mg/24 h)	v_r (mg/24 h)	P (mg)	v_o+ (mg/24h)	v_o+/kg (mg/24 h/kg)
O.M.	Pseudo untreated	M	47	64.3	162	4.70	5.6	3.4	12.7	14.3	37.7	395	5	74	2,707	234	3.64
	+ vit D			65.7		9.47	4.0	2.1	13.3	13.0	25.7	395	60	67	3,753	344	5.24
M.A.	Pseudo untreated	F	46	55.8	157	6.67	3.9	3.3	—	—	36.6	161	2	75	2,641	347	6.22
	+ vit D			51.1		10.07	2.3	3.1	16.3	20.4	29.2	161	51	93	3,320	262	5.13
M.B.	Pseudo + vit D	M	47	54.5	160	9.36	3.5	2.8	23.1	28.6	31.6	147	87	61	2,866	317	5.82
K.D.	Pseudo untreated	M	13	56.8	172	8.83	5.6	12.6	155.5	172.0	7.0	118	18	78	5,040	4,944	87.04
R.M.	Pseudo untreated	M	25	52.9	143	7.40	4.5	3.2	28.4	25.7	29.9	224	5	221	3,069	321	6.07
	+ NaF			52.7		6.75	5.2	2.3	34.6	31.3	29.8	224	8	360	2,936	262	4.97
	+ vit D			55.3		9.36	3.6	2.1	26.2	22.8	28.1	224	36	232	3,509	136	2.46
E.G.	Hypopara untreated	F	72	57.4	159	6.50	4.2	5.7	—	—	29.4	—	12	61	4,389	247	4.30
M.L.	Hypopara + vit D	F	57	51.2	160	8.55	3.3	2.0	18.8	21.8	27.6	237	252	62	3,441	352	6.88
J.P.	Latent Hypopara	M	58	81.0	168	8.70	4.0	8.2	—	—	20.2	200	17	139	4,663	679	8.28
7 Normal[a]		F	26	58.7	167	9.50	3.8	2.0	23.2	—	25.8	—	115	63	3,586	468	7.98
S.D.				7.2		—	—	—	—	—	3.4	—	49	21	463	80	1.18
23 Normal[a]		M + F	50	66.7	166	—	—	—	—	—	20.3	—	115	103	4,853	522	7.83

[a] Details on the normal subjects are given elsewhere (Nagant de Deuxchaisnes and Krane, 1967).

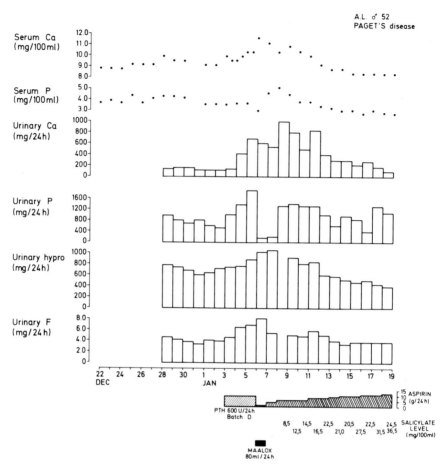

Fig. 18. Response of a patient with Paget's disease of bone to PTH, magnesium-aluminum hydroxide gel (Maalox) and aspirin.

mg/24 hours. The further experimental results in this case have been explained in detail elsewhere (Nagant de Deuxchaisnes and Krane, 1974). Undoubtedly, batch "D" of PTE had appreciable biologic potency.

The second patient with PHP in whom we tested the responsiveness to PTE prior to and after vitamin D was R.M., case no. 3 of the original publication by Albright *et al.* (1942), who was born at full term, weighing 3.8 kg. He had suffered from laryngospasm from the age of two, and had convulsions at the age of 2½ years. Serum calcium was 7.1 and serum P 10.0 mg/dl. A tracheotomy had to be performed because of severe laryngospasm following an upper respiratory infection. Fig. 19 shows the

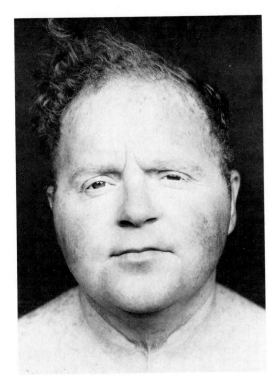

Fig. 19.   Photograph of patient R.M. with PHP, at age 25. Note tracheotomy scar.

patient at the age of 25, when he first entered the metabolic ward. The tracheotomy scar can be seen. He is a typical case of PHP, with the full-blown picture of short stature (1.43 m), obesity (53 kg), round face, mental retardation, brachydactyly at the upper (short, stubby fingers with particularly short thumbs) and lower (Fig. 20) extremities, radius curvus, platyspondyly, and subcutaneous bone formation which not only could be seen roentgenologically (two forearms, right trochanter, legs, knees, ankles, feet), but which could also be felt, especially over his back and abdomen. Roentgenograms also showed generalized radiolucency, with among others, a femur score of 53. Combined cortical thickness was 7 mm for the humerus and 5 mm for the radius. Fig. 20 shows a dystrophic right great toe nail, but moniliasis has been ruled out. On the Wechsler Adult Intelligence Scale, at age 25, he was rated as having a "defective" general ability (IQ 67).

Both his sisters were in good health. One was 1.54 m and the other 1.73 m. The mother was short (1.50 m) and died at the age of 29, while

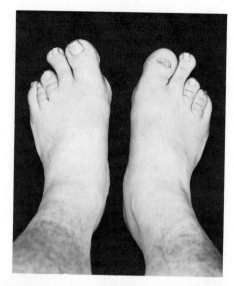

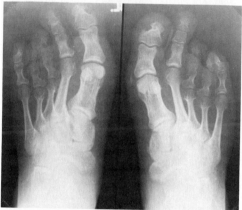

Fig. 20. Photographs of the feet and corresponding roentgenograms in patient R.M. with PHP at age 25. Note particularly shortening of digits 3 and 4 due to brachymetatarsia III and IV.

pregnant. She was diabetic, as were her own mother (R.M.'s maternal grandmother) and one of her five sisters (R.M.'s maternal aunts), while her brother is in good health, another brother having died when he was young. Propositus and his two sisters were delivered by Caesarean section. This is reminiscent of the family history obtained in patient O.M. and of what one of us has described (Nagant de Deuxchaisnes *et al.*, 1960b) as a general finding in the families with PHP and PPHP. Between the age of 4 and 9, the patient did well except for his school performances. He had been taking 1.2 g of calcium lactate three times daily and 150,000 U/d of vitamin D_2. At that time his serum calcium was 7.2 and serum P 7.6 mg/dl. The alkaline phosphatase was 4.8 Bodansky Units. At the age of 16, he was readmitted to the hospital because of repeated attacks (every 2–3 days) of numbness of his left leg, and occasionally of his left arm, often appearing after some degree of excessive exertion, but also unexpectedly at any time. He also had spells of carpal spasm and twitching of both eyes. He had not had convulsions. His vision was diminished and teeth were carious. Since the age of 9, he had discontinued medications. Chvostek's sign had been repeatedly positive, and Trousseau's sign negative. Symptoms of tetany were absent despite lack of therapy between age 9 and 15. His serum calcium on admission was again 7.2 and serum P 9.2 mg/dl, with an alkaline phosphatase value of 6.4 Bodansky Units. Typical cataracts were not found at the age of 16 but were present when the eyes were re-examined at the age of 24, at which time calcifications of the basal ganglia were observed. He had resumed his treatment at age 16, but stopped it again at age 22. The studies were performed as shown in Fig. 21 at age 22, the patient being untreated (R.M.I). Serum calcium was 7.4 and serum P 4.6 mg/dl. Upon PTE administration, 600 U/day for 3 days, the highest recorded serum calcium was 8.2 and the lowest serum P 4.3 mg/dl. Urinary calcium and P did not appreciably change, nor did the urinary output of total hydroxyproline (maximum: 33.7 mg/24 hours, from an average of 28.4 mg/24 hours).

Almost one year later, when the serum calcium had been corrected (9.4 mg/dl), as well as the serum P (3.6 mg/dl) through the administration of vitamin D_2 100,000 U/day, the same test was performed (R.M.II) with the same parathyroid extract (Batch B). Highest serum calcium was 10.4, lowest serum P 3.6 mg/dl, while the urinary calcium rose from an average of 36 to a high 99 mg/24 hours, without any noticeable change in phosphaturia. Again the total hydroxyproline in the urine increased from an average 26.2 to a high 32.5 mg/24 hours. That Batch "B" of PTE was an active one can be seen from Figs. 10 and 11.

Normalization of serum calcium and P through vitamin D therapy was not accompanied either by an increase in calcium deposition rate in bone (v_{o+}) or by an increase in the urinary excretion of total hydroxyproline (see Table IX). Only the calcium pool (P) increased, owing to the increase of the serum calcium level. The same pattern was seen in M.A. as far as calcium kinetic data are concerned, and in O.M. for the urinary hydroxyproline excretion data. From Table VIII it can be seen that no

difference in the results of the Ellsworth–Howard test could be observed
when comparing pretreatment and posttreatment values obtained with
Batch "B" PTE.

Another trial of vitamin D was attempted to demonstrate its action and
another test performed 14 months later with another batch of PTE, using
as control a patient with postoperative hypoparathyroidism. The dosage
of vitamin D_2 had been reduced to 50,000 U/day which proved sufficient.
Fig. 21 (R.M. III) shows that little effect followed this new prolonged test
with PTE. Average pretreatment values for serum calcium and P were

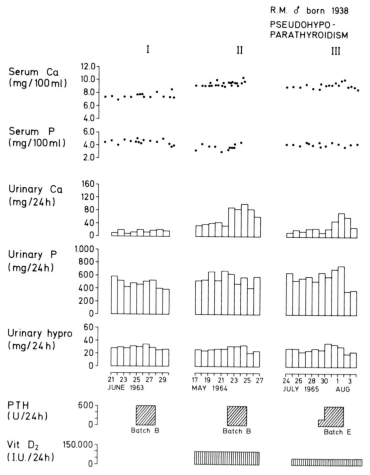

Fig. 21. Response to prolonged administration of PTH in patient R.M. with PHP, before
and during treatment with varying doses of vitamin D_2.

respectively 9.0 and 4.2 mg/dl. Peak level for serum calcium during PTE administration was 10.0 mg/dl, while the nadir for serum P was 3.8 mg/dl. Urinary calcium rose from an average of 19 to a maximum of 74 mg/24 hours, while urinary P increased from an average 576 to a maximum of 753 mg/24 hours. Increase in total hydroxyproline excretion in the urine was from an average of 26.4 to a maximum of 35.9 mg/24 hours.

The activity of Batch E of PTE was assayed in patient M.L. who had postoperative hypoparathyroidism following surgery for Graves' disease in 1930. She was inadequately treated for this complication and intracranial calcifications were documented in 1950. Tremor was first observed in 1953 and Parkinson's disease was diagnosed in 1960. Cataracts had been present since 1941 as well. Fig. 22 (M.L. II) shows the effect of PTE while patient M.L. was undertreated (50,000 U/day). The serum calcium rose from an average 7.5 to a peak of 10.6 mg/dl and serum P fell from an average of 4.2 to a low 1.8 mg/dl. These changes were accompanied by striking modifications in the urinary excretion of calcium (from an average 73 to a peak 269 mg/24 hours) and P (from an average 451 to a peak 1399 mg/24 hours with a marked subsequent negative rebound excretion). Total hydroxyproline excretion in the urine increased from an average of 17.6 to a peak 29.1 mg/24 hours.

An earlier test (M.L. I) had been performed in this patient 17 months previously with Batch C of PTE, the same as that used on retesting M.A. and M.B. The serum calcium was higher (8.6 mg/dl) to start with since patient was receiving 100,000 U/day of vitamind D_2 and 1 ml/day of AT 10. The reason for later reducing the dosage of vitamin D_2 and for withdrawal of AT 10 had been an episode of toxicity between test I and II of Fig. 22, when the patient was readmitted with a serum calcium of 13.9 mg/dl. Upon PTE administration, serum calcium rose from an average 8.6 mg/dl to a peak 11.4 mg/dl, while serum P dropped from an average 3.3 to a low 2.0 mg/dl. The urinary calcium rose from a mean 271 mg/24 hours to a high 387 mg/24 hours, while the urinary P increased from an average 498 to a peak 1473 mg/24 hours, with a subsequent negative rebound excretion. The increase in the urinary output of total hydroxyproline had been from an average 22.0 to a peak 37.7 mg/24 hours. Whatever her treatment, M.L. seemed to represent the ideal control patient who responded maximally to PTE administration. From Table VIII, the Ellsworth-Howard test of M.L. with both batches of PTE can be seen in contrast sharply with the results of the same test with Batch "E" in R.M.

In summary, all three patients in whom serum calcium was normalized with vitamin D_2, from 6.7 to 9.2 mg/dl (M.A.), from 4.6 to 9.5 mg/dl (O.M.), and from 7.4 to 9.4 or 9.0 mg/dl (R.M.), did not show any significant difference as far as their response to three day administration

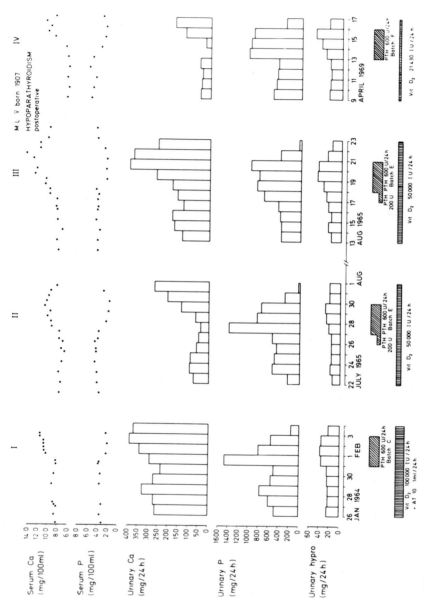

Fig. 22. Response to prolonged administration of PTH in patient M.L. with postoperative hypoparathyroidism during treatment with vitamin D₂. Tests M.L. II, III, and IV correspond, respectively, to R.M. III, IV, and VI, and serve as controls.

of PTE is concerned. The hypercalcemic response was respectively
+ 1.1(M.A.) + 1.2(O.M.) and + 0.8(R.M.I.) mg/dl, prior to treatment,
and + 0.6 (M.A.), + 0.5 (O.M.), + 1.0 (in both R.M. II and R.M. III) mg/dl,
once the serum calcium was corrected. This is in contrast with M.A.'s twin
sister, in which responses of +3.6 and +4.6 mg/dl were observed, comparable to the increases of patient M.L. with postoperative hypoparathyroidism (+2.8 and +3.1 mg/dl respectively, in M.L. I and M.L. II). A
summary of all the data is shown in Table X. In patient J.T. (Fig. 11) with
cirrhosis of the liver, the increase in serum calcium had been +2.3 mg/dl,
and in patient A.L. (Fig. 18) with Paget's disease of bone, it was +2.6
mg/dl.

The urinary calcium excretion data could not adequately be compared,
because of fluctuations in the basal level coinciding with fluctuations in
the serum calcium. However, monitoring the urinary excretion of total
hydroxyproline is possibly a better reflection of the turnover of bone
collagen, because it is not significantly affected by therapy. The PTE-
induced increase amounted to a factor of 1.4 prior to and 1.5 after
treatment with vitamin D in O.M. In R.M. it was 1.2 prior to and respectively 1.2 (R.M. II) and 1.4 (R.M. III) after therapy. In patient M.A. this
was not determined prior to treatment. The changes produced in hydroxyproline excretion after therapy with vitamin D are therefore not
significantly different as compared with those initially observed.

Finally, the phosphaturic action of PTE did not seem to be affected
either by normalization of the serum calcium or serum phosphorus by
vitamin D. PTE-induced increase was by a factor of 1.4 in M.A., versus a
factor of 1.5 after treatment. Similar increases were of 1.2 versus 1.5
respectively prior to and during vitamin D therapy in O.M. In R.M. the
increase was initially nil, and became 1.1 (R.M. II) and 1.3 (R.M. III) after
therapy. All these increments are negligible, as compared with the 2.0 to
2.5 increase in M.B., and the 3.0 to 3.1 increase in M.L.

Patient M.B. therefore remained unique in her very high degree of
responsiveness towards PTE. It was concluded that the very fact she was
treated with vitamin D or AT 10 could not account for this different type
of response as compared to the other patients. The hypothesis was considered that as a result of the neck exploration which had been performed
in search of the parathyroids and the biopsy of the only parathyroid gland
that had been found, the patient indeed might have become a case of
postoperative hypoparathyroidism. The fact that her response to PTE
administration was more similar to that of M.L. than to that of M.A.,
O.M. and R.M. lent some weight to the hypothesis that in the other
patients vitamin D had not suppressed all of the supposedly abnormal
hormone (the working hypothesis) that might be circulating. The putative

TABLE X

Summary of Responses to Parathyroid Extract (PTE) in Patients with Hypoparathyroidism and Pseudohypoparathyroidism[a]

Subject	Treatment/24 hr	Batch of PTE	Serum levels (mg/dl)				Urinary excretion (mg/24 h)						
			Calcium		Phosphorus		Calcium		Phosphorus		Total hydroxyproline	
			Av.	Peak	Av.	Nadir	Av.	Peak	Av.	Peak	Av.	Peak
M.A.	None	A	6.7	7.8	3.8	N.D.	20	39	404	580	N.D.	N.D.
M.A.	Vit.D 100,000[b]	C	9.2	9.8	2.4	2.5	48	94	227	348	15.3	32.3
M.B.	AT 10 1 ml	A	9.4	13.0	3.5	N.D.	80	214	337	833	N.D.	N.D.
M.B.	Vit.D 150,000	C	9.2	13.8	3.8	2.2	51	244	353	713	23.1	60.8
O.M.	None	D	4.6	5.8	5.6	4.8	5	12	344	423	14.4	20.2
O.M.	Vit.D 100,000	D	9.5	10.0	4.0	4.0	68	128	500	786	13.3	20.3
R.M. I	None	B	7.4	8.2	4.6	4.3	16	33	509	520	28.4	33.7
R.M. II	Vit.D 100,000	B	9.4	10.4	3.6	3.6	36	99	581	619	26.2	32.5
R.M. III	Vit.D 50,000	E	9.0	10.0	4.2	3.8	19	74	576	753	26.4	35.9
R.M. IV[e]	Vit.D 100,000[c]	E	9.2	12.3	4.7	4.2	203	343	431	623	16.6	22.1
R.M. V[e]	None	E	7.1	9.2	5.8	4.7	120	N.D.	809	1016	N.D.	N.D.
R.M. VI[e]	Vit.D 150,000	F	7.8	11.0	5.0	3.9	154	293	588	995	23.1	42.2
M.L. I	Vit.D 100,000[d]	C	8.6	11.4	3.3	2.0	271	387	498	1473	22.0	37.7
M.L. II	Vit.D 50,000	E	7.5	10.6	4.2	1.8	73	269	451	1399	17.9	29.1
M.L. III	Vit.D 50,000	E	8.3	14.4	4.2	2.4	182	391	442	989	24.2	47.1
M.L. IV	Vit.D 21,430	F	6.3	10.6	5.4	2.8	47	127	486	1096	23.8	43.9

[a] See text for details. Vitamin D dosage refers to IU/24 h.
[b] Stopped 6 days prior to testing, because of toxicity.
[c] + AT 10 2ml.
[d] + AT 10 1ml.
[e] Postoperatively.

abnormal hormone would be ineffective (or partially so), but compete (partially) with exogenous extract and therefore impede the normal response. To check this hypothesis and possibly improve medical management, it was decided to perform total parathyroidectomy in a patient with PHP. The most typical and the best studied case was R.M., and consent was obtained from the propositus and his parents.

3. Total Parathyroidectomy in a Patient with PHP

The studies prior to parathyroidectomy have been described and are summarized in Fig. 21. In Fig. 22 are shown the studies performed simultaneously with the same Batch of PTE in M.L., the patient with postoperative hypoparathyroidism, who served as a control (M.L. II, M.L. III and M.L. IV). In Fig. 23 are shown the studies performed immediately before and after parathyroidectomy.

Total parathyroidectomy was performed by Dr. John W. Raker on August 5, 1965. Four hyperplastic parathyroid glands were removed. The normal size of a parathyroid gland is usually $3-6 \times 2-4 \times 0.5-2$ mm (Bruining, 1971). The right upper parathyroid in this case measured $4 \times 2 \times 2$ mm, the left upper $6 \times 4 \times 4$ mm and the right lower $12 \times 6 \times 6$ mm. The left lower was not measured since it was embedded in a tongue of the thymus. It was estimated as being "quite large." The glands showed hyperplasia histologically (Dr. S. I. Roth). Their content of iPTH, as measured by Dr. John T. Potts, Jr. (see Chapter 1), was excessive. Simultaneously, a right subtotal thyroidectomy was performed and tissue was assayed for calcitonin (see Chapter 4). This was found to be excessive in amount. Bioassay of the thyroid specimen (Aliapoulios *et al.*, 1966) was indicative of a CT concentration of approximately 100 times greater than the average in the normal thyroid tissue obtained in control patients (4,700 U/g of thyroid tissue versus an average of 42 U/g).

Following parathyroidectomy, several biological consequences ensued almost immediately. First, the serum calcium level, despite continued vitamin D_2 therapy (50,000 U/day), fell from 8.7–9.0 to 7.8 mg/dl in 24 hours, reached 7.4 mg/dl the next day and, when it reached 6.7 mg/dl after 3 days, the patient experienced the first clear-cut attack of tetany he could remember in his life. Trousseau's sign had been observed from the first postoperative day, an unusual finding in this patient. The dosage of vitamin D_2 was increased from 50,000 to 100,000 U/d, AT 10 was given in dosages indicated in Fig. 23, and oral calcium supplements were given as calcium lactate, providing 1.17 g of elemental calcium daily. It took nine days under this regimen before reaching the initial value of 9.0 mg/dl serum calcium. The serum P had initially fallen from 4.2 to 3.5 mg/dl on the first post-operative day, and 3.7 mg/dl on the second post-operative

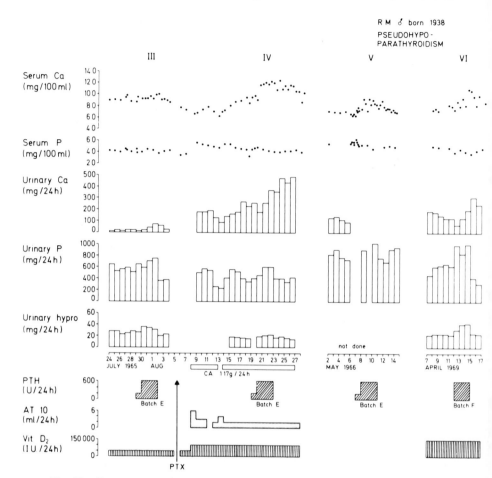

Fig. 23. Response to prolonged administration of PTH in patient R.M. with PHP following parathyroidectomy. See text for details.

day. It thereafter rose to levels above 5.0 mg/dl and finally plateaued at an average 4.7 mg/dl when the serum calcium level had normalized. The conclusion of this study was that by removing the parathyroid glands' the source of a partially active hormone had been eliminated. The finding that cases of PHP have a serum calcium which is on the average 1.0 mg/dl higher (Tables III and IV) than that of classic cases of IHP is, therefore, not surprising.

Moreover, the synergistic action between vitamin D and PTH is demonstrated, as stressed in the animal by Carlsson (1954) and Crawford *et al.* (1957). The latter authors showed that in rats deprived of vitamin D and calcium, the serum calcium was 4.9 mg/dl. When supplemented with 10,000 U/day of vitamin D (and no calcium), the serum calcium level rose to 8.5 mg/dl. If the animals fed 10,000 U/day without calcium were parathyroidectomized, their serum calcium again fell to 4.6 mg/dl. The operation performed in R.M. provided somewhat unexpectedly the human counterpart of this experiment. Not only does PTH require the presence of vitamin D to be active on bone, but vitamin D action requires the presence of PTH, a point which is better appreciated now that its role as a "trophic" factor is better known, since it has been shown to increase the concentrations of $1,25\text{-}(OH)_2D_3$ in blood and tissues (see Chapters 2 and 5, Volume I). No wonder the dosage of vitamin D_2 had to be increased from 50,000 to 150,000 U/day, AT 10 had to be added and calcium supplements had to be given to restore the initial serum calcium level. The slight but definite drop in the urinary excretion of total hydroxyproline (Fig. 23 and Table X) further substantiates the fact that endogenous PTH does affect the turnover of bone collagen as well. The alkaline phosphatase also fell slightly, but significantly ($p < 0.05$), from 3.1 ($n = 9$) to 2.7 ($n = 10$) Bodansky Units. Endogenous parathyroid hormone therefore had bone remodeling effects as well as calcium replacement activity.

The fact that the serum P increased, a finding which was repeatedly confirmed over the subsequent years (Table X), as a consequence of parathyroidectomy also shows that endogenous hormone did exert some spontaneous, albeit discrete, phosphaturic action. It is therefore not surprising that in PHP, the serum P level is lower (and not higher) than in IHP, as shown in Tables III, IV, and V, a finding that persists even if one selects the patients with the very lowest serum calcium values.

Finally, one of the most striking immediate biological consequences of the operation was the instantaneous rise in urinary calcium excretion after parathyroidectomy. From Table X it can be concluded that in this patient the corresponding urinary calcium values for the normocalcemic range (9.0 to 9.4 mg/dl) was approximately 20–40 mg/24 hours prior to parathyroidectomy versus approximately 200 mg/24 hours after parathyroidectomy, whereas in the hypocalcemic state (7.1 to 7.8 mg/dl), they were approximately 15 mg/24 hours prior to parathyroidectomy and 120–160 mg/24 hours after parathyroidectomy. Clearly, the endogenous hormone exerted a normal calcium-sparing action on the kidney tubule and it is not surprising that hypocalcemic hypercalciuria is not a feature of PHP, but one of IHP (or of the postoperative state). This could be deduced from the circumstantial evidence collected by Litvak et al. (1958). The data are comparable to those obtained by Talmage and Kraintz (1954) in the rat. Thus, patients with PHP are protected by their endogenous secretion from developing vitamin D-induced nephrocalcinosis.

There remained to be determined what the response would be to exogenous PTE administration now that the patient had been deprived of his endogenous hormone. This had been attempted on three occasions. The first time PTE was administered after parathyroidectomy, only 14 days had elapsed from the time of the operation. The serum calcium had returned to normal levels for a period of 4 days. From Fig. 23 (R.M. IV) and Table X, it can be seen that a normal response was obtained as far as the elevation of the serum calcium level is concerned ($+3.1$ mg/dl) but that the phosphaturic action had remained suppressed. Admittedly, the test performed when the new steady state was not yet completely achieved. A simultaneous test with the same batch of PTE was performed in the control patient (M.L. III in Fig. 22), demonstrating a vigorous hypercalcemic and a striking phosphaturic response. cAMP response to PTE remained nil.

A second test was performed eight months later when the patient was without medication and was frankly hypocalcemic. Once more (R.M. V in Fig. 23 and Table X), the hypercalcemic response to the same parathyroid extract was normal ($+2.0$ mg/dl), while the phosphaturic response was poor, but the dietary conditions of this experiment were different, in that the patient's diet was not as low in phosphate. Under those circumstances, the response was blunted.

A third test was performed (R.M. VI in Fig. 23 and Table X) with Batch F of PTE four years after the operation. Despite the intake of 150,000 U/d of vitamin D_2 the serum calcium was still 7.8 mg/dl, versus a requirement of 50,000 to 100,000 U of vitamin D_2 daily before parathyroidectomy for normalization of serum calcium to occur. When PTE was given for the third time the calcemic response was normal ($+3.2$ mg/dl), and a more striking effect was obtained on the urinary total hydroxyproline excretion, which increased by a factor of 1.8, versus 1.2 to 1.4 prior to the operation. This is similar to the response obtained repeatedly in patient M.L., who upon PTE administration increased her urinary output of total hydroxyproline by a factor of 1.6 to 1.9. On a low P diet, some phosphaturic response was obtained. However, when the test was simultaneously performed in M.L. with the same batch of PTE (M.L. IV in Fig. 22 and Table X), the phosphaturic response was more striking (increase in urinary P by factor of 2.3) and the subsequent fall in serum P was more impressive (-2.6 mg/dl, versus -1.1 mg/dl in R.M. VI).

From the results of the Ellsworth–Howard test (Table VIII), it is clear that no effect had been obtained in R.M. prior to parathyroidectomy on three occasions, if one excludes the 4th test where purified PTH had been used. On two occasions after parathyroidectomy, a "normal" response was obtained, but not to the level observed on three occasions in patient M.L. with hypoparathyroidism.

G. Pathogenesis of Pseudohypoparathyroidism

The conclusions from the studies following parathyroidectomy in R.M. are that the patient's excessive endogenous hormone had (1) a striking though insufficient calcium mobilizing action on bone, (2) a barely detectable, but nonetheless indisputable phosphaturic action on the kidney, and (3) a perfectly normal calcium-sparing action on the kidney tubule. In the absence of endogenous hormone, exogenous parathyroid extract in physiological doses was able to mobilize calcium from bone in a normal fashion, and elicited an improved, though subnormal, phosphaturic response. These observations suggest (1) that the endogenously produced hormone is an abnormal one, as postulated, (2) that the response to PTH in bone is not dependent upon the adenylate cyclase system, and (3) that full expression of the phosphaturic response to PTH requires a normally functioning adenylate cyclase system.

That vitamin D metabolism was not critical for the response of bone to PTE is suggested from the following points: (1) the calcium-mobilizing action was demonstrated after parathyroidectomy when the blood chemistries were similar to those prior to parathyroidectomy, especially high P values which inhibit the 1α-hydroxylase in the kidney tubule (Tanaka and DeLuca, 1973); (2) the response of bone was an immediate one, so that bone was not altered, whatever its state as a possible consequence of lack of $1,25$-$(OH)_2D_3$; (3) the response of bone was obtained during periods of administration of high doses of vitamin D as well as during periods when the patient was off medication. The blunted phosphaturic response prior to parathyroidectomy can partially be explained on the basis of high levels of circulating hormone (normal or abnormal), as has been shown in the Ellsworth–Howard test (Becker et al., 1964; Gershberg et al., 1966; Purnell et al., 1968).

From the scanty information available (Evanson, 1966; Purnell et al., 1968), it seems that the hypercalcemic response to PTE infusion is similar in primary hyperparathyroidism and in normal subjects. If these observations are consistently obtained and adenylate cyclase does not play a crucial role in the calcium-mobilizing action from bone, then the blunted hypercalcemic response observed in patients with PHP upon PTE administration is due the presence of the abnormal hormone, secondary to competition at the effector site.

Adenylate cyclase also does not play a critical role in this disease as far as the feedback response of the parathyroid glands to the circulating levels of the calcium ion is concerned. Not only can the secretion of PTH readily be suppressed by calcium infusions (Chase et al., 1969; Potts and Deftos, 1974; Stögmann and Fischer 1975), but in a case of PHP studied by one of us (C.N.) PTH release was stimulated upon a disodium-EDTA

(70 mg/kg) infusion (Devogelaer *et al.*, unpublished). The levels rose as they did in cases of primary hyperparathyroidism.

Thus it seems that in this disease there are two abnormalities, one in the adenylate cyclase system (lack of production and/or release of cAMP, or excessive destruction of cAMP), and possibly one in the parathyroid hormone molecule and/or its metabolism, and/or interaction with receptors. Whether there is a connection between these two abnormalities remains a matter of speculation and would involve another, as yet unknown, point of interaction between the adenylate cyclase system and either PTH synthesis or PTH metabolism. If these two abnormalities and unconnected, we favor the hypothesis that abnormal PTH metabolism and/or molecule is the more important pathogenetic mechanism. Indeed, if the adenyl cyclase system is operating effectively only at the kidney level as far as P excretion is concerned, all this would eventually produce would be hyperphosphatemia. Whether hyperphosphatemia *per se* can produce permanent hypocalcemia in the absence of an active circulating PTH is doubtful.

Fig. 24 shows the experiment conducted by one of us (C.N.) in a patient with IHP (Rombouts-Lindemans *et al.*, unpublished). After baseline observations, oral calcium supplements were given up to 6 g/24 hours of elemental calcium during two weeks. The serum calcium rose from a base-line level of 5.0 to a high 8.5 mg/dl. The serum P value was not affected. When the last six values of serum P are considered, which correspond to the period when serum calcium had risen to values higher than 7.9 mg/dl, the mean fasting serum P was 4.2 mg/dl, compared with the initial mean 4.5 mg/dl pre-treatment value. Calcium supplements were then continued at the same dosage, but aluminum hydroxide was given by mouth in doses of 180 ml/24 hours (60 ml t.i.d. before meals) for one week. The serum P level dropped to a low 1.7 mg/dl, with no appreciable rise in serum calcium level (peak level: 8.8 mg/dl). Within 48 hours of withdrawal of the aluminum hydroxide and diminution of oral calcium supplementation from 6 g/24 hours to 1 g/24 hours of elemental calcium, the serum P rose to 5.8 mg/dl (withdrawal of Al(OH)$_3$) and serum calcium dropped to 7.1 mg/dl (withdrawal of calcium supplements). Further fall of the latter was prevented by the administration of crystalline dihydrotachysterol orally and a further increase in the oral calcium supplements.

Thus, in patients lacking endogenous PTH, no reciprocal changes in calcium and P levels occur. An illustrative case is that of postoperative hypoparathyroidism reported by Lordon *et al.* (1966). Hypocalcemia and hyperphosphatemia treated with vitamin D over two years resulted in hypercalcemia (serum calcium constantly around 12.1–13.5 mg/dl). As a result, a tubular leak of phosphate developed, and when all medication

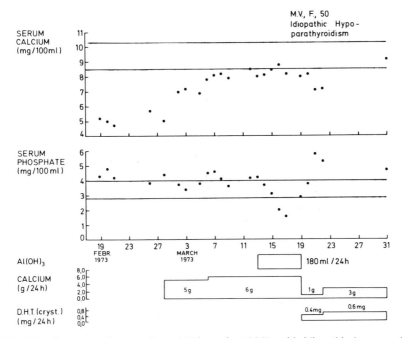

Fig. 24. Response of serum Ca and P in patient M.V. with idiopathic hypoparathyroidism to the administration of oral calcium supplements, aluminum hydroxide gel [Al(OH)₃] and crystalline dihydrotachysterol (D.H.T.). See text for details.

was withdrawn, the serum P level was 2.7 mg/dl, when the serum calcium level fell to 6.2 mg/dl. Certainly hyperphosphatemia is not necessary for the serum calcium level to fall strikingly, a situation well known following parathyroidectomy in patients with renal azotemic osteodystrophy, where both plasma calcium and P fall simultaneously (Stanbury, 1962) (see Chapter 2). In normal subjects, reciprocal changes do not necessarily occur either (Philpot, 1958). When sudden hypocalcemia is produced by means of sodium-EDTA infusions, the serum P level falls. In the disease entity known as tumoral calcinosis, hyperphosphatemia (at times higher than 10.0 mg/dl) is a consistent finding, but the serum calcium levels are normal in all cases, as are levels of PTH (Morgan *et al.*, 1975). It is unlikely therefore that a chronically elevated serum P level *per se* is sufficient to produce permanent hypocalcemia of the type found in PHP. Perhaps in tumoral calcinosis, the cAMP response towards PTE is impaired, but endogenous hormone is normal.

Secretion of an abnormal parathyroid hormone would mimic the state of hypoparathyroidism, with both hypocalcemia and hyperphosphatemia.

That the action of the endogenous hormone on bone is not impeded by the absence of a cofactor, or by the presence of an antagonist or an antibody, is shown by the experience in R.M. That antibodies are capable of producing hypoparathyroidism has been shown experimentally by Kooh and Fraser (1968), who injected antibodies produced in the guinea pig against bovine PTH in rats and rabbits. These experiments have been confirmed in the rat, using a PTH antiserum produced in the guinea pig (Monchik *et al.*, 1976), which neutralized endogenous circulating PTH. No such antibody has ever been shown to exist in PHP (Elrick *et al.*, 1950; Wise and Hart, 1952; Arnstein *et al.*, 1966), although Harell-Steinberg *et al.* (1957) felt they had some evidence for inactivation of normal PTH by incubation with PTH from an (atypical) case of PHP. The possibility that an antagonist could counteract the action of PTH rose when huge amounts of calcitonin were shown to be present in R.M.'s thyroid gland. This problem will be dealt with later.

It is a reasonable possibility that an abnormal endogenous parathyroid hormone could compete with exogenous parathyroid hormone for receptors. Martin *et al.*, (1974) showed for example that bovine PTH (2–34) inhibited the response to bovine PTH (1–34) in its action on chick kidney, as measured by the adenyl cyclase activity in crude plasma membranes. The analogue was capable of achieving this inhibitory action at concentrations which were ineffective in stimulating the adenyl cyclase system, suggesting that it could bind to the PTH receptor but not initiate subsequent events. More recently, Goltzman *et al.* (1975) demonstrated that two synthetic analogues of bovine PTH with amino-terminal modifications, PTH (3–34) and [desamino-Ala-1] PTH (1–34), also were devoid of activity in the adenyl cyclase system of the rat renal cortex *in vitro*, but inhibited the action of the native hormone or of bovine PTH (1–34). The degree of inhibition was proportional to the dose of inhibitor and reversible by the addition of an excess of active hormone. If an analogous situation were to exist in PHP, this could account for the fact that some response has been obtained by some authors either because they used huge doses of exogenous PTE or because the inhibitor might not have been present in high enough concentration.

How all this pertains to the problem of PHP is uncertain, except that it demonstrates that a dichotomy may exist between receptor binding and expression of the biological response, with inhibition by inactive analogues of receptor binding by active components. In these experiments, the biological activity was evaluated in terms of renal adenyl cyclase function, which may or may not be the most adequate measurement. However, other actions of PTH might exhibit the same properties of receptor binding, competition, effectiveness or lack of activity at the site of the target-organs.

More pertinent are the findings of Weinstein *et al.*, (1974), who demonstrated that sera from two patients with PHP contained immunoreactive fragments of PTH, which differed from sera from patients with primary hyperparathyroidism. The glandular hormone, with an estimated 9,500 molecular weight, was detected (see Chapter 1), but the fragment with M.Wt. 7,000–7,500 was conspicuously absent and replaced by two previously undescribed fragments with estimated molecular weights of 5,000 and 3,000–4,000. The authors concluded that abnormal circulating fragments of PTH may account for the apparent end-organ resistance in PHP. Clearly, confirmation of this important piece of information as well as further characterization of the abnormal fragments as to their action on adenyl cyclase is needed.

If cAMP production is essential to obtain a normal phosphaturic response, inhibitors of the enzyme phosphodiesterase might be of help in correcting the abnormality by increasing the intracellular concentration of cAMP. Indeed, Weitzman and Murad (1973a) succeeded in increasing the phosphaturic response to PTE in three patients with PHP (as well as in normal subjects) by administering aminophylline. Using chlorpropamide, McDougal and Lukert (1974) were able in PHP to increase the basal cAMP output in the urine (unaffected by PTE administration) by a factor of two. Addition of PTE to chlorpropamide increased the urinary cAMP by a factor of four. The blood chemistries, and urinary excretion of P, however, remained unaffected. Coulson and Moses (1975) could not confirm the effects of chlorpropamide on cAMP excretion in PHP. The phosphaturic response to PTE also remained unaffected when this drug was administered, confirming the findings of Weitzman and Murad (1973a). How useful inhibitors of phosphodiesterase might be in the treatment of PHP remains to be determined. If their effects are restricted to normalization of the phosphaturic response, their usefulness should be limited.

Having discussed our findings in respect to the pathogenesis of the condition, some questions remain to be resolved. One may wonder why a normal response was not obtained after normalization of the serum calcium level in patients M.A., O.M., and R.M., whereas this would have eliminated most of the "evil" circulating hormone. It is possible that all of the hormone had not been eliminated, and was still blocking receptor sites in the target-organs. After we had conducted these studies, we were comforted in observing that other authors had achieved normalization of serum calcium values in this condition and found that the patients had remained resistant towards PTE (Mautalen *et al.*, 1967; Felitti and McAfee, 1968; McDonald, 1972; Birkenhäger *et al.*, 1973). This was also true when the serum calcium was normalized with $1,25(OH)_2D_3$ (Coburn *et al.*, 1974). However, there were exceptions to this rule. Suh *et al.* (1970) demonstrated that their patient became responsive upon correction of the serum calcium level. After 4 months of treatment with vitamin D_2 (100,000 U/24 hours), the serum calcium rose upon PTH administration (800 U/24 hours) from 10.0 to 14.4 ($+4.4$) mg/dl within a 48-hour period, and although the urinary excretion of phosphate increased more than 2-fold, the serum P level did not change. This is in contrast to the results obtained with the same batch of PTE in a patient with IHP in whom the serum calcium rose from 6.6 to 12.1 ($+5.5$) mg/dl, and the serum P fell from 9.4 to 3.6 (-5.8) mg/dl within a 72-hour period. The results are similar to those in R.M. after parathyroidectomy: normalization of the calcium-mobilizing effect from bone and improvement of the phosphaturic action owing to decrease in secondary hyperparathyroidism, but the phosphaturia remained short of what can be observed in IHP and did not affect the serum P level significantly.

The results obtained by Stögmann and Fischer (1975) are comparable. After treatment with vitamin D_3 (120,000–160,000 U/24 hours during 10 months) the hypercalcemic response, from 9.5 to 14.4 ($+4.9$) mg/dl, obtained after 4 days of PTE administration (700 U/24 hours), was perfectly normal whereas it had been nil prior to therapy. The normalization of the phosphaturic response, however, consisted in the demonstration of an improved Ellsworth-Howard response. From the same test performed after 2 months of vitamin D therapy and published by Stögmann (1973), it can be seen that if the Ellsworth-Howard test was normalized and a hypercalcemic response obtained, the effect on the serum P level was superimposable on that obtained prior to the initiation of vitamin D therapy.

Frame *et al.* (1972), in a case of "hypo–hyperparathyroidism" obtained similar results after raising the serum calcium level with huge doses of vitamin D. When the patient was retested, the serum calcium rose from 10.0 to 13.0 mg/dl on the fourth day of PTE administration (400 U/24 hours). In an Ellsworth-Howard test, the average hourly P excretion rose from 7.0 to 25.3 mg upon PTE injection, whereas in a control patient, tested previously, the rise had been from 9 to 50 mg/hour.

Finally, Drezner *et al.* (1976) also obtained a normal hypercalcemic response in 4 patients with PHP whose serum calcium had been normalized with ergocalciferol. Unfortunately they did not verify the phosphaturic response in these patients. These four reports therefore reinforce our conclusions that the hypercalcemic response can be normalized, but that the phosphaturic response, albeit improved, remains subnormal. The question remains why these groups of workers obtained an improved response after vitamin D whereas others did not. It possibly depends on the degree or duration of inhibition of PTH obtained by elevation of the ionized calcium fraction. Although the serum Ca may be rapidly increased, it may take longer than 7 months (Birkenhäger et al., 1973; Stögmann and Fischer, 1975) before normal iPTH levels are obtained. There might be a critical level of inhibition of endogenous PTH necessary for the normal or improved response to be observed, a critical level that might not have been achieved in nonresponsive cases.

A second problem is that of calcium infusion experiments in which lowering of the circulating levels of PTH should restore PTE responsiveness. Authors who attempted this were unable to obtain a normal response toward PTE (Suh et al., 1969; Drezner et al., 1976), although more work is needed along these lines. It is not known how much time is required for the binding sites of the target-organs to be freed of the putative competitive hormone fragment.

A third point that should be dealt with is the possibility of abnormal vitamin D metabolism. (See Chapters 2 and 5, Vol. I.) It has been suggested that refractoriness of renal 1α-hydroxylase to the action of PTH could be an additional factor in the pathogenesis of PHP (Kooh et al., 1975), or even account entirely for the abnormal calcium metabolism in this condition (Sinha and Bell, 1976). The last statement is untenable in view of two facts: (1) our experience in R.M. showing that parathyroidectomy alone restored the responsiveness of bone toward PTE (whether vitamin D was given or not), makes it hard to accept that bone resistance in PHP is a problem of intrinsic refractoriness of renal 1α-hydroxylase, and (2) equating the problem of hypocalcemia and bone disease to vitamin D deficiency [i.e., a deficiency of its active metabolite $1,25\text{-(OH)}_2 D_3$] implies that all patients with PHP should have histological osteomalacia, and that all infants, children and adolescents with the disease would suffer from rickets. Not one case of adult PHP has ever demonstrated clinical signs of osteomalacia, nor have Looser's zones been observed radiologically. Not one infant, child or adolescent has been shown to have clinical or radiological signs of rickets, excluding cases with florid radiological hyperparathyroid bone lesions, as reviewed by Frame et al., 1972.

This is not to say that vitamin D metabolism is normal in PHP, or for that matter in IHP. Mawer et al., (1975) injected double-isotope-labeled cholecalciferol in two patients with postoperative hypoparathyroidism and found that labeled $25\text{-(OH)}D_3$ was formed appropriately, although labeled $1,25\text{-(OH)}_2 D_3$ failed to appear in the serum. If elevated P levels inhibit transformation of 25-(OH)D$_3$ to 1,25-(OH)$_2$D$_3$ and if normal PTH promotes this transformation, it may be assumed that high levels of serum P and a supposedly abnormal PTH are two factors impeding normal production of 1,25-(OH)$_2$D$_3$ in PHP. If the hormone is ineffective in its action on bone, it may be equally ineffective in promoting high concentrations of the active vitamin D metabolite, but in a non-specific fashion. This may not require supposition of an additional kidney defect, unless adenyl cyclase is necessary for this transformation to occur, as has been suggested (MacAuley et al., 1975). However, enough 1,25-(OH)$_2$D$_3$ is present to prevent florid rickets and/or osteomalacia. Perhaps, the development of rickets and/or osteomalacia is prevented by the high serum P level, which maintains the driving force for mineralization. Available measurements of circulating levels of 1,25-(OH)$_2$D$_3$, as determined by radioreceptor assay (Brumbaugh et al., 1974) have shown patients with PHP and IHP to have lower levels than a control population, although the values are not undetectable as in cases of end-stage renal failure (Haussler et al., 1975). In another report (Haussler, 1975), circulating levels of 1,25-(OH)$_2$D$_3$ were found to be "low" in 4 patients with IHP, "low" in 7 patients with postoperative hypoparathyroidism, "low-normal" in 4 patients with PHP, and "undetectable" in 3 cases of vitamin D-deficient osteomalacia as well as in 1 case of vitamin D-deficient rickets. Thus, among all these patients those with PHP seem to be rather privileged as far as 1,25-(OH)$_2$D$_3$ plasma concentrations are concerned.

Mild histological osteomalacia may occasionally be present in PHP, as well as in IHP, which could result from the diminished availability of 1,25-(OH)$_2$D$_3$ concentrations in blood and tissues. Erdheim (1906) showed that parathyroidectomy in the rat resulted in newly formed dentinoid that was inadequately calcified. The evidence that this could also occur in bone soon followed (Erdheim, 1911). Burkhart and Jowsey (1966) showed in dogs that parathyroidectomy was followed by an increased mean width of osteoid borders, which averaged 12.6 μm, versus 6.5 $\pm$ 0.6 μm in normal dogs. The first description of osteomalacia in hypoparathyroid man was that by Albright (1956) in a case of postoperative hypoparathyroidism and this was soon followed by that of Mathieu et al. (1961) in a case of IHP. The most dramatic case of IHP and osteomalacia was reported recently (Drezner and Neelon, 1976).

Jowsey (1968) also reported studies of 5 patients with hypoparathyroidism (2 cases of IHP and 3 postoperative cases) and 3 patients with PHP. In hypoparathyroidism, there was an increase in the amount of surface covered by osteoid tissue, as well an increase in the thickness of the osteoid. In PHP, the average width of the osteoid borders was "slightly larger than normal, although not in the range characteristic of osteomalacia."

Other data from the literature minimize the importance of an osteomalacic component in PHP and IHP. Frost *et al.* (1968) studied four patients with each entity. The "number of osteoid seams" as well as the "circumference per osteoid-seam" were found to be decreased in both conditions. In isolated case reports of PHP, the absence of excessive osteoid seams has been specifically commented upon (Schüpbach and Courvoisier, 1949; Gsell, 1950; Schwarz and Loewe, 1966; Cohen and Vince, 1969). In other cases, the bone biopsy was interpreted as "normal," without further comment (Klotz and Kahn, 1957; Zisman *et al.*, 1969). Finally in the case described by Spech and Olah (1974), the relative osteoid surface was increased, but the mean thickness of osteoid seams was normal; osteoblastic surface was satisfactory and calcification fronts were normal.

Whenever osteomalacia has been found, another cause could be incriminated, such as consumption of anticonvulsant drugs (Birkenhäger *et al.*, 1973), the initial diagnosis of PHP was thought to be incorrect as in the interpretation by Arnstein *et al.* (1967) of a case of Tashjian *et al.* (1966), or florid hyperparathyroidism was present (Frame *et al.*, 1972). No comment concerning osteoid tissue was made in the case with radiological and histological hyperparathyroidism reported by Bell *et al.* (1963).

More recently, Drezner *et al.* (1976) reported osteomalacia in two patients with PHP. The biopsies were analyzed by Jowsey and osteoid width was found to be respectively 20.8 μm (age 32) and 16.9 μm (age 29). Control values are given as 13.8 $\pm$ 1.4 μm, but in other papers from the same Center it is given as 12–22 μm (Johnson *et al.*, 1971) or 16.2 $\pm$ 2.3 μm (Brickman *et al.*, 1975). From these values it appears as if the osteoid width is not much increased in PHP, and not much different from what was found in a group of osteoporotic patients (Jowsey *et al.*, 1969), despite the higher average age (47; range 36–51). Osteoid width in these 6 patients with osteoporosis was 16.7 μm (range: 12.0–20.2). Calcification fronts could be analyzed in only one patient with PHP and were found to be abnormal (either absent or broad and diffuse), but this case with the highest osteoid width also had radiological changes typical of secondary hyperparathyroidism. It is also known that in primary hyperparathyroidism, when roentgenologic changes are florid, rickets, or osteomalacia may be present (Lloyd *et al.*, 1965; Lomnitz *et al.*, 1966; Boyce and Jowsey, 1966; Bordier *et al.*, 1973; Seedat, 1974).

More complete histomorphometric measurements have seldom been performed in cases of IHP or PHP. It may therefore be appropriate to review the experience of one of us (C.N.) with this technique as applied to undecalcified sections of trabecular bone of a transiliac biopsy specimen. Measurements on four patients with IHP and one with PHP, all five prior to the onset of therapy, have been performed in the Department of Pathology (Prof. F. Meerseman), Louvain University. Results are given in Table XI. The bone in three patients with IHP was normal. Patient K.N. had considerable osteoid tissue. Both relative osteoid volume (percent of trabecular bone occupied by osteoid) and relative osteoid surface (extent of trabecular surface covered with osteoid) were increased by more than two standard deviations above the means, which are respectively 1.85 ± 1.25% (Courpron et al., 1973) and 17.7 ± 9.7% (Meunier and Edouard, 1976). However, the osteoid seams were not increased (normal values at that age: 6.7 ± 2.2 μ according to Merz and Schenk, 1970), nor was the thickness index of osteoid layers, as defined by Meunier et al. (1975). It follows that the osteoblastic appositional rate is equal to the calcification rate. Patient J.G. with PHP had only increased osteoid surface, but the relative osteoid volume was only one standard deviation above the normal

TABLE XI

Biological and Histomorphometric Data in Four Cases of IHP and One Case of PHP

	Normal values	J.P.	R.S.	M.V.	K.N.	J.G.
Diagnosis		IHP	IHP	IHP	IHP	PHP
Sex		M	M	F	M	M
Age		16	25	52	75	29
Weight (kg)		51	46	46	68	80
Serum calcium (mg/dl)	8.5–10.5	5.3	6.3	5.0	6.2	8.2
Serum phosphorus (mg/dl)	2.8– 4.0	5.9	6.5	4.5	5.1	4.4
Alkaline phosphatase (U/liter)	20–60	70	25	26	22	52
Urinary total hydroxyproline (mg/24 h)	15–40	106	30	11	N.D.[d]	42
Absolute bone volume (%)	Var.[c]	20.9	N.D.	17.6	16.0	25.0
Relative resorption surface (%)[a]	<4	1.9	N.D.	2.0	0.8	2.3
Mean surface periosteocytic lacunae (μm^2)	50.6 ± 5.2	53.1	59.9	35.9	50.4	71.7
Relative osteoid volume (%)[b]	<4	1.0	1.6	0.6	6.1	3.2
Relative osteoid surface (%)	<25	8.3	9.3	3.8	49.2	39.9
Absolute osteoid volume (%)	<1.0	0.2	N.D.	0.1	1.0	0.8
Mean thickness osteoid seams (μm)	<12	6.6	5.8	8.0	7.3	10.3
Thickness index of osteoid layers	<25	12.0	17.2	15.8	12.4	8.0
Calcification fronts	+ +	+ +	+	+ +	±	+ +

[a] According to Courpron et al. (1973) 3.6 ± 1.1.
[b] Same reference 1.85 ± 1.26 for M; 1.05 ± 0.91 for F.
[c] Too variable according to age and sex for normal values to be given.
[d] N.D. = not determined.

mean, and calcification fronts were normal, extending over 83.1% of the osteoid surface. The osteoblastic surface was 7.4% (normal value: 5.0 ± 2.9% according to Merz and Schenk, 1970). The mean thickness of osteoid seams was 10.4 μ (normal values for that age are 10.9 ± 3.6 μ according to Merz and Schenk, 1970). The thickness index of osteoid layers was lower than in any of the other patients. If anything, the calcification process was relatively faster than the appositional rate in this patient with PHP, as compared with the patients with IHP.

Thus, osteomalacia is seldom present in IHP or PHP. When present, it is manifested only histologically, and does not provide the reason for skeletal resistance to PTH. From the available data, there is no difference between IHP and PHP. Bone histology (as far as osteoid tissue is concerned) and $1,25(OH)_2D_3$ availability are comparable in both conditions.

Inasmuch as osteoid tissue in IHP is related to the abnormal basic chemistries and/or the lack of PTH, corrections of this should result in a decrease of osteoid tissue. In patient M.V., two bone biopsies were performed 26 months apart after treatment with crystalline dihydrotachysterol. Table XII shows that although all measurements pertaining to osteoid tissue were normal to start with, changes observed after two years of therapy moved in the direction of a decrease, usually by a factor of about two to four.

A final factor that should be considered with regard to the possible pathophysiological mechanisms intervening in the biochemical abnormalities of PHP is hypercalcitonism. Since the demonstration by Aliapoulious

TABLE XII

Morphometric (and Biological) Data on Repeated Bone Biopsies in M.V.

	Normal values	2/22/1973	4/24/1975
Serum calcium (mg/dl)	8.5–10.3	5.0	9.3
Serum phosphorus (mg/dl)	2.8– 4.0	4.5	3.9
Alkaline phosphatase (U/liter)	20–60	26	35
Urinary total hydroxyproline (mg/24 hour)	15–40	11	15
Absolute bone volume (%)	19.9 ± 3.6[a]	16.9	16.4
Relative osteoid volume (%)	1.05 ± 0.91[a]	0.6	0.3
Relative osteoid surface (%)	10.3 ± 5.3[b]	3.8	1.0
Absolute osteoid volume (%)	0.2 ± 0.1[a]	0.10	0.05
Mean thickness osteoid seams (μm)	8.8 ± 3.8[c]	8.0	4.7
Calcification fronts	+ +	+ +	+ +

[a] According to Courpron et al. (1973).
[b] According to Meunier and Edouard (1976).
[c] According to Merz and Schenk (1970).

et al. (1966) of a striking excess of calcitonin in R.M.'s thyroid gland, this subject has stirred interest and initially was considered as "a possible factor of importance" in the pathogenesis of PHP (Aliapoulios *et al.*, 1966). The well-known antagonistic action of calcitonin versus PTH at the bone level seemed to give some support to this theory, but the synergism between calcitonin and PTH as far as phosphaturia is concerned should result in hypophosphatemia not hyperphosphatemia, which is so characteristic of PHP. Furthermore, the inhibitory action on bone resorption reinforces the tendency toward hypophosphatemia by inhibiting the release of phosphate from bone (see review by Queener and Bell [1975]). These considerations made it unlikely that calcitonin excess would play any significant role in the pathogenesis of PHP. It has been amply confirmed that calcitonin levels in the thyroid gland of patients with PHP are high (Tashjian *et al.*, 1966; Mazzuoli *et al.*, 1966 and 1967; Suh *et al.*, 1969). So striking were these findings that several authors performed surgical total thyroidectomy (Suh *et al.*, 1969) or subtotal thyroidectomy in addition to treatment with radioiodine (Mazzuoli *et al.*, 1967; Lee *et al.*, 1968). It was initially felt that in one case a definite improvement had been obtained by the procedure (Mazzuoli *et al.*, 1966 and 1967) and the syndrome was considered as a "thyrocalcitonin-excess syndrome" (Mazzuoli *et al.*, 1966). When it appeared that the results were only transient (Mazzuoli *et al.*, 1968) and that no changes were observed in other cases (Lee *et al.*, 1968; Suh *et al.*, 1969), it was concluded that calcitonin excess in the thyroid glands of patients with PHP was the consequence rather than the cause of hypocalcemia. Indeed, Gittes *et al.* (1966 and 1968) had shown that calcitonin accumulated in glands of PTX-rats, because of continuing synthesis in the absence of the normal (hypercalcemic) stimuli governing release of the hormone. In humans, Tashjian and Voelkel (1967) have shown that in the glands of patients with hyperparathyroidism, the reverse situation exists and decreased calcitonin contents are found by bioassay. This corresponds to data collected in animals after parenteral or oral administration of calcium (Gittes *et al.*, 1968) or pharmacologic doses of vitamin D (Young and Capen, 1970).

A proper perspective could not be achieved until reliable methods for assaying circulating levels of calcitonin were available. A bioassay (Gudmundsson *et al.*, 1970) had first been applied, but its specificity raised some questions. When radioimmunoassays later became available, it could be shown that unusually high amounts of calcitonin could be released into the circulation following calcium infusions in all hypocalcemic patients, whatever the etiology of the hypocalcemia. Using relatively insensitive radioimmunoassays, high levels of immunoreactive calcitonin (iCT) (in the range of the values found in medullary carcinoma of the thyroid) could be measured in hypocalcemic patients at the end of a calcium infusion, whereas no iCT could be detected in normal or hypercalcemic subjects under the same circumstances (Deftos *et al.*, 1973; Chapter 4). Thus, thyroidal storage had occurred and accumulated hormone was available for release if the proper stimulus was applied whether calcium or pentagastrin. Why the hypercalcemic-induced iCT release was statistically higher in patients with PHP ($n = 9$) than in patients with IHP ($n = 7$) or hypocalcemia of other origin ($n = 6$) is unknown.

H. Special Forms of Pseudohypoparathyroidism and Related Conditions

1. Pseudohypoparathyroidism with Intermittently Normal Serum Calcium Values, and Considerations to the Natural History of Pseudohypoparathyroidism

It has been emphasized in previous sections that normocalcemia occurs in patients with PHP. Resistance to exogenous PTE as well as endogenous PTH is only partial in PHP. The severity of the manifestations may vary from one case to the other and the serum calcium may vary considerably during the lifespan of any one patient. What is not usually appreciated is that the serum calcium may approach or even reach normal values and eventually remain so for long periods of time despite persistence of the underlying abnormalities, as illustrated in the following case presentation.

Patient K.D. was aged 13 when he was first studied. Dr. Anne P. Forbes suggested the diagnosis of PHP on the basis of the association of ectopic ossifications, brachymetatarsia, and a serum calcium value of 8.0 mg/dl. At the time of our initial study a serum calcium was 8.8 (range: 8.6–9.0) mg/dl with a serum P level of 5.6 mg/dl and a serum alkaline phosphatase value of 12.5 Bodansky Units. He was tall (1.72 m) and not obese (56.8 kg), although he had been a fat baby. In Fig. 25 he is shown at the age of 10 months. On the Wechsler Adult Intelligence Scale his general mental ability measured within the "dull-normal" range. On roentgenograms, brachymetatarsia IV was noted on the right, and ectopic ossifications were noted in several areas. Platyspondyly was present as well. Numerous Schmorl's nodes could be seen in the dorsal vertebrae. On eye examination, no lenticular opacities could be seen. Father was diabetic (late onset), as was patient's paternal grandmother (diabetes mellitus, late onset). K.D. has two siblings, both well and tall.

As can be seen in Fig. 26, he proved resistant to the administration of PTE. Serum calcium rose from an average 8.8 to a maximum 10.0 ($+ 1.2$) mg/dl. The same batch of PTE was employed as in R.M. I. and R.M. II (Fig. 21), as well as in patient J.T. (Fig. 11) with cirrhosis of the liver, whose serum calcium rose from 8.3 to 10.6 ($+ 2.3$) mg/dl. Urinary calcium

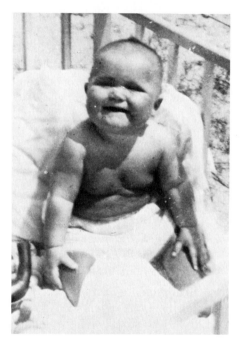

Fig. 25. Photograph of patient K.D. with PHP taken at the age of 10 months.

rose from an average 13 to a high 59 mg/24 hours, whereas the urinary excretion of total hydroxyproline, high to start with, did not increase further. Urinary phosphate output increased from an average 559 to a high 755 mg/24 hours.

He was retested five years later, in April 1969 (not 1964 as indicated in Fig. 26). His height had increased to 1.79 m and his weight to 71.5 kg. During the entire period he consumed 50,000 U of vitamin D_2 3 times weekly. The serum calcium was still 8.3 mg/dl, with a serum P of 4.7 mg/dl. PTE administration (same batch as R.M. VI and M.L. IV) increased the serum calcium to a maximum of 9.0 (+ 0.7) mg/dl, while the urinary calcium rose from an average 33 to a maximum of 45 mg/24 hours. Urinary total hydroxyproline output rose from an average 53.8 to a high 61.4 mg/24 hours. Urinary phosphate output increased from an average 665 to a high 878 mg/24 hours, a 1.3 maximal increase, whereas the lowest serum P achieved amounted to 4.3 mg/dl.

It is concluded that patients with PHP unresponsive to PTE as far as cAMP is concerned may occasionally be normocalcemic, as well as normophosphatemic. Very large amounts of hormone are required to reach this normal or near-normal state, as was later demonstrated in a similar

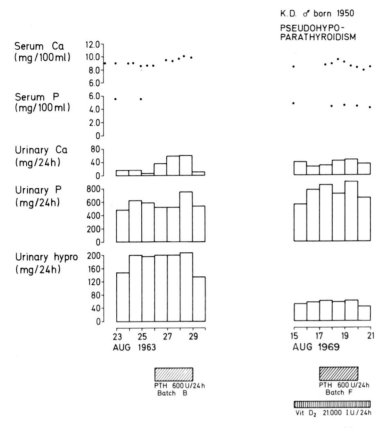

Fig. 26. Response to prolonged administration of PTH of patient K.D. with normocalcemic PHP before (1963) and after (1969) treatment with vitamin D_2.

case (Balachandar *et al.*, 1975). This could have been predicted, however, from the existence of the roentgenologic signs of subperiosteal bone resorption in a case with normocalcemia (Cohen and Vince, 1969). This state of normality may only be intermittent, and these patients are still subject to the effects of hypocalcemia. Therefore patients who have typical lesions of osteochondrodystrophy and are normocalcemic should not automatically be considered as examples of PPHP, unless their acute response of cAMP and P to PTE has been tested. A prolonged test of PTE administration will also show that bone and kidney are indeed resistant to PTE. Several cases in the literature substantiate the entity of "intermittently normocalcemic PHP," demonstrating large swings of serum calcium values. The shift from hypocalcemia (6.5–7.0 mg/dl) to normocalcemia (9.1 mg/dl) has been particularly well documented by Hinkle *et al.*,

(1965), concomitantly with a shift from hyperphosphatemia (6.8–7.5 mg/dl) to normophosphatemia (4.5 mg/dl at the age of 9). Under both circumstances the patient remained resistant to protracted administration of a potent PTE extract.

Most instructive is the case reported by Gershberg and Weseley (1960), who was hypocalcemic (6.7–8.4 mg/dl) and hyperphosphatemic (7.0 mg/dl) and had convulsions at age 14. Treatment was provided, but stopped by the patient at age 20. She remained relatively well (occasional tingling) with a higher serum calcium (8.3–8.5 mg/dl) and a lower serum P level (5.0–5.5 mg/dl), until she became pregnant, at which time both serum calcium (9.0–11.9 mg/dl) and P (3.5–3.9 mg/dl) were normal. Serum calcium decreased in the second trimester of pregnancy (8.7 mg/dl) with associated tingling in hands and feet. In this case, therefore, the periods of hypocalcemia coincided with periods of increased calcium demand, i.e., growth and pregnancy. A similar pattern was followed by case 3 of Palubinskas and Davies (1959) and case 2 of Rosenberg et al. (1967). Conversely, an initially normal calcium level may decrease in later years [Steinbach et al., 1965; Ray and Gardner, 1959 (plus follow-up by Papadatos and Alivisatos, 1960); Enthoven, 1960].

From many case histories there emerges a pattern as to the natural evolution in patients with "intermittently normocalcemic PHP." Gershberg and Weseley (1960) were the first to stress the point that most cases of PHP appear in childhood, whereas most cases of so-called PPHP are reported in adults. It furthermore seems clear that hypocalcemia is usually not present in infants (with notable exceptions), but appears in childhood. In a recent abstract, Kind et al. (1974) report the results of cAMP response to PTE in 5 children belonging to two families in both of which one other member suffered from PHP. All 5 had normal blood chemistries at the time of testing and never had symptoms suggestive of hypocalcemia. Yet 2 out of 5, aged respectively 5 days and 13 months, did not respond. These infants were most probably in the presymptomatic state of the disease, a situation the authors referred to as "latent pseudohypoparathyroidism." This fits the pattern that first symptoms of hypocalcemia in PHP usually appear at the average of 8.5 years, as commented on earlier.

Not all patients follow this "logical" sequence of events of calcium homeostatic failure in periods of greater requirements for this element. The best example is that of Mautalen et al. (1967) in a male patient with, at age 15, a serum calcium of 7.2 (serum P: 6.4) mg/dl, lenticular opacities, and calcifications of the basal ganglia. At age 19 he suffered from paresthesias and pain in the extremities (serum calcium 6.8 and serum P 6.7 mg/dl), and was treated adequately until age 24, when all therapy was discontinued. Despite this, his serum calcium remained normal, as well as his serum P level, from age 24 till age 30. At age 30, however, he again suffered from paresthesias, and his serum calcium dropped to 7.8 mg/dl. He was treated from age 30 to 32, and once more therapy was withheld. At age 41, his serum calcium was found to be 4.8 mg/dl. This all happened, the authors insist, without any demonstrable changes in the patient's medical, dietary or environmental conditions. Large swings of serum calcium values were observed in the adult period, witnessing repeated homeostatic failure. Such large swings have aso been found in case 3 of Bader *et al.* (1968), and in the case described by Cohen and Vince (1969). If periods of hypocalcemia are overlooked PPHP will be the (erroneous) diagnosis unless the patients are tested with PTE. The possibility of intermittently normocalcemic PHP should at least be considered, especially in those cases of "PPHP" with possible stigmata of prior hypocalcemia, such as calcifications of the basal ganglia (Tanz, 1960; Dudley and Hawkins, 1970), typical dental defects, or lenticular opacities "of the endocrine type" (Miles and Elrick, 1955; Casey *et al.*, 1959; Smulyan and Raisz, 1959; Papadatos and Alivisatos, 1960; Dickson *et al.*, 1960), in cases with a past history suggestive of hypocalcemia (case 4 of Palubinskas and Davies 1959), as well as in the cases who did not show an adequate response in the Ellsworth-Howard test (case 4 of Palubinskas and Davies, 1959; Smulyan and Raisz, 1959; Tanz, 1960).

PPHP should be defined as a genotypic condition with no biochemical abnormalities of the type that can be found in PHP, and with normal response to PTE. PHP is a genetic osteochondrodystrophy in individuals with typical somatic hallmarks and permanent or intermittent hypocalcemia and hyperphosphatemia who demonstrate a defective response of adenyl cyclase to PTE and secondary, ineffective hyperparathyroidism. In this sense, of course, PPHP is not a milder form of PHP, as has often been stated. It is a different disorder.

Numerous cases of PHP exist without osteochondrodystrophy as shown by the description of cases of so-called hypo–hyperparathyroidism. Several patients without roentgenologic osteitis fibrosa probably also belong to this group, especially those described by Harell-Steinberg *et al.* (1957) and Felitti and McAfee (1968) among many others (cases 3 and 4 of Elrick *et al.*, 1950). The term PHP would only be justified because absence of PTH is not the cause of the condition. In this regard, one may speak of typical PHP, nontypical PHP, and more or less typical PHP.

The age at which symptoms may arise is variable. It may be very early in life, as in patient R.M. (age 2), or as in the case described by Oberst and Tompkins (1955), where a 16-month-old girl was admitted for a generalized clonic convulsive seizure. If most cases do manifest themselves in childhood or adolescence, a rare patient may present symptoms later. A patient of Baer *et al.* (1957) developed first symptoms of tetany at age 22, but already had intracranial calcifications "presumably of the basal ganglia." Our patient J.G. had first symptoms of epilepsy at age 27, and patient O.M. suffered his first attacks of tetany at age 32. Dental examination did not show evidence of disturbances of calcium metabolism prior to the ages of 8 to 9, but was consistent with such derangement at ages 17 to 20. Yet the hypocalcemia was the most pronounced of all our patients and produced disabling bilateral cataracts. At times the disease may pass unnoticed, and be discovered by serendipity. This was such in the case reported by Surks and Levenson (1962), in whom hypocalcemia (6.4–7.1 mg/dl) and hyperphosphatemia (4.8–5.8 mg/dl) were discovered at age 52. Multiple lenticular opacities were observed, as well as calcifications of the basal ganglia and unerupted teeth, in a short patient with round face, mental retardation, and brachymetacarpia. There is no reason, therefore, to consider that because of onset of symptoms in the third decade, and because of the absence of skeletal abnormalities characteristic of PHP, the defect in responsiveness to PTE is an acquired one as postulated by Bell *et al.* (1963) in their case, unless one of the other causes, described in previous sections, is found to account for this resistence. Presentation of symptoms and course of the disease is variable.

2. Pseudohypoparathyroidism with Roentgenologic Osteitis Fibrosa (Pseudohypophyperparathyroidism and Hypo–hyperparathyroidism)

The hypocalcemia of PHP represents a potent stimulus to the parathyroid glands. Since they are able to respond, secondary hyperparathyroidism ensues as it does in all cases of hypocalcemia not due to absence, atrophy, or ischemia of the parathyroid glands. The parathyroid glands in PHP are either grossly normal macroscopically (Albright *et al.*, 1942; Mann *et al.*, 1962; Arnstein *et al.*, 1966; Lee *et al.*, 1968), and microscopically (Albright *et al.*, 1942; Arnstein *et al.*, 1966; Lee *et al.*, 1968), slightly enlarged (Mazzuoli *et al.*, 1967) or "hyperplastic" (Elrick *et al.*, 1950; Schwarz and Loewe, 1966). The latter was found in the cases of R.M. and M.B., the latter one of the two cases explored by Elrick *et al.* (1950). In the case of Mann *et al.* (1962), two upper parathyroid glands were removed, measuring, respectively, $9 \times 6 \times 4$ and $5 \times 3 \times 2$ mm. Histological examination showed predominance of large, clear cells and a general appearance of cellular hyperactivity. Hypercellularity of the parathyroid glands was described in the case of Bell *et al.* (1963). The case of Frame *et al.* (1972) had chief cell hyperplasia and signs of hyperfunction were seen by electron microscopy studies. This gland measured $10 \times 7 \times$

5 mm. The contrast between the glands of a case of PHP (Schwarz and Loewe, 1966) versus those of a case of PPHP (Schwarz, 1965), both examined on autopsy, is interesting. In PPHP, 3 normal glands were identified, with maximal diameter of 4 mm, and signs of normal age-related involution (age 60). In PHP, 3 parathyroid glands were found, one of which was hyperplastic. These findings only provide evidence of hyperparathyroidism.

Nakajima et al. (1966) attempted to demonstrate the presence in the urine of their patient of PTH-like activity using a rat bioassay. The calcium mobilizing activity was higher than in controls, although the phosphaturic action was not increased. Bell et al. (1963) also demonstrated excess PTH-like activity in the urine of their patient, using the rat bioassay. The problem of interpreting levels of circulating PTH determined by immunoassay has been discussed in detail (Chapter 1). Nevertheless, iPTH is increased in patients with PHP. The first samples were obtained from thyroid venous plasma (Tashjian et al., 1966) in two cases, in one of which the diagnosis has been questioned (Arnstein et al., 1967). Since then, numerous cases have been reported, all with elevated levels (Lee et al., 1968; Chase et al., 1969; Okano et al., 1969; Lequin et al., 1970; Preece, 1971; Frame et al., 1972; Birkenhäger et al., 1973; Roof et al., 1973; Stogmann and Fischer, 1975; Van der Veen et al., 1975; Drezner et al., 1976). Only Zisman et al. (1969) were unable to detect iPTH in their case 1. By analogy to other, acquired, PTH-refractory conditions, such as vitamin D deficiency and renal azotemic osteodystrophy, in which secondary hyperparathyroidism also exists with an equally ineffective hormone, it would be expected that histological signs of osteitis fibrosa would develop and roentgenologic signs of hyperparathyroidism appear.

This is the case in PHP with longstanding and severe hypocalcemia with or without typical osteodystrophy. Such instances have been termed "PHP with secondary hyperparathyroidism and osteitis fibrosa" (Kolb and Steinbach, 1962), "PHP with bone changes simulating hyperparathyroidism" (Singleton and Teng, 1962), "PHP with osteitis fibrosa cystica" (Bell et al., 1963) or, less convincingly, "PHP with raised plasma alkaline phosphatase" (Cohen and Vince, 1969). Costello and Dent (1963) described hypo-hyperparathyroidism, followed by Watson (1968) and Allen et al. (1968). But it is quite clear that the cases described by Singleton and Teng (1962), Bell et al. (1963) and Cohen and Vince (1969) had neither typical features of osteochondrodystrophy, nor ectopic ossifications. Only one of the cases of Kolb and Steinbach (1962) had typical brachymetacarpia, brachymetatarsia and brachyphalangia, as well as a typical physiognomy, whereas the other patient had ectopic ossifications only. Franconi et al. (1964) reported three patients from one family with and one patient belonging to another family without signs of osteochondrodystrophy typical of PHP. They discussed "clinical and biochemical hypoparathyroidism with radiological hyperparathyroidism." Finally, Frame *et al.*, (1972) reported two cases of hypo-hyperparathyroidism describing them as "renal resistance to PTH with osteitis fibrosa." They reviewed most cases of the literature and assembled them under the term of pseudohypohyperparathyroidism (PHHP), as proposed by Kolb and Steinbach (1962).

It is reasonable to consider all patients as one single disease entity. Frame *et al.*, (1972) provided evidence that one of their two cases had renal resistance to PTE administration as far as cAMP is concerned. We have had access to a case in the Department of Pediatrics (Leuven University) with chemical findings typical of PHP or IHP, radiological findings typical of hyperparathyroidism (Fig. 27) and renal resistance to PTE as far as cAMP is concerned. There are no typical lesions of osteochondrodystrophy. A recent case of Malpuech *et al.* (1975) also showed no increase in cAMP output upon PTE administration.

We do not feel that this "entity" of PHHP is other than a logical by-product of PHP. It should not be considered as a distinct disorder "in which the bones are sensitive to PTH", representing a different type, i.e. type I of Frame *et al.* (1972) of "renal resistance", as opposed to type II, where PHP is not accompanied by roentgenologic signs of hyperparathyroidism ("skeletal and renal resistance"), and to type III, where isolated skeletal resistance would be present, to account for an intriguing observation of Frame *et al.* (1962), which will be commented on later.

The pathogenetic mechanism proposed by Kolb and Steinbach (1962) and supported by others (Frame *et al.*, 1972) is that renal resistance to PTH is the primary and sole defect and the resultant hyperphosphatemia in some way produces hypocalcemia, the stimulus for hyperparathyroidism. Since bone is sensitive, osteitis fibrosa ensues, but the calcemic effect of this is blocked by the hyperphosphatemia. This sequence of events is not tenable, since (1) hyperphosphatemia is as striking, or more so, in IHP as in PHP, yet the calcemic response to PTE can easily be demonstrated, and (2) bone is not unduly sensitive to PTH, since upon administration of PTE no hypercalcemic response is observed in these cases (Bell *et al.*, 1963; Franconi *et al.*, 1964; Frame *et al.*, 1972; Malpuech *et al.*, 1975). Furthermore, the hyperphosphatemia which is supposed to inhibit the bone response is not striking in several of the reported cases; levels were reported of 2.5–5.0 mg/dl in the case of Bell *et al.*, (1963) and 4.7–5.8 mg/dl in case 1 of Frame *et al.* (1972).

Histologically osteitis fibrosa would be the expected finding. In the only

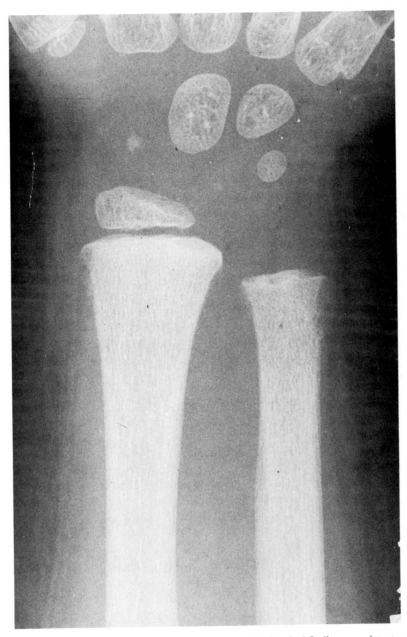

Fig. 27. Roentgenograms of the wrist in a child with chemical findings consistent with either PHP or IHP and renal resistance to PTH (cAMP). Note subperiosteal resorption at the distal ends of ulna and radius, particularly the lateral margins.

bone specimen (J.G.) we were able to analyze using decalcified sections and histomorphometric methods, the relative osteoclastic resorption surface was not increased (although it was higher than in any of the 4 patients with IHP), but the mean size of periosteocytic lacunae was increased to an extent we have not seen even in the most severe case of primary hyperparathyroidism. It was 71.7 μm^2, versus 50.6 ± 5.2 μm^2 in normal subjects, compared with 59 ± 9.1 μm^2 in patients with renal azotemic osteodystrophy (n = 14) and 65.6 ± 8.5 in patients with primary hyperparathyroidism (n= 41) according to the values reported by Meunier *et al.* (1972). Comparison of our data with those of these authors is reasonable since we use the same methods. Jowsey (1968), utilizing a different method of quantitative microradiography, also contrasted hypoparathyroidism, a disease characterized by diminished osteoclastic bone resorption (by an average of 4.0 standard deviations below the mean in her experience) with PHP, a disease characterized by a "strikingly increased osteoclastic bone resorption." The latter finding was also made by Spech and Olah (1974). We would therefore expect to find the entire spectrum of bone lesions characteristic of secondary hyperparathyroidism in patients with PHP from the more subtle alterations to the most striking, including some cases with typical roentgenologic stigmata (see Chapters 1 and 2).

Before these occur, some bone atrophy may be seen radiologically. This was not the case in patient J.G., who also had a normal bone mineral content of the radius as measured by ^{125}I photon absorptiometry (0.93 g/cm^2 at the shaft, versus 0.89 ± 0.07 for that age in males and 0.56 g/cm^2 at the distal epiphysis, versus 0.60 ± 0.08 in controls). However, 14% of the patients with PHP have bone atrophy on roentgenograms according to Bronsky *et al.* (1958), versus 5% of the patients with IHP, and in many individual cases this has been a striking finding (Reynolds *et al.*, 1952; Alterman and Lieber, 1965; Zampa and Zucchelli, 1965; Felitti and McAfee, 1968).

The existence of roentgenologic hyperparathyroidism would not be more than a curiosity, were it not accompanied by a greater degree of morbidity (bone pain, gait disturbances). Children and adolescents are more likely to develop this picture than adults, probably owing to their already increased bone turnover. Among the 14 patients (5 males, 9 females) thus far recorded, only 1 adult was affected (Bell *et al.*, 1963), the mean age of the other 13 patients being 9.2 years (range: 5.5–17). Slipped capital epiphysis is a common complication in these young patients with PHHP (Kolb and Steinbach, 1962; Fanconi *et al.*, 1964; Cohen and Vince, 1969; Frame *et al.*, 1972; Malpuech *et al.*, 1975). This might be prevented by appropriate therapy to correct hypocalcemia as early as possible. This complication is also seen in infants and children suffering from renal azotemic osteodystrophy (Mehls *et al.*, 1975) and has occasionally been described as well in primary hyperparathyroidism (Chiroff *et al.*, 1974).

There is no reason to separate PHP from PHHP, as suggested by Frame and Parfitt (1973), on the basis that the bone remodeling (osteoclastic) action of PTH would be maintained in PHHP and impaired in classical PHP, while in both conditions osteocytic calcium transfer would be deficient. [Distinction between these two modes of action of PTH on bone fits the concepts developed by Park and Talmage (1968)]. From the above it follows that there is a spectrum of bone remodeling activity in PHP, of which PHHP represents one extreme, as is also the case in primary hyperparathyroidism with or without roentgenologic signs of osteitis fibrosa. Not enough is known of the intimate mechanism of PTH failure at the bone level to be able to pinpoint the defect more accurately than in the most general terms.

One point should be resolved before it can be admitted that the bone is both just as sensitive and as resistant towards PTH in patients with pseudo-hypohyperparathyroidism as in classic PHP. On two occasions (Kolb and Steinbach, 1962; Frame *et al.*, 1972) the serum calcium level could be normalized by lowering the plasma P level using a low phosphate diet and aluminum hydroxide, as well as probenecid (Kolb and Steinbach, 1962). This hypophosphatemic effect, however, may not have been accomplished through the action of PTH. When bone turnover is very high, as in these studies, with serum levels of alkaline phosphatase of 14 and 15–16.1 Bodansky Units, in girls (aged 6.5 and 9 years), and phosphate deprivation is induced, reutilization of the calcium derived from bone resorption may be impaired (Nagant de Deuxchaisnes and Krane, 1964). Simply by lowering the P intake for only 3 days in patients with primary hyperparathyroidism, Eisenberg (1968) was able to increase the serum calcium level significantly. Administration of phosphate resulted in the opposite effect.

3. Pseudohypoparathyroidism, Type II

Drezner *et al.*, (1973) described a 22-month-old male who suffered from grand mal seizures since the age of 4 months. Serum calcium was decreased (5.7 mg/dl) and iPTH was increased. The infant had no phosphaturic response to the administration of a single injection of PTE, nor did he demonstrate any hypercalcemic or hypophosphatemic response to a trial of PTE administered over 4 days. Since the patient was small in stature (10th percentile), and was mentally slow (IQ 51), the diagnosis of PHP seemed obvious. However, the acute response of urinary cAMP to the administration of PTE was normal which should exclude the diagnosis of classical PHP. These findings presented a new pattern of biochemical abnormalities, with the possible exception of one of the patients originally studied by Chase et al. (1969). Drezner et al. (1973) hypothesized that this patient's disorder was representative of an abnormality in the chain of events which lead from the second messenger (cAMP) to the desired physiological effect. The existence of a block in the action of PTH distal to the cAMP step was postulated to account for this state of refractoriness towards both exogenous PTE and endogenous PTH. The same pattern of response was also observed in one of the 12 patients studied by Kind et al. (1973), with biochemical abnormalities characteristic of IHP or PHP. In this series, 4 patients had a response characteristic of IHP, whereas 7 fitted the pattern for PHP, type I, and 1 for PHP, type II.

Another patient was reported soon thereafter by Rodriguez et al. (1974). This was a 26-year-old woman who developed tetanic features during the fifth month of her first pregnancy, as well as after delivery. Biochemical characteristics were similar with a serum calcium of 8.0 mg/dl, a high iPTH level, no phosphaturic response to acute administration of PTE, and no hypercalcemic response on a protracted trial with the extract. The patient was short, moderately obese, stockily built, had a round face and, on examination of roentgenograms, an "area of calcification was found in the soft tissue adjacent to the right medial humeral condyle." cAMP response to acute PTE infusion was perfectly normal. As has been demonstrated several times in PHP, type I, the authors were able to normalize phosphorus excretion by the acute administration of PTE in an Ellsworth-Howard test after the serum calcium level had been normalized by a constant 4 day-infusion of calcium and the level of iPTH had decreased from 60 to 6 μlEq/ml. The same result was achieved after acute calcium infusion for 10 minutes. It was not shown whether the hypercalcemic response had been restored, or whether a more than transient phosphaturic response to PTE could be achieved as well. The two cases, which have been described in detail (Drezner et al., 1973; Rodriguez et al., 1974) have one salient feature in common, which the authors did not emphasize, a normal serum phosphorus value, a rare finding in classical PHP. The 22-month-old patient had a serum P of 5.0 (normal range for that age in that laboratory: 4.0–6.0 mg/dl) and a serum calcium of 5.7 mg/dl (Drezner et al., 1973), whereas the serum P of the 26-year-old patient was 4.3 mg/dl, and on initiation of the studies ranged between 3.8 and 4.0 mg/dl (Rodriguez et al., 1974). An alternative hypothesis to explain the findings is that there is no defect in the adenyl cyclase-generated metabolic steps. PHP, type II, would then be a condition sharing with PHP, type I, endogenous defective PTH, but would be devoid of the renal manifestation represented by a defective adenyl cyclase-cAMP system. In this situation the serum P would be normal. In PHP, type I, the high serum P level presumably would result from two abnormalities: a defective hormone and a defective adenyl cyclase-cAMP system. In PHP, type II, with an intact adenyl cyclase-cAMP system but an ineffective hormone, the P level is neither elevated as in PHP, type I, nor low as in secondary hyperparathyroidism. Since less hormone is necessary to obtain a normal phosphaturic effect than to mobilize calcium from bone, the latter action is not accomplished efficiently, whereas the former is achieved.

One may speculate whether the case of a woman who had tetany since age 8, reported by Frame et al. (1962), also represents one of the first cases of PHP, type II. In this instance hypocalcemia (7.4 mg/dl) was not associated with hyperphosphatemia (serum P: 2.6 mg/dl; normal range in that laboratory: 2.6–4.0 mg/dl), in a female at age 31. When restudied at age 49, serum calcium and P were respectively 6.6 and 3.2 mg/dl. Clear-cell hyperplasia was found on parathyroid biopsy and histologic examination. No widened osteoid seams were found on undecalcified bone sections. No hypercalcemic response was elicited by the protracted administration of PTE on two occasions and no physical or roentgenologic signs of PHP were present. However, there was an adequate phosphaturic response to the administration of PTE during an Ellsworth-Howard test, although a control study to evaluate spontaneous P excretion was not performed. No data were provided in regard to the two protracted periods of PTE administration as far as urinary or serum P are concerned. Frame et al. (1972) subsequently considered this case as an example of selective skeletal resistance to PTH, advancing the hypothesis that the PTH-dependent adenyl cyclase-cAMP system in the skeleton was defective but that in the kidney normal. It remains to be proven that the kidney tubule would be as responsive to protracted PTE administration as the single Ellsworth-Howard test suggested it could be.

One may wonder how many other subjects, previously considered classical examples of PHP, actually represent cases of PHP, type II. If our assumptions are correct, several might be found among the cases of PHP with a serum P value within the normal range. An example is the case reported by Sjaastad (1963). Whether the case reported by Marcus et al. (1971), whose renal cortex was assayed post mortem for adenyl cyclase activity, and found to possess such activity, might have been a case of PHP, type II, as suggested by Drezner et al. (1973), is not known but unlikely in view of the fact that the sister of the propositus had well documented PHP, type I.

These cases of PHP, type II, are also instructive in that they further demonstrate that in PHP high P levels are not the cause either of the development of hypocalcemia or the refractoriness of the skeleton toward PTH. The demonstration by Rodriguez *et al.* (1974) that calcium infusions restore the tubular responsiveness toward PTE-induced phosphaturia is in accord with the hypothesis of the existence of an abnormal, partially ineffective PTH competing efficiently at receptors with normal PTE, although it is surprising that this could be accomplished by infusing calcium for only 10 minutes. However feedback mechanisms are known to operate rapidly, and the most important biologically active (and therefore receptor site-occupying) fragments of the amino-terminal region of the PTH molecule have very short survival times (Arnaud, 1973; Chapter 1). If *N*-specific immunoassays could measure precisely the putative abnormal PHP-fragment responsible for competition with exogenous PTE, it would also have to be shown whether an acute calcium infusion would rapidly alter circulating amounts of this hormone or hormone fragment to permit exogenous PTE to operate at the kidney level. The distinction between types I and II of PHP may be envisioned in terms of what would happen if parathyroidectomy were performed in PHP type II. In PHP, type I, this resulted in restoring calcemic response to PTE toward normal, whereas the phosphaturic response, albeit improved, remained subnormal, because of the persistent defect in the adenyl cyclase receptor site. It is anticipated that if parathyroidectomy were performed in PHP, type II, the response to PTE would mimic that of patients with postoperative hypoparathyroidism.

The hormone in PHP, type II, is probably only partially inactive, as it is in PHP, type I, as shown by the serum calcium values in the patient described by Rodriguez *et al.* (1974) which were 8.0 mg/dl on first examination and 8.7 mg/dl when studies were started. From the two cases described in detail up until now, it is impossible to conclude whether a "pattern" exists in the evolution of the level of the serum calcium values.

The description of syndromes with the prefix "pseudo," as well as the addition of the prefix hypo to hyper, whether one likes it or not, is more likely to continue as a trend than to disappear, because of well established custom and because no alternatives which are both concise and precise are as yet available, and may not be in the near future. As of now, however, it is useful to establish a glossary of the existing terms and to pinpoint the major corresponding biochemical abnormalities, as well as the eventual clinical signs (Table XIII).

4. Conditions Related to or Possibly Related to PHP

An additional possible congenital defect of the kidney tubule-cAMP system has been suggested by Weitzman and Murad (1973b). These authors described a patient with PHP who was PTE resistant with respect to cAMP excretion. The response to PTE was restored, however, by the administration of the phosphodiesterase inhibitors, chlorpropamide and aminophylline, suggesting that in this patient the underlying defect was enhanced cAMP hydrolysis, which could be reversed by appropriate therapy. This patient is unique, and attempts to reproduce this response in 3 other patients with PHP failed. The patient described by Weitzman and Murad (1973b) is also unique in that PHP was associated with acromegaly. How this pertains to the above-mentioned abnormalities is uncertain and may not represent more than a coincidence. Patients with acromegaly do respond to PTE administration with an appropriate urinary cAMP excretion (Weitzman and Murad, 1973b).

Another group of conditions which bear some resemblance to PHP are those diseases in which the phosphaturic response to the administration of PTE is blunted, i.e., gonadal dysgenesis with a 45 X0 karyotype (Zisman et al., 1967; Szczepski et al., 1971), Gardner's syndrome (Trygstad et al., 1968) and the multiple basal cell nevi syndrome (Block and Clendenning, 1963; Gorlin et al., 1965; Murphy, 1969; Chopra and Nugent, 1970; Murphy, 1975). Only Aurbach et al. (1970) observed an appreciable phosphaturic response to acute PTE administration in the multiple basal cell nevi syndrome. There are no abnormalities of the blood chemistries in these syndromes, and the hypercalcemic action of protracted PTE administration is maintained (Zisman et al., 1967; Trygstad et al., 1968; Chopra and Nugent, 1970). In all these syndromes (gonadal dysgenesis was not tested) the cAMP response was normal (Aurbach et al., 1970; Murphy, 1975; Moriarty et al., 1975).

Although normal PTE-induced cAMP excretion may be present, P excretion may still be impaired. The best examples of this are the cases of PHP, type II. Some of the data presented are convincing, especially those in which PTE was administered consecutively for several days (Zisman et al., 1967; Trygstad et al., 1968). It could be that there is a defect in these syndromes beyond the cAMP activation step, the hypothesis advanced by Drezner et al. (1973), Kind et al. (1973) and Rodriguez et al. (1974) to explain PHP, type II. This explanation, however, better fits the status of the syndromes under discussion.

Patients with gonadal dysgenesis have many somatic features and osteochondrodystrophic abnormalities (including brachydactyly) in common with PHP or PPHP. This is also true for multiple basal cell nevi syndrome. Only Gardner's syndrome (''multiple cutaneous and subcutaneous lesions occurring simultaneously with hereditary polyposis and osteomatosis'' (Gardner and Richards, 1953) shows few features in common.

A different problem is that of familial calcification of the basal ganglia. Indeed, calcification, or ''mineralization'' (Dudley and Hawkins, 1970) of the basal ganglia is a feature of PHP, not of true PPHP, as it is of IHP, and therefore is ascribed to hypocalcemia. As pointed out by Bennett *et al.*, (1959), two thirds of the patients presenting with calcifications of the basal ganglia have IHP or PHP, and approximately half of the patients with IHP and PHP have such calcifications.

Nichols *et al.* (1961) reported an unusual family with basal ganglia calcification. Out of the 13 members of the family consisting of three generations, 9 had calcifications of the basal ganglia, 7 of whom had definite hypocalcemia and hyperphosphatemia, as well as latent tetany (all had a positive Trousseau sign), one patient having in addition epileptiform seizures. The affected individuals were short, obese, mentally dull and had short, stubby fingers (but not selective brachydactyly). The association with mild hypocalcemia (average in the hypocalcemic members of the family: 6.9, range 6.5–8.2 mg/dl) and mild hyperphosphatemia (average 4.6, range 3.2–6.3 mg/dl) favors the diagnosis of PHP rather than that of IHP, an hypothesis endorsed by Mann *et al.* (1962). On the other hand, a normal response in the Ellsworth-Howard test in case 1, the absence of demonstrable parathyroid tissue at autopsy of case 13, and the consistent finding of hypocalcemic hypercalciuria when four of the patients were treated with vitamin D favor the diagnosis of IHP. Patients with normal serum calcium levels and familial calcification of the basal ganglia usually show a normal PTE-induced urinary cAMP increase (Aurbach *et al.* 1970; Moskowitz *et al.*, 1971).

Two reported patients have had suboptimal or absent phosphaturic responses to PTE administration: case 4 of Palubinskas and Davies (1959) and case 1.4 of Matthews (1957). In the latter, 5-day administration of PTE (300 U/day) was insufficient to raise the (normal) serum calcium level, whereas it did in a control subject. This patient could have had PHP with normal serum calcium levels at the time of investigation.

I. Associated Endocrinopathies

One of us (C.N.) has emphasized the association of PHP or PPHP with diabetes mellitus and hypothyroidism in the propositi as well as in their families (Nagant de Deuxchaisnes, 1959; Nagant de Deuxchaisnes, *et al.*, 1960a and 1960b). Several cases of concomitant diabetes have also been described by others (Moehlig and Gerish, 1950, Berardinelli, 1951; Azerad *et al.*, 1953; Buchs, 1954; Smulyan and Raisz, 1959; Tanz, 1960, Nagant de Deuxchaisnes *et al.*, 1960a and 1960b; Mann *et al.*, 1962, Emanuelli and Pellegrini, 1968; Voog *et al.*, 1972). Several cases fit the pattern of prediabetes (Seringe and Tomkiewicz, 1957; Fabbrini *et al.*, 1958; Nagant de Deuxchaisnes *et al.*, 1960b). In addition there has been a high incidence of diabetes in the families of affected patients described in previous sections (M.A., M.B., O.M., R.M., K.D.). Similar findings have been made by Forbes and Engel (1963) in gonadal dysgenesis. These authors recorded a high incidence of diabetes mellitus in patients with gonadal dysgenesis ($n = 41$) and in their families. The birth weight of the propositi (Nagant de Deuxchaisnes *et al.*, 1960b) was found to be above 4 kg in 38% of the cases of PHP in which it was recorded (versus approximately 10% in the normal population).

The association of hypothyroidism with PHP and PPHP has also been emphasized (Nagant de Deuxchaisnes *et al.*, 1960b). The diagnosis was usually made only on clinical grounds, in addition to a low basal metabolic rate and a high serum cholesterol level. Since the early report (Nagant de Deuxchaisnes, 1960b), more cases have been described (Barr *et al.*, 1960; Tanz, 1960; Hortling *et al.*, 1960; Cohen and Donnell, 1960; Mann *et al.*, 1962; Denniston and Son, 1963; Voog *et al.*, 1972). Several cases were mentioned as having received thyroid replacement therapy (Palubinskas and Davies, 1959; Mautalen *et al.*, 1967). In more recent studies TSH stimulation in 3 cases produced a striking increase of ^{131}I uptake, suggesting secondary rather than primary hypothyroidism (Turner and Takamura, 1962; Kieffer *et al.*, 1965; Winnacker *et al.*, 1967). Marx *et al.* (1971) subsequently pointed out that TSH release under the influence of TRH, as well as iodothyronines under the influence of TSH, are mediated through the adenyl cyclase-cAMP system respectively in the pituitary and thyroid. An abnormal receptor-adenyl cyclase complex in the central nervous system, anterior pituitary and thyroid might therefore account for ultimate thyroid hypofunction. This attractive hypothesis has, however, not been substantiated. In any event, TSH was undetectable by bioassay and radioimmunoassay; this was confirmed in two cases by Zisman *et al.* (1969). TSH stimulation in each case induced an increase of ^{131}I uptake, as it did in the case of Aubert and Arroyo (1968), and later in the cases of Birkenhäger *et al.* (1973) and Van der Veen *et al.* (1975). Zisman *et al.* (1969), however, properly stressed that the radioimmunoassay for thyrotropin in human serum at that time lacked sensitivity and basal TSH levels were detectable in only about 50% of normal subjects. The sensitivity of the assay over a few years did improve and when retested by Marx *et al.* (1971), the patient described by Winnacker *et al.* (1967) had detectable levels of TSH in the basal state. However the diagnosis of secondary hypothyroidism was maintained, based upon diminished release of TSH upon TRH infusion. In the case reported by Birkenhäger *et al.* (1973), the basal TSH level was also normal.

All patients with hypothyroidism do not have thyroid dysfunction of pituitary or hypothalamic origin as shown by Marx *et al.* (1971). In two cases (mother and daughter), hypothyroidism was associated with high basal TSH levels, and in the only patient tested with TRH, the expected exaggerated response in terms of TSH levels, which is characteristic of primary hypothyroidism, was found. This was probably also the abnormality in the case described by Cohen and Donnell (1960).

Werder et al. (1975) compared 10 patients with PHP and 8 patients with IHP. Basal TSH levels were elevated in 7 of the 10 patients with PHP but in none of those with IHP. Excessive TSH response to TRH was noticed in 8 of 10 patients with PHP, and in none with IHP. Clinical signs of hypothyroidism were absent, but in 3 cases of 10 with PHP plasma T4 concentrations were below the normal range. The group of patients with PHP was so strikingly different in this respect from those with IHP that these authors even suggested that TRH stimulation of TSH release might serve as an adjunctive diagnostic tool in the differential diagnosis between the two conditions.

Occasionally, this abnormality may be of more clinical importance. A patient described by Malvaux and Beckers (1973) as having increased TRH-induced TSH response with normal thyroid function at age 10 has since become hypothyroid, as indicated by Werder et al. (1975). Hypothyroidism was detected by Marx et al. (1971) in 3 of 13 patients (23%). Spech and Olah (1974) found specific information on thyroid function in 85 cases of PHP. They estimated hypothyroidism was present in 20% of these cases. As far as latent hypothyroidism is concerned, this might be the rule rather than the exception (Werder et al., 1975). Primary hypothyroidism probably predominates, although secondary hypothyroidism has been documented on several occasions.

The abnormality in TSH release upon TRH administration was examined in case J.G. of Table XI. He also showed an exaggerated response, from a normal basal level of 5.3 to levels of 26.0 and 16.0 μU/ml, respectively, 20 and 60 minutes after TRH administration. This response is moderately exaggerated, although definitely abnormal as compared to a control population. The prolactin response to TRH may also be abnormal. Carlson and Brickman (1976) recently showed minimal prolactin responses upon TRH infusion in 3 patients with PHP. This abnormality was also confirmed in patient J.G. (Devogelaer et al., 1976). Carlson and Brickman (1976) showed that hypocalcemia may impede the release of TSH as well as thyroid hormone. Thus, one patient was found to have a normal basal TSH level and normal TRH-induced TSH response prior to treatment. When hypocalcemia was corrected, both basal and post-TRH levels of TSH were high.

Other endocrinopathies associated with PHP are probably chance occurrences. Acromegaly has been mentioned (Weitzman and Murad, 1973b). Diabetes insipidus has been recorded (Emanuelli and Pellegrini,

1968), as well as multiple pheochromocytomas (Nagant de Deuxchaisnes *et al.*, 1960a), and hyperthyroidism (Uchimura *et al.*, 1974). Forbes (1962) speculated that patients with PHP had abnormal responses toward hormones other than PTH, specifically thyroxine and growth hormone. She administered thyroxine to a patient with PHP and found a normal metabolic response. She also reviewed the metabolic balances performed by Pechet (unpublished observations), in 2 patients treated with growth hormone (GH). The data were indicative of a normal response to exogenous GH (Forbes, 1962). These studies were extended recently by Urdanivia *et al.* (1975) who determined that fasting GH levels were normal and responded normally to provocative tests of GH secretion, i.e., insulin-induced hypoglycemia and 1-dopa, in two adults with PHP and short stature; normal amounts of GH-dependent sulfation factor were also found. End-organ resistance to both endogenous GH and sulfation factor such as that described in the African pygmy (Merimee *et al.*, 1972) remains a remote possibility in PHP. Children with lack of or resistance to GH usually have a retarded bone age. This has not been observed in children with PHP, where the bone age has often been advanced (Ray and Gardner, 1959; Steinbach and Young, 1966) rather than retarded, unless hypothyroidism is present.

As far as PTH is concerned, all of its actions do not seem to be impaired in PHP. Recent information concerning the lipolytic action of PTH suggests that this is maintained. PTE administration to patients with PHP increased the serum concentration of free fatty acids to the same extent in normal subjects and patients with hypoparathyroidism (Thajchayapong *et al.*, 1976).

J. Typical Signs of Pseudohypoparathyroidism

The signs characteristic of this condition were described by Albright and his co-workers (Albright *et al.*, 1942; Elrick *et al.*, 1950). As Albright was well aware (Elrick *et al.*, 1950; Albright *et al.*, 1952; Forbes, 1962), in any one case these signs (from a single one to all of them) may be present in almost any combination. In some instances all signs may be absent. Therefore, we distinguish "typical," "more or less typical," or "nontypical" cases of PHP. These are listed in Table XIV as a modification of Table 3 from Spech and Olah (1974). The latter reviewed 186 cases of PHP in the literature and recorded the symptoms and signs only when their presence or absence was specifically mentioned in the case reports. This is the correct way to proceed but introduces a bias in terms of percentages. Another problem with signs listed in Table XIV is the precision of the information provided. Probably short stature is the only objective

TABLE XIII

Characteristics of Various Forms of Hypoparathyroidism[a]

Condition	Response to PTE				Roentgenological hyperparathyroidism	Classic signs PHP	Serum[b]	
	iPTH levels	Cyclic AMP	Phospha-turia	Hyper-calcemia			Ca	P
Normal subject	+	+++	+++	+++	(−)	(−)	N	N
Idiopathic (or postoperative) hypoparathyroidism (IHP)	(−)	+++	++++	++++	(−)	(−)	LL	HH
Pseudohypoparathyroidism (PHP)	+++	(−) to +	+	+	(−)	(−) to ++++	L	H
Pseudopseudohypoparathyroidism (PPHP)	+	+++	+++	+++	(−)	++ to ++++	N	N
PHP with normal serum Ca	+++	(−) to +	+	+	(−)	(−) to ++++	N	N
Pseudohypohyperparathyroidism (PHHP)	+++	(−) to +	+	+	+ to +++	(−) to ++++	L	H
Hypo-hyperparathyroidism	+++	(−) to +	+	+	+ to +++	(−)	L	H
Pseudohypoparathyroidism, type II	+++	+++	+	+	(−)	(−) to ++++	L	N
Pseudoidiopathic hypoparathyroidism	+++	+++	++++	++++	(−)	(−)	L	H
PHP following parathyroidectomy	(−)	(−) to +	++ to +++	++++	(−)	(−) to ++++	LL	HH

[a] Classic signs of PHP include short stature, obesity, round face, typical osteochondrodystrophy, and/or ectopic ossifications. PHP is also called "PHP, type 1," according to the latest classification of PHP types, or "classic PHP" (as opposed to PHP, type II). It may be "typical" (when clinical signs are present) or "atypical" (when classic signs are absent). PHP with normal serum Ca levels has been referred to in the text as "intermittently normocalcemic PHP." When detected prior to onset of symptoms, it has been called "latent PHP."

As can be seen, there is very little difference between hypohyperparathyroidism and pseudohypohyperparathyroidism. These two conditions should be grouped under the latter term, unless (and more conveniently) the descriptive term of "PHP with roentgenologic signs of hyperparathyroidism" is used.

[b] N, normal; H, high; L, low; HH, somewhat higher than H; LL, somewhat lower than L.

finding, although the sexes and races are mixed and no consideration is given to the height of the (unaffected) parents. It is obvious that the commonest reason for being short and normal is to be the child of short parents. Furthermore, other causes of shortness may be present in individual patients, such as described by Garceau and Miller (1956).

Some signs, as they are recorded, are (unconsciously) overemphasized or underemphasized. The incidence of short metacarpals may be overemphasized for at least two reasons. Brachymetacarpia is sometimes taken to mean that all metacarpals are short which may characterize "short hands" in short patients. True brachymetacarpia almost never includes all ten digits. We prefer the terms "selective brachymetacarpia or brachymetatarsia". Even selective brachymetacarpia may be overemphasized, especially since the publication of the paper by Archibald et al. (1959) on "short fourth metacarpals" measured by a straight edge held tangential to the distal ends of the fourth and fifth metacarpals, which should normally pass distal to the distal end of the third metacarpal. If the edge intersects the third metacarpal proximal to its distal end, the sign is considered positive ("metacarpal sign"). Subsequently it has been found to be positive in 10.5% of normal women and 12.6% of normal men in a Finnish population (Vartio and Meronen, 1961), 13.6% of normal men and 16.1% of normal women in an American population (Slater, 1970), and 10.4% of infants, children and adolescents in a German population (Willich and Englert, 1973). This sign is therefore of little interest but has been used to mean that the fourth metacarpal is short. When the metacarpals are short in PHP, they are stubby as well. There is a correlation between the shortness of a metacarpal bone and the lack of tubulation, as pointed out by Steinbach and Young (1966). This is not true for metatarsal bones.

An important finding which has been systematically underrated in most reports is brachyphalangia. Distal phalanges (brachytelephalangia), especially of the thumb, middle phalanges (brachymesophalangia), as well as proximal phalanges (brachybasophalangia) are often shortened, as originally observed by Elrick et al. (1950). The recorded incidence of 25% (Table XIV) is probably a minimal one. We have seen instances of isolated brachyphalangia without brachymetapodia (= brachymetacarpia and/or brachymetatarsia). The most reliable finding probably is brachydactyly. Alleged absence of brachyphalangia in true PHP or PPHP has been used to differentiate those cases of PPHP with male-to-male transmission of the disease from true PPHP, on the basis that these cases had phalangeal shortening (Hertzog, 1968).

A final problem with estimates of the incidence of these signs is that some patients are described early in life and (1) may not undergo exten-

TABLE XIV

Incidence of Signs and Symptoms in Pseudohypoparathyroidism

Signs and symptoms	%	(*n*)
1. Typical somatotype		
Short stature (<1.55 m)[a]	80	(87)
Round face	92	(158)
Thickset, stocky, or obese	50	(40)
2. Mental retardation	75	(161)
3. Typical osteochondrodystrophy		
Brachymetacarpia	68	(169)
Brachymetatarsia	43	(105)
Brachyphalangia	25	(91)
Thickened calvaria	62	(68)
Exostoses	51	(33)
4. Ectopic ossifications	56	(155)
5. Hypocalcemic symptoms or signs		
Tetany	86	(169)
Convulsive seizures	59	(114)
Lenticular opacities	44	(144)
Intracranial calcifications	45	(148)
Dental hypoplasia, enamel defects	51	(67)
Unerupted teeth	56	(93)

[a] Only those cases above age 16.

sive radiographic evaluation as an adult patient, or (2) may not show classical signs which have yet to develop. Thus, in a patient with PPHP, a costal exostosis, which was not present on roentgenograms at age 13, could be seen on similar roentgenograms at age 26 (Nagant de Deuxchaisnes *et al.*, 1960a).

Short stature, with round face and thickset, stocky body habitus, is best illustrated by patient R. M. (Fig. 28), at age 27 (1.43 m, 53kg). His growth chart has been published as Fig. 8 in Forbes' paper (1962). It can be seen that R. M. was not dwarfed as compared to his peers until the age of 13. From age 6 to 13, velocity of growth had almost been normal. However, height velocity decreased from age 13 to 17, and adult height was reached at age 19. For unknown reasons he did not experience a growth spurt at the critical age. His condition was not treated between age 9 and 16 but it is doubtful that this plays the determining role as suggested by Alterman and Lieber (1965), since other patients with untreated IHP would be dwarfed as well, which is not the case.

Short digits arise from early closure of the epiphyses, preceded by

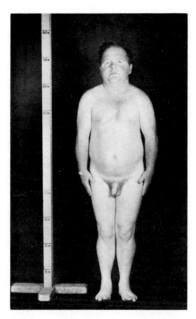

Fig. 28.   Photograph of patient R.M. with PHP taken at age 27.

earlier decrease in longitudinal growth (Steinbach and Young, 1966). At times, cone-shaped epiphyses are formed (Elrick *et al.*, 1950) and at the phalanges rudimentary or pseudoepiphyses (without growth cartilage) or absent epiphyses may occur (Steinbach *et al.*, 1965). In Fig. 29 are shown roentgenograms of the hands of patients R. M. at the age of 10 and at the age of 27. Cone-shaped epiphyses may be seen at the bases of both first metacarpals, whereas premature closure of the epiphyses is observed in both fourth metacarpals and both distal first phalanges. The result of this is bilateral brachymetacarpia I-IV and brachytelephalangia I. Not all cases are as symmetrical as this.

Not all metacarpals and metatarsals show equal propensity to shorten and broaden. Table XV gives the pattern of metapodial shortening, according to Spech and Olah (1974). Fourth and fifth digits are most often involved in that (decreasing) order, while the second digit is most often spared and is never the only one involved. These changes have given rise to at least two physical signs. The first was described by Albright *et al.* (1952), and refers to metacarpal shortening: "If the patient makes a fist, knuckles will appear at the distal ends of the normal metacarpals, whereas dimples will appear at the ends of the shortened metacarpals". The other physical sign refers to brachytelephalangia I and was described by Ray and Gardner (1959). The ratio of width to length of the thumb nail should

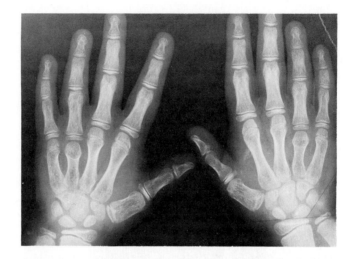

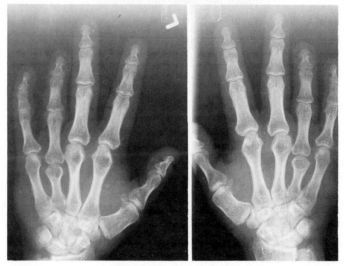

Fig. 29. Roentgenograms of the hands of patient R.M. with PHP taken at age 10 (upper) and age 27 (lower). See text for description of findings.

be approximately equal or not superior to 1.5-2.0. The patient described in their paper had a width/length ratio of almost 3. When evaluating the respective length of the different bones of the hands, comparison can be made with well established tables of standard measurements, such as those of Parish (1967) and Garn *et al.* (1972).

Other typical features of osteochondrodystrophy not listed in Table

TABLE XV

Incidence of Brachymetapodia in Pseudohypoparathyroidism according to Digit and Extremity

	Brachymetacarpia ($n = 169$)					Brachymetatarsia ($n = 105$)				
	I	II	III	IV	V	I	II	III	IV	V
%	30	6	19	57	51	14	7	19	39	21

XIV include radius curvus, cubitus valgus, coxa vara, coxa valga, genu varum and genu valgum deformities. We have been impressed by the incidence of radius curvus (Fig. 30) which gives rise to another physical sign, the inability to supinate completely. The vertebral abnormalities of platyspondyly also occur (Fig. 31). The last problem to be considered is ectopic (or soft-tissue) ossifications, often called "soft-tissue calcifications." It has not been established that calcification (i.e., deposition of the solid, inorganic mineral phase containing calcium and P ions, not organized in the manner that characterizes bone as a tissue) must precede the formation of ectopic bone (i.e., deposition of the mineral phase in well-formed bone, consisting of either spicules of spongy bone or sheets of compact bone), nor is soft-tissue calcification, once formed, necessarily converted into true (ecotopic) bone. The fundamental mechanisms responsible for the deposition of the mineral phase in these two forms (calcification and ossification) are probably different (Miller and Krane, 1971).

There is little evidence, at least on histological grounds, that soft-tissue "calcification" occurs as a rule in PHP. On the other hand, biopsies of subcutaneous "calcifications," plaques or nodules have repeatedly shown organized bony structure (Sprague *et al.*, 1945; Alexander and Tucker, 1949; Elrick *et al.*, 1950; Albright *et al.*, 1952). Alexander and Tucker (1949) described "extensive soft tissue calcinosis" on roentgenograms but provided photomicrographs showing trabeculae of bone with osteoblastic activity. Albright *et al.* (1952) found "miliary ossification of deep subcutaneous tissue and plaques of cutaneous ossification" and demonstrated histologically both well-formed adult bone and primitive fiberbone. The ratio of calcium to phosphorus was analyzed from "two calcareous plaques excised from the abdominal wall" and found to be 2.07:1 (Sprague *et al.*, 1945). The entity of osteoma cutis, when idiopathic (i.e., not following trauma or acne) is disputed as an isolated finding. It has been linked to PPHP by Piesowicz (1965) and to PHP by Eyre and Reed

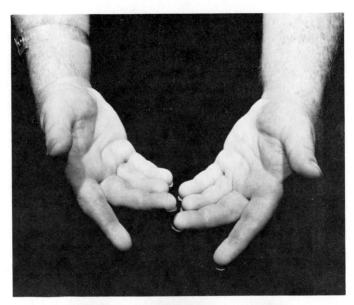

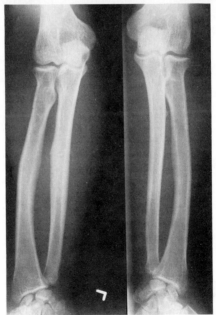

Fig. 30. Photographs of hands (upper) and roentgenograms of forearms (lower) of patient R.M. with PHP, age 27.

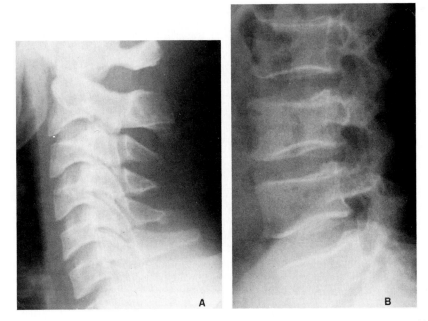

Fig. 31. Roentgenograms of cervical spine (A) and lumbar spine (B) in patient K.D. with PHP taken at age 19 to demonstrate platyspondyly.

(1971) and Barranco (1971). Brook and Valman (1971), as well as Hermier *et al.* (1972), concluded that most if not all cases of osteoma cutis were in fact associated with PHP or PPHP. Ectopic bone of osteoma cutis has been studied in detail by Peterson *et al.* (1963). Despite these observations the terms soft-tissue or subcutaneous calcifications are still the most widely used to refer to the ectopic ossifications of PHP or PPHP. They should be abandoned. Ectopic ossifications (as distinct from calcifications of the basal ganglia) usually appear early in life. When patient R. M. was seen at the age of 3 years "many small, hard, palpable, calcified masses in the subcutaneous tissue of the trunk and extremities" were described (Elrick *et al.*, 1950). Fig. 32 shows bony spicules with a trabecular pattern at the lower extremity of the tibia in patient R. M. at age 27. Typically, ossifications may be located anywhere, but preferential sites are in the extremities and around large joints. They present as hard non-tender nodules or plaques which are palpable if superficial and sometimes visible. They never involve muscles, an important differential from myositis ossificans progressiva, nor do they affect viscera.

The typical features of osteochondrodystrophy (Table XIV), as well as ectopic ossifications, are not features of IHP unless the two diseases

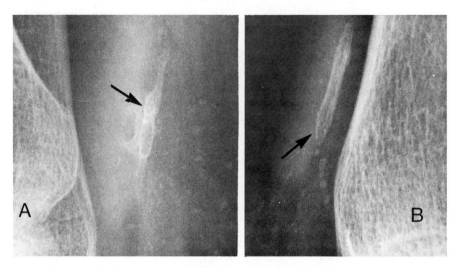

Fig. 32. Roentgenograms of the lower tibia of patient R.M. with PHP, age 27. Ectopic ossifications (arrows) are located posterior to the tibia (A) and anterior to the tibia (B).

occur by chance in the same patient (Moses *et al.*, 1974). The somatotype characteristic for PHP or PPHP also is not present in IHP, except by chance. The only debatable point is that of mental retardation, which was present in 20% of IHP versus 68% of PHP, according to one comparative table (Beaudoing *et al.*, 1970) and in 18% of IHP versus 63% of PHP in another comparative table (Bronsky *et al.*, 1958). Although the differences are statistically significant, some patients with IHP probably have subnormal intelligence in a greater number of propositi than would be expected by chance. If so, early treatment of hypocalcemia might be of considerable importance. Alterman and Lieber (1965) gained the impression that correction of the low serum calcium level between age 12 and 17 in their case of PHP produced a moderate but significant improvement in IQ. This is substantiated by a study in IHP. The IQ in 10 children with this condition averaged 104.9 (S. D. ± 19.1), with no difference between Verbal and Performance IQ. Serial IQs performed in 3 of these cases showed a definite elevation when the serum calcium was corrected (Money and Ehrhardt, 1966).

Reference should be made to other abnormalities in patients with PHP. Henkin (1968) pointed out that these patients had gustatory abnormalities, consisting of elevated detection and recognition thresholds for sour and bitter (normal for salt and sweet). Detection and recognition thresholds of olfaction for all vapors tested were significantly elevated ("type II hyposmia"). These abnormalities of taste and smell sensitivity were not unlike those found by other authors in chromatin-negative gonadal dysgenesis. They did not improve upon correction of hypocalcemia. Forbes (1964) found another abnormality which patients with PHP and PPHP shared with those affected by gonadal dysgenesis. Fingerprints and palmprints as well as palmar-flexion creases in both groups were characterized by fine, crowded lines of the long, vertically oriented loops. Two to five times as many distally placed axial triradii with increased ATD angles were found in both conditions compared with the control population, as well as an increased frequency of hypothenar patterns with more than the usual proportion of whorls and S patterns, and few radial loops on index fingers. The pattern in patients with Klinefelter's syndrome is different from that in PHP, PPHP and gonadal dysgenesis.

X. SIGNS AND SYMPTOMS OF HYPOCALCEMIA

Forbes (1956), referring to IHP in children, stated: "The clinical picture is both confusing and fascinating; an insidious onset, coupled with a bizarre symptomatology as manifestations of a rare disease, cannot fail to tax the ingenuity of even the most astute diagnostician."

When typical, the symptoms seldom cause difficulty as to the diagnosis. In other instances hypocalcemia may not be easily recognized, accounting for long delays in establishing the diagnosis, which in IHP is on the average 6.3 years from the onset of symptoms (Robins, 1963). An awareness of these symptoms is thus of utmost importance. In PHP, the physical signs, when typical, are likely to draw attention to the underlying abnormal chemistries.

A. Neurologic Features

Tetany is the single most common mode of presentation of hypocalcemia, as an expression of increased neuromuscular irritability. It manifests itself essentially as muscle cramps. A typical attack is often preceded by paresthesias in hands and feet or around the mouth. Muscular stiffness may follow. The hands characteristically assume a position with forced adduction of the thumb, the fingers being firmly pressed together, with extension at the proximal and distal interphalangeal joints, and flexion at the metacarpalphalangeal joints (cf. Fig. 33), known as "main d'accoucheur" (or "obstetrical hand"). The palm of the hand is hollowed. Other muscles may contract, and give rise to plantar flexion of the toes resulting in pedal spasm. Other manifestations are bronchospasm,

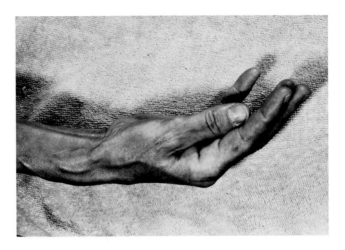

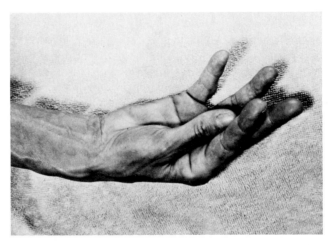

Fig. 33. Photographs of the typical position of the hands in tetany, the "main d'ac-coucheur."

perioral spasm, spasm of the sphincter of Oddi (giving rise to biliary colic), or laryngospasm, giving rise to laryngeal stridor and occasionally to obstruction of the airways in children. Spasm of smooth muscles may also result in mydriasis, abdominal cramps, urinary frequency, or tenesmus.

It has been suggested that hypocalcemia may act centrally on the spinal motor neurons, exciting the peripheral receptors through efferent motor innervation. These impulses to the peripheral receptors also stimulate respiration, and the resulting hyperventilation aggravates the situation through respiratory alkalosis and lowering of the calcium ion concentration. A vicious cycle is initiated that will only be interrupted by correction of hypocalcemia or cessation of hyperventilation. The importance of hypocapnic alkalosis has recently been reinvestigated by Edmondson *et al.* (1975), who showed that the calcium ion concentration in extracellular fluid and alkalosis act synergistically in the etiology of tetany. Experimental lowering of the calcium ion concentration in the cerebrospinal fluid, by infusion of sodium citrate or EDTA, or by exchange perfusion of the brain with calcium-free synthetic cerebrospinal fluid, will produce tetany, emphasizing the role played by the central nervous system. If spinal cord transection at Ll is performed in dogs on a low calcium diet followed by thyroparathyroidectomy, tetany will occur in the forelimbs yet be absent in the hindlimbs (Kirk *et al.*, 1973). The time necessary for equilibration of calcium between extracellular and cerebrospinal fluids is greater than 4 hours, and the calcium ion concentration falls much more slowly and to a lesser extent in cerebrospinal than in the extracellular fluid (Kirk *et al.*, 1973). However, with prolonged hypocalcemia, the calcium ion concentration in the cerebrospinal fluid will fall progressively. Since this decrease alters the sensitivity to CO_2 of the central mechanism for the regulation of respiration (Berkenbosch and Adan, 1974), respiratory alkalosis results. This may therefore be a cause of hyperventilation and respiratory alkalosis, as pointed out by Edmondson *et al.* (1975). In addition patients with hypoparathyroidism may have systemic alkalosis (Barzel, 1969), ascribed to a direct effect of PTH on renal tubular reabsorption of bicarbonate.

Tetany is often precipitated by exertion, emotional distress, menstruation, pregnancy and lactation, or by repeated vomiting. Latent tetany, and the signs to detect it, have been described in a previous section. Manifestations characteristic of central nervous system involvement other than tetany may be seen (Greene and Swanson, 1941; Bartter, 1953; Sugar, 1953; Grant, 1953; Kyle *et al.*, 1954; Dickson *et al.*, 1960; Clark *et al.*, 1962; McKinney, 1962; Vincent *et al.*, 1962; Rose and Vas, 1966; Fonseca and Calverly, 1967; Muenter and Whisnant, 1968; Basser *et al.*, 1969; Fourman, 1969; Hossain, 1970a; Ritter *et al.*, 1970; Rubenstein and Brust, 1974; Eraut, 1974; Dahlmann and Prill, 1974; Sollberg, 1975). First, hypocalcemic seizures may occur which resemble syncopal attacks. Patients lose consciousness, "black out," may be in trance-like states with feelings of marked unreality. This may be accompanied by tonic rigidity and varying degrees of mental awareness. These hypocalcemic seizures differ from true epilepsy in that there is no warning, no aura (except occasionally in the form of paresthesias or muscular twitching), no urinary or fecal incontinence, no tongue biting and no postictal confusion. Second, true epileptiform attacks, which may be typical of grand mal convulsions, may occur and present with characteristic electroencephalographic tracings. Petit mal may also occur, as well as focal attacks. It is probable in these cases that hypocalcemia precipitates seizures in susceptible patients, predisposed to idiopathic epilepsy. Under those circumstances, aura may be present, as well as tongue biting, incontinence and postconvulsive coma. Idiopathic epilepsy is the most frequent single erroneous diagnosis which is made prior to recognition of hypoparathyroidism or PHP. A systematic determination of serum calcium and P should always be performed in all "epileptic" patients. It is our experience that with correction of hypocalcemia, the typical hypocalcemic seizures disappear and the frequency of the epileptic attacks is reduced, but they are not always eliminated. These patients with epilepsy do not respond well to anticonvulsant therapy (which may aggravate hypocalcemia). Third, papilledema with increased spinal fluid pressure has been reported in IHP and in postoperative hypoparathyroidism, but to our knowledge not in PHP. The papilledema has been ascribed to cerebral edema (pseudotumor cerebri). The most common diagnosis, especially when these findings coexist with convulsions may be that of an intracranial tumor.

Fourth, all kinds of mental derangements from depression to acute or chronic psychosis, paranoid reactions, dementia, schizophrenic behavior, hallucinations, and delusions may be encountered, all of which may be reversed by correction of hypocalcemia. Minor symptoms in this category include irritability, emotional lability, anxiety, apathy, and impairment of memory and intellectual capacity (especially concentration).

Fifth, extrapyramidal symptoms may be present, such as chorea, athetosis, dystonia, tremors, oculogyric crises and parkinsonism. These usually occur in patients with calcifications of the basal ganglia. The symptoms may or may not revert upon correction of serum calcium level. In a recent case of kinesiogenic (i.e., occurring during periods of activity or exercise) choreoathetosis, Tabaeeh-Zadeh *et al.* (1972) stressed the disappearance of symptoms upon therapy. Frame (1965) described the occurrence of parkinsonism in postoperative hypoparathyroidism; this complication is less amenable to therapy. Calcifications of the basal ganglia, which accompany these complications, are irreversible. Their progression, however, can be arrested by correction of the hypocalcemia (Alterman and Lieber, 1965). These calcifications appear in low incidence in postoperative cases (Danowski *et al.*, 1960), as in idiopathic ones.

B. Ectodermal Changes

Ectodermal changes in hypoparathyroidism are classical (Simpson, 1954; Dent and Garretts, 1960; Risum, 1973; Hirano *et al.*, 1974). The skin is frequently dry and scaly. Eczema and psoriasis may appear, or be aggravated by hypocalcemia. The nails are brittle and hair is coarse and dry. Eyebrows may be sparse (Fig. 34). Treatment of hypocalcemia often

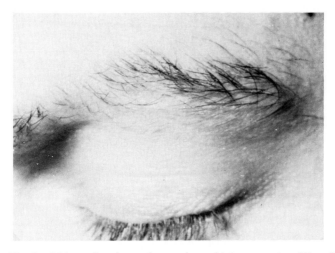

Fig. 34.   Partial loss of eyebrows in a patient with hypoparathyroidism (IHP).

brings dramatic relief. Hair growth may be a salient feature of the response to vitamin D administration in these patients. Superficial moniliasis is a feature of IHP only, with a single possible exception (Frech and McAlister, 1970).

C. Dental Abnormalities

Whether IHP or PHP is the underlying condition, the dental abnormalities are identical. They consist of enamel hypoplasia (pitting and defects), depending upon the age of onset and treatment, dentin defects which parallel enamel malformation in severity, short and blunted roots (especially of the premolars), and delay or absence of eruption. Pulp chambers are often found to be normal, although they at times may be large and sometimes nearly occluded by calcified deposits. The jaws themselves are short and wide (Ritchie, 1965). Hypoplastic teeth are prone to caries. Some patients eventually become edentulous. Careful correlation of the dental abnormalities with respect to the chronological development of the teeth can provide useful information concerning the time of onset of the disease (Ritchie, 1965; Witkop, 1966; Frensilli *et al.*, 1971). Lamina dura may be present, thickened or normal. In PHP with sufficient secondary hyperparathyroidism, lamina dura may eventually disappear. Fig. 35 shows dental roentgenograms of a patient with typical PHP.

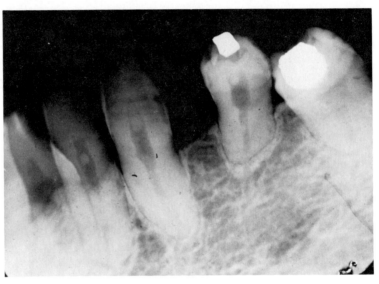

Fig. 35. Roentgenograms of the teeth of an adult with PHP. Dr. Norman Trieger's interpretation was as follows: irregular spacing secondary to lost teeth, and relatively high incidence of dental sepsis. Upper r. and lower l. third molars, though not impacted, are unerupted. The clinical crowns of most teeth show enamel hypoplasia. These hypoplastic areas are best seen in the middle third of the canine crowns and the occlusal third of the premolars. This would place the time of onset of the metabolic derangement at approximately +2 years of age. Rootwise, there is generalized blunting and arrested development. This is particularly well demonstrated in the lower pre-molars. These findings would indicate that the basic defect was present throughout formative years and still operative at age 9–11 years.

D. Ocular Findings

Subcapsular (especially posterior but also anterior zonular) cataracts are a common complication of hypoparathyroidism. Postoperatively, typical lenticular opacities may appear within one year after surgery (Bell and Bartels, 1951; Wijnbladh, 1952; Buckwalter *et al.*, 1955; Painter, 1960; Watkins *et al.*, 1962; Dent and Friedman, 1964). O'Brien (1932), Pohjola

(1962), Ireland *et al.* (1968b), and Segal and Lichtig (1974) have reviewed the subject. Typical lenticular opacities are located in one or more cortical layers which are separated from each other and from the lens capsule by zones of clear cortex (Ireland *et al.*, 1968b). They are usually visible with the naked eye or with the ophthalmoscope (Ireland *et al.*, 1968b). Although these opacities are irreversible, their progression can be stopped by adequate therapy. If the serum calcium remains low, the opacities will usually continue to grow. Thus, macroscopic opacities were present in 28% of postoperative patients who had remained hypocalcemic for 4 years or less, versus 73% of the patients who remained hypocalcemic for 15 years or longer (Ireland *et al.*, 1968b). The pathogenesis of hypocalcemic cataracts is not known. It is believed that a low calcium ion concentration in fluids surrounding the lens inhibits ion transport mechanisms in the lens epithelium. The result would be inward flux of Na^+ and outward flux of K^+. Low intralenticular Na^+ concentrations are necessary for normal lenticular hydration. Firschein (1962) suggested that hypoparathyroidism may lead to cataract formation because of the loss of the stimulating effects of PTH on carbohydrate metabolism. If this were so, one would have to suppose that in PHP ocular end organ resistance to PTH would also exist.

E. Cardiac Disease

That hypocalcemia alters the electrocardiogram has long been known and repeatedly emphasized (Bronsky *et al.*, 1961; Parkin, 1964; Conrad and Baxter, 1966). The major abnormality is in the Q-oTc interval (Colletti *et al.*, 1974), i.e., the interval from the origin of the Q wave to the origin of the T wave, which has been recommended as a rapid screening test for hypocalcemia in the neonate. Corrected QT interval (Q-Tc) i.e., the electrical systole, is classically prolonged, whereas the contractibility of the heart is diminished.

Cardiomegaly and congestive heart failure associated with hypocalcemia have also been described (Boothby *et al.*, 1931; Ranke and Holinger, 1955; Parfitt, 1967a; Gatau-Pelanchon *et al.*, 1969; Dorra *et al.*, 1971; Roche *et al.*, 1972; Aryanpur *et al.*, 1974). One case reported by Buckwalter *et al.* (1955) actually died from cardiac failure postoperatively at the age of 38. Several types of cardiac arrythmias have been reported in connection with hypocalcemia (Johnson and Jennings, 1968), particularly heart block (Griffin, 1965; Sidiropoulos and Schneider, 1972). These cardiac complications of chronic hypocalcemia usually respond dramatically to correction of the hypocalcemia.

XI. BIOLOGICAL FINDINGS

In previous sections, the essential biological findings of IHP and PHP have been emphasized, i.e., serum calcium and phosphorus values. Although the alkaline phosphatase level is usually normal, an occasional patient has an elevated level, which decreases upon treatment. This has been noted in cases of PHP with osteitis fibrosa, and occasionally in other forms of hypoparathyroidism as well (Berezin and Stein, 1948; Jordan and Kelsall, 1951; Dimich et al., 1967). In some of these cases histological osteomalacia may also be present. Hypomagnesemia, a feature of some instances of severe primary hyperparathyroidism, is not an associated biochemical finding in hypoparathyroidism. The reported cases are open to question.

Hypocalcemia is the prerequisite for uncorrected hypoparathyroidism of any etiology. The proportion of the ultrafiltrable (non protein-bound) calcium fraction has been found to be reduced (Prasad and Flink, 1958; Prasad, 1960; Freeman and Breen, 1960) or normal (Terepka et al., 1958; Leighton et al., 1964) and the calcium-binding affinity of the plasma proteins does not differ (Wills and Lewin, 1971) from other groups of patients. There is a correlation between the ultrafiltrable and ionized calcium concentrations in the serum when considerations are made for the differences in total plasma protein concentrations (Wills and Lewin, 1971). When rats are parathyroidectomized, the total, protein-bound and ionized calcium levels are all significantly and proportionally reduced, whereas PTH administration reverses this trend (Raman, 1972). Since the serum calcium values are of paramount importance, especially in the evaluation of patients with postoperative hypoparathyroidism or with PHP, it should be emphasized that care must be taken in the technique of drawing blood samples, especially considering the effect of posture (Smeenk and van den Brand, 1965; Husdan et al., 1973) and venous occlusion (Radcliff et al., 1962; Dent, 1962; Berry et al., 1973; Payne et al., 1973; Parfitt, 1974a; Husdan et al., 1974). Several formulas are available based on the measurement of either the specific gravity (plasma relative density) or of serum albumin or protein concentrations. For every 0.001 unit of specific gravity above 1.027, 0.25 mg/dl (Dent, 1962) or 0.23 mg/dl (Berry et al., 1973) is subtracted from the measured total calcium. For serum albumin and/or total protein, the following have been proposed: for every 0.1 g/dl of albumin above 4.6 mg/dl, 0.09 mg/dl is subtracted from the measured total calcium, and vice versa if the serum albumin level is lower than 4.6 g/dl (Berry et al., 1973), or for every 0.1 g/dl of albumin above 4.0 g/dl, 0.1 mg/dl is subtracted from the measured calcium value and vice versa if the serum calcium level is lower than

4.0 g/dl (Payne *et al.*, 1973). Another formula is adjusted calcium (mg/dl) = measured calcium (mg/dl) (0.55 + total protein (g/dl/16). (Parfitt, 1974a). Adjusted total serum calcium values show no sex-related differences. They do correct for variations in serum calcium levels accounted for by postural changes or venous occlusion.

Phosphate clearance is low in hypoparathyroidism (Kyle *et al.*, 1958) and tubular reabsorption of phosphate (T.R.P.) is high. Phosphate excretion index (P.E.I.) is low (Nordin and Fraser, 1960; Nordin and Bulusu, 1968), and TmP/GFR (i.e., the theoretical tubular maximum for the reabsorption of phosphate per liter of glomerular filtrate, or "theoretical renal phosphate threshold") is elevated (Bijvoet and Morgan, 1971).

When an intravenous calcium load is administered (15 mg/kg body weight over 4 hours) the 24 hour urinary excretion of phosphate increases, as compared with baseline urinary P excretion (Baylor *et al.*, 1950; Howard *et al.*, 1953b; Nordin and Fraser, 1954), whereas calcium is avidly retained (Courvoisier *et al.*, 1956). Total hydroxyproline excretion in the urine does not decrease during this test (Keiser(1964). In a normal person, during a similar calcium load, the 24 hour urinary P excretion decreases, total hydroxyproline excretion in the urine also decreases, and calcium retention amounts to approximately 50% of the infused calcium, versus 80–90% in the two patients tested by Courvoisier *et al.* (1956). High calcium retention should not be equated with osteomalacia.

During the same intravenous calcium load, the relationship between serum and urinary calcium can be studied. In the basal state, "absolute hypocalciuria" characterizes hypoparathyroidism, ascribable to the hypocalcemia. However, when calcium is administered intravenously, the urinary excretion of calcium increases at a rate comparable with that in the controls, but this occurs at much lower levels of serum calcium (Peacock *et al.*, 1969). In other words, at all levels of filtered load, tubular reabsorption of calcium is diminished. The reverse may be seen in primary hyperparathyroidism. Thus, the theoretical calcium threshold (theoretical intercept of concentration threshold on the plasma calcium axis of the linear progression of urinary calcium during intravenous calcium load), which is 9.0 (Peacock *et al.*, 1969) or 9.3 (Nordin *et al.*, 1975) mg/dl in normal subjects, is about 6.5 mg/dl in hypoparathyroidism, and 12.0 mg/dl in hyperparathyroidism. Peacock *et al.* (1969) maintain there would be sufficient calcium passing through the circulation ("calcium throughput") of most patients with hypoparathyroidism to sustain a normal level of serum calcium were the renal threshold for calcium normal. According to these authors, this lowered renal threshold accounts largely or wholly for the hypocalcemia of hypoparathyroidism. This theory has recently been reemphasized by Nordin *et al.* (1975), who showed in addition that the urinary calcium in the fasting state (after 12 hours of fasting), a reflection of bone resorption, is well within normal limits in most hypoparathyroid subjects (this is true at least for 8 of the 15 patients studied, but not so for the 7 other patients). The authors hypothesized that this reflected the activity of a calcium pump in the bone cells, able to draw upon the bone mineral reserves by some "as yet undiscovered mechanism."

No such calcium infusion studies have been performed in patients with PHP, but it might be expected that the renal threshold for calcium would be much higher. If it were normal, this would demonstrate that the hypocalcemia of hypoparathyroidism is not accounted for by reduced tubular reabsorption of calcium. This mechanism might account for the fact that the serum calcium is significantly lower in IHP than in PHP.

Kinetic studies with labeled calcium have shown low rates of bone turnover (Krane *et al.*, 1956; Heaney and Whedon, 1958; Bell and Bartter, 1963; Dymling, 1964; Milhaud and Bourichon, 1964). Calcium absorption from the gut is decreased (Milhaud *et al.*, 1961; Avioli *et al.*, 1965), as measured with labeled calcium.

Total hydroxyproline excreted in the urine is diminished (Benoit *et al.*, 1963; Kivirikko *et al.*, 1965; Gruson *et al.*, 1967; Mautalen, 1970). When normal rats are parathyroidectomized, the urinary output of total hydroxyproline decreases from 1.58 ± 0.3 to 1.11 ± 0.22 and 0.60 ± 0.14 mg/100 g body weight/24 hours 7 and 14 days respectively after parathyroidectomy (Goulding *et al.*, 1973). In the interpretation of hydroxyproline excretion in humans growth must be considered, since the absence of endogenous PTH (or of normal PTH) will not impair the action of growth hormone. The absence of PTH also does not impair the osteoclastic activity of pagetic bone as shown in a case of simultaneous occurrence of IHP and Paget's disease of bone (Genuth and Klein, 1972).

The findings described so far fit all cases with IHP and postoperative hypoparathyroidism, as well as most patients with PHP. If in PHP with secondary hyperparathyroidism bone turnover is high, this may be reflected in the urinary excretion of total hydroxyproline (which then may be normal or slightly elevated), as well as in ^{47}Ca kinetic studies of calcium deposition rate in and resorption rate from bone. Patient J.G. (Table XI) probably belongs to this group. Basal cAMP output in the urine is low. It may occasionally approach low-normal levels in PHP and be high in PHP type II. The presence of metabolic alkalosis (Barzel, 1969) has been mentioned previously and probably relates to renal tubular function (Hellman *et al.*, 1965; Muldowney *et al.*, 1971; Rodman and Heinemann, 1975).

Finally, elevated levels of creatine phosphokinase (CPK) have been reported in a number of patients with hypoparathyroidism or with PHP (Cape, 1969; Wolf and Lusk, 1972; Hower *et al.*, 1972, 1974a and 1974b; Goto, 1974). Other enzymes of muscular origin may be elevated as well, especially aldolase (Cape, 1969; Hower *et al.*, 1972). The elevations may be striking and correlate inversely with hypocalcemia (Hower *et al.*, 1974a). Correction of the latter is followed by a fall of CPK values to normal, or at least to lower levels. Goto (1970), who separated CPK isoenzymes by agar gel electrophoresis, showed that in this situation only the MM isoenzyme was present, thus providing evidence that CPK elevation originates in skeletal muscle. Whether this was due to "hypocalcemic myopathy," the term coined by Wolf and Lusk (1972), is unknown. Muscle biopsy provided evidence of "non-specific" alterations (Wolf and Lusk, 1972) or was suggestive of myopathy (Hower *et al.*, 1974b). Cape (1969) has shown by histochemical staining complete absence of phosphorylase a with a normal phosphorylase b in specimens of resting muscle of a patient with untreated PHP. However, muscular work *in vivo*, as well as addition of calcium *in vitro*, produced activation of phosphorylase b to phosphorylase a. The author theorized that the presence of low calcium ion concentration induces a failure in activation of phosphorylase b kinase. Many of our patients with IHP have high CPK values. Total CPK activity in serum, however, is one of the least specific tests performed in the laboratory (Nevins *et al.*, 1973).

XII. TREATMENT

The treatment of hypoparathyroidism has been recently reviewed in detail (Avioli, 1974). The main objective of therapy is to normalize the serum calcium level sufficiently to prevent all complications of hypocalcemia; hypercalciuria should be avoided. There are several principles useful to guide therapy and avoid the hypercalcemia of overtreatment. Undertreatment, maintaining the serum calcium level between 8.6 and 9.4 mg/dl, is the best safeguard against possible toxicity. Chronic levels as high as 9.6–10.2 mg/dl are to be avoided to prevent hypercalcemic episodes. Patients should be kept under strict supervision, once adequate dosage has been determined. Determination at intervals of 3–6 months of serum calcium, P, Mg, and (if necessary) creatinine levels, as well as 24 hour urinary calcium and creatinine determinations, are useful since the sensitivity of an individual patient to a given dose and form of calcium-elevating principle may vary from time to time. Phosphorus levels may be diminished, if necessary, by replacement of calcium-(and P-) containing foods by oral calcium supplements, so that phosphate binding agents will seldom be necessary. Once equilibrium has been achieved and a convenient dosage of one drug has been found, another "equivalent" drug should not be introduced. Individual sensitivity to these drugs is variable and cannot be predicted. Intoxication has occurred, for example, when vitamin D_3 was substituted for vitamin D_2 in equivalent dosages (Parfitt, 1970), when changing from old to new AT 10 preparations in so-called equivalent dosages (Parfitt, 1967b) or when changing from a preparation of vitamin D_2 in oily solution to a preparation of the same vitamin solubilized in water (Fahraeus et al., 1973).

The problems of potential intoxication in chronic therapy of hypoparathyroidism have been described by Hossain (1970b). In a series of 20 patients treated for 1 to 5 years, 29 episodes of hypercalcemia (i.e., serum Ca levels > 11.3 mg/dl) occurred in 13. Renal function was temporarily impaired in 22 of 29 episodes where the average serum calcium level had been 14.2 mg/dl. Five of these patients developed permanent renal damage. The daily dose of vitamin D administered to these individuals was 0.5–5.0 mg and of DHT 0.3–8 mg. However, it is unusual that doses of more than 1.0 mg/24 hours of DHT are required (Harrison et al., 1967; Dymling and Ryd, 1968; Parfitt, 1970). Parfitt (1970) reported in 29 patients treated for 2 to 8 years an incidence of 8 hypercalcemic episodes occurring in 7 patients. Although this seems much more "reasonable," it still illustrates the difficulties of management; half of the episodes were accounted for by substantial increases in the consumption of milk or ice cream. Since it is difficult to keep patients for long periods on a constant intake of milk and dairy products, we have permitted them to consume liberal amounts of high calcium-containing foods, encouraging milk drinking, so that any deviation from their usual habits results in a tendency toward hypocalcemia rather than toward hypercalcemia. Whether episodes of toxicity account for the hypertension in one series (Krane, 1961), occurring after several decades of therapy, remains to be shown. In the series of 33 patients followed by Parfitt (1972b), in which relatively little toxicity occurred (Parfitt, 1970), at least 5 patients suffered from hypertension and were treated with thiazide diuretics. Patients should be warned to report all symptoms, usually general malaise, lassitude, polydypsia, polyuria, anorexia and nausea, which may herald any episode of toxicity, and to take steps accordingly. Most episodes of toxicity, however, pass unnoticed (Sevringhaus and John, 1943; Hossain, 1970b).

Calcium-raising agents have been available since the 1930's, when irradiated ergosterol became available, allowing treatment with vitamin D_2 (ergocalciferol), and later with vitamin D_3 (cholecalciferol). Simultaneously Holtz et al. (1934) introduced his Antitetanisches Präparat 10, under the name AT 10, which rapidly became popular (Albright, 1939), despite its increased cost. It also is derived from irradiated ergosterol in which vitamin D is eliminated, and represents a mixture of various sterols presented in an oily solution, the active principle of which has always been stated to be dihydrotachysterol (DHT). Its standardization was achieved through bioassays which unfortunately have been changed repeatedly over the years, apparently without re-evaluation of its clinical effect (Parfitt, 1967b). Therefore, the potency of the preparation has strikingly decreased over the years (giving rise to cases of "resistance" to AT 10) (Dent and Friedman, 1964). Furthermore, this compound has often been marketed as a liquid preparation which deteriorates on exposure to air and light. Encapsulated preparations are preferable for more constant activity. Terepka *et al.* (1961) showed by chromatography that the principal component of Hytakerol, the commercial preparation of AT 10 in the United States (Winthrop Laboratories), did not contain DHT but dihydrovitamin D_2 II (hydrocalciferol), another (active) isomer. As a result of this, the manufacturer of Hytakerol first relabeled the product as a brand of hydrocalciferol in June 1964 (Reilly, 1967), but subsequently replaced the material for encapsulation with crystalline DHT (Kaye *et al.*, 1971). This led in England to relabeling of the preparation from "1 ml of AT 10 is equivalent to 1.25 mg pure DHT" to "1 ml of AT 10 contains 0.25 mg of DHT" (Dent and Friedman, 1964). In continental Europe, the material is provided as an oily solution, non-encapsulated, and labeled 1 ml = 1 mg. This is probably correct, but it is not known when the change in potency was introduced. These variations in potency, formulation, and geographic distribution have contributed to the disrepute of this excellent medication, and some authors indeed have switched from the use of AT 10 back to vitamin D. Pure crystalline DHT is now available in most countries, as capsules, tablets or a solution in oil (containing for Hytakerol^R, respectively, 0.125 mg/caps, 0.2 mg/tablet and 0.25 mg/ml solution).

The reason for preferring pure crystalline DHT over vitamin D_2 and D_3 is that the former can be administered in exact dosage, of importance in the lifelong therapy of a chronic disorder with a potentially dangerous medication. Furthermore, the desired therapeutic effect is more quickly achieved than with vitamin D and since the biological half-life is shorter with DHT, either through more rapid inactivation or excretion, any episode of intoxication will spontaneously regress much more rapidly, thus enhancing the margin of safety. It has been observed that intoxication with vitamin D may be long lasting (Howard and Meyer, 1948; Spaulding and Yendt, 1964). Vitamin D, as well as 25-(OH)D_3, is stored in many tissues, but mainly in skeletal muscle and in adipose tissue (Mawer *et al.*, 1972). Thomas *et al.* (1959) noted that antirachitic activity of the serum remained elevated for many months after administration of vitamin

D, confirmed by more recent determination of levels of 25-(OH)D$_3$ by a specific competitive protein-binding assay. Avioli and Haddad (1973), after having administered 1 mg/24 hours of vitamin D to a normal subject during a period of 25 days, found upon withdrawal a biological half-life of 4 to 5 weeks. Bouillon *et al.* (1976) found in renal azotemic osteodystrophy that upon withdrawal of vitamin D$_3$ (15 mg weekly) the 25-(OH)D$_3$ levels in the serum remained elevated for several months. Another point of interest is that, if the main action of DHT is on intestinal absorption of calcium (Hunt and Morgan, 1970), there undoubtedly is a powerful calcium-mobilizing action on bone, which renders the effect of this medication more independent of the dietary intake of calcium than vitamin D. Toxic doses of DHT produced hypercalcemia, even with a calcium-free diet, whereas little hypercalcemia was produced by toxic doses of vitamin D when calcium was withdrawn from the diet (Kaye *et al.*, 1971). This demonstrates, at least in this model, the predominant action of DHT on mobilization of calcium from bone. 25-(OH)DHT is fully active in stimulating bone resorption in tissue culture as well (Trummel *et al.*, 1971). That vitamin D also has calcium-mobilizing properties was shown earlier by Carlsson (1952). The plasma concentrations of the active form of DHT, i.e., 25-(OH)DHT, is proportional to the intake of DHT (Bhattacharyya and DeLuca, 1973). Hepatic 25-hydroxylation occurs in a fashion that is not product-regulated (Hallick and DeLuca, 1971). Moreover, no further renal hydroxylation is required for full biological activity (Harrison and Harrison, 1972). It is not surprising that in the treatment of renal azotemic osteodystrophy, where dosages of at least 2.5 mg/24 hours of vitamin D are required to improve the bone disease, the same may be accomplished with 0.25–0.375 mg/24 hours of DHT (Kaye *et al.*, 1970) (Chapter 2). Under similar circumstances, DHT may show activity at dosages 1/5 to 1/10 those of vitamin D which still proved to be ineffectual (Sagar *et al.*, 1972). Whether 1 α-hydroxylation is required for the activity of 25-(OH)DHT is not known.

Harrison *et al.* (1967) had the impression that control of hypoparathyroidism was much easier to achieve with DHT than with vitamin D$_2$ and that 1 mg of crystalline DHT corresponded to approximately 3 mg (120,000 IU) of vitamin D$_2$. Furthermore, patients "resistant" to conventional vitamin D therapy could be adequately controlled with the same dose of DHT as those patients who were not resistant to the usual doses of vitamin D$_2$ used under these circumstances. A maximum of 1 mg/24 hours of DHT was found to be needed to control such patients, unless steatorrhea was present. In the latter cases, doses as high as 5 mg/24 hours have been required for short periods of time, until fat malabsorption improved and lower doses were required (Harrison, 1970).

Dymling and Ryd (1968) treated 26 patients with DHT, using doses of 0.2 to 2.0 mg/24 hours with an average of 0.77 mg/24 hours. Only 4 patients of 26 required daily doses above 1.0 mg, and in only 2 above 1.2 mg/24 hours. Parfitt (1970) in a series of 22 patients used on the average 0.6 mg/24 hours of DHT, with a maximum of 1.0 mg/24 hours, whereas one of us used 3.75 to 8.75 mg per week (Krane, 1961).

Vitamins D_2 and D_3 are still widely used in the treatment of hypoparathyroidism, owing to their low cost, effectiveness and the long experience with their use. Ireland *et al.* (1968a) reviewed their experiences in 30 patients controlled with this medication (vitamin D_2). The mean controlling dose was 2.12 mg/24 hours (84,000 IU), compared with 0.77 mg/24 hours used by Dymling and Ryd (1968) in terms of crystalline DHT. None of the patients followed by Ireland *et al.* (1968a) was controlled on less than 1.25 mg/24 hours (50,000 IU). All patients who received vitamin D in daily dosages greater than 2.5 mg/24 hours (100,000 U/day) suffered from episodes of hypercalcemia (16/30), the mean dose producing hypercalcemia being 3.28 mg/24 hours (131,200 IU). When hypocalcemic episodes occurred, the mean dosage of vitamin D was 1.73 mg/24 hours (69,200 IU). Variations of sensitivity in the same patient were difficult to explain. As a rule, adequate therapy should be provided by doses ranging between 1.25 and 2.50 mg/24 hours of vitamin D, with little chance of toxicity. These authors also determined that the vitamin D requirements were independent of the thyroid function in their patients. Parfitt (1970) used a mean dosage of 1.93 mg/24 hours of vitamin D for optimal control, with highest dosage 3.0 mg/24 hours.

Vitamin D toxicity occasionally reduces the further requirements for vitamin D, an observation made by Leeson and Fourman (1966). One hypothesis is that the intoxicating dosage had been too high to start with for proper equilibration, but there is evidence supporting an increased sensitivity to vitamin D following an episode of poisoning (Chertow *et al.*, 1974). In any event, this possibility of increased sensitivity after an episode of toxicity should be kept in mind in the practical management of these patients. There is another circumstance when patients are more sensitive to the administered vitamin D, i.e., when thiazide diuretics are given concomitantly. In the year 1970, Parfitt (1972b) observed 3 episodes of vitamin D toxicity in 5 hypoparathyroid patients receiving a thiazide diuretic, versus 1 such episode in 25 hypoparathyroid patients not receiving thiazides. There may also be variability in the potency of vitamin D preparations. Tablets of vitamin D are particularly unreliable (Parfitt, 1968). If capsules are utilized, containing an oily solution of pure vitamin D_2 or D_3 (usually 0.625 or 1.25 mg per capsule), the reliability will be increased, although Parfitt (1968) questioned the stability of the preparations used, since most capsules are translucent and devoid of an antioxidant, and therefore liable to deterioration upon exposure to light (Chen et al., 1965). However, significant decrease of vitamin D_3 activity (at least 20%) occurs only after several years (Fisher et al., 1969).

Whether vitamin D-resistance or DHT-resistance occurs in the absence of steatorrhea, hypomagnesemia, the high bone turnover of "hungry" bone disease following operation for hyperthyroidism (Blohm et al., 1953; Dent and Harper, 1958) or an associated treatment with anticonvulsant agent is not certain. The case of Homer (1961) responded dramatically to the administration of magnesium sulfate, possibly indicative of hypomagnesemia which however was not measured. Dent et al. (1955) have shown that some patients become insensitive to vitamin D_2 but respond to corresponding dosages of vitamin D_3 or DHT. Subsequently such patients have been found to be sensitive to 25-$(OH)D_3$ (Pak et al., 1970).

Whether 25-$(OH)D_3$ offers advantages over D_3 or DHT remains to be shown. However, patients have been successfully treated with this metabolite of vitamin D in dosages of 5,000 U/24 hours or less (Pak et al., 1970), or in dosages of 25–200 μg/day (Konopka et al., 1971; Klotz and Konopka, 1972; Codaccioni et al., 1974; Kooh et al., 1975). Its potency compared to vitamin D_2 is increased ten- to fifteenfold and compared to DHT, about 4- to 5-fold.

More recent modes of therapy include treatment with the biologically active form of vitamin D, i.e., 1,25-$(OH)_2D_3$ or its synthetic analog 1α-$(OH)D_3$. 1α-$(OH)D_3$ is rapidly metabolized to 1,25-$(OH)_2D_3$ and probably functions by conversion to 1,25-$(OH)_2D_3$ (Zerwekh et al., 1974; DeLuca et al., 1975). This mode of therapy, especially the use of 1,25-$(OH)_2D_3$ theoretically obviates the difficulties encountered with the use of the parent vitamins D_2 and D_3. Furthermore, the onset of action is rapid and the biological half-life is short, so that many of the advantages of pure crystalline DHT are met. The doses necessary to achieve this action have been 0.7–2.7 μg/24 hours (Russell et al., 1974), 1 μg/24 hours (Kind et al., 1975), 1.3–2.5 μg/24 hours (Kooh et al., 1975), 1.0–2.5 μg/24 hours (Neer et al., 1975), 5 μg/24 hours in a patient on diphenylhydantoin and phenobarbital (Neer et al., 1975), and 0.5–1.0 μg/24 hours (Davies, 1976). Occasionally, lower doses have proven sufficient (0.25 μg/24 hours) (Evans et al., 1975). Serum calcium is normalized in 1–2 weeks, and upon withdrawal of therapy, returns to hypocalcemic levels in 2–3 weeks (Kooh et al., 1975; Evans et al., 1975). Disturbing is the finding by Evans et al. (1975) that in one case the serum P level did not change and in the other serum P actually rose by 1.0 mg/dl on the 0.25 μg/24 hours calcium-normalizing dosage. Lowering of serum P has been striking in other cases so treated, but normalization has been the exception rather than the rule.

It is probable, however, that this depends more on the short duration of treatment than on intrinsic inability to normalize serum P levels. The action of 25-(OH)D_3 on P excretion is much the same as that of 1,25-(OH)$_2$$D_3$ (Popovtzer et al., 1974; Jelonek, 1975). The time factor, however, does play a crucial role.

That lowering of the P level is not achieved earlier is not surprising, since 1,25-(OH)$_2$$D_3$ does not increase P clearance but produces decreases (Puschett et al., 1972) or no change in the absence of PTH (Popovtzer et al., 1974). Probably normalization of serum calcium level per se may be the determining factor (Eisenberg, 1965).

Kooh et al. (1975) established that treatment should be given on a body weight-basis, amounting to 0.04–0.08 μg/24 hours in PHP, IHP or postoperative hypoparathyroidism. They also compared in one patient with IHP and one with PHP, the relative dosages of 25-(OH)D_3 and 1,25-(OH)$_2$$D_3$ required to normalize the serum calcium values. This ratio was of the order of 100 in favor of 1,25-(OH)$_2$$D_3$. It also corresponds to the ratio of potency of these two metabolites on bone resorption, as studied in vitro (Raisz et al., 1972a; Reynolds et al., 1973). However, in one patient (Kooh et al., 1975) with IHP and steatorrhea (an "unexplained complication of the case"), this ratio was unexpectedly 2000, showing normal sensitivity to 1,25-(OH)$_2$$D_3$, but insensitivity to 25-(OH)D_3. This finding was not discussed by the authors. However, since the 25-(OH)D_3 was administered by mouth, and the 1,25-(OH)$_2$$D_3$ was given intravenously, the logical explanation would be that 25-(OH)D_3 had not been appropriately absorbed. The authors, who measured 25-(OH)D_3 concentrations in the plasma of their patients after treatment, unfortunately did not report the levels achieved in this particular patient.

The doses of 1α-(OH)D_3 used were almost equivalent to those of 1,25-(OH)$_2$$D_3$ (Russell et al., 1974; Neer et al., 1975). Brenton et al. (1976) used 2–10 μg/24 hours, a slightly higher dose. Russell et al. (1974) also concluded that dose for dose, 1,25-(OH)$_2$$D_3$ appeared to be more potent than 1α-(OH)D_3. If we neglect this (slight) difference in potency between 1,25-(OH)$_2$$D_3$ and 1 α-(OH)D_3, and assign an arbitrary value of 1 to the potency of vitamin D (D_2 or D_3), then approximate values for the other related compounds would be DHT 2–3, 25-(OH)D_3 10–15, 1,25-(OH)$_2$$D_3$ and 1α-(OH)D_3 1000–1500. Parfitt (1974b) also assigned a factor of 3 to DHT, but gave 25-(OH)D_3 and 1,25-(OH)$_2$$D_3$ a factor of 15 and 1α(OH)D_3 a factor of 2500.

These factors are useful for the clinician to more easily master changes from one compound to the other, when this becomes necessary. However, it should be stressed that these factors are only pertinent to the condition described, i.e., hypoparathyroidism, as well as PHP. In cases of slight postoperative hypoparathyroidism where the serum calcium is not very low owing to remaining but diminished PTM secretion, the factors might already be different, i.e., smaller than when PTH is not playing its role as a "trophic" factor.

The exact mechanism whereby all these agents act to achieve normalization of serum calcium is not known, nor is it known whether there are major differences between them. All promote intestinal absorption of calcium (Bauer *et al.*, 1932). Whether an important renal action is involved, as suggested by Nordin (1973) for vitamin D and DHT, remains to be shown. Studies in rats have shown that PTH activity is necessary for the mobilization of bone, at least as induced by physiological doses of $1,25\text{-}(OH)_2 D_2/D_3$, whereas PTH is not necessary for the action on calcium absorption from the intestine (Garabedian *et al.*, 1974). According to Seymour and DeLuca (1974), DHT as well as 25-(OH)DHT does not produce calcium mobilization from bone in the absence of PTH. Both $1,25\text{-}(OH)_2 D_3$ and DHT remain fully active under these circumstances as far as calcium transport in the intestine is concerned. Most probably, the mode of action in hypoparathyroid man is similar to that in the rat when PTH is completely absent.

It is therefore not surprising that vitamin D or its metabolites and/or analogues do not increase total urinary hydroxyproline excretion (Mautalen, 1970; Neer *et al.*, 1975), as can also be seen in Table IX, in contrast to the action of PTE. In isolated cases where hydroxyproline excretion rose after therapy [case No. 1 of Russell *et al.* (1974), case No. 1 of Pak *et al.* (1960) and two cases of Hunt and Morgan (1970)] it is possible that some PTH secretion was retained.

Calcium supplements may also have a role in therapy of hypoparathyroidism. We often suggest a high calcium diet ($\sim$ 1 g of elemental calcium/day). The alternative, especially if the upper limit of the "safe" range for vitamin D ($\sim$ 2.5 mg/24 hours) or for DHT ($\sim$ 1.2 mg/24 hours) has been reached, is to provide supplemental calcium orally. To provide 1.0 g of elemental calcium requires 2.5 g of calcium carbonate, 3.7 g of calcium chloride, 4 g of calcium acetate, 5 g of calcium citrate, 5.7 g of calcium glycerophosphate, 7.7 g of calcium levulinate, 7.7 g of calcium lactate, 9 g of calcium orthophosphate, 11.1 g of calcium gluconate or 15.2 g of calcium glubionate. Phosphate salts of calcium should not be administered for this purpose. Calcium carbonate may induce metabolic alkalosis. Calcium chloride, on the other hand, produces metabolic acidosis as well as gastric irritation. If administered by gavage to children, it may even cause necrosis or ulceration of the gastrointestinal tract. Calcium lactate does not alter acid-base equilibrium and is non-irritating to the gastrointestinal tract. However, when compressed into tablets, calcium lactate may be poorly solubilized and absorbed. Calcium lactate therefore is more effective as a powder to be dissolved and taken in solution (Watkins *et al.*, 1962). Many details of oral calcium therapy may be found in the review by Harrison (1970) and by Peach (1975).

Huge amounts of calcium are eventually successful in correcting the serum calcium level without other agents even in the most severe cases of IHP. Some authors are of the opinion that cases of mild postoperative hypoparathyroidism may be treated with oral calcium supplements only. Parfitt (1970) recommends this treatment when serum calcium levels are not lower than 8.5 mg/dl, and finds that patients with levels between 7.5 and 8.5 mg/dl can usually be maintained on this therapy alone, an opinion shared by Woodhouse (1974).

Calcium therapy is mandatory when acute hypocalcemia supervenes, such as may occur in the days following parathyroid or thyroid surgery. A single injection of 10–20 ml of calcium gluconate (10% solution, providing 9 mg of elemental calcium/ml) should be administered at a slow rate (over a 10-minute period) to avoid high intracardiac concentrations of calcium. An infusion of 15 mg/kg body weight over 4 hours (or 6 hours) can be used subsequently. An alternative to calcium gluconate is to inject calcium gluceptate (glucoheptonate) 5–10 ml (18 mg of elemental Ca/ml). Whatever preparation is used, the serum calcium level should be closely monitored. If symptoms recur, slow intravenous infusions of 1 g of calcium gluconate can be repeated every 6 or 8 hours. Other therapeutic measures, for example the administration of high doses of the rapidly-acting DHT (for example 2 mg q.i.d.), may be used simultaneously, as well as oral calcium therapy when practical. Special care should be taken as far as intravenous calcium administration is concerned in patients consuming digitalis, since hypercalcemia may provoke digitalis toxicity, especially cardiac arrhythmias. Treatment of infants is essentially the same as adults (Harrison, 1970), except that lower doses of injected calcium should be used and the heart rate should be monitored and not be decrease during the intravenous infusion.

It is desirable in postoperative hypoparathyroidism to attempt periodically to decrease substitution therapy to determine whether the remaining parathyroid glands have resumed their activity. However, in patients receiving vitamin D, a long period of time may elapse (7–18 months), due to storage of this vitamin in body fat, before the serum calcium level eventually falls, demonstrating the continued need for substitution therapy (Krane, 1961). "Recovery" from surgical hypoparathyroidism is always a possibility as previously discussed. "Recovery" in PHP is also a possibility although therapy should be withdrawn cautiously since these patients (1) may develop severe episodes of relapse; (2) have secondary hyperparathyroidism which is best eliminated if bone atrophy is to be avoided; and (3) tolerate therapy better as far as possible development of nephrocalcinosis is concerned. IHP, however, does not recover. Any spontaneous normalization of the serum calcium, on the contrary, heralds a new complication such as the development of Addison's disease. Postoperative hypocalcemia would be anticipated in patients with hyperparathyroidism and florid osteitis fibrosa. Woodhouse *et al.* (1971) have shown that giving small doses of vitamin D (0.025 mg/24 hours) for 2 to 8 weeks prior to surgery, with forced fluid intake, will hasten healing of the bone lesions and prevent postoperative hypocalcemia. A similar program of preventive therapy prior to parathyroidectomy has been recommended by Jackson and Dancaster (1962) and Davies and Friedman (1966). We also recommend monitoring the serum Mg level, since patients with prominent primary osteitis fibrosa are usually hypomagnesemic or become so postoperatively. Magnesium sulfate, administered intramuscularly (2 ml of 50% $MgSO_4$ using the hydrated salt $MgSO_4 \cdot 7H_2O$, 1 g of which provides 97.4 mg of elemental Mg, i.e., 4.06 mmoles) will rapidly restore the serum magnesium level to normal.

There is no substantial difference between the therapy of PHP and that of IHP, if allowance is made for the problems with associated diseases. Most patients with PHP can be successfully treated with relatively small dosages of vitamin D_2.

Barzel (1976) has claimed that metabolic alkalosis in IHP is not affected by vitamin D and calcium therapy alone. He found elevated arterial blood pH with normal or elevated pCO_2 as often in treated as in untreated patients. Acid therapy has long been considered as a possible adjuvant in the therapy of hypoparathyroidism, since Aub *et al.* (1932) reported improvement in tetany with the use of HCl or NH_4Cl, as reviewed by Freyberg *et al.* (1936). Acidifying agents produce undesirable hypercalciuria (Lemann *et al.*, 1967; Reidenberg *et al.*, 1968) and we do not recommend their use. Thomas *et al.* (1967) actually treat their patients with large doses of alkalinizing calcium carbonate alone or supplemented with 1.25–3.75 mg/24 hours of vitamin D per week.

Treatment of hypoparathyroidism with parathyroid hormone might be considered to be the most physiological, therapeutic approach to therapy. However, because of antibody response to non-human forms of PTE, resistance invariably develops during chronic treatment (Collip, 1935; Freyberg *et al.*, 1936; Melick *et al.*, 1967). Additional problems with PTE are its expense, the requirement for parenteral administration and the tendency to provoke allergic reactions, and even anaphylaxis (O'Rourke *et al.*, 1973). PTE has still been advocated in exceptional circumstances as an adjuvant therapeutic agent in those cases who are "resistant" to the usual modes of therapy (Raymond and Klotz, 1971).

Jacob and Dunphy (1963) have reviewed the earlier literature on the subject of implantation and transplantation of parathyroid tissue, demonstrating that homologous and heterologous parathyroid tissue implanted in man may function for several months. Longterm benefit, however, has not been conclusively shown and the good results in the reported cases probably could be explained by "adaptation" to the hypoparathyroid state.

Parathyroid glands have been transplanted successfully, and physiologic proof of function and response to the double negative feedback mechanism has been demonstrated. Parathyroid allografts function adequately only if the host is immunosuppressed (Wells et al., 1974), which has been achieved in humans (Groth et al., 1973; Wells et al., 1974). Parathyroid autotransplantation, however, can be performed in a non-immunosuppressed host. A number of small pieces of parathyroid glands have been implanted intramuscularly in the forearm, while several other small pieces are frozen in liquid nitrogen at the time of total PTX in patients with primary or secondary hyperplasia of the parathyroids. If control of parathyroid function proves inadequate, delayed implantation can be carried out. On the contrary, if too much tissue has been implanted, pieces of the grafted material can be removed from the forearm under local anesthesia (Wells et al., 1975 and 1976).

XIII. CONCLUDING REMARKS

It is apparent from the material presented here that considerable information can be gleaned from the study of patients with deficient parathyroid function. Interactions of mineral ions in plasma, the intestinal, skeletal, and renal control of the metabolism of these ions, the relationships between structure and function of parathyroid hormone and vitamin D and their metabolites, as well as mechanisms of action of other skeletal hormones, are all pertinent to the interpretation of the pathophysiology. Aspects of the alterations in normal physiology pertain to almost all of the disorders discussed in these volumes.

ACKNOWLEDGMENTS

A portion of the original work reported here was supported by USPHS grants AM-04501 and AM-03564.

REFERENCES

Abrams, H. L., Spiro, R., and Goldstein, N. (1950). *Cancer* **3,** 74.
Aceto, T., Jr., Batt, R. E., Bruck, E., Schultz, R. B., and Perez, Y. R. (1966). *J. Clin. Endocrinol. Metab.* **26,** 487.

Adams, P. H., Chalmers, T. M., Peters, N., Rack, J. H., and Truscott, B. M. (1965). *Ann. Int. Med.* **63**, 454.

Adams, H. D., and Murphy, R. (1963). *Surg. Gynecol. Obstet.* **116**, 45.

Adams, P., and Jowsey, J. (1967). *Endocrinology* **81**, 735.

Adams, P. H., and Chalmers, T. M. (1965). *Clin. Sci.* **29**, 391.

Adams, P. H., Jowsey, J., Kelly, P. J., Riggs, B. L., Kinney, V. R., and Jones, J. D. (1967). *Q. J. Med.* **36**, 1.

Adie, R. (1973). *Aust. N.Z. J. Surg.* **43**, 299.

Agus, Z. S., Puschett, J. B., Senesky, D., Goldberg, M. (1971). *J. Clin. Invest.* **50**, 617.

Aida, M., Hurukawa, Y., Miura, K., Mihara, A., Kato, K., Tano, T., Ojima, M., Haniw, K., Murakami, O., Lee, S. C., and Yoshinaga, K. (1975). *Tohoku J. Exp. Med.* **115**, 319.

Alajouanine, T., Contamin, F., Cathala, H. P., Scherrer, J. (1954). *Presse Med.* **62**, 339.

Albright, F. (1939). *J. Am. Med. Assoc.* **112**, 2592.

Albright, F. (1941). *J. Am. Med. Assoc.* **117**, 527.

Albright, F. (1956). *J. Clin. Endocrinol. Metab.* **16**, 419.

Albright, F., and Reifenstein, E. C., Jr. (1948). "The Parathyroid Glands and Metabolic Bone Disease." Williams & Wilkins, Baltimore, Maryland.

Albright, F., Burnett, C. H., Smith, P. H., and Parson, W. (1942). *Endocrinology* **30**, 922.

Albright, F., Forbes, A. P., and Henneman, P. H. (1952). *Trans. Assoc. Am. Physicians* **65**, 337.

Alexander, S. B., and Tucker, H. S. G. (1949). *J. Clin. Endocrinol.* **9**, 862.

Aliapoulios, M. A., Voelkel, E. F., and Munson, P. L. (1966). *J. Clin. Endocrinol. Metab.* **26**, 897.

Allen, E. H., Millard, F. J. C., and Nassim, J. R. (1968). *Arch. Dis. Child.* **43**, 295.

Altenähr, E., and Jenke, W. (1974). *Virchows Arch. A* **363**, 333.

Altenähr, E., and Leonhardt, F. (1972). *Virchows Arch. A.* **355**, 297.

Alterman, S. L., and Lieber, A. L. (1965). *Ann. Intern. Med.* **63**, 140.

Alveryd, A. (1968). *Acta Chir. Scand., Suppl.* **389**.

Anast, C. S. (1964). *Pediatrics* **33**, 969.

Anast, C. S., Mohs, J. M., Kaplan, S. L., and Burns, T. W. (1972). *Science* **177**, 606.

Anderson, J., Bannister, D. W., and Tomlinson, R. W. S. (1965). *Clin. Sci.* **29**, 583.

Anderson, T. J., and Ewen, S. W. B. (1974). *J. Clin. Pathol.* **27**, 656.

Anderson, R. H., Bouton, J., Burrow, C. T., and Smith, A. (1974). *Br. Med. J.* **2**, 135.

Aperia, A., Broberger, O., Bergstrand, C. G., and Zetterström, R. (1967). *Acta Paediatr. Scand.* **56**, 357.

Archibald, R., Finby, N., and De Vito, F. (1959). *J. Clin. Endocrinol. Metab.* **19**, 1312.

Arkless, R., and Graham, C. B. (1967). *Am. J. Roentgenol., Radium Ther. Nucl. Med.* [N.S.] **99**, 724.

Arnaud, C. D. (1973). *Am. J. Med.* **55**, 577.

Arnaud, C. D., Tsao, H. S., and Littledike, T. (1971). *J. Clin. Invest.* **50**, 21.

Arnstein, A. R., Frame, B., Frost, H. M., and Block, M. A. (1966). *Ann. Intern. Med.* **64**, 996.

Arnstein, A. R., Frame, B., and Frost, H. M. (1967). *Ann. Intern. Med.* **67**, 1296.

Aryanpur, I., Farhoudi, A., and Zangeneh, F. (1974). *Am. J. Dis. Child.* **127**, 738.

Au, W. Y. W., and Raisz, L. G. (1967). *J. Clin. Invest.* **46**, 1572.

Aub, J. C., Albright, F., Bauer, W., and Rossmeisl, E. J. (1932). *J. Clin. Invest.* **11**, 211.

Aubert, L., and Arroyo, H. (1968). *Marseille Med.* **105**, 709.

Aurbach, G. D. (1971). *Birth Defects, Orig. Artic. Ser.* **6**, 24.

Aurbach, G. D. (1971). *In* P. B. Beeson, and W. McDermott (eds.), "Textbook of Medicine" 13th ed., pp. 1846–1855. Saunders, Philadelphia.

Aurbach, G. D., and Chase, L. R. (1970). *Fed. Proc., Fed. Am. Soc. Exp. Biol.* **29,** 1179.

Aurbach, G. D., and Heath, D. A. (1974). *Kidney Int.* **6,** 331.

Avery, S. H., Bell, N. H., and Stern, P. H. (1971). *Endocrinology* **89,** 951.

Avioli, L. V. (1974). *Am. J. Med.* **57,** 34.

Avioli, L. V., and Haddad, J. G. (1973). *Metab., Clin. Exp.* **22,** 507.

Avioli, L. V., McDonald, J. E., Singer, R. A., and Henneman, P. H. (1965). *J. Clin. Invest.* **44,** 128.

Avioli, L. V., Birge, S. J., and Lee, S. W. (1968). *J. Clin. Endocrinol. Metab.* **28,** 1341.

Axelrod, D. R. (1959). *J. Clin. Endocr.* **19,** 590.

Azerad, E., Gatha, J., and Raverdy, P. (1953). *Bull. Soc. Med. Hop. Paris* **69,** 199.

Aziz, E. M. (1972). *Clin. Res.* **20,** 92.

Babka, J. C., Czerwinski, C. L., Miller, R. C., Cefalo, R. C., and Sode, J. (1974). *Clin. Res.* **22,** 708A.

Bader, J. C., Canlorbe, P., Lambertz, J., Poitout, M., and Lelong, M. (1968). *Sem. Hop. Paris* (Ann. Pediat.) **44,** 1061.

Baer, R. B., Benedek, T., Rosenthal, I. M., and Zimmerman, H. J. (1957). *Arch. Intern. Med.* **99,** 14.

Bakwin, H. (1937). *Am. J. Dis. Child.* **54,** 1211.

Balachandar, V., Pahuja, J., Maddaiah, V. T., and Collipp, P. J. (1975). *Amer. J. Dis. Child.* **129,** 1092.

Barr, D. G. D., Prader, A., Esper, U., Rampini, S., Marrian, V. J., and Forfar, J. O. (1971). *Helv. Paediatr. Acta* **26,** 507.

Barr, S. E., Taylor, E. F., and Rabkin, B. (1960). *Arch. Intern. Med.* **105,** 492.

Barranco, V. P. (1971). *Arch. Dermatol.* **104,** 643.

Bartels, E. C. (1952). *Ann. Intern. Med.* **37,** 1123.

Bartley, P. C., Lloyd, H. M., and Willgoss, D. (1975a). *Aust. N. Z. J. Med.* **5,** 32.

Bartley, P. C., Willgoss, D., and Lloyd, H. M. (1975b). *Aust. N. Z. J. Med.* **5,** 36.

Bartter, F. C. (1953). *Res. Publ., Assoc. Res. Nerv. Ment. Dis.* **32,** 1.

Bartter, F. C. (1966). *In* J. B. Stanbury, J. B. Wyngaarden, and D. S. Fredrickson (eds.), "The Metabolic Basis of Inherited Disease" 2nd ed., pp. 1024–1031. McGraw-Hill, New York.

Barzel, U. S. (1969). *J. Clin. Endocrinol. Metab.* **29,** 917.

Barzel, U. S. (1976). *N.Y. State J. Med.* **76,** 579.

Basser, L. S., Neale, F. C., Ireland, A. W., and Posen, S. (1969). *Ann. Intern. Med.* **71,** 507.

Bauer, W., Marble, A., and Claflin, D. (1932). *J. Clin. Invest.* **11,** 47.

Baxter, J. D., and Bondy, P. K. (1966). *Ann. Intern. Med.* **65,** 429.

Baylor, C. H., Van Alstine, H. E., Keutmann, E. H., and Bassett, S. H. (1950). *J. Clin. Invest.* **29,** 1167.

Beahrs, O. H., and Pasternak, B. M. (1969). *Curr. Probl. Surg.* **1,** 38.

Beahrs, O. H., Ryan, R. F., and White, R. A. (1956). *J. Clin. Endocrinol. Metab.* **16,** 1456.

Beaudoing, A., Jalbert, P., Jaillard, M., Bost, M., and Nigri, M. M. (1970). *Ann. Pediatr.* **17,** 245.

Beck, A. (1928). *Arch. Klin. Chir.* **152,** 123.

Beck, N., and Davis, B. B. (1975). *Am. J. Physiol.* **228,** 179.

Beck, N., Kim, H. P., Moody, E. L., and Davis, B. B. (1974a). *Clin. Res.* **22,** 460A.

Beck, N., Singh, H., Reed, S. W., and Davis, B. B. (1974b). *J. Clin. Invest.* **53,** 717.

Becker, K. L., Purnell, D. C., and Jones, J. D. (1964). *J. Clin. Endocrinol. Metab.* **24,** 347.

Bell, G. O., and Bartels, E. C. (1951). *Lahey Clin. Bull.* **7,** 105.
Bell, N. H., and Bartter, F. C. (1963). *Trans. Assoc. Am. Physicians* **76,** 163.
Bell, N. H., Gerard, E. S., and Bartter, F. C. (1963). *J. Clin. Endocrinol. Metab.* **23,** 759.
Bell, N. H., Avery, S., Sinha, T., Clark, L. C., Jr., Allen, D. O., and Johnston, C., Jr. (1972). *J. Clin. Invest.* **51,** 816.
Bennett, J. C., Maffly, R. H., and Steinbach, H. L. (1959). *Am. J. Roentgenol., Radium Ther. Nucl. Med.* [N.S.] **72,** 368.
Bennett, T. I., Hunter, D., and Vaughan, J. M. (1932). *Q. J. Med.* **1,** 603.
Benoit, F. L., Theil, G. B., and Watten, R. H. (1963). *Metab. Clin. Exp.* **12,** 1072.
Benson, P. F., and Parsons, V. (1964). *Q. J. Med.* **33,** 197.
Benzonana, G. (1968). *Biochim. Biophys. Acta* **151,** 137.
Berardinelli, W. (1951). *Acta Endocrinol. Copenhagen* (Kbh) **7,** 7.
Berdjis, C. C. (1972). *Strahlentherapie* **143,** 48.
Berezin, S. W., and Stein, J. D. (1948). *J. Pediatr.* **33,** 346.
Bergman, L., Kjellmer, I., and Selstam, U. (1974). *Biol. Neonate* **24,** 151.
Berkenbosch, A., and Adan, A. J. M. (1974). *Pfluegers Arch.* **348,** 33.
Berry, E. M., Gupta, M. M., Turner, S. J., and Burns, R. R. (1973). *Br. Med. J.* **4,** 640.
Berson, S. A., and Yalow, R. S. (1966). *Science* **154,** 907.
Berson, S. A., and Yalow, R. S. (1967). *N. Engl. J. Med.* **277,** 640.
Berson, S. A., and Yalow, R. S. (1968). *J. Clin. Endocrinol. Metab.* **28,** 1037.
Bertelsen, A., and Bruun, E. (1947). *Acta Chir. Scand., Suppl.* **133,** 33.
Bethune, J. E., Smith, L. F., and Inoue, H. (1964). *J. Clin. Endocrinol. Metab.* **24,** 1103.
Betro, M. G., and Pain, R. W. (1972). *Br. Med. J.* **1,** 273.
Better, O. S., Garty, J., Brautbar, N., and Barzilai, D. (1969). *Isr. J. Med. Sci.* **5,** 419.
Beumer, H., and Falkenheim, C. (1926). *Muench. Med. Wochenschr.* **78,** 818.
Bhatia, S. K., Hadden, D. R., Montgomery, D. A. D., and Weaver, J. A. (1968). *Ir. J. Med. Sci.* **7,** 449.
Bhattacharyya, M. H., and DeLuca, H. F. (1973). *J. Biol. Chem.* **248,** 2974.
Bianchi, G. S., Meunier, P., Courpron, P., Edouard, C., Bernard, J., and Vignon, G. (1972). *Rev. Rhum. Mal. Osteo-Articulaires* **39,** 19.
Bijvoet, O. L. M. (1969). *Clin. Sci.* **37,** 23.
Bijvoet, O. L. M., and Morgan, D. B. (1971). (D. J. Hioco, ed.), *In* "Phosphate et Métabolisme Phosphocalcique" Sandoz, Paris. pp. 153–180.
Birkenhäger, J. C., Saldenrath, H. J., Hackeng, W. H. L., Schellekens, A. P. M., van der Veer, A. L. J., and Roelfsema, F. (1973). *Eur. J. Clin. Invest.* **3,** 27.
Birtwell, W. M., Magsamen, B. F., Fenn, P. A., Torg, J. S., Tourtelotte, C. D., and Martin, J. H. (1970). *J. Bone Jt. Surg., Am. Vol.* **52,** 1222.
Black, W. C., III. (1969). *Arch. Pathol.* **88,** 225.
Blalock, J. B. (1971). *Surg., Gynecol. Obstet.* **133,** 627.
Bland, J. H., Kirschbaum, B., O'Connor, G. T., and Whorton, E. (1973). *Arch. Intern. Med.* **132,** 209.
Blizzard, R. M., and Gibbs, J. H. (1968). *Pediatrics* **42,** 231.
Blizzard, R. M., Chee, D., and Davis, W. (1966). *Clin. Exp. Immunol.* **1,** 119.
Block, J. B., and Clendenning, W. E. (1963). *N. Engl. J. Med.* **268,** 1157.
Block, M. A., Greenawald, K., Horn, R. C., Jr., and Frame, B. (1967). *Am. J. Surg.,* **114,** 530.
Block, M. A., Miller, J. M., and Horn, R. C. (1966). *Surg., Gynecol. Obstet.* **123,** 501.
Block, M. B., Pachman, L. M., Windhorst, D., and Goldfine, I. D. (1971). *Am. J. Med. Sci.* **261,** 213.

Blohm, R. W., Jr., Wurl, O. A., Gillespie, J. O., and Escamilla, R. F. (1953). *J. Clin. Endocrinol. Metab.* **13**, 519.

Blonde, L., Wehmann, R. E., and Steiner, A. L. (1974). *J. Clin. Invest.* **53**, 163.

Blondeau, P., Brocard, M., and René, L. (1973). *Ann. Chir.* **27**, 1121.

Blumgart, H. L., Freedberg, A. S., and Kurland, G. S. (1955). *J. Am. Med. Assoc.* **157**, 1.

Bocquentin, F., Safar, A., Aicardi, J., and Job, J. C. (1973). *Arch. Fr. Pediatr.* **30**, 989.

Boonstra, C. E., and Jackson, C. E. (1965). *Ann. Intern. Med.* **63**, 468.

Boonstra, C. E., and Jackson, C. E. (1971). *Am. J. Clin. Pathol.* **55**, 523.

Boothby, W. M., Haines, S. F., and Pemberton, J. D. (1931). *Am. J. Med. Sci.* **181**, 81.

Bordier, P. J., Arnaud, C., Hawker, C., Tun Chot, S., and Hioco, D. (1973). *In* "Clinical Aspects of Metabolic Bone Disease." (B. Frame, A. M. Parfitt, and H. Duncan, eds.) *Int. Congr. Ser. No. 270*, pp. 222–228. Excerpta Med. Found., Amsterdam.

Bordier, P., Miravet, L., Matrajt, H., Hioco, D., and Ryckewaert, A. (1967). *Proc. R. Soc. Med.* **60**, 1132.

Borle, A. B. (1968). *In* "Parathyroid Hormone and Thyrocalcitonin (Calcitonin)" (R. V. Talmage and L. F. Bélanger, eds.). Int. Congr. Ser. No. 159, pp. 258–272. Excerpta Med. Found., Amsterdam.

Borle, A. B. (1970). *Fed. Proc., Fed. Am. Soc. Exp. Biol.* **29**, 646.

Borle, A. B. (1974). *J. Mem. Biol.* **16**, 207.

Borowy, Z. Y. (1969). *Can. J. Surg.* **12**, 104.

Bottazzo, G. F., Pouplard, A., Florin-Christensen, A., and Doniach, D. (1975). *Lancet* **2**, 97.

Burckhardt, P., Boillat, A. M., Ruedi, B., Felber, J. P., and Courvoisier, B. (1975). *Schweiz. Med. Wschr.* **105**, 1692.

Bouillon, R., and De Moor, P. (1973). *Ann. Endocrinol.* **34**, 657.

Bouillon, R., Koninckx, P., and De Moor, P. (1974). "Methods and Clinical Evaluation," Vol. I. pp. 353–365. IAEA, Vienna.

Bouillon, R., Van Kerkhove, P., and De Moor, P. (1976). *Clin. Chem.* **22**, 364.

Bowser, E. N., Hargis, G. K., Henderson, W. J., and Williams, G. A. (1975). *Proc. Soc. Exp. Biol. Med.* **148**, 344.

Boyce, D., and Jowsey, J. (1966). *Mayo Clin. Proc.* **41**, 836.

Brailsford, J. F. (1945). *Brit. J. Radiol.* **18**, 167.

Bremner, W. F., McDougall, I. R., and Greig, W. R. (1973). *Lancet* **2**, 281.

Brenton, D. P., Dent, C. E., and Gertner, J. M. (1976). *Abstr. Eur. Symp. Calcif. Tissues, 12th*, 4–8 July 1976, p. 145.

Brickman, A. S., Jowsey, J., Sherrard, D. J., Friedman, G., Singer, F. R., Baylink, D. J., Maloney, N., Massry, S. G., Norman, A. W., and Coburn, J. W. (1975). *In* "Vitamin D and Problems Related to Uremic Bone Disease" (A. W. Norman, K. Schaeffer, H. G. Grigoleit, D. von Herrath, and E. Ritz, eds.), pp. 241–247. de Gruyter, Berlin.

Broadus, A. E., Kaminsky, N. I., Hardman, J. G., Sutherland, E. W., and Liddle, G. W. (1970). *J. Clin. Invest.* **49**, 2222.

Bronner, F., Harris, R. S., Maletskos, C. J., and Benda, C. E. (1954). *J. Nutr.* **54**, 523.

Bronsky, D., Kushner, D. S., Dubin, A., and Snapper, I. (1958). *Medicine* (Baltimore) **37**, 317.

Bronsky, D., Dubin, A., Kushner, D. S., and Waldstein, S. S. (1961). *Am. J. Cardiol.* **7**, 840.

Bronsky, D., Kiamko, R. T., Moncada, R., and Rosenthal, M. (1968). *Pediatrics* **42**, 606.

Bronsky, D., Weisbery, M. G., Gross, M. C., and Barton, J. J. (1970). *Am. J. Med. Sci.* **260**, 160.

Brook, C. G. D., and Valman, H. B. (1971). *Br. J. Dermatol.* **85**, 471.

Brown, D. M., Boen, J., and Bernstein, A. (1972a). *Pediatrics* **49**, 841.
Brown, J. K., Cockburn, F., and Forfar, J. O. (1972b). *Lancet* **1**, 135.
Bruce, J., and Strong, J. A. (1955). *Q. J. Med.* **24**, 307.
Bruining, H. A. (1971). "Surgical Treatment of Hyperparathyroidism, with an Analysis of 267 Cases." Royal Van Gorcum Ltd., Assen.
Brumbaugh, P. F., Haussler, D. H., Bressler, R., and Haussler, M. R. (1974). *Science* **183**, 1089.
Brünner, H., and Rothmund, M. (1973a). *Dtsch. Med. Wochenschr.* **98**, 426.
Brünner, H., and Rothmund, M. (1973b). *Muench. Med. Wochenschr.* **115**, 1208.
Buchs, S. (1954). *Ann. Paediatr.* **183**, 65.
Buck, B. A., and Robertson, R. D. (1971). *Surg., Gynecol. Obstet.* **133**, 218.
Buckle, R. M. (1969). *Br. Med. J.* **2**, 789.
Buckle, R. M., Care, A. D., Cooper, C. W., and Gitelman, H. J. (1968). *J. Endocrinol.* **42**, 529.
Buckwalter, J. A., Soper, R. T., Davies, J., and Mason, E. E. (1955). *Surg., Gynecol. Obstet.* **101**, 657.
Burkhart, J. M., and Jowsey, J. (1966). *Mayo Clin. Proc.* **41**, 663.
Butler, A. M. (1957). Discussion after DiGeorge and Paschkis (1957).
Caffey, J. (1952). *Am. J. Roentgenol., Radium Ther. Nucl. Med.* [N.S] **68**, 875.
Cantarow, A., Stewart, H. L., and Morgan, D. R. (1939). *Endocrinology* **24**, 556.
Canterbury, J. M., Levey, G. S., and Reiss, E. (1973). *J. Clin. Invest.* **52**, 524.
Canterbury, J. M., Levy, G., Ruiz, E., and Reiss, E. (1974). *Proc. Soc. Exp. Biol. Med.* **147**, 366.
Cape, C. A. (1969). *Neurology* **19**, 167.
Capen, C. C., Cole, C. R., and Hibbs, J. W. (1968). *Fed. Proc. Fed. Am. Soc. Exp. Biol.* **27**, 142.
Carlson, H. E., and Brickman, A. S. (1976). *Clin. Res.* **24**, 99A.
Carlsson, A. (1952). *Acta Physiol. Scand.* **26**, 212.
Carlsson, A. (1954). *Acta Physiol. Scand.* **31**, 308.
Carré, M., Ayigbedé, O., Miravet, L., and Rasmussen, H. (1974). *Proc. Natl. Acad. Sci. U.S.A.* **71**, 2996.
Carson, R. J., Schubert, W. K., and Partin, J. C. (1973). *J. Pediatr.* **83**, 150.
Carter, A. C., Kaplan, S. A., DeMayo, A. P., and Rosenblum, D. J. (1959). *J. Clin. Endocrinol. Metab.* **19**, 1633.
Case Records of the Massachusetts General Hospital. (1954). *N. Engl. J. Med.* **251**, 442 (Case 40361).
Casey, T. R., Fast, B. B., and Cherniak, R. M. (1959). *J. Am. Med. Ass.* **169**, 1988.
Cassar, J., and Joseph, S. (1969). *Clin. Chim. Acta* **23**, 33.
Cathala, H. P., and Contamin, F. (1957). *Rev. Fr. Etud. Clin. Biol.* **2**, 358.
Cattell, R. B. (1949). *J. Clin. Endocrinol.* **9**, 999.
Cattell, R. B. (1953). *Surg. Clin. North Am.* **33**, 867.
Cederbaum, S. D., and Lippe, B. M. (1973). *Am. J. Hum. Genet.* **25**, 638.
Chamberlin, J. A., Fries, J. G., and Allen, H. C., Jr. (1964). *Surgery* **55**, 787.
Chaptal, J., Jean, R., Bonnet, H., Guillaumot, R., and Morel, G. (1960). *Arch. Fr. Pediatr.* **17**, 866.
Chase, L. R., and Aurbach, G. D. (1967). *Proc. Natl. Acad. Sci. U.S.A.* **58**, 518.
Chase, L. R., and Aurbach, G. D. (1968). *Science* **159**, 545.
Chase, L. R., and Aurbach, D. G. (1970). *J. Biol. Chem.* **245**, 1520.
Chase, L. R., and Slatopolsky, E. (1974). *J. Clin. Endocrinol. Metab.* **38**, 363.
Chase, L. R., Melson, G. L., and Aurbach, G. D. (1969). *J. Clin. Invest.* **48**, 1832.

Chen, P. S., Jr., Terepka, A. R., Lane, K., and Marsh, A. (1965). *Anal. Biochem.* **10,** 421.

Chertow, B. S., Plymate, S. R., and Becker, F. O. (1974). *Arch. Intern. Med.* **133,** 838.

Chiroff, R. T., Sears, K. A., and Slaughter, W. H., III. (1974). **56,** 1063.

Chisari, F. V., Hochstein, D., Kirchstein, R. L., and Seligmann, E. B. (1972). *Am. J. Pathol.* **68,** 461.

Chodack, P., Attie, J. N., and Groder, M. G. (1965). *Arch. Intern. Med.* **116,** 416.

Chopra, I. J., and Nugent, C. A. (1970). *Am. J. Med. Sci.* **260,** 171.

Christiaens, L., Fontaine, G., Farriaux, J. P., and Biserte, G. (1967). *Acta Paediatr. Belg.* **21,** 5.

Chu, L. L. H., Forte, L. R., Anast, C. S., and Cohn, D. V. (1975). *Endocrinology* **97,** 1014.

Clain, A. (1965). *Br. J. Cancer* **19,** 15.

Clark, J. A., Davidson, L. J., and Ferguson, H. C. (1962). *J. Ment. Sci.* **108,** 811.

Clark, L. C., Jr., and Beck, E. (1950). *J. Pediatr.* **36,** 335.

Clark, R. L., Ibañez, M. L., and White, E. C. (1966). *Arch. Surg. (Chicago)* **92,** 23.

Clarkson, B., Kowlessar, O. D., Horwith, M., and Sleisinger, M. H. (1960). *Metab. Clin. Exp.* **9,** 1093.

Coburn, J. W., Brickman, A. S., Kurokawa, K., Massry, S. G., Bethune, J. E., Harrison, H. H., and Norman, A. W. (1974). *In Endocrinology 1973* (S. Taylor, ed.), pp. 385–392. Heinemann, London.

Cochrane, W. A., Morse, W. I., and Landrigan, P. (1960). *Am. J. Dis. Child.* **100,** 544.

Cockburn, F., Brown, J. K., Belton, N. R., and Forfar, J. O. (1973). *Arch. Dis. Child.* **48,** 99.

Codaccioni, J. L., Payalodan, A., Saier, J., and Gastaut, H. (1974). *Ann. Endocrinol.* **35,** 591.

Coenegracht, J. M., and Houben, H. G. J. (1974). *Clin. Chim. Acta* **50,** 349.

Coffey, R. J., Potter, J. F., and Canary, J. J. (1965). *Ann. Surg.* **161,** 732.

Cohen, M. L., and Donnell, G. N. (1960). *J. Pediatr.* **56,** 369.

Cohen, R. D., and Vince, F. P. (1969). *Arch. Dis. Child.* **44,** 96.

Colletti, R. B., Pan, M. W., Smith, E. W. P., and Genel, M. (1974). *N. Engl. J. Med.* **290,** 931.

Collins-Williams, C. (1950). *Pediatrics* **5,** 998.

Collip, J. B., and Backus, P. L. (1920). *Am. J. Physiol.* **51,** 568.

Collip, J. B. (1935). *Ann. Intern. Med.* **9,** 150.

Comin, D. B., Hines, J. D., and Wieland, R. G. (1969). *J. Am. Med. Assoc.* **207,** 1147.

Conaway, H. H., and Anast, C. S. (1974). *J. Lab. Clin. Med.* **83,** 129.

Connelly, J. P., Crawford, J. D., and Watson, J. (1962). *Pediatrics* **30,** 425.

Connor, T. B., Toskes, P., Mahaffey, J., Martin, L. G., Williams, J. B., and Walser, M. (1972). *Johns Hopkins Med. J.* **131,** 100.

Conrad, L. L., and Baxter, D. J. (1966). *Am. J. Physiol.* **210,** 831.

Cook, P. B., Nassim, J. R., and Collins, J. (1959). *Q. J. Med.* **28,** 505.

Cope, O. (1960). *Am. J. Surg.* **99,** 394.

Cope, O. (1966). *N. Engl. J. Med.* **274,** 1174.

Copp, D. H., Moghadam, H., Mensen, E. D., and McPherson, G. D. (1961). *In* "The Parathyroids" (R. O. Greep and R. V. Talmage, eds.), pp. 203–219. Thomas Springfield, Illinois.

Corvilain, J., and Abramow, M. (1962). *J. Clin. Invest.* **41,** 1230.

Costello, J. M., and Dent, C. E. (1963). *Arch. Dis. Child.* **38,** 397.

Coulson, R., and Moses, A. M. (1975). *J. Pharmacol. Exp. Ther.* **194,** 603.

Courpron, P., Meunier, P., Edouard, C., Bernard, J., Bringuier, J. P., and Vignon, G. (1973). *Rev. Rhum.* **40,** 469.

Courvoisier, B., Martin, E., Bopp, J., and Vernet, A. (1956). *Sem. Hop.* **32,** 2127.

Craig, J. M., Schiff, L. H., and Boone, J. E. (1955). *Am. J. Dis. Child.* **89,** 669.

Crawford, J. D., Gribetz, D., Diner, W. C., Hurst, P., and Castleman, B. (1957). *J. Clin. Endocrinol. Metab.* **61,** 59.

Curtis, J. C., Dodge, W. F., and Daeschner, C. W. (1962). *Pediatrics* **29,** 52.

Cushard, W. G., Jr., Creditor, M. A., Canterbury, J. M., and Reiss, E. (1972). *J. Clin. Endocrinol. Metab.* **34,** 767.

Czekalski, S., Loreau, N., Paillard, F., Ardaillou, R., Fillastre, J. P., and Mallet, F. (1974). *Europ. J. Clin. Invest.* **4,** 85.

Dahl, J. R., McFadden, S. D., and Eisenberg, E. (1962). *Ann. Intern. Med.* **57,** 635.

Dahlmann, W., and Prill, A. (1974). *Z. Neurol.* **206,** 223.

Dancaster, C. P., Schendel, H. E., and Jackson, W. P. U. (1960). *Clin. Sci.* **19,** 563.

Danowski, T. S., Lasser, E. C., and Wechsler, R. L. (1960). *Metab. Clin. Exp.* **9,** 1064.

David, L., and Anast, C. S. (1973). *Clin. Aspects Metab. Bone Dis. Proc. Int. Symp., 1972* (Int. Congr. Ser. No. 270), pp. 661–666.

Davies, D. R., and Friedman, M. (1966). *J. Bone Jt. Surg.* **48,** 117.

Davies, M. (1976). *Abstr. Eur. Symp. on Calcified Tissues, 12th,* 4–8 July, *1976* York, p. 19.

Davis, R. H. (1961). *Proc. R. Soc. Med.* **54,** 970.

Davis, R. H., Fourman, P., and Smith, J. W. G. (1961). *Lancet* **2,** 1432.

De Backer, M., Manderlier, T., Nijs-Dewolf, N., Six, R., and Corvilain, J. (1974). *Biomedicine* **21,** 338.

Deftos, L. J., Powell, D., Parthemore, J. G., and Potts, J. T., Jr. (1973). *J. Clin. Invest.* **52,** 3109.

Deftos, L. J., Swenson, K., and Bode, H. (1972). *Clin. Res.,* **20,** 424.

DeGroote, J. W. (1969). *J. Am. Med. Assoc.* **208,** 2160.

Delong, A., Feinblatt, J., and Rasmussen, H. (1971). *Calcif. Tissue Res.* **8,** 87.

Delore, X., and Alamartine, H. (1910). *Rev. Chir.* *(Paris)* **30,** 540.

DeLuca, H. F., Morii, H., and Melancon, M. J., Jr. (1968). *In* "Parathyroid Hormone and Thyrocalcitonin Calcitonin" (R. V. Talmage and L. F. Bèlanger, eds.), Int. Congr. Ser. No. 159, pp. 448–454. Excerpta Med. Found., Amsterdam.

DeLuca, H. F., Holick, S. A., and Holick, M. F. (1975). *Calcified Tissues 1975. In* "Calcified Tissues 1975." (S. P. Nielsen and E. Hjorting-Hansen, eds.), pp. 128–135. Fadl's Forlag, Copenhagen.

Denniston, J. C., and Son, C. D. (1963). *J. Tenn. Med. Assoc.* **56,** 436.

Dent, C. E. (1953). *Proc. R. Soc. Med.* **46,** 291.

Dent, C. E. (1962). *Br. Med. J.* **2,** 1495.

Dent, C. E., and Friedman, M. (1964). *Lancet* **2,** 164.

Dent, C. E., and Garretts, M. (1960). *Lancet* **1,** 142.

Dent, C. E., and Harper, C. M. (1958). *Proc. R. Soc. Med.* **51,** 489.

Dent, C. E., and Harper, C. M. (1962). *Lancet* **1,** 559.

Dent, C. E., Harper, C. M., Morgans, M. E., Philpot, G. R., and Trotter, W. R. (1955). *Lancet* **2,** 687.

de Quervain, F. (1923). *Bruns' Beitr. Klin. Chir.* **128,** 197.

Deren, J. J., Williams, L. A., Muench, H., Chalmers, T., and Zamcheck, N. (1964). *N. Engl. J. Med.* **270,** 1277.

de Sèze, S., Hioco, D., Hubault, A., Solnica, J., Rouaud, J. P., and Degavre, D. (1972a). *Rev. Rhum. Mal. Osteo-Articulaires* **39,** 50.

de Sèze, S., Solnica, J., Mitrovic, D., Miravet, L., and Dorfmann, H. (1972b). *Semin. Arthritis Rheum.* **2,** 71.

Diaz-Buxo, J. A., and Knox, F. G. (1975). *Mayo Clin. Proc.* **50,** 537.

Dickson, L. G., Morita, Y., Cowsert, E. J., Graves, J., and Meyer, J. S. (1960). *J. Neurol., Neurosurg. Psychiatry* **23**, 33.

DiGeorge, A. M. (1965). *J. Pediatr.* **67**, 907.

DiGeorge, A. M. (1968). *Birth Defects, Orig. Artic. Ser.* **4**, 116.

DiGeorge, A. M., and Paschkis, K. (1957). *Am. J. Dis. Child.* **94**, 476.

Dimich, A., Bedrossian, P. B., and Wallach, S. (1967). *Arch. Intern. Med.* **120**, 449.

Dohan, P. H., Yamashita, K., Larsen, P. R., Davis, B., Deftos, L., and Field, J. B. (1972). *J. Clin. Endocrinol. Metab.* **35**, 775.

Doppman, J. L., Marx, S. J., Spiegel, A. M., Mallette, L. E., Wolfe, D. R., Aurbach, G. D., and Geelhoed, G. (1975). *Radiology* **115**, 37.

Dorra, M., Waynberger, M., Lardy, P., Normand, J. P., Bordier, P., and Bouvrain, Y. (1971). *Presse Med.* **79**, 1381.

Dousa, T. B. (1974). *Am. J. Physiol.* **226**, 1193.

Dousa, T., and Rychlik, I. (1968). *Biochim. Biophys. Acta* **158**, 484.

Drake, T. G., Albright, F., Bauer, W., and Castleman, B. (1939). *Ann. Intern. Med.* **12**, 1751.

Drezner, M. K., and Neelon, F. A. (1976). *Clin. Res.* **24**, 28A.

Drezner, M., Neelon, F. A., and Lebovitz, H. E. (1973). *N. Engl. J. Med.* **289**, 1056.

Drezner, M. K., Neelon, F. A., Hanssler, M., McPherson, H. T., and Lebovitz, H. E. (1976). *J. Clin. Endocrinol. Metab.* **42**, 621.

Drury, M. I., Keelan, D. M., Timoney, F. J., and Irvine, W. J. (1970). *Clin. Exp. Immunol.* **7**, 125.

Dudley, A. W., and Hawkins, H. (1970). *J. Neurol., Neurosurg. Psychiatry* **33**, 147.

Dudley, H. R., Ritchie, A. C., Schilling, A., and Baker, W. H. (1955). *N. Engl. J. Med.* **252**, 331.

Dufresne, L. R., and Gitelman, H. J. (1972). *In* "Calcium Parathyroid Hormone and the Calcitonins," (R. V. Talmage and P. L. Munson, eds.), Int. Congr. Ser. No. 243, pp. 202–206. Excerpta Med. Found., Amsterdam.

Dull, T. A., and Henneman, P. H. (1963). *N. Engl. J. Med.* **268**, 132.

Durlach, J., and Lebrun, R. (1959). *C. R. Sciences Soc. Biol.* **153**, 1973.

Durlach, J., Gremy, F., and Metral, S. (1967). *Rev. Neurol.* **117**, 177.

Durlach, J., Cordier, M. L., and Henrotte, J. G. (1971). *In* "Le déficit magnésique en pathologie humaine" (J. Durlach, ed.), pp. 135–162. S.G.E.M.V., Vittel.

Dymling, J. F. (1964). *Acta Med. Scand.* **175**, Suppl. 408.

Dymling, J. F., and Ryd, H. (1968). *Acta Med. Scand.* **184**, 333.

Dziak, R., and Stern, P. H. (1975). *Endocrinology* **97**, 1281.

Edmondson, J. W., Brashear, R. E., and Li, T. K. (1975). *Am. J. Physiol.* **228**, 1082.

Eipe, J., Johnson, S. A., Kiamko, R. T., and Bronsky, D. (1968). *Arch. Intern. Med.* **121**, 270.

Eisenberg, E. (1965). *J. Clin. Invest.* **44**, 942.

Eisenberg, E. (1968). *J. Clin. Endocrinol. Metab.* **28**, 651.

Eisinger, J., Dell'anno, R., and Laponche, A. M. (1969). *Rhumatologie* **21**, 47.

Eliel, L. P., Thomsen, C., and Chanes, R. (1965). *J. Clin. Endocrinol. Metab.* **25**, 457.

Eliel, L. P., Palmieri, G. M. A., Thompson, J. S., Bird, P. C., and Hawrylko, J. (1971). *Pediatrics* **47**, 229.

Ellsworth, R., and Howard, J. E. (1934). *Bull. Johns Hopkins Hosp.* **55**, 296.

Ellwood, M. G., and Robb, G. H. (1971). *Postgrad. Med. J.* **47**, 129.

Elrick, H., Albright, F., Bartter, F. C., Forbes, A. P., and Reeves, J. D. (1950). *Acta Endocrinol. Copenhagen (Kbh)* **5**, 199.

Emanuelli, G., and Pellegrini, A. (1968). *Minerva Med.* **59**, 681.

Emerson, K., Jr., Walsh, F. B., and Howard, J. E. (1941). *Ann. Intern. Med.* **14,** 1256.

Engel, E., Haenni, A., and Ducommun, P. (1956). *Schweiz. Med. Wochenschr.* **86,** 1260.

Enthoven, R. (1960). *Ned. T. Geneeskd.* **104,** 1994.

Eraut, D. (1974). *Br. Med. J.* **1,** 429.

Erdheim, J. (1906). *Mitt. Grenzgeb. Med. Chir.* **16,** 632.

Erdheim, J. (1911). *Frankfurt. Z. Path.* **7,** 175.

Ertel, N. H., Reiss, J. S., and Spergel, G. (1969). *N. Engl. J. Med.* **280,** 260.

Esselstyn, C. B., Jr., and Popowniak, K. L. (1971). *Surg. Clin. North Am.* **51,** 1211.

Estep, H., Shaw, W. A., Watlington, C., Hobe, R., Holland, W., and Tucker, S. G. (1969). *J. Clin. Endocrinol. Metab.* **29,** 842.

Estep, H. L., Gardner, C. T., Jr., Taylor, J. P., Minott, A., and Tucker, H. S. G., Jr. (1965). *J. Clin. Endocrinol. Metab.* **25,** 1385.

Esterly, N. B., Brammer, S. R., and Crounse, R. G. (1967). *J. Invest. Dermatol.* **49,** 246.

Evans, I. M. A., Boulton-Jones, M., Doyle, F. H., Joplin, G. F., Lockwood, M., Matthews, E. W., and MacIntyre, I. (1975). *Calcified Tissues 1975. In* "Calcified Tissues 1975" (S. P. Nielsen and E. Hjorting-Hansen, eds.), Fadl's Forlag, Copenhagen, pp. 236–241.

Evans, W. E., Armstrong, R. G., and Dawson, R. G. (1968). *Am. J. Surg.* **116,** 456.

Evanson, J. M. (1966). *Clin. Sci.* **31,** 63.

Eyre, W. G., and Reed, W. B. (1971). *Arch. Dermatol.* **104,** 632.

Fabbrini, A., Ramorino, M. L., and Naccarato, R. (1958). *Folia Endocrinol.* **11,** 545.

Fahraeus, B., Andersson, L., Bergdahl, L., and Westling, P. (1973). *Acta Chir. Scand.* **139,** 437.

Fairney, A., and Weir, A. A. (1970). *J. Endocrinol.* **48,** 337.

Fairney, A., Jackson, D., and Clayton, B. E. (1973). *Arch. Dis. Child.* **48,** 419.

Fanconi, A. (1969). *Ergeb. Inn. Med. Kinderheilk.* **28,** 54.

Fanconi, A., and Prader, A. (1967). *Helv. Paediatr. Acta* **4,** 342.

Fanconi, A., and Rose, G. A. (1958). *Q. J. Med.* **27,** 463.

Fanconi, A., Henrich, H. G., and Prader, A. (1964). *Helv. Paediatr. Acta* **19,** 181.

Farriaux, J. P., Delmas, Y., Ropartz, C., and Fontaine, G. (1975). *Nouv. Presse Med.* **4,** 589.

Favus, M. J., Kimberg, D. V., Millar, G. N., and Gershon, E. (1973a). *J. Clin. Invest.* **52,** 1328.

Favus, M. J., Walling, M. W., and Kimberg, D. V. (1973b). *J. Clin. Invest.* **52,** 1680.

Felitti, V. J., and McAfee, L. L. (1968). *Johns Hopkins Med. J.* **123,** 271.

Felman, A. H., and Kirkpatrick, J. A., Jr. (1969). *Radiology* **93,** 1037.

Felts, J. H., Whitley, J. E., Anderson, D. D., Carpenter, H. M., and Bradshaw, H. H. (1965). *Ann. Intern. Med.* **62,** 1272.

Ferris, J. A. J. (1973). *Brit. Med. J.* **2,** 23.

Ferris, J. A. J., Aherne, W. A., Locke, W. S., McQuillin, J., and Gardner, P. S. (1973). *Br. Med. J.* **2,** 439.

Fichman, M. P., and Brooker, G. (1972). *J. Clin. Endocrinol. Metab.* **35,** 35.

Fields, J. P., Fragola, L., and Hadley, T. P. (1971). *Arch. Dermatol.* **103,** 687.

Fine, R. N., Rosoff, L., Grushkin, C. M., Donnell, G. N., and Lieberman, E. (1970). *J. Pediatr.* **76,** 32.

Firschein, H. E. (1962). *Invest. Ophtal.* **1,** 788.

Fischer, J. A., Blum, J. W., and Binswanger, U. (1973). *J. Clin. Invest.* **52,** 2434.

Fisher, M., and Fitzpatrick, T. B. (1970). *Arch. Dermatol.* **102,** 110.

Fisher, A. L., Parfitt, A. M., and Lloyd, H. M. (1969). *Calcif. Tissue Res.* **4,** 283.

Fonseca, O. A., and Calverly, J. R. (1967). *Arch. Intern. Med.* **120,** 202.

Forbes, A. P. (1962). *Endocrinol. Nutr.* **6**, 111.

Forbes, A. P. (1964). *N. Engl. J. Med.* **270**, 1268.

Forbes, A. P., and Engel, E. (1963). *Metab.* **12**, 428.

Forbes, G. B. (1956). *Ann. N.Y. Acad. Sci.* **64**, 432.

Ford, C. E., Jones, K. W., Polani, P. E., de Almeida, J. C., and Briggs, J. H. (1959). *Lancet* **1**, 711.

Fourman, P. (1969). *Acta Clin. Belg.* **24**, 129.

Fourman, P., Davis, R. H., Jones, K. H., Morgan, D. B., and Smith, J. W. G. (1963). *Brit. J. Surg.* **50**, 608.

Fourman, P., Rawnsley, K., Davis, R. H., Jones, K. H., and Morgan, D. B. (1967). *Lancet* **2**, 914.

Fragola, L. (1971). Discussion, in Field's *et al.* (1971).

Frame, B. (1965). *Arch. Intern. Med.* **116**, 424.

Frame, B., Fruchtman, M., and Smith, R. W., Jr. (1962). *N. Engl. J. Med.* **267**, 1112.

Frame, B., Hanson, C. A., Frost, H. M., Block, M., and Arnstein, A. R. (1972). *Am. J. Med.* **52**, 311.

Frame, B., and Parfitt, A. M. (1973). *In* "Clinical Aspects of Metabolic Bone Disease." (B. Frame, A. M. Parfitt, and H. Duncan, eds.) Int. Congr. Ser. No. 270, pp. 454–464. Excerpta Med. Found., Amsterdam.

Fraser, R., Harrison, M., and Ibbertson, K. (1960). *Q. J. Med.* **29**, 85.

Fratkin, M., Smith, P., and Estep, H. (1972). *Clin. Res.* **20**, 426.

Frech, R. S., and McAlister, W. H. (1970). *Am. J. Dis. Child.* **119**, 447.

Freeman, G. C. (1970). *Surg. Clin. North Am.* **70**, 409.

Freeman, M., Giuliani, M., Schwartz, E., and Gomprecht, R. F. (1969). *N.Y. State J. Med.* **69**, 2036.

Freeman, S., and Breen, M. (1960). *Clin. Orthop. Relat. Res.* **17**, 186.

Frensilli, J. A., Stoner, R. E., and Hinrichs, E. H. (1971). *J. Oral Surg.* **29**, 727.

Freyberg, R. H., Grant, R. L., and Robb, M. A. (1936). *J. Am. Med. Assoc.* **107**, 1769.

Friderichsen, C. (1938). *Monatsschr. Kinderheilkd.* **75**, 146.

Friderichsen, C. (1939). *Lancet* **1**, 85.

Friderichsen, C., and Rosendal, T. (1968). *Lancet* **1**, 757.

Friedlaender, A. (1930). *Acta Paediatr. Scand.* **9**, 129.

Friedman, M., Hatcher, G., and Watson, L. (1967). *Lancet*, **1**, 703.

Friis, T., and Hahnemann, S. (1964). *Acta Med. Scand.* **176**, 711.

Froeling, P. G. A. M., and Bijvoet, O. L. M. (1974). *Neth. J. Med.* **17**, 174.

Frost, H. M., Villanueva, A. R. and Ilnicki, L. (1968). *In* "Parathyroid Hormone and Thyrocalcitonin (Calcitonin)" (R. V. Talmage, and L. F. Bélanger, eds.) Int. Congr. Ser. No. 159, pp. 123–136. Excerpta Med. Found., Amsterdam.

Fujita, T., Orimo, H., Okano, K., Yoshikawa, M., Shimo, R., Inoue, T., and Itami, Y. (1972). *Endocrinol. Jpn.* **19**, 571.

Fujita, T., Orimo, H., and Yoshikawa, M. (1966). *Endocrinol Jpn.* **13**, 338.

Funk, C., Ammann, R., Binswanger, U., Mayor, G., Bihrer, R., Clavadetscher, P., Fumagalli, I., Leemann, A., Seiler, P., and Stuby, K. (1974). *Schweiz. Med. Wochenschr.* **104**, 1060.

Gallagher, J. C., and Nordin, B. E. C. (1972). *Lancet* **1**, 503.

Gallagher, J. C., and Wilkinson, R. (1973). *Clin. Sci. Mol. Med.* **45**, 785.

Garabedian, M., Tanaka, Y., Holick, M. F., and DeLuca, H. F. (1974). *Endocrinology* **94**, 1022.

Garceau, G. J., and Miller, W. E. (1956). *J. Bone Jt. Surg. Am. Vol.* **38**, 131.

Gardner, E. J., and Richards, R. C. (1953). *Am. J. Hum. Genet.* **5**, 139.

Gardner, L. I. (1970). *Lancet* **2**, 879.
Garn, S. M., Hertzog, K. P., Poznanski, A. K., and Nagy, J. M. (1972). *Radiology* **105**, 375.
Gass, J. D. M. (1962). *Am. J. Ophthalmol.* **54**, 660.
Gatau-Pelanchon, J., Bernard, P. M., and Gèrard, R. (1969). *Marseille Med.* **106**, 175.
Gay, J. D. L., and Grimes, J. D. (1972). *Can. Med. Assoc. J.* **107**, 54.
Geertinger, P. (1967). *Pediatrics* **39**, 43.
Genuth, S. M., and Klein, L. (1972). *J. Clin. Endocrinol. Metab.* **35**, 693.
George, W. K., Smith, J. P., George, W. D., Jr., Baird, E. E., Gordon, F. T., and Fisher, R. G. (1963). *N. Engl. J. Med.* **268**, 958.
Gerloczy, F., and Farkas, K. (1953). *Acta Med. Acad. Sci. Hung.* **4**, 73.
Gershberg, H., and Weseley, A. C. (1960). *J. Pediatr.* **56**, 383.
Gershberg, H., Mari, S., and St. Paul, H. (1966). *Metab. Clin. Exp.* **15**, 206.
Gibson, R. (1961). *Can. Med. Assoc. J.* **85**, 70.
Gilbert-Dreyfus, Zara, M., and Gali, P. (1958). *Sem. Hop.* **34**, 1301.
Gill, J. R., Jr., and Casper, A. G. T. (1971). *J. Clin. Invest.* **50**, 1231.
Gilmour, J. R. (1938). *J. Pathol. Bacteriol.* **46**, 133.
Giraud, J., Atlan, D., et Giudicelli, P. (1967). *Electrodiagnostic-Thérapie* **4**, 221.
Girling, J. A., and Murley, R. S. (1963). *Br. Med. J.* **1**, 1323.
Gitelman, H. J., Kukoly, S., and Welt, L. G. (1968). *Am. J. Physiol.* **215**, 483.
Gittes, R. F., Munson, P. L., and Toverud, S. U. (1966). *Fed. Proc., Fed. Am. Soc. Exp. Biol.* **25**, 496.
Gittes, R. F., Toverud, S. U., and Cooper, C. W. (1968). *Endocrinology* **82**, 83.
Gittleman, I. F., Pinkus, J. B., and Schmertzler, E. (1964). *Am. J. Dis. Child.* **107**, 119.
Giudicelli, P., Atlan, D., and Jacquin-Cotton, L. (1967). *Marseille Med.* **104**, 463.
Gley, E. (1891). *C. R. Sciences Soc. Biol. Ses.* **3**, 843.
Goeminne, L. (1965). *Acta Genet. Med. Gemellol.* **14**, 226.
Goldring, S. R., Dayer, J.-M., Russell, R. G. G., Mankin, H. J., and Krane, S. M. (1978). *J. Clin. Endocrinol. Metab.* **36**, 425.
Goldsmith, R. E., King, L. R., Zalme, E., and Bahr, G. K. (1968). *Acta Endocrinol. Copenhagen (Kbh)* **58**, 565.
Goldsmith, R. S., Siemsen, A. W., Mason, A. D., Jr., and Forland, M. (1965). *J. Clin. Endocrinol. Metab.* **25**, 1649.
Golonka, J. E., and Goodman, A. D. (1968). *J. Clin. Endocrinol. Metab.* **28**, 79.
Goltzman, D., Peytremann, A., Callahan, E., Tregear, G. W., and Potts, J. T., Jr. (1975). *J. Biol. Chem.* **250**, 3199.
Gomez, M. R., Engel, A. G., and Dyck, P. J. (1972). *Neurology* **22**, 849.
Gorbman, A. (1950). *J. Clin. Endocrinol.* **10**, 1177.
Gordon, H. E., Coburn, J. W., and Passaro, E., Jr. (1972). *Arch. Surg. (Chicago)* **104**, 520.
Gorlin, R. J., and Sedano, H. O. (1971). *Mod. Med (Minneapolis)* **39**, 166.
Gorlin, R. J., Vickers, R. A., Kelln, E., and Williamson, J. J. (1965). *Cancer* **18**, 89.
Gorman, C. A., Hermans, P. E., Martin, W. J., and Kelly, P. J. (1962). *Proc. Staff Meet. Mayo Clin.* **37**, 530.
Gorodischer, R., Aceto, T., Jr., and Terplan, K. (1970). *Am. J. Dis. Child.* **119**, 74.
Goto, I. (1974). *Clin. Chim. Acta* **52**, 27.
Goulding, A., Jukes, C., McChesney, R., and Irvine, R. O. H. (1973). *J. Endocrinol.* **58**, 127.
Gounelle, H., Gulat-Marnay, C., Fauchet, M., and Mollereau, M. (1970). *Ann. Med. Interne* **121**, 471.
Graham, S. G., and Anderson, G. H. (1924). *Lancet* **1**, 1307.
Granström, K. O., and Hed, R. (1965). *Acta Med. Scand.* **178**, 417.
Grant, D. K. (1953). *Q. J. Med.* **22**, 243.
Gray, T. K., and Gitelman, H. J. (1973). *Clin. Res.* **21**, 43.

Greene, J. A., and Swanson, L. W. (1941). *Ann. Intern. Med.* **14**, 1233.

Greenwald, I. (1913). *J. Biol. Chem.* **14**, 369.

Greenwald, I. (1922). *J. Biol. Chem.* **54**, 285.

Griffin, J. H. (1965). *Am. J. Dis. Child.* **110**, 672.

Grosser, P., and Betke, R. (1911). *Z. Kinderheilkd.* **1**, 458.

Groth, C. G., Popovtzer, M., Hammond, W. S., Cascardo, S., Iwatsuki, S., Halgrimson, C. G., and Starzl, T. E. (1973). *Lancet* **1**, 1082.

Gruson, M., Miravet, L., and Hioco, D. (1967). *Ann. Biol. Clin. (Paris)* **25**, 711.

Gsell, O. (1950). *Dtsch. Med. Wschr.* **75**, 1117.

Gudmundsson, T. V., Galante, L., Horton, R., Matthews, E. W., Woodhouse, N. J. Y., MacIntyre, I., and Nagant de Deuxchaisnes, C. (1970). *Calcitonin 1969. In* "Endocrinology 1969 (S. Taylor and G. Foster, eds.), pp. 102–109. Heinemann, London.

Guilleminault, C., Peraita, R., Souquet, M., and Dement, W. C. (1975). *Science* **190**, 677.

Haff, R. C., Black, W. C., and Ballinger, W. F., II (1970). *Ann. Surg.* **171**, 85.

Hagen, G. A., Hoffman, D. L., and Rosevear, J. W. (1964). *J. Clin. Endocrinol. Metab.* **24**, 1244.

Hahn, T. J., Chase, L. R., and Avioli, L. (1972). *J. Clin. Invest.* **51**, 886.

Haljamäe, H., and MacDowall, I. G. (1972). *Acta Paediatr. Scand.* **61**, 591.

Hallick, R. B., and DeLuca, H. F. (1971). *J. Biol. Chem.*, **246**, 5733.

Hällström, T. (1967). *Heredität* **58**, 325.

Halmos, V., Kendall, J. M., and Ogryzlo, M. A. (1962). *Can. Med. Assoc. J.* **87**, 173.

Halsted, W. S., and Evans, H. M. (1907). *Ann. Surg.* **46**, 489.

Halver, B. (1966). *Acta Med. Scand.* **180**, 377.

Halver, B. (1967). *Acta Med. Scand.* **181**, 209.

Harden, R. M., Harrison, M. T., and Alexander, W. D. (1963). *Clin. Sci.* **25**, 27.

Hardin, W. J., and Hardy, J. D. (1971). *Surg., Gynecol. Obstet.* **132**, 450.

Harell-Steinberg, A., Ziprkowski, L., Haim, S., Gafni, J., and Levin, M. (1957). *J. Clin. Endocrinol. Metab.* **17**, 1099.

Harris, M., Jenkins, M. V., and Wills, M. R. (1974). *Br. J. Pharmacol.* **50**, 405.

Harrison, H. E. (1970). *Mod. Treat.* **7**, 636.

Harrison, H. E., and Harrison, H. C. (1972). *J. Clin. Invest.* **51**, 1919.

Harrison, H. E., Lifshitz, F., and Blizzard, R. M. (1967). *N. Engl. J. Med.* **276**, 894.

Harrold, C. C., and Wright, J. (1966). *Am. J. Surg.* **112**, 482.

Hartemann, P., Leclere, J., Mollet, E., Wiolland, M., Weyland, M., and Thomas, J. L. (1971). *Ann. Med. Nancy* **10**, 1349.

Haussler, M. R. (1975). *In* "Vitamin D and Problems Related to Uremic Bone Disease" (A. W. Norman *et al.*, eds.), pp. 25–42. de Gruyter, Berlin.

Haussler, M. R., Lightner, E. S., Brumbaugh, P. F., Hughes, M. R., and Bursac, K. (1975). *Clin. Res.* **23**, 155A.

Hawker, C. D. (1975). *Ann. Clin. Lab. Sci.*, **5**, 383.

Heaney, R. P., and Whedon, G. D. (1958). *J. Clin. Endocrinol. Metab.* **18**, 1246.

Heath, D. A., Palmer, J. S., and Aurbach, G. D. (1972). *J. Clin. Endocrinol. Metab.* **90**, 1589.

Heaton, F. W., and Fourman, P. (1965). *Lancet* **2**, 50.

Heaton, L. D., Beisel, W. R., Sprinz, H., and Forsee, J. H. (1962). *Ann. Surg.* **155**, 90.

Heersche, J. N. M., Fedak, S. A., and Aurbach, G. D. (1971). *J. Biol. Chem.* **246**, 6770.

Heidbreder, E., Kappel, W., and Heidland, A. (1975). *Res. Exp. Med.* **165**, 93.

Hellman, D. E., Au, W. F., and Bartter, F. C. (1965). *Am. J. Physiol.* **209**, 643.

Hellström, J., and Ivemark, B. I. (1962). *Acta Chir. Scand.*, *Suppl.* **294**.

Hélou, A., Tyan, E., and Zara, M. (1964). *Ann. Endocrinol.* **25**, 238.

Henkin, R. I. (1968). *J. Clin. Endocrinol. Metab.* **28**, 624.

Henneman, P. M., Carroll, E. L., and Albright, F. (1956). *Ann. N.Y. Acad. Sci.* **64**, 343.

Hermans, P. E., Gorman, C. A., Martin, W. J., and Kelly, P. J. (1964). *Mayo Clin. Proc.* **39**, 81.

Hermans, P. E., Ulrich, J. A., and Markowitz, H. (1969). *Am. J. Med.* **47**, 503.

Hermier, M., Moulin, G., Pouillaude, J. M., Hermier, C., Frederich, A., and François, R. (1972). *Arch. Fr. Pediatr.* **29**, 771.

Herrmann-Erlee, M. P. M., and Konijn, T. M. (1970). *Nature (London)* **227**, 177.

Herrmann-Erlee, M. P. M., and van der Meer, J. M. (1974). *Endocrinology* **94**, 424.

Herrmann-Erlee, M. P. M., Hekkelman, J. W., Heersche, J. N. M., and Nijweide, P. J. (1975). *J. Endocrinol.* **64**, 69P.

Hertzog, K. P. (1968). *Acta Genet. Med. Gemellol.* **17**, 428.

Hiatt, H. H., and Thompson, D. D. (1957). *J. Clin. Invest.* **36**, 557.

Hillman, L. S., and Haddad, J. G. (1974). *J. Pediatr.* **84**, 742.

Himsworth, H. P., and Maizels, M. (1940). *Lancet* **1**, 959.

Hinkle, D. O., Travis, L. B., and Dodge, W. F. (1965). *Tex. Rep. Biol. Med.* **23**, 463.

Hioco, D. (1974). *Concours Med.* **96**, 3461.

Hirano, K., Ishibashi, A., and Yoshino, Y. (1974). *Arch. Dermatol.* **109**, 242.

Hoesch, K. (1937). *Dtsch. Med. Wochenschr.* **63**, 1582.

Höffken, B., Parkinson, D. K., Storms, P., and Radde, I. C. (1971). *Clin. Orthop. Relat. Res.* **78**, 30.

Hoffman, E. (1958). *Am. J. Surg.* **96**, 33.

Holt, M., and Oram, S. (1960). *Br. Heart J.* **22**, 236.

Holtz, F., Gissel, H., and Roszmann, R. (1934). *Dtsch. Z. Chir.* **242**, 521.

Homer, L. (1961). *J. Clin. Endocrinol. Metab.* **21**, 219.

Hooper, M. J., Carter, J. N., and Stiel, J. N. (1973). *Med. J. Aust.* **1**, 990.

Hortling, H., Puupponen, E., and Koski, K. (1960). *J. Clin. Endocrinol. Metab.* **20**, 466.

Horwitz, C. A., Myers, W. P. L., and Foote, F. W., Jr. (1972). *Am. J. Med.* **52**, 797.

Hossain, M. (1970a). *J. Neurol., Neurosurg. Psychiatry* **33**, 153.

Hossain, M. (1970b). *Lancet* **1**, 1149.

Howard, J. E., and Meyer, R. J. (1948). *J. Clin. Endocrinol.* **8**, 895.

Howard, J. E., Hopkins, T. R., and Connor, T. D. (1953a). *J. Clin. Endocrinol. Metab.* **13**, 1.

Howard, J. E., Follis, R. H., Jr., Yendt, E. R., and Connor, T. B. (1953b). *J. Clin. Endocrinol. Metab.* **13**, 997.

Hower, J., Struck, H., Tackmann, W., and Stolecke, H. (1972). *N. Engl. J. Med.* **287**, 1098.

Hower, J., Maruhn, D., and Struck, H. (1974a). *Dtsch. Med. Wochenschr.* **99**, 14.

Hower, J., Struck, H., Tackmann, W., and Bohlmann, H. G. (1974b). *Z. Kinderheilkd.* **116**, 193.

Hsien-Yi, C., Chün, C., and Wei, Y. (1964). *Chin. Med. J.* **83**, 723.

Huber, J., Cholnoky, P., and Zoethout, H. E. (1967). *Arch. Dis. Child.* **42**, 190.

Hung, W., Migeon, C. J., and Parrot, R. H. (1963). *N. Engl. J. Med.* **269**, 658.

Hunt, G., and Morgan, D. B. (1970). *Clin. Sci.* **38**, 713.

Hurvitz, R. J., Perzik, S. L., and Morgenstern, L. (1968). *Arch. Surg. (Chicago)* **97**, 723.

Hurwitz, L. J. (1956). *Lancet* **1**, 234.

Husdan, H., Rapoport, A., and Locke, S. (1973). *Metab. Clin. Exp.* **22**, 787.

Husdan, H., Rapoport, A., Locke, S., and Oreopoulos, D. (1974). *Clin. Chem.* **20**, 529.

Ikkala, E., Siurala, M., and Viranko, M. (1964). *Acta Med. Scand.* **176**, 73.

Imbert, M., Chabardés, D., and Morel, F. (1974). *Mol. Cell. Endocrinol.* **1**, 295.

Ireland, A. W., Clubb, J. S., Neale, F. C., Posen, S., and Reeve, T. S. (1968a). *Ann. Intern. Med.* **69**, 81.

Ireland, A. W., Hornbrook, J. W., Neale, F. C., and Posen, S. (1968b). *Arch. Intern. Med.* **122**, 408.

Irvine, W. J., and Barnes, E. W. (1972). *Clin. Endocrinol. Λetab.* **1**, 549.

Irvine, W. J., and Scarth, L. (1969). *Clin. Exp. Immunol.* **4**, 505.

Irvine, W. J., Chan, M. M. W., Scarth, L., Kolb, F. O., Hartog, M., Bayliss, R. I. S., and Drury, M. I. (1968). *Lancet* **2**, 883.

Iversen, K., Friis, T., Fuchs, F., and Hansen, T. S. (1957). *Dan. Med. Bull.* **4**, 4.

Jackson, W. P. U. (1957). *Lancet* **1**, 1086.

Jackson, W. P. U., and Dancaster, C. P. (1962). *Metab. Clin. Exp.* **11**, 123.

Jackson, W. P. U., Hanelin, J., and Albright, F. (1954). *Arch. Intern. Med.* **94**, 886.

Jackson, W. P. U., Hoffenberg, R., Linder, G. C., and Irwin, L. (1956). *J. Clin. Endocrinol. Metab.* **16**, 1043.

Jacob, S. W., and Dunphy, J. E. (1963). *Am. J. Surg.* **105**, 196.

Jaffe, H. L. (1943). *Arch. Pathol.* **36**, 335.

Jancar, J. (1965). *J. Med. Genet.* **2**, 32.

Jeandelize, P. M. P. (1902). "Insuffisance Thyroïdienne et Parathyroïdienne." Humblot et Simon, Nancy.

Jehanne, M. and Guirvarch, J. (1974). *Ouest Med.* **27**, 313.

Jellinek, (1971). Discussion, in Fields *et al.* (1971).

Jelonek, A. (1975). *Calcified Tissues 1975 In* "Calcified Tissues 1975" (S. P. Nielsen and E. Hjorting-Hansen, eds.), pp. 160–165. Fadl's Forlag, Copenhagen.

Jenkins, M. V., Harris, M., and Wills, M. R. (1974). *Calcif. Tissue Res.* **16**, 163.

Jesserer, H. (1958). "Tetanie," Georg Thieme, Stuttgart.

Johansson, H., and Segerström, A. (1972). *Acta Chir. Scand.* **138**, 397.

John, H. T., and Wills, M. R. (1964). *Brit. J. Surg.* **51**, 586.

John, H. T., Wills, M. R., and Marcus, R. T. (1966). *Brit. J. Surg.* **53**, 685.

Johnson, J. D., and Jennings, R. (1968). *Am. J. Dis. Child.* **115**, 373.

Johnson, K. A., Riggs, B. L., Kelley, P. J., and Jowsey, J. (1971). *J. Clin. Endocrinol. Metab.* **33**, 745.

Johnston, C. C., Jr., and Schnute, R. B. (1961). *J. Clin. Endocrinol. Metab.* **21**, 196.

Johnstone, R. E., II, Kreindler, T., and Johnstone, R. E. (1972). *Obstet. Gynecol.* **40**, 580.

Joly, J. B. (1973). *Arch. Franc. Pediatr.* **30**, 1037.

Jones, C. R., Bergman, M. W., Kittner, P. J., and Pigman, W. (1964). *Proc. Soc. Exp. Biol. Med.* **116**, 931.

Jones, K. H., and Fourman, P. (1963a). *Lancet* **2**, 119.

Jones, K. H., and Fourman, P. (1963b). *Lancet* **2**, 121.

Jordan, A., and Kelsall, A. R. (1951). *Arch. Intern. Med.* **87**, 242.

Jowsey, J. (1968). *In* Parathyroid Hormone and Thyrocalcitonin (Calcitonin) (R. V. Talmage and L. F. Bèlanger, eds.), Int. Congr. Ser. No. 159, pp. 137–151. Excerpta Med. Found., Amsterdam.

Jowsey, J., Hoye, R. C., Pak, C. Y. C., and Bartter, F. C. (1969). *Am. J. Med.* **47**, 17.

Judd, D. R., Heimburger, I., and Johnston, C., Jr. (1966). *Ann. Surg.* **164**, 1077.

Kahn, A., Snapper, I., and Drucker, A. (1964). *Arch. Intern. Med.* **114**, 434.

Kaiser, W., Loewe, I., and Ponsold, W. (1960). *Klin. Monatsbl. Augenheilkd.* **136**, 65.

Kaiser, W., and Ponsold, W. (1959). *Klin. Wschr.* **22**, 1183.

Kalliomäki, J. L., Markkanen, T. K., and Mustonen, V. A. (1961a). *Acta Med. Scand.* **170**, 211.

Kalliomäki, J. L., Turunen, M., and Viikari, S. J. (1961b). *Acta Chir. Scand.* **122**, 57.

Kalu, D. N., Hadji-Georgopoulos, A., Sarr, M. G., Salomon, B. A., and Foster, G. V. (1974). *Endocrinology* **95**, 1156.

Kaminsky, N. I., Broadus, A. E., Hardman, J. G., Jones, D. J., Jr., Ball, J. H., Sutherland, E. W., and Liddle, G. W. (1970). *J. Clin. Invest.* **49**, 2387.
Kaufman, R. L., Rimoin, D. L., McAlister, W. H., and Hartmann, A. F. (1974). *Am. J. Dis. Child.* **127**, 21.
Kaye, M., Chatterjee, G., Cohen, G. F., and Sagar, S. (1970). *Ann. Intern. Med.* **73**, 225.
Kaye, M., Just, G., and Wilson, M. (1971). *Can. J. Physiol. Pharmacol.* **49**, 857.
Keen, J. H., and Lee, D. (1973). *Arch. Dis. Child.* **48**, 542.
Keipert, J. A. (1969). *Med. J. Aust.* **2**, 242.
Keiser, H. R., Gill, J. R., Jr., Sjoerdsma, A., and Bartter, F. C. (1964). *J. Clin. Invest.* **43**, 1073.
Kenny, F. M., and Holliday, M. A. (1964). *N. Engl. J. Med.* **271**, 708.
Keynes, M. (1963). *Lancet* **2**, 418.
Kieffer, S. A., Peterson, D. H., and Aurelius, J. R. (1965). *Minnesota Med.* **48**, 9.
Kind, H. P., Parkinson, D. K., Kooh, S. W., and Fraser, D. (1974). *Pediatr. Res.* **8**, 128.
Kind, H. P., Prader, A., DeLuca, H. F., and Gugler, E. (1975). *Lancet.* **1**, 1145.
Kind, H. P., Parkinson, D. K., Suh, S. M., Fraser, D., and Kooh, S. W. (1973). *Pediatr. Res.* **7**, 324.
King, L. R., and Goldsmith, R. E. (1964). *Acta Endocrinol. Copenhagen (Kbh)* **47**, 121.
King, L. R., Portnoy, R. M., and Goldsmith, R. E. (1965). *J. Clin. Endocrinol. Metab.* **25**, 577.
Kirk, G. R., Breazile, J. E., and Kenny, A. D. (1963). *Fed. Proc.* **32**, 269.
Kirkpatrick, C. H., Rich, R. R., and Bennett, J. E. (1971). *Ann. Intern. Med.* **74**, 955.
Kleeman, C. R., and Cooke, R. E. (1951). *Endocrinology* **38**, 112.
Kleeman, C. R., Bernstein, D., Rockney, R., Dowling, J. T., and Maxwell, M. H. (1961). *Yale J. Biol. Med.* **34**, 1.
Kleerekoper, M., Basten, A., Penny, R., and Posen, S. (1974). *Arch. Intern. Med.* **134**, 944.
Klein, D. C., and Raisz, L. G. (1971). *Endocrinology* **89**, 818.
Klein, R. (1957). Discussion, see DiGeorge and Paschkis (1957).
Klopper, P. J., and Moe, R. E. (1966). *Surgery* **59**, 1101.
Klotz, H. P., and Fiks, Mme. (1962). *Probl. Actuels Endocrinol. Nutr.* **6**, 245.
Klotz, H. P., and Jungers (1959). *Ann. Endocrinol.* **20**, 283.
Klotz, H. P., and Kahn, F. (1957). *Sem. Hôp.* **33**, 3772.
Klotz, H. P., and Konopka, P. (1972). *Ann. Endocrinol.* (Paris) **33**, 156.
Klotz, H. P., and Witchitz, S. (1963). *Sem. Hop. Paris* **39**, 2493.
Klotz, H. P., Tomkiewicz, S., Witchitz, S., Weil, F., and Massin, J. P. (1962). *Probl. Actuels Endocrinol. Nutr.* **6**, 173.
Klotz, H. P., Witchitz, S., and Kleinman, Mme. (1963). *Ann. Endocrinol.* **24**, 1068.
Kohn, A. (1895). *Arch. Mikr. Anat.,* **44**, 366.
Kolb, F. O., and Steinbach, H. L. (1962). *J. Clin. Endocrinol. Metab.* **22**, 59.
Kooh, S. W., and Fraser, D. (1968). (R. V. Talmage and L. F. Bélanger, eds.), Int. Congr. Ser. No. 159, pp. 442–444. Excerpta Med. Found., Amsterdam.
Kooh, S. W., Fraser, D., DeLuca, H. F., Holick, M. F., Belsey, R. E., Clark, M. B., and Murray, T. M. (1975). *N. Engl. J. Med.* **293**, 840.
Konopka, P., Benhamou, R., and Klotz, H. P. (1971). *Ann. Endocrinol.* **32**, 906.
Kopin, I. J., and Rosenberg, I. N. (1960). *Ann. Intern. Med.* **53**, 1238.
Kopp, L. E., Lin, T., and Tucci, J. R. (1972). *Clin. Res.* **20**, 866.
Kössling, F. K., and Emmrich, P. (1971). *Verh. Dtsch. Ges. Pathl.* **55**, 155.
Kraintz, L. (1969). *Can. J. Physiol. Pharmacol.* **47**, 477.
Kramer, F. (1936). *Fortschr. Ther.* **12**, 521.
Kramer, P. H. (1936). *Ned. Tijdschr. Geneeskd.* **30**, 3008.
Krane, S. M. (1957). *J. Clin. Endocrinol.* **17**, 386.

Krane, S. M. (1961). *J. Amer. Med. Assoc.* **178,** 472.

Krane, S. M., Brownell, G. L., Stanbury, J. B., and Corrigan, H. (1956). *J. Clin. Invest.* **35,** 874.

Kreines, K., and DeVaux, W. D. (1971). *Pediatrics* **47,** 516.

Kugelberg, E. (1948). *Arch. Neurol. Psychiat.* **60,** 153.

Kugelberg, E., and Cobb, W. (1951). *J. Neurol., Neurosurg. Psychiat.* **14,** 88.

Kukreja, S. C., Hargis, G. K., Bowser, E. N., Henderson, W. J., Fisherman, E. W., and Williams, G. A. (1975). *J. Clin. Endocrinol.* **40,** 478.

Kunin, A. S., and Krane, S. M. (1965). *Endocrinology* **76,** 343.

Kunin, A. S., MacKay, B. R., Burns, S. L., and Halberstam, M. J. (1963). *Am. J. Med.* **34,** 856.

Kurokawa, K., and Massry, S. G. (1973). *Proc. Soc. Exp. Biol.* **143,** 123.

Kurokawa, K., and Rasmussen, H. (1973). *Biochim. Biophys. Acta* **313,** 59.

Kurokawa, K., Nagata, N., Sasaki, M., and Nakane, K. (1974). *Endocrinology* **94,** 1514.

Kurth, K. H. (1972). *Helv. Chir. Acta* **39,** 737.

Kyle, L. H., Schaaf, M., and Meyer, R. J. (1954). *J. Clin. Endocrinol.* **14,** 579.

Kyle, L. H., Schaaf, M., and Canary, J. J. (1958). *Am. J. Med.* **24,** 240.

Lachmann, A. (1941). *Acta Med. Scand., Suppl.* **121.**

Lamberg, B. A., Gordin, R., Kuhlbäck, B., and Björkenheim, G. (1960). *Acta Endocrinol. Copenhagen (Kbh.)* **33,** 317.

Lamy, M., and Maroteaux, P. (1960). *Presse Med.* **68,** 1977.

Landing, B. H., and Kamoshita, S. (1970). *J. Pediatr.* **77,** 842.

Lange, M. J. (1963). *Lancet* **2,** 1007.

Larson, E., and Elkourie, L. A. (1928). *Amer. J. Physiol.* **85,** 387.

Laymon, C. W., and Zelickson, A. (1959). *Arch. Dermatol.* **79,** 194.

Layzer, R. B., and Rowland, L. P. (1971). *N. Engl. J. Med.* **285,** 31.

Lee, J. B., Tashjian, A. H., Jr., Streeto, J. M., and Frantz, A. G. (1968). *N. Engl. J. Med.* **279,** 1179.

Leeson, P. M., and Fourman, P. (1966). *Lancet* **1,** 1182.

Lefebvre, J., and Lerique, J. (1962). *Probl. Actuels Endocrinol. Nutr.* **6,** 209.

Leifer, E., and Hollander, W., Jr. (1953). *J. Clin. Endocrinol. Metab.* **13,** 1264.

Leighton, G. A., Holland, R., and Frame, B. (1964). *Henry Ford Hosp. Med. Bull.* **12,** 37.

Lelong, M., Canlorbe, P., Le Tan Vinh, Paupe, J., Gentil, C., Colin, J., Houllemare, L., and Courtecuisse, V. (1962). *Ann. Pediatr.* **38,** 222.

Lelong, M., Canlorbe, P., Lagrue, G., and Bader, J. C. (1968). *Ann. Pediatr.* **44,** 253.

Lemann, J., Jr., and Donatelli, A. A. (1964). *Ann. Intern. Med.* **60,** 447.

Lemann, J., Jr., Litzow, J. R., and Lennon, E. J. (1967). *J. Clin. Invest.* **46,** 1318.

Leonard, M. F. (1946). *J. Clin. Endocrinol.* **6,** 493.

Lequin, R. M., Hackeng, W. H. L., and Schopman, W. (1970). *Acta Endocrinol. Copenhagen (Kbh)* **63,** 655.

Léri, A. (1926). "Les Affections des Os et des Articulations" Masson, et Cie, Paris.

Léri, A., and Weill, J. (1929). *Bull. Soc. Med. Hop. Paris* **53,** 1491.

Leriche, R. and Jung, A. (1936). *Presse Med.* **44,** 777.

Lerner, S., and Lukert, B. (1974). *Clin. Res.* **22,** 650A.

Levi, J., Massry, S. G., Coburn, J. W., Llach, F., and Kleeman, C. R. (1974). *Metabolism Clin. Exp.* **23,** 323.

Levin, P., Kunin, A. S., Donaghy, R. M. P., Hamilton, W. V., and Maurer, J. J. (1961). *Neurology* **11,** 1076.

Levy, R. L., Huang, S. W., Bach, M. L., Bach, F. H., Hong, R., Ammann, A. J., Bortin, M., and Kay, H. E. M. (1971). *Lancet* **2,** 898.

Lieberman, A., and DeLellis, R. A. (1973). *Arch. Pathol.* **95,** 422.

Lieschke, H. J., and Witkowski, R. (1968). *Arch. Gynäkol.* **206**, 25.

Linarelli, L. G., Bobik, J., and Bobik, C. (1972). *Pediatrics* **50**, 14.

Linarelli, L. G., Bobik, J., and Bobik, C. (1973). *Pediatr. Res.* **7**, 878.

Lindgärde, F. (1972). *Clin. Chim. Acta* **40**, 477.

Lischner, H. W., Punnett, H. H., and DiGeorge, A. M. (1967). *Nature* (London) **214**, 580.

Litvak, J., Moldawer, M. C., Forbes, A. P., and Henneman, P. H. (1958). *J. Clin. Endo-crinol. Metab.* **18**, 246.

Lloyd, H. M., Aitken, R. E., and Ferrier, T. M. (1965). *Br. Med. J.* **2**, 853.

Lobdell, D. H. (1959). *Arch. Pathol.* **67**, 412.

Lockefeer, J. H. M., Hackeng, W. H. L., and Birkenhäger, J. C. (1973). *Proc. Eur. Symp. Calcif. Tissues, 9th, 1973,* Vienna, pp. 237–240.

Lockefeer, J. H., Hackeng, W. H. L., and Birkenhäger, J. C. (1974). *In* "Calcified Tissue 1972," (H. Czitober and J. Eschberger, eds.). pp. 237–240. Facta-Publication Vienna.

Lomnitz, E., Sepulveda, L., Stevenson, C., and Barzelatto, J. (1966). *J. Clin. Endocrinol. Metab.* **26**, 309.

Lordon, R. E., McPhaul, J. J., Jr., and McIntosh, D. A. (1966). *Ann. Intern. Med.* **64**, 1066.

Lorentz, W. B., Jr. (1974). *J. Clin. Invest.* **53**, 1250.

Lorenz, R., and Burr, I. M. (1974). *J. Pediatr.* **85**, 522.

Louria, D. B., and Brayton, R. G. (1964). *Nature (London)* **201**, 309.

Lowe, C. U., and Calcagno, P. L. (1955). *Helv. Paediatr. Acta* **10**, 117.

Lowe, C. U., Ellinger, A. J., Wright, W. S., and Stauffer, H. M. (1950). *J. Pediatr.* **36**, 1.

Lubell, D. (1957). *Helv. Paediatr. Acta* **12**, 179.

Ludwig, G. D. (1962). *N. Engl. J. Med.* **267**, 637.

Lukert, B. P., Stanbury, S. W., and Mawer, E. B. (1973). *Endocrinology* **93**, 718.

Lumb, G. A., and Stanbury, S. W. (1974). *Amer. J. Med.* **56**, 833.

Lund, B., Hindberg, I., and Sorensen, O. H. (1975). *Horm. Metab. Res.* **7**, 176.

Lupulescu, A., Poe, A., Merculiev, E., Neacsu, C., and Heitmanek, C. (1965). *Nature (London)* **206**, 415.

Lupulescu, A., Potorac, E., Pop, A., Heitmanek, C., Merculiev, E., Chisiu, N., Oprisan, R., and Neacsu, C. (1968). *Immunology* **14**, 475.

Lyon, M. F. (1961). *Nature (London)* **190**, 372.

Lyon, M. F. (1962). *Am. J. Human Genet.* **14**, 135.

Lyon, M. F. (1963). *Genet. Res.* **4**, 93.

MacAuley, S. J., Larkins, R. G., Rapoport, A., Martin, T. J., and MacIntyre, I. (1975). "Calcium Metabolism, Bone and Metabolic Bone Diseases," (F. Kuhlencordt and H. P. Kruse, eds.), pp. 91–96. Springer-Verlag, Berlin and New York.

MacCallum, W. G., and Voegtlin, C. (1909). *J. Exp. Med.* **11**, 118.

McCormack, K. R. (1966). *Cancer* **19**, 181.

McCrory, W. W., Forman, C. W., McNamara, H., and Barnett, H. L. (1952). *J. Clin. Invest.* **31**, 357.

McDonald, K. M. (1972). *Metabolism* **21**, 521.

McDougal, B., and Lukert, B. (1974). *Clin. Res.* **22**, 619A.

McDougall, I. R., Greig, W. R., and Gillespie, F. C. (1971). *N. Engl. J. Med.* **285**, 1099.

McGeown, M. G. (1965). *Urol. Int.* **19**, 137.

McGeown, M. G., and Field, C. M. B. (1960). *Lancet* **2**, 1268.

MacGregor, M. E., and Whitehead, T. P. (1954). *Arch. Dis. Child.* **29**, 398.

MacIntyre, I., Boss, S., and Troughton, V. A. (1963). *Nature (London)* **198**, 1058.

McKenzie, A. D. (1971). *Arch. Surg.* **102**, 274.

McKinney, A. S. (1962). *Neurology* **12**, 485.

Mackler, H., Fouts, J. R., and Birsner, J. W. (1952). *Calif. Med.* **77**, 332.

McKusick, V. A. (1966). ''Mendelian Inheritance in Man,'' Baltimore, The Johns Hopkins Press, Baltimore, Maryland.

McMahon, F. G., Cookson, D. U., Kabler, J. D., and Inhorn, S. L. (1959). *Ann. Intern. Med.* **51,** 371.

MacManus, J., Heaton, F. W., and Lucas, P. W. (1971). *J. Endocrinol.* **49,** 253.

McNeill, A. D., and Thomson, J. A. (1968). *Brit. Med. J.* **3,** 643.

Madelung, O. W. (1878). *Verh. Dtsch. Ges. Chir.* **7,** 259.

Magladery, J. W., McDougal, D. B., Jr., and Stoll, J. (1950). *Bull. Johns Hopkins Hosp.* **86,** 313.

Maillard, E., Farriaux, J. P., Deminatti, A., Walbaum, R., and Fontaine, G. (1966). *Lille. Med.* **11,** 462.

Malpuech, G., Gaillard, G., Merle, P., Pailloncy, J. M., and Raynaud, E. J. (1975). *Arch. Franc. Pediatr.* **32,** 235.

Malvaux, P., and Beckers, C. (1973). *Clin. Endocrinol.* **2,** 219.

Mandl, F. (1933). *Dtsch. Z. Chir.* **240,** 362.

Mann, J. B., Alterman, S., and Hills, A. G. (1962). *Ann. Intern. Med.* **56,** 315.

Marcus, R. (1975). *Endocrinology* **96,** 400.

Marcus, R., Wilber, J. F., and Aurbach, G. D. (1971). *J. Clin. Endocrinol.* **33,** 537.

Margolis, C. I., and Goldenberg, V. E. (1969). *N.Y. St. J. Med.* **69,** 702.

Marieb, N. J., Melby, J. C., and Lyall, S. S. (1974). *Arch. Intern. Med.* **134,** 424.

Marks, J. F., Mize, C. E., and Carruth, D. M. (1973). *Clin. Res.* **21,** 110.

Maroteaux, P., and Malamut, G. (1968). *Presse Med.* **76,** 2189.

Maroteaux, P., Martinelli, B., and Campailla, E. (1971). *Press. Med.* **79,** 1839.

Martin, T. J., Vakakis, N., Eisman, J. A., Livesey, S. J., and Tregear, G. W. (1974). *J. Endocrinol.* **63,** 369.

Marx, S. J., Hershman, J. M., and Aurbach, G. D. (1971). *J. Clin Endocrinol.* **33,** 822.

Marx, S. J., Woodard, C. J., and Aurbach, G. D. (1972). *Science* **178,** 999.

Marx, S. J., Doppman, J. L., Spiegel, A. M., Wolfe, D., and Aurbach, G. D. (1974). *J. Clin. Endocrinol. Metab.* **39,** 1110.

Massry, S. G., Coburn, J. W., and Kleeman, C. R. (1970). *J. Clin. Invest.* **49,** 1619.

Mathieu, H., de Menibus, C. H., Frederich, A., Lestradet, H., and Royer, P. (1961). *Sem. Hop. Paris (Ann. Pediat.)* **37,** 921.

Matsuzaki, S., and Dumont, J. E. (1972). *Biochim. Biophys. Acta* **284,** 227.

Matthews, W. B. (1957). *J. Neurol., Neurosurg. Psychiatry* **20,** 172.

Mauro, C. (1950). *G. Ital. Chir.* **6,** 384.

Mautalen, C. A. (1970). *J. Clin. Endocrinol. Metab.* **31,** 595.

Mautalen, C. A., Dymling, J. F., and Horwith, M. (1967). *Amer. J. Med.* **42,** 977.

Mawer, E. B., Backhouse, J., Holman, C. A., Lumb, G. A., and Stanbury, S. W. (1972). *Clin. Sci.* **43,** 413.

Mawer, E. B., Backhouse, J., Hill, L. F., Lumb, G. A., de Silva, P., Taylor, C. M., and Stanbury, S. W. (1975). *Clin. Sci. Mol. Med.* **48,** 349.

Mazzuoli, G. F., and Naccarato, R. (1959). *Folia Endocrinol.* **12,** 366.

Mazzuoli, G. F., Coen, G., and Baschieri, L. (1966). *Lancet* **2,** 1192.

Mazzuoli, G. F., Coen, G., and Antonozzi, I. (1967). *Isr. J. Med.* **3,** 627.

Mazzuoli, G. F., Coen, G., and Antonozzi, I. (1968). *In* ''Calcitonin'' (S. Taylor, ed.), pp. 364–372. Heinemann, London.

Medalle, R., and Waterhouse, C. (1973). *Ann. Intern. Med.* **79,** 76.

Meersseman, F. P. (1973). *J. Belge Rhumatol. Med. Phys.* **28,** 303.

Mehls, O., Ritz, E., Krempien, K., Gilli, G., and Schärer, K. (1975). *In* Norman, A. W.,

Schaeffer, K., Grigoleit, H. G., von Herrath, D. and Ritz, E. (Eds.), "Vitamin D and Problems Related to Uremic Bone Disease" pp. 553–560. de Gruyter, Berlin.

Melick, R. A., Gill, J. R., Jr., Berson, S. A., Yalow, R. S., Bartter, F. C., Potts, J. T., Jr., and Aurbach, G. D. (1967). *N. Engl. J. Med.* **276**, 144.

Mellanby, E. (1949). *J. Physiol. (London)* **109**, 488.

Melson, G. L., Chase, L. R., and Aurbach, G. D. (1970). *Endocrinology* **86**, 511.

Merimee, T. J., Rimoin, D. L., and Cavalli-Sforza, L. L. (1972). *J. Clin. Invest.* **51**, 395.

Merz, W. A., and Schenk, R. K. (1970). *Acta Anat.* **76**, 1.

Messer, H. H., Armstrong, W. D., and Singer, L. (1973). *Calcif. Tissue Res.* **13**, 217.

Meunier, P., Vignon, G., Bernard, J., Edouard, C., Courpron, P., and Porte, J. (1972). *Rev. Rhum.* **39**, 635.

Meunier, P., and Courpron, P. (1976). *In* "Bone Morphometry" (Z. F. G. Jaworski, ed.), pp. 100–105. University of Ottawa Press, Ottawa.

Meunier, P., Edouard, C., Courpron, P., and Toussaint, F. (1975). *In* "Vitamin D and Problems Related to Uremic Bone Disease" (A. W. Norman, K. Schaefer, H. G. Grigoleit, D. von Herrath, and E. Ritz, eds.), pp. 149–155. de Gruyter, Berlin.

Meyer, R. A., Jr., and Meyer, M. H. (1974). *Endocrinology* **94**, 1331.

Michie, W., Stowers, J. M., Frazer, S. C., and Gunn, A. (1965). *Br. J. Surg.* **52**, 503.

Michie, W., Stowers, J. M., Duncan, T., and Pegg, C. A. S. (1971). *Lancet* **1**, 508.

Miettinen, T. A., and Perheentupa, J. (1971). *Scand. J. Clin. Lab. Invest.* Suppl. 116, **27**, 36.

Miles, J., and Elrick, H. (1955). *J. Clin. Endocr.,* **15**, 576.

Milhaud, G., and Bourichon, J. (1964). *C. R. Hebd. Science, Acad. Sci.* **258**, 3398.

Milhaud, G., Aubert, J. P., Bourichon, J., and Klotz, H. P. (1959). *Ann. Endocrinol.* (Paris) **20**, 288.

Milhaud, G., Aubert, J. P., and Bourichon, J. (1961). *Pathol. et Biol.* **9**, 1761.

Milhaud, G., Bourichon, J., and Aubert, J. P. (1962). *Probl. Actuels Endocrinol. Nutr.* **6**, 237.

Miller, J. Q., Rostafinski, M. J., and Hyde, M. S. (1965). *Arch. Intern. Med.* **116**, 940.

Miller, L. H., and Krane, S. M. (1971). *In* "Dermatology in General Medicine" (T. R. Fitzpatrick et al., eds.), p. 1204–1211. McGraw-Hill, New York.

Miller, M. J., Frame, B., Poznanski, A. K., Jackson, C. E., and Bermudez, G. (1972). *Henry Ford Hosp. Med. J.* **20**, 3.

Mills, J. N., and Stanbury, S. W. (1952). *J. Physiol. (London)* **117**, 22.

Minaire, P., Meunier, P., Edouard, C., Bernard, J., and Courpron, P. (1975). *Rev. Rhum.,* **42**, 479.

Minkin, C. (1973). *Calcif. Tissue Res.* **13**, 249.

Minozzi, M., Faggiano, M., Bianco, A., Brizzi, G., and Coligianni, A. (1963). *Folia Endocrinol.* **16**, 168.

Minozzi, M., Faggiano, M., Bianco, A., and Vitale, A. (1964). *Endocrinol. Sci. Cost.* **28**, 3.

Mitschke, H., Altenähr, E., Delling, G., and Wiebel, J. (1973). *Dtsch. Med. Wochenschr.* **98**, 1666.

Moehlig, R. C., and Gerish, R. A. (1950). *J. Clin. Endocrinol.* **10**, 1609.

Moehlig, R. C., and Steinbach, A. L. (1954). *J. Amr. Med. Assoc.* **154**, 42.

Monchik, J. M., Gemma, F. E., Bond, H., and Wray, H. L. (1976). *Am. J. Surg.* **131**, 471.

Money, J., and Ehrhardt, A. A. (1966). *Amer. J. Mental. Defic.* **71**, 237.

Monod, H., Rosa, M., Borlone, M., and Scherrer, J. (1970). *Rev. Neurol.* **122**, 487.

Moore, W. T., and Smith, L. H., Jr. (1963). *Metabolism* **12**, 447.

Morel, L. (1912). "*Les Parathyroïdes.*" Hermann, & Fils. Paris.

Morgan, H. G., Dryburgh, F. J., and Mills, E. A. (1975). *In* "Calcium Metabolism, Bone and

Metabolic Bone Disease'' (E. Kuhlencordt, and H. P. Kruse, eds.), pp. 356–361. Springer-Verlag, Berlin and New York.

Moriarty, M. J., Powell, D., and Burgess, D. (1975). *Ir. J. Med. Sci.* **144**, 212.

Morse, W. I., Cochrane, W. A., and Landrigan, P. L. (1961). *N. Engl. J. Med.* **264**, 1021.

Moseley, J. M., Martin, T. J., Robinson, C. J., Reit, B. W., and Tregéar, G. W. (1975). *Clin. Exper. Pharmacol. Physiol.* **2**, 549.

Moses, A. M., Breslau, N., and Coulson, R. (1976). *Amer. J. Med.,* **61**, 184.

Moses, A. M., Rao, K. J., Coulson, R., and Miller, M. (1974). *J. Clin. Endocrinol. Metab.* **39**, 496.

Moskowitz, M. A., Winickoff, R. N., and Heinz, E. R. (1971). *N. Engl. J. Med.* **285**, 72.

Mosonyi, L., and Szilagyi, G. (1964). *Acta Med. Acad. Sci. Hung.* **20**, 113.

Moulias, R., Goust, J. M., and Muller-Berat, C. N. (1971). *Lancet* **1**, 1239.

Muenter, M. D., and Whisnant, J. P. (1968). *Neurology* **18**, 1075.

Muldowney, F. P., McKenna, T. J., Kyle, L. H., Freaney, R., and Swan, M. (1970). *N. Engl. J. Med.* **282**, 61.

Muldowney, F. P., Carroll, D. V., Donohoe, J. F., and Freaney, R. (1971). *Q. J. Med.* **40**, 487.

Murad, F., and Pak, C. Y. C. (1972). *N. Engl. J. Med.* **286**, 1382.

Murad, F., Brewer, H. B., Jr., and Vaughan, M. (1970). *Proc. Nat. Acad. Sci. [N.S.]* 4 **65**, 446.

Murley, R. S., and Peters, P. M. (1961). *Proc. R. Soc. Med.* **54**, 487.

Murphy, K. J. (1969). *Clin. Radiol.* **20**, 287.

Murphy, K. J. (1975). *Clin. Radiol.* **26**, 37.

Murray, T. M., Peacock, M., Powell, D., Monchik, J. M., and Potts, J. T., Jr. (1972). *Clin. Endocrinol.* **1**, 235.

Myers, W. P. L. (1960). *Arch. Surg. (Chicago)* **80**, 308.

Myers, W. P. L., and Lawrence, W., Jr. (1958). *J. Clin. Invest.* **37**, 919.

Naeye, R. L. (1974). *Science* **186**, 837.

Nagant de Deuxchaisnes, C. (1959). *Schweiz. Med. Wochenschr.* **89**, 1239.

Nagant de Deuxchaisnes, C., and Krane, S. M. (1964). *Medicine (Baltimore)* **43**, 233.

Nagant de Deuxchaisnes, C., and Krane, S. M. (1967). *Am. J. Med.* **43**, 508.

Nagant de Deuxchaisnes, C., and Krane, S. M. (1971). Paper delivered to the Journèes d'Endocrinologie et de Nutrition Paris (Maison des Centraux), October 1st–2nd, Paris.

Nagant de Deuxchaisnes, C., and Krane, S. M. (1974). *In* "La Maladie de Paget" (D. J. Hioco, ed.), pp. 196–213. Sandoz, Paris.

Nagant de Deuxchaisnes, C., Fanconi, A., Alberto, P., Rudler, J. C., and Mach, R. S. (1960a). *Schweiz. Med. Wochenschr.* **90**, 886.

Nagant de Deuxchaisnes, C., Isaac, G., Jacquet, A., and Hoet, J. J. (1960b). *Rev. Fr. and Clin. Biol.* **5**, 153.

Nagata, N., Sasaki, M., Kimura, N., and Nakane, K. (1975). *Endocrinology* **96**, 725.

Nakajima, H., Fukumoto, Y., and Nakata, M. (1966). *Endocrinol. Jpn.* **13**, 1.

Nedok, A. S., Garzicic, B. S., and Soldatovic, B. M. (1968). *J. Clin. Endocrinol. Metab.* **28**, 1513.

Neelon, F. A., Drezner, M., Birch, B. M., and Lebovitz, H. E. (1973). *Lancet* **1**, 631.

Neer, R. M., Holick, M. F., DeLuca, H. F., and Potts, J. T., Jr. (1975). *Metab. Clin. Exp.* **24**, 1403.

Nerup, J. (1974). *Dan. Med. Bull.* **21**, 201.

Neuman, W. F., Neuman, M. W., Sammon, P. J., Simon, W., and Lane, K. (1975c). *Calcif. Tissue Res.* **18**, 251.

Neuman, W. F., Meidam, M. W., Sammon, P. J., and Casarett, G. W. (1975b). *Calcif. Tissue Res.* **18**, 263.

Neuman, W. F., Neuman, M. W., Lane, K., Miller, L., and Sammon, P. J. (1975a). *Calcif. Tissue Res.* **18**, 271.

Nevins, M. A., Madhukar, S., Bright, M., and Lyon, L. J. (1973). *J. Amer. Med. Assoc.* **224**, 1382.

Newcombe, D. S., and Keats, T. E. (1969). *Am. J. Roentgenol., Radium Ther. Nucl. Med.* [N.S.] **106**, 176.

Newns, G. H. (1973). *Acta Paediatr. Scand.,* **62**, 91.

Newton, N. C., and Sumich, M. G. (1968). *Med. J. Aust.* **2**, 394.

Nézelof, C., Satge, P., Lavaud, J., and Le Sec, G. (1975). *Arch. Fr. Pediatr.* **32**, 161.

Nichols, F. L., Holdsworth, D. E., and Reinfrank, R. E. (1961). *Am. J. Med.* **30**, 518.

Nicholson, W. F. (1969). *Br. J. Surg.* **56**, 106.

Nielsen, H. (1952). *Acta Med. Scand., Suppl.* **266**, 783.

Niklasson, E. (1970). *Acta Paediatr. Scand.* **59**, 715.

Nilsson, F., and Segerström, A. (1973). *Acta Chir. Scand.* **139**, 60.

Nordin, B. E. C. (1973). "Metabolic Bone and Stone Disease." Churchill, London.

Nordin, B. E. C., and Bulusu, L. (1968). *Postgrad. Med. J.* **44**, 93.

Nordin, B. E. C., and Fraser, R. (1954). *Clin. Sci.* **13**, 477.

Nordin, B. E. C., and Fraser, R. (1960). *Lancet* **1**, 947.

Nordin, B. E. C., and Peacock, M. (1969). *Lancet* **2**, 1280.

Nordin, B. E. C., Marshall, D. H., Peacock, M., and Robertson, W. G. (1975). *In* "Calcium-Regulating Hormones" (R. V. Talmage, M. Owen, and J. A. Parsons, eds.), Int. Congr. Ser. No. 346, pp. 239–253. Excerpta Med. Found., Amsterdam.

Nordio, S., Donath, A., Macagno, F., and Gatti, R. (1971). *Acta Paediatr. Scand.* **60**, 441.

Norris, E. H. (1946). *Arch. Pathol.* **42**, 261.

Northcutt, R. C., Levinson, J. D., and Earnest, J. B. (1969). *Ann. Intern. Med.* **70**, 353.

Numann, P. J., and Moses, A. M. (1974). *Surgury* **75**, 869.

Nusynowitz, M. L., and Klein, M. H. (1973). *Am. J. Med.* **55**, 677.

Oberklaid, F., and Seshadri, R. (1975). *Med. J. Aust.,* **1**, 304.

Obertst, B. B., and Tompkins, C. A. (1955). *Amer. J. Dis. Child.,* **90**, 205.

O'Brien, C. S. (1932). *Arch. Ophthalmol.* **7**, 71.

O'Donovan, D. K. (1948). *Br. Med. J.* **2**, 900.

Ogg, C. S. (1967). *Br. Med. J.* **4**, 331.

Okano, K., Fujita, T., Orimo, H., and Yoshikawa, M. (1969). *Endocrinol. Jpn.* **16**, 423.

Olin, R., and Poindexter, M. H. (1972). *Minn. Med.* **55**, 701.

Ollayos, R. W., and Winkler, A. W. (1943). *J. Clin. Invest.* **22**, 147.

O'Malley, B. W., and Kohler, P. O. (1968). *Postgrad. Med.* **44**, 71(4), 182(5), 77(6).

Orme, R. L. E. (1971). *Proc. R. Soc. Med.* **64**, 727.

Orme, R. L. E., and Conolly, M. E. (1971). *Ann. Intern. Med.* **75**, 136.

O'Rourke, J. N., Booth, B. H., and Patterson, R. (1973). *J. Allergy Clin. Immunol.* **52**, 55.

Orr, R. J., and Graham, B. C. (1972). *Clin. Res.* **20**, 283.

Osborn, D. A., and Jones, W. I. (1968). *Br. J. Surg.* **55**, 277.

Painter, N. S. (1960). *Br. J. Surg.* **48**, 291.

Pak, C. Y. C., DeLuca, H. F., Chavez de los Rios, J. M., Suda, T., Ruskin, B., and Delea, C. S. (1970). *Arch. Intern. Med.* **126**, 239.

Paloyan, E., Lawrence, A. M., Baker, W. H., and Straus, F. H. (1969). *Surg. Clin. North Am.* **49**, 43.

Palubinskas, A. J., and Davies, H. (1959). *Am. J. Roentgenol., Radium Ther. Nucl. Med.* [N.S.] **82**, 806.

Papadatos, C., and Alivisatos, J. G. (1960). *J. Pediat.*, **57**, 436.

Papadatos, C., and Klein, R. (1954). *J. Clin. Endocrinol. Metab.* **14**, 653.

Parfitt, A. M. (1965). *J. Bone Jt. Surg., Br. Vol.* **47B**, 137.

Parfitt, A. M. (1967a). *Med. J. Aust.* **1**, 702.

Parfitt, A. M. (1967b). *Australas. Ann. Med.* **16**, 114.

Parfitt, A. M. (1968). *Australas. Ann. Med.* **17**, 56.

Parfitt, A. M. (1969). *J. Clin. Endocrinol. Metab.* **29**, 569.

Parfitt, A. M. (1970). *Lancet* **2**, 614.

Parfitt, A. M. (1971). *Med. J. Aust.* **1**, 1103.

Parfitt, A. M. (1972a). *J. Clin. Endocrinol. Metab.* **34**, 152.

Parfitt, A. M. (1972b). *Ann. Intern. Med.* **77**, 557.

Parfitt, A. M. (1974a). *Br. Med. J.* **1**, 520.

Parfitt, A. M. (1974b). *Lancet* **2**, 360.

Parish, J. G. (1967). *J. Med. Genet.* **4**, 227.

Park, H. Z. and Talmage, R. V. (1968). *In* "Parathyroid Hormone and Thyrocalcitonin (Calcitonin)" (R. V. Talmage, and L. F. Bélanger, eds.), Int. Congr. Ser. No. 159, pp. 203–215. Excerpta Med. Found., Amsterdam.

Parkin, T. W. (1964). *Postgrad. Med.* **35**, 638.

Parrott, M. W., Johnston, M. E., and Durbin, P. W. (1960). *Endocrinology* **67**, 467.

Parrott, R. H. (1957). Discussion, see DiGeorge and Paschkis (1957).

Parsons, J. A., and Reit, B. (1974). *Nature (London)* **250**, 254.

Parsons, J. A., and Robinson, C. J. (1971). *Nature (London)* **230**, 581.

Paunier, L., Radde, I., Kooh, S. W., Conen, P. F., and Fraser, D. (1968). *Pediatrics* **41**, 385.

Pawlotsky, Y., Marcheteau, M., Simon, M., Ferrand, B., and Bourel, M. (1972). *Rev. Rhum. Mal. Osteo-Artisulaires* **39**, 259.

Payne, R. B., Little, A. J., Williams, R. B., and Milner, J. R. (1973). *Br. Med. J.* **4**, 643.

Peach, M. J. (1975). *In* "The Pharmacological Basis of Therapeutics" (L. S. Goodman, and A. Gilman, eds.), 5th ed., pp. 782–797. Macmillan, New York.

Peacock, M., Robertson, W. G., and Nordin, B. E. C. (1969). *Lancet* **1**, 384.

Pechet, M. M., Rasmussen, H., Carroll, E. L., and Gramer, I. (1961). *J. Clin. Invest.* **40**, 1070.

Peck, W. A., Carpenter, J., and Messinger, K. (1974a). *Endocrinology* **94**, 148.

Peck, W. A., Messinger, K., Kimmich, G., and Carpenter, J. (1974b). *Endocrinology* **95**, 289.

Peden, H. (1960). *Am. J. Hum. Genet.* **12**, 323.

Pendras, J. P. (1969). *Arch. Intern. Med.* **124**, 312.

Peng, T. C., and Gitelman, H. J. (1974). *Endocrinology* **94**, 608.

Pergament, E., Pietra, G. C., Kadotani, T., Sato, H., and Berlow, S. (1970). *J. Pediatr.* **76**, 745.

Perlmutter, M., Ellison, R. R., Norsa, L., and Kantrowitz, A. R. (1956). *Am. J. Med.* **21**, 634.

Peterson, W. C., Jr., Carlson, C. H., Singer, L., and Armstrong, W. D. (1963). *Arch. Dermatol.* **88**, 540.

Phang, J. M., and Downing, S. J. (1973). *Am. J. Physiol.* **224**, 191.

Phang, J. M., Hahn, T. J., Chase, L. R., and Ramberg, C. F. (1968). *J. Clin. Invest.* **47**, 78a.

Philpot, G. R. (1958). Ph.D. Thesis, London (quoted by Dent, 1962).

Piesowicz, A. T. (1965). *Proc. R. Soc. Med.* **58**, 126.

Pohjola, S. (1962). *Acta Ophthalmol.* **40**, 255.

Pool, E. H. (1907). *Ann. Surg.*, **46**, 507.

Popovtzer, M. M., Robinette, J. B., DeLuca, H. F., and Holick, M. F. (1974). *J. Clin. Invest.* **53**, 913.

Potts, J. T., Jr. (1972). In "The Metabolic Basis of Inherited Disease" (J. B. Stanbury, J. B., Wyngaarden, and D. S. Fredrickson, eds.), 3rd ed. pp. 1305–1319. McGraw-Hill, New York.

Potts, J. T., Jr., and Deftos, L. J. (1974). "Duncan's Diseases of Metabolism, Endocrinology and Nutrition." (P. K. Bondy, and L. E. Rosenberg, eds.), 7th Ed., pp. 1225–1430. W. B. Saunders, Philadelphia, Pennsylvania.

Potts, J. T., Jr., Tregéar, G. W., Keutmann, H. T., Niall, H. D., Sauer, R., Deftos, L. J., Dawson, B. F., Hogan, M. L., and Aurbach, G. D. (1971). *Proc. Natl. Sci. U.S.A.* **68**, 63.

Powles, T. J., Easty, D. M., Easty, G. C., Bondy, P. K., and Munro-Neville, A. (1973). *Nature (London), New Biol.* **245**, 83.

Prasad, A. S. (1960). *Arch. Intern. Med.* **105**, 560.

Prasad, A. S., and Flink, E. B. (1958). *J. Lab. Clin. Med.* **52**, 1.

Pratley, S. K., Posen, S., and Reeve, T. S. (1973). *Med. J. Aust.* **1**, 421.

Preece, M. A. (1971). *Proc. R. Soc. Med.* **64**, 730.

Preisman, R. A., and Mehnert, J. H. (1971). *Arch. Surg.* **103**, 12.

Prentice, R. J. (1954). *J. Clin. Endocr.* **14**, 1069.

Presley, S. J., and Paul, J. T. (1960). *Ill. Med. J.* **118**, 298.

Puissant, F., Williame, E., and Van Coppenolle, B. (1975). *J. Belge Rhumatol. Med. Phys.* **30**, 164.

Purnell, D. C., Jones, J. D., and Becker, K. L. (1968). *J. Clin. Endocrinol. Metab.* **28**, 567.

Purnell, D. C., Smith, L. H., Scholz, D. A., Elveback, L. R., and Arnaud, C. D. (1971). *Am. J. Med.* **50**, 670.

Puschett, J. B., Fernandez, P. C., Boyle, I. T., Gray, R. W., Omdahl, J. L., and DeLuca, H. F. (1972). *Proc. Soc. Exp. Biol. Med.* **141**, 379.

Puschett, J. B., Beck, W. S., Jr., Jelonek, A., and Fernandez, P. C. (1974). *J. Clin. Invest.* **53**, 756.

Pyrah, L. N., Hodgkinson, A., and Anderson, C. K. (1966). *Br. J. Surg.* **53**, 245.

Queener, S. F., and Bell, N. H. (1975). *Metab., Clin. Exp.* **24**, 555.

Quichaud, J., Le Bozec, R., Frison, B., Galez, A., Massy, B., and Blanchard, J. (1969). *Ann. Endocrinol.* **30**, 682.

Quinto, M. G., Leikin, S. L., and Hung, W. (1964). *J. Pediat.,* **64**, 241.

Radcliff, F. J., Baume, P. E., and Jones, W. O. (1962). *Lancet* **2**, 1249.

Radde, I. C., Parkinson, D. K., Höffken, B., Appiah, K. E., and Hanley, W. B. (1972). *Pediatr. Res.* **6**, 43.

Raisz, L. G., and Klein, D. C. (1969). *Fed. Proc., Fed. Am. Soc. Exp. Biol.* **28**, 320.

Raisz, L. G., and Niemann, I. (1969). *Endocrinology* **85**, 446.

Raisz, L. G., Trummel, C. L., Holick, M. F., and DeLuca, H. F. (1972a). *Science* **175**, 768.

Raisz, L. G., Trummel, C. L., Wener, J. A., and Simmons, H. (1972b). *Endocrinology* **90**, 961.

Raisz, L. G., Holtrop, M. E., and Simmons, H. (1973). *Endocrinology* **92**, 556.

Raman, A. (1972). *Horm. Metab. Res.* **4**, 104.

Rameis, K., Kurz, R., and Glatzl, J. (1972). *Paediatr. Paedol.* **7**, 279.

Ranke, E. J. and Holinger, P. H. (1955). *J. Am. Med. Assoc.* **158**, 543.

Rao, K. J., Tomar, R. H., and Moses, A. M. (1974). *Clin. Res.* **22**, 704A.

Rasmussen, H., and Tenenhouse, A. (1968). *Proc. Natl. Acad. Sci.* **59**, 1364.

Rasmussen, H., Pechet, M., and Fast, D. (1968). *J. Clin. Invest.* **47**, 1843.

Ray, E. W., and Gardner, L. I. (1959). *Pediatrics* **23**, 520.

Raymond, J. P., and Klotz, H. P. (1971). *Ann. Endocrinol.* **32**, 460.

Rayssiguier, Y., and Larvor, P. (1974). *Horm. Metab. Res.* **6**, 91.

Reddy, C. R., Coburn, J. W., Hartenbower, D. L., Friedler, R. M., Brickman, A. S., Massry, S. G., and Jowsey, J. (1973). *J. Clin. Invest.* **52**, 3000.

Reeve, T. S. (1967). *Surgery* **62**, 493.

Reeve, T. S., Hales, I. B., White, B., Thomas, I. D., and Hunt, P. S. (1969). *Surgery* **65**, 694.

Reik, L., Petzold, G. L., Higgins, J. A., Greengard, P., and Barrnett, R. J. (1970). *Science* **168**, 382.

Reilly, M. J. (1967). *N. Engl. J. Med.* **27**, 1207.

Reidenberg, M. M., Sevy, R. W., and Cucinotta, A. J. (1968). *Proc. Soc. Exp. Biol.*, **127**, 1.

Reiner, L., Klayman, M. J., and Cohen, R. B. (1962). *Jew. Mem. Hosp. Bull.* **7**, 103.

Reinhart, R., Brickman, A. S., Kurokawa, K., Coburn, J. W., and Massry, S. G. (1973). *Clin. Res.* **21**, 255.

Reisner, D. J., and Ellsworth, R. M. (1955). *Ann. Intern. Med.* **43**, 1116.

Reiss, E., and Canterbury, J. M. (1968). *Proc. Soc. Exp. Biol. Med.* **128**, 501.

Relkin, R. (1974). *Fed. Proc., Fed. Am. Soc. Exp. Biol.* **33**, 241.

Reynolds, J. J., Holick, M. F., and DeLuca, H. F. (1973). *Calcif. Tissue Res.* **12**, 295.

Reynolds, T. B., Jacobson, G., Edmondson, H. A., Martin, H. E., and Nelson, C. H. (1952). *J. Clin. Endocrinol. Metab.* **12**, 560.

Riccardi, V. M., and Holmes, L. B. (1974). *J. Pediatr.* **84**, 251.

Riddick, F. A., Jr., and Reiss, E. (1962). *Ann. Intern. Med.* **56**, 183.

Risum, G. (1973). *Br. J. Dermatol.* **89**, 309.

Ritchie, G. M. (1965). *Arch. Dis. Child.* **40**, 565.

Ritter, G. (1970). *Dtsch. Z. Nervenheilkd.* **197**, 1.

Rixon, R. H., and Whitfield, J. F. (1972). *Proc. Soc. Exp. Biol. Med.* **141**, 93.

Rixon, R. H., and Whitfield, J. F. (1974). *Proc. Soc. Exp. Biol.*, **146**, 926.

Robins, M. M. (1963). *Clin. Pediatr. (Philadelphia)* **2**, 43.

Robins, P. R., and Jowsey, J. (1973). *J. Lab. Clin. Med.* **82**, 576.

Robinson, C. J., Rafferty, B., and Parsons, J. A. (1972). *Clin. Sci.* **42**, 235.

Roche, P., Carli, A., Benhamou, R., and Macrez, C. (1972). *Ann. Med. Interne* **123**, 23.

Rodan, S. B., and Rodan, G. A. (1974). *J. Biol. Chem.* **249**, 3068.

Rodman, J. S., and Heinemann, H. O. (1975). *Am. J. Med. Sci.* **270**, 481.

Rodriguez, H. J., Walls, J., Yates, J., and Klahr, S. (1974). *J. Clin. Invest.* **53**, 122.

Roof, B. S., Gordan, G. S., Goldman, L., and Piel, C. F. (1973). *Mt. Sinai J. Med., N.Y.* **40**, 433.

Rose, G. A., and Vas, C. J. (1966). *Acta Neurol. Scand.* **42**, 537.

Rose, N. (1963). *Lancet* **2**, 116.

Rosen, F., Roginsky, M., Nathenson, G., and Finberg, L. (1974). *Am. J. Dis. Child.* **127**, 220.

Rosenbaum, J. L. (1965). *J. Clin. Endocrinol. Metab.* **25**, 767.

Rosenbaum, J. L. (1966). *Am. J. Med. Sci.* **251**, 297.

Rosenberg, D., Moreau, P., Salle, B., Gauthier, J., and Monnet, P. (1967). *Sem. Hop. Paris (Ann. Pediat.)* **43**, 2785.

Rösli, A., and Fanconi, A. (1973). *Helv. Paediatr. Acta* **28**, 443.

Rosselle, N., and De Doncker, K. (1959). *Acta Clin. Belg.* **14**, 162.

Rossier, A., Caldera, R., and Le-Oc-Mach, A. (1973). *Ann. Pediatr.* **20**, 869.

Rössle, R. (1932). *Virchows Arch. Pathol. Anat. Physiol.* **283**, 41.

Rössle, R. (1938). *Schweiz. Med. Wochenschr.* **68**, 848.

Roth, F. J., Jr., Boyd, C. C., Sagami, S., and Blank, H. (1959). *J. Invest. Dermatol.* **32,** 549.
Roth, S. I., and Munger, B. L. (1962). *Virchows Arch. Pathol. Anat. Physiol.* **335,** 389.
Royer, P., Lestradet, H., de Menibus, C. H., and Frederich, A. (1959). *Rev. Fr. Etud. Clin. Biol.* **4,** 1007.
Rubenstein, A., and Brust, J. C. M. (1974). *N.Y. State J. Med.* **74,** 2029.
Rude, R. K., Oldham, S. B., and Singer, F. R. (1975). Program of the Endocr. Soc. 57th Annual Meeting, p. 74.
Russell, R. G. G., Smith, R., Walton, R. J., Preston, C., Basson, R., Henderson, R. G., and Norman, A. W. (1974). *Lancet* **2,** 14.
Russell, R. I. (1967). *Br. Med. J.* **3,** 781.
Sagar, S., Estrada, R. L., and Kaye, M. (1972). *Arch. Intern. Med.* **130,** 768.
Sagel, J., Colwell, J. A., Loadholt, C. B., and Lizzaralde, G. (1973). *J. Clin. Endocr.,* **37,** 570.
Sagel, J., Epstein, S., Kalk, J., and Van Mieghem, W. (1972). *Postgrad. Med. J.* **48,** 308.
Salet, J., Polonovski, C., de Guyon, F., Pean, G., Melekian, B., and Fournet, J. P. (1966). *Arch. Fr. Pediatr.* **23,** 749.
Sallis, J. D. (1970). *J. Endocrinol.* **46,** 185.
Sallis, J. D., Hopcroft, S. C., and Opit, L. J. (1967). *J. Appl. Physiol.* **23,** 316.
Saltzman, H. A., Heyman, A., and Sieker, H. O. (1963). *N. Engl. J. Med.* **268,** 1431.
Salvesen, H. A., and Böe, J. (1953). *Acta Med. Scand.* **146,** 290.
Salz, J. L., Daum, F., and Cohen, M. I. (1973). *J. Pediatr.* **82,** 536.
Sandström, I. (1880). Upsala Läk.-Fören. Förh., **40,** 441.
Sarda, L., Marchis-Mouren, G., Constantin, M. J., and Desnuelle, P. (1957). *Biochim. Biophys. Acta* **23,** 264.
Saxena, K. M., Crawford, J. D., and Talbot, N. B. (1964). *Br. Med. J.* **2,** 1153.
Scaletta, S., and Consolo, F. (1960). *Boll. Soc. Ital. Biol. Sper.* **36,** 529.
Schlack, H. G. (1969). *Arch. Kinderheilkd.* **179,** 72.
Schmidt-Gayk, H., and Röher, H. D. (1973). *Surg., Gynecol. Obstet.* **137,** 439.
Schüpbach, A., and Courvoisier, B. (1949). *Schweiz. Med. Wschr.,* **79,** 887.
Schwartz, M. K., Kessler, G., and Bodansky, O. (1960). *Am. J. Clin. Pathol.* **33,** 275.
Schwarz, G. (1960). *Acta Endocrinol.* (Copenhagen) **34,** 399.
Schwarz, G. (1964). "Pseudohypoparathyreoidismus and Pseudo-pseudohypoparathyreoidismus' Heidelberg," Springer-Verlag.
Schwarz, G. (1965). *Acta Endocrinol.* (Copenhagen) **49,** 331.
Schwarz, G., and Bahner, F. (1963). *Dtsch. Med. Wochenschr.* **88,** 240.
Schwarz, G., and Loewe, K. R. (1966). *Acta Endocrinol.* (Copenhagen) **51,** 341.
Scurry, M. T., and Pauk, G. L. (1974). *Acta Endocrinol.* (Copenhagen) **77,** 282.
Seedat, Y. K., Angorn, I. B., and Pillay, N. (1974). *S. Afr. Med. J.* **48,** 2267.
Seelig, M. S. (1971). *In* "Le Déficit Magnésique en Pathologie Humaine" (J. Durlach, ed.), pp. 11–38. S.G.E.M.V., Vittel.
Seelig, M. S., Berger, A. R., and Spielholz, N. (1975). *Dis. Nerv. Syst.* **36,** 461.
Seemann, N. (1967). *Dtsch. Med. Wochenschr.* **92,** 106.
Segal, N., and Lichtig, A. (1974). *Otorinolaringol. Oftalmol.* **18,** 167.
Segerström, A. (1973). *Acta Chir. Scand.* **139,** 55.
Selle, J. G., Altemaier, W. A., Fullen, W. D., and Goldsmith, R. E. (1972). *Arch. Surg. (Chicago)* **105,** 369.
Seringe, P., and Tomkiewicz, S. (1957). *Sem. Hop. Paris (Ann. Pediat.)* **33,** 1092.
Sevringhaus, E. L., and John, R. S. (1943). *J. Clin. Endocrinol.* **3,** 635.
Seymour, J. L., and DeLuca, H. F. (1974). *Endocrinology* **94,** 1009.

Shaw, J. W., Oldham, S. B., Rosoff, L., Fichman, M. P., and Bethune, J. E. (1974). *Clin. Res.* **22**, 167A.

Shearman, B. T., Clubb, J. S., Neale, F. C., and Posen, S. (1965). *Br. Med. J.* **2**, 619.

Sheldon, J. H. (1935). "Haemochromatosis." Oxford University Press, London and New York.

Sherman, L. A., Pfefferbaum, A., and Brown, E. B., Jr. (1970). *Ann. Intern. Med.* **73**, 259.

Sherwood, L. M., Potts, J. T., Jr., Care, A. D., Mayer, G. P., and Aurbach, G. B. (1966). *Nature (London)* **209**, 52.

Sherwood, L. M., Mayer, G. P., and Ramberg, C. F., Jr. (1968). *Endocrinology* **83**, 1043.

Sherwood, L. M., Herrman, I., and Bassett, C. A. (1970). *Nature (London)* **225**, 1056.

Sherwood, L. M., Abe, M., Rodman, J. S., Lundberg, W. B., Jr., and Targovnik, J. H. (1972). *In* "Calcium Parathyroid Hormone and the Calcitonins" (R. V. Talmage and P. L. Munson, eds.), Int. Congr. Ser. No. 243, pp. 183–196. Excerpta Med., Amsterdam.

Sidiropoulos, D., and Schneider, H. (1972). *Z. Kinderheilkd.* **112**, 226.

Siersbaek-Nielsen, K., Skovsted, L., Hansen, J. M., Kristensen, M., and Christensen, L. K. (1971). *Acta Med. Scand.* **189**, 485.

Sigurdsson, G., Woodhouse, N. J. Y., Taylor, S., and Joplin, G. F. (1973). *Br. Med. J.* **1**, 27.

Silverberg, S. G., Hutter, R. V. P., and Foote, F. W., Jr. (1970). *Cancer* **25**, 792.

Simpson, J. A. (1954). *Br. J. Dermatol.* **66**, 1.

Sinclair, J. G. (1942). *J. Nutr.* **23**, 141.

Singleton, A. O., Jr., and Allums, J. (1970). *Arch. Surg. (Chicago)* **100**, 372.

Singleton, E. B., and Teng, C. T. (1962). *Radiology* **78**, 388.

Sinha, T. K., and Bell, N. H. (1976). *N. Engl. J. Med.* **294**, 612.

Sisson, G. A., and Vander Aarde, S. B. (1971). *Arch. Otolaryngol.* **93**, 249.

Siurala, M., Varis, K., and Lamberg, B. A. (1968). *Acta Med. Scand.* **184**, 53.

Sjaastad, O. (1963). *Nord. Med.* **70**, 924.

Sjöberg, K. H. (1966). *Acta Med. Scand.* **179**, 157.

Skjoldborg, H., and Nielsen, H. M. (1971). *Acta Chir. Scand.* **137**, 213.

Skyberg, D., Stromme, J. H., Nesbakken, R., and Harnaes, K. (1968). *Scand. J. Clin. Lab. Invest.* **21**, 355.

Slater, S. (1970). *Pediatrics* **46**, 468.

Smales, O. R. C. (1974). *Proc. Roy. Soc. Med.*, **67**, 759.

Smeenk, D., and van den Brand, I. B. A. M. (1965). *Ned. Tijdschr. Geneeskd.* **109**, 1799.

Smith, D. M., and Johnston, C. C., Jr. (1974). *Endocrinology* **95**, 130.

Smith, J. W. G., Davis, R. H., and Fourman, P. (1960). *Lancet* **2**, 510.

Smulyan, H., and Raisz, L. G. (1959). *J. Clin. Endocrinol. Metab.* **19**, 478.

Snodgrass, G. J. A. I., Stimmler, L., Went, J., Abrams, M. E., and Will, E. J. (1973). *Arch. Dis. Child.* **48**, 279.

Snodgrass, R. W., and Mellinkoff, S. M. (1962). *Am. J. Dig. Dis.* **7**, 273.

Sollberg, G. (1975). *Dtsch. Med. Wochenschr.* **100**, 2213.

Spaulding, W. B., and Yendt, E. R. (1964). *Can. Med. Assoc. J.* **90**, 1049.

Spech, H. J., and Olah, A. J. (1974). *Med. Klin. (Munich)* **69**, 387.

Spinner, M. W., Blizzard, R. M., and Childs, B. (1968). *J. Clin. Endocrinol. Metab.* **28**, 795.

Spinner, M. W., Blizzard, R. M., Gibbs, J., Abbey, H., and Childs, B. (1969). *Clin. Exp. Immunol.* **5**, 461.

Sprague, R. G., Haines, S. F., and Power, M. H. (1945). *J. Lab. Clin. Med.* **30**, 363.

Spranger, J. W. (1969). *Birth Defects,* Orig. Artic. Ser. **5**, 122.

Spranger, J. W., and Rohwedder, J. (1965). *Med. Welt* **41**, 2308.

Sraer, J., Ardaillou, R., Loreau, N., and Sraer, J. D. (1974). *Mol. Cell. Endocrinol.* **1**, 285.

Stanbury, S. W. (1962). *Schweiz. Med. Wochenschr.* **92,** 883.

Steinbach, H. L., and Young, D. A. (1966). *Am. J. Roentgenol., Radium Ther. Nucl. Med.* [N.S.] **97,** 49.

Steinbach, H. L., Rudhe, U., Jonsson, M., and Young, D. A. (1965). *Radiology* **85,** 670.

Steinberg, H., and Waldron, B. R. (1952). *Medicine (Baltimore)* **31,** 133.

Stögmann, W. (1973). *Klin. Paediatr.* **185,** 146.

Stögmann, W., and Fischer, J. A. (1975). *Am. J. Med.* **59,** 140.

Stowers, J. M., Michie, W., and Frazer, S. C. (1967). *Lancet* **1,** 124.

Streeto, J. M. (1969). *Metab., Clin. Exp.* **18,** 968.

Stromme, J. H., Nesbakken, R., Normann, T., Skjorten, F., Skyberg, D., and Johannessen, B. (1969). *Acta Paediatr. Scand.* **58,** 433.

Sugar, O. (1953). *Arch. Neurol. Psychiatry* **70,** 86.

Suh, S. M., Kooh, S. W., Chan, A. M., Fraser, D., and Tashjian, A. H., Jr. (1969). *J. Clin. Endocrinol. Metab.* **29,** 429.

Suh, S. M., Fraser, D., and Kooh, S. W. (1970). *J. Clin. Endocrinol. Metab.* **30,** 609.

Suh, S. M., Csima, A., and Fraser, D. (1971). *J. Clin. Invest.* **50,** 2668.

Suh, S. M., Tashjian, A. H., Jr., Matsuo, N., Parkinson, D. K., and Fraser, D. (1973). *J. Clin. Invest.* **52,** 153.

Surks, M. I., and Levenson, D. (1962). *Ann. Intern. Med.* **56,** 282.

Sutphin, A., Albright, F., and McCune, D. J. (1943). *J. Clin. Endocrinol.* **3,** 625.

Suzuki, H., Ogata, E., Eto, S., Fujimoto, Y., and Fukumitsu, M. (1968). *Endocrinol. Jpn.* **15,** 251.

Swinton, N. W. (1937). *N. Engl. J. Med.* **217,** 165.

Szczepski, O., Walczak, M., Maciejewski, J., Bittner, K., Czekalski, S., and Waligora, A. (1971). *Acta Paediatr. Scand.* **60,** 73.

Tabaeeh-Zadeh, M. J., Frame, B., and Kapphahn, K. (1972). *N. Engl. J. Med.* **286,** 762.

Taitz, L. S., and de Lacy, C. D. (1962). *Pediatrics* **30,** 884.

Taitz, L. S., Zarate-Salvador, C., and Schwartz, E. (1966). *Pediatrics* **38,** 412.

Talbott, J. H., Cobb, S., Coombs, F. S., Cohen, M. E., and Consolazio, W. V. (1938). *Arch. Neurol. Psychiatry* **39,** 973.

Talmage, R. V., and Kraintz, F. W. (1954). *Proc. Soc. Exp. Biol. Med.* **87,** 263.

Tan, C. M., Raman, A., and Sinnathyray, T. A. (1972). *J. Obstet. Gynaecol. Br. Cwlth.* **79,** 694.

Tanaka, Y., and DeLuca, H. F. (1973). *Arch. Biochem. Biophys.* **154,** 566.

Tanz, S. S. (1960). *Am. J. Med. Sci.* **239,** 453.

Tardy, M. E., Jr., and Tenta, L. T. (1971). *Laryngoscope* **81,** 1455.

Targovnik, J. H., Rodman, J. S., and Sherwood, L. M. (1971). *Endocrinology* **88,** 1477.

Tashjian, A. H., Jr., and Voelkel, E. F. (1967). *J. Clin. Endocrinol. Metab.* **27,** 1353.

Tashjian, A. H., Jr., Frantz, A. G., and Lee, J. B. (1966). *Proc. Natl. Acad. Sci. U.S.A.* **56,** 1138.

Taybi, H., and Keele, D. (1962). *Am. J. Roentgenol., Radium Ther. Nucl. Med.* [N.S.]. **88,** 432.

Taylor, A. L., Davis, B. B. Pawlson, L. G., Josimovich, J. B., and Mintz, D. H. (1970). *J. Clin. Endocrinol. Metab.* **30,** 316.

Terepka, A. R., Toribara, T. Y., and Dewey, P. A. (1958). *J. Clin. Invest.* **37,** 87.

Terepka, A. R., Chen, P. S., and Jorgensen, B. (1961). *Endocrinology* **68,** 996.

Tettenborn, D., Hobik, H. P., and Luckhaus, G. (1970). *Arzneimittel-Forsch.* **20,** 1753.

Thajchayapong, P., Queener, S. F., McClintock, R., Allen, D. O., and Bell, N. H. (1976). *Horm. Metab. Res.* **8,** 190.

Thew, R. F., and Goulston, S. (1962). *Australas. Ann. Med.* **11,** 275.

Thiele, J., Ries, P., and Georgii, A. (1975). *Virchows Arch. A.* **367**, 195.

Thomas, W. C., Jr., and Tilden, M. T. (1972). *Johns Hopkins Med. J.* **131**, 133.

Thomas, W. C., Jr., Morgan, H. G., Connor, T. B., Haddock, L., Bills, C. E., and Howard, J. E. (1959). *J. Clin. Invest.* **38**, 1078.

Thomas, W. C., Jr., Lewis, A. M., and Bird, E. D. (1967). *J. Clin. Endocrinol. Metab.* **27**, 1328.

Thompson, D. D., and Hiatt, H. H. (1957). *J. Clin. Invest.* **36**, 550.

Thorén, L., and Werner, I. (1969). *Acta Chir. Scand.* **135**, 395.

Tighe, W. J. (1952). *J. Clin. Endocrinol. Metab.* **12**, 1220.

Todd, J. N., III, Hill, S. R., Jr., Nickerson, J. F., and Tingley, J. O. (1961). *Am. J. Med.* **30**, 289.

Tomlinson, S., Barling, P. M., Albano, J. D. M., Brown, B. L., and O'Riordan, J. L. H. (1974). *Clin. Sci. Mol. Med.* **47**, 481.

Townsend, J. D. (1961). *Ann. Intern. Med.* **55**, 662.

Treusch, J. V., and Cohen, S. (1962). *Ann. Intern. Med.* **56**, 484.

Trummel, C. L., Raisz, L. G., Hallick, R. B., and DeLuca, H. F. (1971). *J. Biol. Chem.* **246**, 5733.

Trygstad, C. W., Zisman, E., Witkop, C. J., Jr., and Bartter, F. C. (1968). *J. Clin. Endocrinol. Metab.* **28**, 1153.

Tsang, R. C., Kleinman, L. I., Sutherland, J. M., and Light, I. J. (1972). *J. Pediatr.* **80**, 384.

Tsang, R. C., Light, I. J., Sutherland, J. M., and Kleinman, L. I. (1973a). *J. Pediatr.* **82**, 423.

Tsang, R. C., Chen, I. W., Friedman, M. A., and Chen, I. (1973b). *J. Pediatr.* **83**, 728.

Tsang, R. C., Chen, I., Hayes, W., Atkinson, W., Atherton, H., and Edwards, N. (1974). *J. Pediatr.* **84**, 428.

Turner, R. W., and Takamura, T. (1962). *Ann. Intern. Med.* **56**, 276.

Turpin, R., and Lefebvre, J. (1943). *Presse Med.* **51**, 338.

Turpin, R., Lefebvre, J., and Lerique, J. (1943). *C.R. Med. Sciences Acad. Sci.* **232**, 552.

Turunen, M., and Saxén, L. (1963). *Acta Chir. Scand.* **126**, 538.

Twycross, R. G., and Marks, V. (1970). *Br. J. Med.* **2**, 701.

Tze, W. J., Saunders, J., and Drummond, G. I. (1975). *Arch. Dis. Child.* **50**, 656.

Uchimura, H., Ariyama, T., Wada, K., Araki, J., Kuwahata, T., Kono, Y., Kawa, A., and Kanchisa, T. (1974). *Calcif. Tissue. Res.* **15**, 161.

Uitto, J., Laitinen, O., Lamberg, B. A., and Kivirikko, K. I. (1968). *Clin. Chim. Acta* **22**, 583.

Ulstrom, R. A. (1957). Discussion, see DiGeorge and Paschkis (1957).

Urdanivia, E., Mataverde, A., and Cohen, M. P. (1975). *J. Lab. Clin. Med.* **86**, 772.

Vachon, A., Vignon, G., Chatin, B., Pansu, D., and Chapuy, N. C. (1970). *Rev. Lyon. Med.* **19**, 543.

Vaes, G. (1968). *Nature (London)* **219**, 939.

Vainsel, M., Vandevelde, G., Smulders, J., Vosters, M., Hubain, P., and Loeb, H. (1970). *Arch. Dis. Child.* **45**, 254.

Valdés-Dapena, M. A., and Weinstein, D. S. (1971). *Acta Pathol. Microbiol. Scand.* **79**, 228.

Van de Casseye, M., and Gepts, W. (1973). *Virchows Arch. A* **361**, 257.

Van Den Berg, C. J., Hill, L. F., and Stanbury, S. W. (1972). *Clin. Sci.* **43**, 377.

Van der Veen, E. A., Van Garsse, L. G. M. M., and Schreuder, H. B. (1975). *Neth. J. Med.* **18**, 262.

van der Werff ten Bosch, J. J. (1959). *Lancet* **1**, 69.

Vartio, T., and Meronen, R. (1961). *Duodecim* **77**, 349.

Vassale, G., and Generali, F. (1896a). *Arch. Ital. Biol.* **25**, 459.

Vassale, G., and Generali, F. (1896b). *Arch. Ital. Biol.*, **26**, 61.

Vazquez, A. M., and Kenny, F. M. (1973). *Obstet. Gynecol.* **41**, 414.

Vesin, P., Milhaud, G., Gamerman, H., and Romeo, R. (1974). *Lancet* **2**, 110.

Vesterhus, P., Eide, J., Froland, S. S., Haneberg, B., and Jacobsen, K. B. (1975). *Acta Paediatr. Scand.* **64**, 555.

Vincent, R. G., Moore, G. E., and Watne, A. L. (1962). *J. Am. Med. Assoc.* **180**, 372.

Visakorpi, J. K., and Gerber, M. (1963). *Ann. Paediatr. Fenn.* **9**, 128.

Vlietstra, R. E. (1973). *N. Z. Med. J.* **2**, 113.

Volpe, J. (1973). *N. Engl. J. Med.* **289**, 413.

Voog, R., Hadjian, A., Nigri, M. M., Perdrix, A., Pallo, D., and Lachaud, P. (1972). *Sem. Hop.* **48**, 3563.

Wacker, W. E. C., and Parisi, A. F. (1968). *N. Engl. J. Med.* **278**, 658.

Wade, J. S. H. (1960). *Br. J. Surg.* **48**, 25.

Wade, J. S. H., Fourman, P., and Deane, L. (1965a). *Br. J. Surg.* **52**, 493.

Wade, J. S. H., Goodall, P., Deane, L., Dauncey, T. M., and Fourman, P. (1965b). *Br. J. Surg.* **52**, 497.

Wagner, G., Transbol, I., and Melchior, J. C. (1964). *Acta Endocrinol. (Copenhagen)* **47**, 549.

Wallach, S., Englert, E., Jr., and Brown, H. (1956). *Arch. Intern. Med.* **98**, 517.

Warwick, O. M., Yendt, E. R., and Olin, J. S. (1961). *Can. Med. Assoc. J.* **85**, 719.

Watkins, E., Jr., Bell, G. O., Snow, J. C., and Adams, H. D. (1962). *J. Am. Med. Assoc.* **182**, 140.

Watson, L. (1968). *Proc. R. Soc. Med.* **61**, 287.

Weinberg, A. G., and Stone, R. T. (1971). *J. Pediatr.* **79**, 997.

Weinstein, R. S. (1974). *Clin. Res.* **22**, 569A.

Weiss, N. (1881). *Samml. Klin. Vortr.* **189**, 1675.

Weiss, N. (1883). *Wien. Med. Wochenschr.* **33**, 683.

Weitzman, R., and Murad, F. (1973a). *Clin. Res.* **21**, 48.

Weitzman, R., and Murad, F. (1973b). *Clin. Res.* **21**, 89.

Wells, H., and Lloyd, W. (1967). *Endocrinology* **81**, 139.

Wells, H., and Lloyd, W. (1968). *Endocrinology* **83**, 521.

Wells, H., and Lloyd, W. (1969). *Endocrinology* **84**, 861.

Wells, S. A., Jr., Burdick, J. F., Hattler, B. G., Christiansen, C., Pettigrew, H. M., Abe, M., and Sherwood, L. M. (1974). *Ann. Surg.* **180**, 805.

Wells, S. A., Jr., Gunnells, J. C., Shelburne, J. D., Schneider, A. B., and Sherwood, L. M. (1975). *Surgery* **78**, 34.

Wells, S. A., Jr., Ellis, G. J., Gunnells, J. C., Schneider, A. B., and Sherwood, L. M. (1976). *N. Engl. J. Med.* **295**, 57.

Welsh, D. A. (1898a). *J. Anat. Physiol. Norm. Pathol. Homme Amm.* **32**, 292.

Weish, D. A. (1898b). *J. Pathol. Bacteriol.* **5**, 202.

Werder, E. A., Illig, R., Bernasconi, S., Kind, H., Prader, A., Fischer, J. A., and Fanconi, A. (1975). *Pediatr. Res.* **9**, 12.

Whitaker, J., Landing, B. H., Esselborn, V. M., and Williams, R. R. (1956). *J. Clin. Endocrinol. Metab.* **16**, 1374.

Wijnbladh, H. (1952). *Acta Endocrinol. (Copenhagen)* **10**, 1.

Wilkins, L. (1957). Discussion, see DiGeorge and Paschkis (1957).

Willi, H., and Baumann, U. (1966). *Arch. Kinderheilkl.* **174**, 263.

Williams, E., and Wood, C. (1959). *Arch. Dis. Child.* **34**, 302.

Williams, G. A., Hargis, G. K., Bowser, E. N., Henderson, W. J., and Martinez, N. J. (1973). *Endocrinology* **92**, 687.

Williams, G. A., Kukreja, S. C., Hargis, G. K., Bowser, E. N., and Henderson, W. J. (1974). *Clin. Res.* **22,** 652A.

Willich, E., and Englert, M. (1973). *Fortschr. Geb. Roentgenstr. Nuklearmed.* **119,** 443.

Wills, M. R., and Lewin, M. R. (1971). *J. Clin. Pathol.* **24,** 856.

Windorfer, A. (1970). Monatsschr. Kinderheilkd. **118,** 103.

Winnacker, J. L., Becker, K. L., and Moore, C. F. (1967). *Metab. Clin. Exp.* **16,** 644.

Wise, B. L., and Hart, J. C. (1952). *Arch. Neurol. Psychiatry* **68,** 78.

Witkop, C. J., Jr. (1966). *J. Den. Res.* **45,** 568.

Wolf, S. M., and Lusk, W. (1972). *Bull. Los Angeles Neurol. Soc.* **37,** 167.

Wölfler, A. (1879). *Wien. Med. Wochenschr.* **29,** 758.

Wong, G. L., and Cohn, D. V. (1975). *Proc. Natl. Acad. Sci. U.S.A.* **72,** 3167.

Woo, J., and Singer, F. R. (1974). *Clin. Chim. Acta,* **54,** 161.

Woodard, J. C., Webster, P. D., and Carr, A. A. (1972). *Am. J. Dig. Dis.* **17,** 612.

Woodhouse, N. J. Y. (1974). *Clin. Endocrinol. Metab.* **3,** 323.

Woodhouse, N. J. Y., Doyle, F. H., and Joplin, G. F. (1971). *Lancet* **2,** 283.

Wuepper, K. D., and Fudenberg, H. H. (1967). *Clin. Exp. Immunol.,* **2,** 71.

Yeghiayan, E., Rojo-Ortega, J. M., and Genest, J. (1972). *J. Anat.* **112,** 137.

Young, D. M., and Capen, C. C. (1970). *Endocrinology* **86,** 1463.

Young, D. M., Olson, H. M., Prieur, D. J., Cooney, D. A., and Reagan, R. L. (1973). *Lab. Invest.* **29,** 374.

Young, M. M., Jasani, C., Smith, D. A., and Nordin, B. E. C. (1968). *Clin. Sci.* **34,** 411.

Zampa, G. A., and Zucchelli, P. C. (1965). *J. Clin. Endocrinol. Metab.* **25,** 1616.

Zerwekh, J. E., Brumbaugh, P. F., Haussler, D. H., Cork, D. J., and Haussler, M. R. (1974). *Biochemistry* **13,** 4097.

Zisman, E., Henkin, R. I., Ross, G. T., and Bartter, F. C. (1967). *Clin. Res.* **15,** 333.

Zisman, E., Lotz, M., Jenkins, M. E., and Bartter, F. C. (1969). *Am. J. Med.* **46,** 464.

Zuyderhoudt, F. M. J., van der Helm, H. J., and Hootsmans, W. J. W. (1974). *Eur. Neurol.* **12,** 377.

4

The Thyroid Gland in Skeletal and Calcium Metabolism

LEONARD J. DEFTOS

I. Introduction 447
II. The Thyroid Hormones: T_3 and T_4 448
    A. Thyroid Hormone Deficiency 448
    B. Thyroid Hormone Excess 452
III. Calcitonin 458
    A. Chemistry 458
    B. Physiology 458
    C. Medullary Thyroid Carcinoma 461
    D. Measurement of Human Calcitonin 473
IV. Recent Developments 479
    References 481

I. INTRODUCTION

The thyroid gland plays a very important role in skeletal metabolism. This effect is mediated by two distinct classes of hormones: the thyroid hormones proper, thyroxine (T_4) and triiodothyronine (T_3), and the peptide hormone of neural crest origin, calcitonin. The effects of T_4 and T_3 on the skeleton have been well known for many years. In contrast, it is only within the past decade that the existence of calcitonin and its influence on skeletal homeostasis have been uncovered. The thyroid hormones and calcitonin exert their effects on each of the three organ systems that influence skeletal metabolism; the skeleton itself, the kidney, and the gastrointestinal tract. By their actions, these hormones affect the growth, maturation, and homeostasis of the skeletal system. In addition, these

447

Copyright © 1978 by Academic Press, Inc.
All rights of reproduction in any form reserved
ISBN 0-12-068702-X

hormones also influence the metabolism of the mineral and organic constituents of bone, especially calcium, phosphate, and collagen.

The importance of the thyroid hormones and calcitonin on skeletal metabolism can be appreciated by considering the effects produced by conditions characterized by hormonal excess and deficiency, respectively.

II. THE THYROID HORMONES: T_3 AND T_4

A. Thyroid Hormone Deficiency

1. Growth and Maturation

One of the most dramatic illustrations of the importance of thyroid hormones in the growth and maturation of the skeleton can be seen in cretins, who are congenitally deficient in thyroid hormone. There is a marked delay in the appearance of ossification in epiphyseal centers. Although all epiphyseal centers are probably involved, the most diagnostically useful in the newborn are the proximal tibial and distal femoral epiphyses (Lowery et al., 1958). Intrauterine thyroid hormone deficiency can be postulated when the distal femoral epiphyses is absent in a newborn who weighs 3000 gm or more or when the distal femoral and proximal tibial epiphyses are absent in a newborn weighing 2500 to 3000 gm at birth (Fisher, 1971). It is of note that infants born of hypothyroid mothers do not exhibit delays in ossification (Krane, 1971b).

Although thyroid hormone deficiency results in delayed skeleton maturation, the skeleton does eventually mature. When an epiphyseal center does ossify in the hypothyroid child, it does so in an irregular pattern of multiple foci. When these foci coalesce there results a "stippled" appearance, which is known as "epiphyseal dysgenesis" (Wilkins, 1955). The onset of thyroid deficiency can be dated by the occurrence of dysgenesis in a particular center of ossification. For example, the finding of stippled epiphyses in the femoral head of a child indicates that thyroid deficiency began before the ninth to twelfth month since this center usually begins to ossify at this time (Wilkins, 1962) (Fig. 1).

In addition to delays in ossification, the hypothyroid dwarf retains infantile skeletal proportions. This is in contrast to the pituitary dwarf who may have proportions consistent with his or her skeletal age. The ratio of bone age to chronological age in hypothyroid infants and children is often less than 0.5. In older children or in patients with a short duration of thyroid deficiency a lesser degree of skeletal retardation will occur (Tapp, 1966).

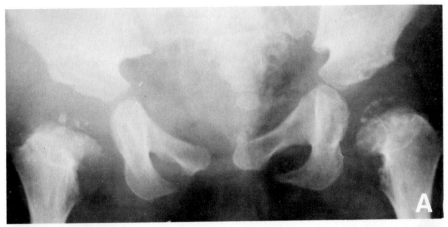
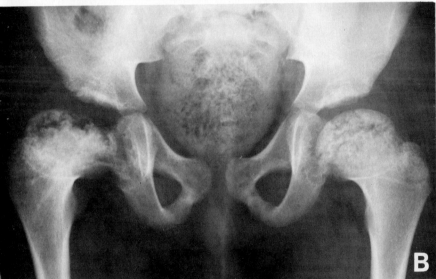

Fig. 1. Epiphyseal dysgenesis in cretins. (A) A 10-year-old girl who never walked. (B) A 15-year-old boy.

The importance of thyroid hormones in skeletal maturation and growth can be further demonstrated by experimental studies. Skeletal maturation in the rat can be accelerated by very small doses of T_3 (Walker, 1957). Furthermore, physiological concentrations of either T_3 or T_4 can promote the maturation in tissue culture of isolated limb buds (Fell and Mellanby, 1956). These effects of the thyroid hormones on skeletal maturation do not require the presence of sex hormones.

The growth retardation of thyroidectomized animals may also be contributed to by a secondary deficiency of secreted growth hormone, due perhaps to "pituitary myxedema." Very little growth can be produced in the hypophysectomized rat by thyroxine alone, whereas growth hormone can stimulate growth in the thyroidectomized rat. However, thyroid hormones do play some primary role in skeletal growth since T_4 can potentiate the growth action of growth hormone (Riekstniece and Asling, 1966).

Thyroid hormones can also affect the growth and maturation of teeth. In rats made thyroid deficient by either thyroidectomy or PTU, the rate of tooth eruption and the size of tooth structures is impaired. Enamel is thinned and there is a decrease in the vascularity of the pulp (Baume *et al.,* 1954). These changes can be reversed by thyroid hormone replacement. In hypothyroid children delayed dentition is characteristic. In addition, the loss of deciduous teeth is delayed and the growth of the roots is also slowed (Jenkins, 1966).

2. Skeletal Metabolism

The metabolism of the skeleton is markedly retarded in thyroid deficiency. This is reflected in most of the parameters that can be used to evaluate skeletal activity.

a. Histopathology. The delay in ossification of epiphyseal centers has been mentioned earlier. When it does occur, epiphyseal ossification takes place in a fragmentary manner which results in a porous appearance of the bone. The decrease in activity of bone cells is also testified to by the low level of alkaline phosphatase in patients with myxedema (Talbot, 1939).

b. Radiological Changes. The characteristic X-ray appearance of epiphyseal dysgenesis has already been discussed. Although there is a generalized decrease in the cellular activity of bone in hypothyroidism, this is not reflected by significant changes in X-ray findings. This is probably due to several reasons. Since bone resorption and bone formation are closely coupled processes, they are both decreased in hypothyroidism and there may be little net change in bone density. Furthermore, there must be substantial changes in bone density before there are any X-ray changes (Whedon *et al.,* 1966). However, in some patients with hypothyroidism an increase in bone density can be demonstrated by X-ray studies.

c. Metabolic Studies. All of the indices that can be used to measure the dynamics of bone turnover demonstrate a decreased activity in hypothyroidism. There is a decrease in the excretion of calcium and phosphorus in both the urine and feces of patients with hypothyroidism (Aub *et al.,* 1929). The excretion of hydroxyproline in the urine of hypothyroid subjects is also reduced (Kivirikko *et al.*, 1965). Experimental studies have demonstrated that the decreased excretion of hydroxyproline is due to a decreased rate of degradation of both soluble and insoluble collagen (Kivirikko, 1971). Injected doses of ^{45}Ca are incorporated into bone more slowly in thyroid-deficient patients (Krane *et al.*, 1956). Finally, essentially all of these abnormalities can be reversed by thyroid hormone replacement (Smith *et al.*, 1973).

3. Calcium Metabolism

Overt disorders of calcium metabolism are not usually seen in patients with hypothyroidism. In most studies, blood calcium has usually been within normal limits despite the fact that there was a decrease in calcium and skeletal turnover (Krane, 1971a). However, a tendency to hypocalcemia can exist and, in a recent study, hypothyroid patients were found to have lower blood calciums than a control group of normal subjects. In addition, increased parathyroid hormone secretion was also observed in these patients, consistent with the presence of secondary hyperparathyroidism due to the hypocalcemia (Figs. 2 and 3). The possibility that such a subtle form of secondary hypoparathyroidism can develop in hypothyroidism awaits further evaluation. If true, this phenomenon might also explain in part the increase in the intestinal absorption of calcium reported in hypothyroidism (Bouillon and DeMoor, 1974).

Although not a consistent finding, in some hypothyroid patients there is a decreased calcium tolerance (Gittes and Irvin, 1966). When challenged with either an oral or intravenous calcium load, hypothyroid subjects exhibit a greater rise in blood calcium than do control subjects. This has been explained on the basis of a decreased calcium deposition in bone due to the decreased skeletal metabolism of thyroid hormone deficiency. However, a concurrent deficiency in calcitonin may also play a role when this phenomenon occurs in thyroidectomized patients who are deficient in calcitonin as well as T_3 and T_4: The absence of the hypocalcemic action of calcitonin may interfere with the subject's ability to regulate a calcium challenge. Finally, hypercalcemia and nephrocalcinosis occasionally have been reported in cretins (Bateson and Chandler, 1965).

4. Clinical Sequelae

The skeletal consequences of hypothyroidism have been mentioned in the preceding sections. To summarize, there is a retardation of growth and maturation of skeleton. Evidence of this is greatest in growing subjects who exhibit short stature, retarded bone age, epiphyseal dysgenesis, and abnormal dentition. In older subjects the skeletal changes are more

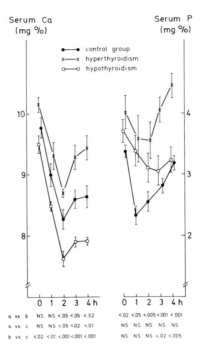

Fig. 2. Serum calcium and serum organic phosphorous levels (mean ±S.E.M.) measured before, during, and after an infusion of EDTA in 13 normal controls (●), 5 hyperthyroid patients (X), and 5 hypothyroid patients (□). The significance of the differences between the groups was assessed by Student's t-test. These results are consistent with a functional decrease in parathyroid hormone secretion in hyperthyroidism and an increase in hypothyroidism. (From Bouillon and DeMoor, 1974.)

subtle and may include an increase in bone density; similarly, overt calcium abnormalities are rare, although there may be a tendency to hypocalcemia and consequent secondary hyperparathyroidism.

B. Thyroid Hormone Excess

The effects of thyroid hormone excess on the skeletal system are essentially the opposite of the effects of thyroid hormone deficiency. There is an increase in the parameters of skeletal metabolism.

1. Growth and Maturation

There is a marked acceleration in the growth and maturation of bone in the young child with hyperthyroidism. Several mechanisms have been suggested as the cause of this process, including increased secretion of growth hormone, increased secretion of insulin, and increased secretion of

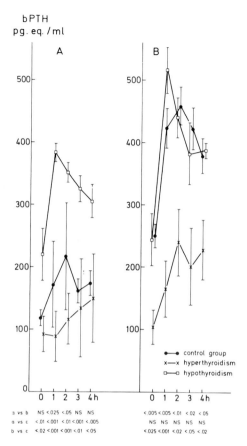

Fig. 3. Serum parathyroid hormone levels (mean ±S.E.M.) measured with two different antisera, A and B, before, during, and after an infusion of EDTA in 13 normal controls (●), 5 hyperthyroid patients (X), and 5 hypothyroid patients (□). The significance of the differences between the groups was assessed by Student's *t*-test. These results are consistent with a functional decrease in parathyroid hormone secretion in hyperthyroidism and an increase in hypothyroidism. (From Bouillon and DeMoor, 1974.)

gonadal steroids. However, the evidence for an increased secretion of these other hormones is not convincing and a primary anabolic effect of the thyroid hormones may be an adequate explanation for the enhanced growth and maturation of bone seen in hyperthyroidism (Silberberg and Silberberg, 1947). In the experimental animal, T_4 stimulates the proliferation of cartilage as well as epiphyseal maturation and closure (Silberberg and Silberberg, 1943).

Although an excess of thyroid hormone does not lead to hypernormal growth in the experimental animal, it can cause an early eruption of teeth and an increased rate of amelogenesis (Karnofsky and Crinkhite, 1939).

2. Skeletal Metabolism

a. Histopathology. An increase in skeletal activity in hyperthyroid states can be demonstrated by many techniques. There is an increase in the number of osteoblasts and osteoclasts and an increase in plasma alkaline phosphatase (Krane, 1971a). Increased cellularity can be accompanied by increased vascularity and connective tissue proliferation to such an extent that, in rare cases, the findings are indistinguishable from those of osteitis fibrosa cystica (von Recklinghausen, 1891). More sophisticated techniques, including microradiography and tetracycline labeling, reveal increased bone resorption as well as increased bone formation; however, the rate of bone resorption seems to exceed the rate of bone formation (Adams *et al.,* 1967). In some patients with hyperthyroidism there is an increase in the number and length of osteoid borders but not the width. However, in contrast to osteomalacia, the increased osteoid is always associated with bone-forming surfaces and these regions are calcified in a normal fashion (Adams *et al.,* 1967). Therefore, the increased osteoid is a result of the increased rate of bone formation (Chapter 4, Volume I).

b. Radiological Changes. With the exception of the changes seen in thyroid acropathy, X-ray findings are not common in hyperthyroidism. Despite the excessive bone resorption and the negative calcium and phosphorous balance, a decrease in bone density is not commonly seen in hyperthyroidism. Hyperthyroidism may exaggerate the development of so-called senile osteoporosis, since the incidence of such bone disease is seen with increased frequency in hyperthyroid women in the older age group (Laake, 1955; Fraser *et al.*, 1971).

A form of hypertrophic osteoarthropathy can be seen in patients with hyperthyroidism (Freedberg, 1971). The bony abnormalities consist of subperiosteal swelling, which can have the radiological appearance of bubbles. There is increased vascularity in the affected regions. In contrast to hypertrophic pulmonary osteoarthropathy, there is no marked new bone formation and the symptoms are minimal except for slight stiffness. The bone changes are usually seen in the metacarpals and proximal phalanges, although the distal phalanges and the proximal ends of the radius and ulna may be involved. A soft, diffuse swelling of adjacent tissues accompanies the bony changes. Although no etiology has been definitely established for thyroid acropachy, this rare syndrome is often associated with pretibial myxedema and exopthalmos. It may occur at any time in relationship to hyperthyroidism, but thyroid acropachy is seldom seen during the active phases of the disease and most commonly occurs weeks to years after the hyperthyroidism has been treated (Gimlett, 1964) (Fig. 4).

c. *Metabolic Studies.* The changes in skeletal turnover that occur in hyperthyroidism can be demonstrated by a wide variety of metabolic parameters. Studies of the effect of thyroid hormone on intestinal calcium absorption are contradictory. In some patients with hyperthyroidism increased absorption has been demonstrated. However, in some patients calcium absorption is normal and in some subjects with clinical and experimental hyperthyroidism calcium absorption is decreased (Adams *et al.*, 1967; Friedlander *et al.*, 1965; Krawitt, 1967; Lewin and Samackson, 1972). These contradictory studies cannot be clearly resolved at this time. The absorption of calcium chloride, which is used in clinical and experimental studies, may not reflect the absorption of food calcium. Furthermore, the absorption of calcium may be influenced by the decreased intestinal transit time seen in hyperthyroidism (Smith *et al.*, 1973).

3. Calcium Metabolism

There is an increase in both urinary and fecal excretion of calcium and phosphorous in both spontaneous and experimental hyperthyroidism (Aub *et al.*, 1929). In some patients the fecal calcium may be higher than the dietary calcium intake. This may represent an increase in the endogenous calcium secretion (Smith *et al.*, 1973). There is even an increase in the calcium excreted by the sweat glands (Harden *et al.*, 1964). The

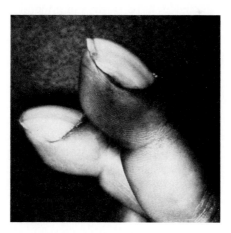

Fig. 4. An example of pachydermoperiostosis of the idiopathic variety that resembles that seen in thyroid achropachy. [Courtesy of D. L. Rimoin (1965) New Engl. J. Med. **272**, 923.]

effect of all of these abnormalities in calcium metabolism is often the negative calcium balance that is commonly seen in hyperthyroidism. Despite the increased urinary excretion of calcium, urinary stones are not common.

Both the plasma level and the urinary excretion of hydroxyproline are increased in spontaneous and experimental hyperthyroidism (Aub *et al.*, 1929). These hydroxyproline indices can be well correlated with indices of thyroid activity in hyperthyroid subjects as well as hypothyroid and normal subjects (Kivirikko *et al.*, 1963; Smith *et al.*, 1973). The increase in the urinary excretion of collagen is caused by increased rates of degradation of both soluble and insoluble collagen (see Chapter 1, Volume I); collagen synthesis does not seem to be increased but may even be decreased (Kivirikko, 1971). Nondialyzable urinary hydroxyproline, which seems to represent the breakdown of the most recently synthesized collagen, contributes less to the total urinary hydroxyproline in hyperthyroidism (Haddad *et al.*, 1969). There may even be tubular secretion of hydroxyproline-containing peptides in hyperthyroidism (Benoit and Watten, 1968).

In hyperthyroidism there is a rapid decrease in the plasma level of administered doses of ^{45}Ca and strontium. This probably reflects a rapid uptake of the isotope by the skeletal system, which is undergoing increased bone formation as well as resorption (Krane *et al.*, 1956). The increased uptake of bone-seeking isotopes gradually returns toward normal after treatment (Smith *et al.*, 1973).

In view of the excessive bone destruction that takes place in hyperthyroidism it is not surprising that disorders of mineral metabolism are not uncommon in hyperthyroid states. The increased urinary and fecal excretion of calcium as well as phosphate have been mentioned. Furthermore, there is a significant occurrence of hypercalcemia in hyperthyroidism. In some series, an incidence of 16 to 23% has been reported. In addition, hyperthyroid patients who are not hypercalcemic tend to have blood calciums toward the upper limits of the normal range (Baxter and Bondy, 1966). In most cases the hypercalcemia is mild and not clinically important and resolves coincident with treatment of the hyperthyroidism (Epstein *et al.*, 1958). In addition, the elevated levels of plasma alkaline phosphatase which are seen in hyperthyroidism (see Chapter 3, Volume I) return toward normal after treatment (Smith *et al.*, 1973).

The hypercalcemia of hyperthyroidism can probably be best explained on the basis of increased bone resorption (Sataline *et al.*, 1962). Alternative explanations have been offered (Parfitt and Dent, 1970), including the view that there is increased parathyroid hormone secretion in hyperthyroidism (Engfeldt and Hertquist, 1954). There is, in fact, a reported incidence of frank hyperparathyroidism in patients with hyperthyroidism with 17 reported cases of an associated parathyroid adenoma (Breuer and McPherson, 1966); however, coincidental occurrence of these two disease states cannot be ruled out. Despite some evidence to support this view, it has been shown that hypercalcemia can occur even in parathyroidectomized animals with experimental hyperthyroidism. In fact, the following evidence suggests that parathyroid function is actually suppressed in hyperthyroidism, presumably due to the tendency toward hypercalcemia.

Although the majority of patients with hyperthyroidism have plasma phosphate levels within the normal range (Smith *et al.*, 1973), the values in hyperthyroid patients tend to be slightly higher. Adams *et al.*(1967) reported a mean plasma phosphorus of 4.01 mg in hyperthyroid patients and a mean value of 3.2 mg in normal subjects. Similar results have been reported by Smith *et al.* (1973). Since serum calcium levels tend to be higher in patients with hyperthyroidism, the decrease in plasma phosphate may be a reflection of suppressed parathyroid hormone secretion by the increased plasma calcium concentrations. This view is also supported by the finding that the tubular reabsorption of phosphorous is increased in patients with hyperthyroidism (Adams *et al.*, 1967; Malamos *et al.*, 1969), and returns toward normal after treatment (Parsons and Anderson, 1964).

Although alternative explanations exist for these findings (Parfitt and Dent, 1970), further support for the concept of functional hypoparathyroidism in hyperthyroidism comes from the observation that patients with hyperthyroidism have increased sensitivity to exogenous parathyroid hormone (Harrison *et al.*, 1964). Although the histology of the parathyroid gland has been reported as normal in patients with hyperthyroidism (Askanazy and Rutishauser, 1933), this may not be a reliable index of secretory activity. In fact, direct support to indicate that there is functional hypoparathyroidism in patients with hyperthyroidism has come from the recent demonstration of decreased levels of PTH (along with increased serum phosphorous) in such patients (Bouillon and DeMoor, 1974) (Figs. 2 and 3).

4. Clinical Sequelae

Clinically significant skeletal disease is uncommon in hyperthyroidism despite the increased rate of bone resorption and compensatory increase in bone formation. Probably because of the relatively mild increase in bone turnover, skeletal sequelae such as severe demineralization, subperiosteal erosions, and cysts are not as commonly seen in hyperthyroidism as they are in hyperparathyroidism. When it does occur, the treatment of clinically significant skeletal disease is the treatment of the hyperthyroidism itself.

III. CALCITONIN

Calcitonin is a potent hypocalcemic peptide whose recent discovery has opened a new chapter in skeletal metabolism (Copp *et al.*, 1962; Hirsch *et al.*, 1963). Its major biological action is to inhibit bone resorption (Hirsch and Munson, 1969). Accordingly, it has been used as a therapeutic agent in disease states that are characterized by increased bone resorption, such as Paget's disease (see Chapter 5). The cells that secrete calcitonin (C cells) in mammals are of neural crest origin (Pearse, 1968; Le Douarin and Le Lievre, 1970). During embryogenesis, these cells migrate to the thyroid anlage and become incorporated into the thyroid gland. They reside adjacent to the thyroid follicles, hence the name parafollicular cells. There is some evidence to suggest that these cells also migrate into other organs such as the thymus and parathyroid, and even more extensively (Galante *et al.*, 1968). In certain submammalian species, the calcitonin-secreting cells form a distinct organ, the ultimobranchial gland (Copp *et al.*, 1967).

A. Chemistry

Human calcitonin is a 32 amino acid peptide. Its amino acid sequence has been determined, as has been the amino acid sequence of six additional calcitonins from four different species (Potts *et al.*, 1970). Examination of all the naturally occurring calcitonins reveals certain common structural features together with a considerable amount of apparent variability. The common features include the 1,7-amino-terminal disulfide bridge and a carboxyl-terminal proline amide residue. Seven of the nine amino-terminal residues are identical in all calcitonins. Residues 28 (glycine) and 32 (proline amide) are the only other sequence positions completely conserved among the calcitonins. There are considerable differences between human calcitonin and the other calcitonins between positions 10 and 27. However, this sequence variability in the middle region of calcitonin is perhaps more apparent than real. Although no single amino acid in this region is constant in all seven calcitonins, there is considerable similarity when the comparison is based on the chemical properties of the amino acid side chains. Acidic, basic, hydrophobic, and hydrophylic residues are distributed in a similar fashion along the peptide chain of all the calcitonins (Potts *et al.*, 1971).

B. Physiology

Calcitonin exerts its effects on calcium and skeletal homeostasis by acting on the three important organ systems that regulate bone mineral metabolism: the skeleton, the kidneys, and the gastrointestinal tract. It is likely that calcitonin exerts its effects through the stimulation of membrane-bound adenyl cyclase (Marx *et al.*, 1973).

1. Effects on Bone and Bone Minerals

The principal effect of calcitonin on the skeleton is blockade of bone resorption (Hirsch and Munson, 1969). The inhibition of bone resorption is the principal mechanism for the hypocalcemic action of calcitonin. This effect is most dramatic in subjects with increased bone resorption, such as patients with Paget's disease or young subjects with rapid bone turnover. In such subjects, the administration of calcitonin can decrease blood calcium by several milligrams. The effectiveness of calcitonin is less marked in older animals, reflecting the gradual reduction in bone turnover that occurs with age. The direct action of calcitonin on bone has been demonstrated *in vitro* (Hirsch and Munson, 1969). Inhibition of bone resorption in experimental preparations occurs when calcitonin alone is added or when the hormone is used to block parathyroid hormone-induced resorption. A few experiments have pointed to a possible stimulation of bone formation, but other studies have indicated that bone formation may be inhibited as well as bone resorption. In general, there has been no conclusive evidence, at least in short-term experiments, of a stimulation of bone formation by calcitonin (Krane *et al.*, 1973). Although inhibition of bone resorption and consequent hypocalcemia have been the most widely studied effects of calcitonin, it should be kept in mind that the hypocalcemia represents the summation of all of the biological effects of calcitonin, including the renal and gastrointestinal effects, which are discussed subsequently.

In addition to being hypocalcemic, calcitonin is also hypophosphatemic. Analogous to its effect on plasma calcium, the inhibition of bone resorption is a principal mechanism of the hypophosphatemic effect of calcitonin (Hirsch and Munson, 1969). Similarly, the hypophosphatemia is the summation of the effects of phosphate transport at all organ systems. However, recent experiments suggest that calcitonin may have an important direct effect on phosphate transport and that the hypophosphatemic effect of the hormone may result from this direct effect of moving phosphate out of plasma (Kennedy and Talmage, 1972; Talmage *et al.*, 1973). These experiments suggest that calcitonin may exert some of its earliest and most prominent effects on phosphorus metabolism. The significance of these observations awaits further elucidation.

In addition to an effect on calcium and phosphorus, the urinary excretion of hydroxyproline, reflecting breakdown of bone matrix, can be inhibited by calcitonin. Moreover, the increased urinary excretion of hydroxyproline brought about by the administration of parathyroid hormone can be blocked by concomitant administration of calcitonin (Hirsch and Munson, 1969; Potts and Deftos, 1974).

2. Effects on Kidney

As noted in detail in Chapter 2, Volume I, the physiological significance of the actions of calcitonin on the kidney has not been established. However, it is clear that administration of pure, synthetic calcitonin causes increased clearance of calcium, phosphate, sodium, potassium, and magnesium through direct renal effect (Bijvoet et al., 1972). Furthermore, calcitonin does affect renal tubular transport of these ions at doses that are within the range of doses effective on bone. The lower concentrations of calcitonin which exert a renal effect have not been studied as well. Although it is definite that calcitonin has renal actions, the physiological significance of these effects of calcitonin on the human kidney remain uncertain, since the circulating concentrations of calcitonin in normal man are generally lower than those that have been attained in most studies by the administration of exogenous calcitonin. In medullary carcinoma of the thyroid with excessive endogenous calcitonin production, no renal abnormalities in either calcium or phosphorous clearance have been reported (Melvin et al., 1972; Potts and Deftos, 1974). It is of interest that patients with this tumor demonstrate resistance to the skeletal but not the renal effects of exogenous calcitonin (Singer and Krane, 1973).

3. Effects on the Gastrointestinal Tract

Most evidence indicates that calcitonin has no dramatic effect on calcium transport in the gastrointestinal tract. Recently, however, it has been shown that calcitonin, in small doses, can cause an inhibition of intestinal calcium absorption. At higher doses, a paradoxical rise in intestinal calcium transport was seen. The presence of vitamin D was required for these effects. The physiological relevance of these findings is still unclear (Olsen et al., 1972).

In addition to having a possible effect on gastrointestinal mineral transport, calcitonin and gastric secretion seem to be related. Gastrin has been shown to stimulate calcitonin secretion and calcitonin has been shown to inhibit the secretory activity of the gastrointestinal tract (Mutt, 1974; Sizemore et al., 1973b; Sizemore et al., 1972). Although gastrin has consequently become a diagnostic calcitonin secretagogue, the physiological significance of these observations remains to be established. It has been suggested that the secretion of gastrin in response to a dietary calcium challenge serves as an important early or even anticipatory regulator of calcitonin secretion (Munson, 1974). Decreased tolerance to an oral calcium challenge has been reported in thyroidectomized patients. However, since this also occurs during parenteral calcium challenge, it cannot be explained on the basis of a gastrointestinal effect of calcitonin (Hirsch and Munson, 1969; Potts and Deftos, 1974).

Although the previously described effects of calcitonin are well documented, the significance of calcitonin in human physiology and pathophysiology remains unclear. This is largely due to the fact that the development of convenient methods that can be applied to the measurement of calcitonin in a wide variety of normal and disease states in humans has been complicated by technical difficulties. Several hypotheses have been advanced regarding the biological role of calcitonin: (1) that the hormone plays an important physiological role in the regulation of calcium and skeletal metabolism which cannot be appreciated until reliable techniques for its measurement have been widely applied; (2) that it constitutes one limb of an enteric-parafollicular cell axis whereby gastrin serves to regulate calcitonin secretion and thereby maintains calcium homeostasis in the face of dietary challenge; (3) that it is an important developmental hormone; (4) and/or that it is a vestigial hormone, having served a function when environmental calcium challenges to our ancestors were more severe (reviewed in Potts and Deftos, 1974). There is currently little decisive data in humans for such views, since the measurement of calcitonin has not been accomplished in a wide variety of physiological and pathophysiologic states. However, a disease state has been described, which is characterized by calcitonin excess: medullary thyroid carcinoma. The study of these patients has not only provided some important information about the control of secretion of this hormone in humans, but, equally important, has posed some important additional questions about calcitonin in human mineral metabolism.

C. Medullary Thyroid Carcinoma

Medullary carcinoma is an unusual thyroid malignancy characterized by calcitonin overproduction; the cancer is associated with other endocrine tumors and there can be a familial incidence of the disease. Although occurring in the thyroid gland, this tumor is a malignancy of the calcitonin-secreting parafollicular cells that have migrated to the thyroid from the neural crest. Medullary carcinoma is, in fact, the first disease of an abnormality in calcitonin secretion that has been described (Hazard *et al.*, 1959; Horn, 1951; Williams, 1967; Milhaud *et al.*, 1968; Meyer and Abdel-Bari, 1968; Melvin and Tashjian, 1968; Cunliffe *et al.*, 1968).

1. Embryology

Medullary thyroid carcinoma is a tumor of cells that are of neural crest origin. These neural crest cells migrate into the developing thyroid anlage in man and other mammals and reside in proximity to the thyroid follicles, and are therefore called parafollicular cells. The parafollicular cells are epithelial in appearance; they are very difficult to identify in the normal human thyroid with standard histological procedures. Using an immunoperoxidase procedure, McMillan *et al.* (1974) demonstrated that these cells reside in the central region of the lobes of the normal thyroid gland (Figures 5–7). In medullary thyroid carcinoma, these calcitonin-secreting cells (C cells) undergo malignant transformation and produce an excess of calcitonin.

2. Histopathology

Medullary carcinoma of the thyroid is made up of sheets and nests of granular cells with eosinophilic staining properties. Most of the cells are

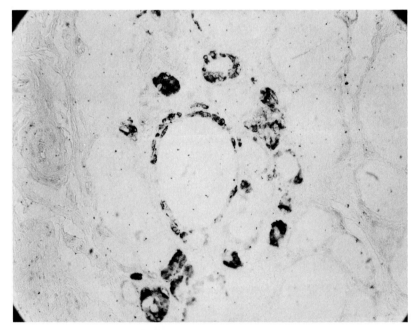

Fig. 5. Calcitonin-containing cells (C cells) in human thyroid gland as demonstrated with an immunoperoxidase procedure using human calcitonin antisera. The photomicrograph shows a cluster of C cells that are associated with both large and small follicles (×175). (From McMillan *et al.*, 1974.)

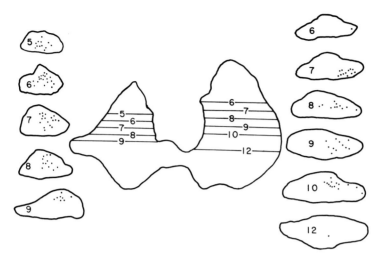

Fig. 6. Map of C cells in the normal human thyroid gland as seen from a ventral view. The gland was laid on a flat surface during fixation so that the dorsal border is lateral in this drawing. Slices were numbered from the superior pole to the inferior pole and only those that stained positively for calcitonin by an immunoperoxidase procedure using anticalcitonin antiserum are represented. Each dot on the transverse sections represents an area of several calcitonin cells. (From McMillan *et al.*, 1974.)

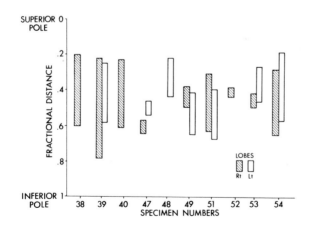

Fig. 7. Chart of the relative location of C cells in a normal human thyroid gland. Each bar extends through the portion of a lobe in which positively stained (immunoperoxidase) cells were found. In all but two glands, the positive slices within a lobe were contiguous. (From McMillan *et al.*, 1974.)

463

closely packed and polygonal in shape. A second type of cell, spindle-shaped, has also been described in these tumors (Williams, 1967). The presence of dense amyloid stroma that separates the cells is one of the most characteristic features of medullary thyroid carcinoma (Fig. 8). The amyloid is usually a conspicuous feature of the tumor, but in some cases may be difficult to find. When detected, however, the presence of amyloid in a thyroid tumor is of great value to the pathologist in establishing the diagnosis. However, since it may be difficult to find, the absence of

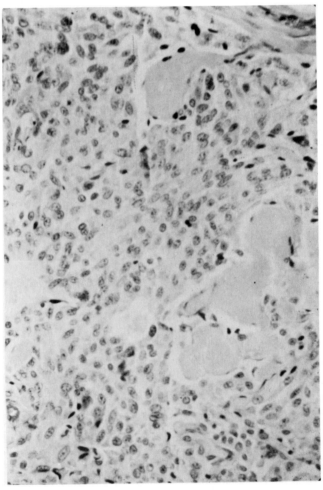

Fig. 8. Histological section of medullary thyroid carcinoma. Prominent amyloid deposits are present.

amyloid, particularly when only small amounts of tissue are available for examination, should not exclude the diagnosis of medullary thyroid carcinoma. Electron photomicrographs show the tumor to be rich in secretory (calcitonin) granules (Fig. 9).

This tumor of the thyroid has been shown to secrete a wide variety of peptides and bioactive substances. In addition to calcitonin, these substances include ACTH, histaminase, prostaglandins, and serotonin. The

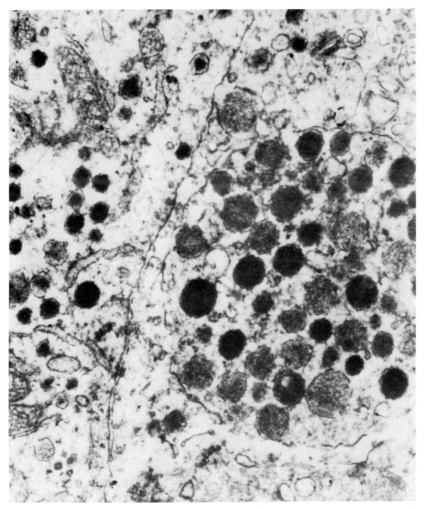

Fig. 9. Electron photomicrograph of human medullary thyroid carcinoma showing prominent secretory (calcitonin) granules (×10,000).

measurement of some of these secretory products in the blood of affected patients is only occasionally useful for the diagnosis of the disease. However, the biological activity of these secreted substances presumably accounts for some of the clinical features seen in patients with medullary thyroid carcinoma (Melvin *et al.*, 1972; Hill *et al.*, 1973; Beylin *et al.*, 1972).

3. Clinical Features

This tumor can occur either sporadically or with a familial incidence. In the sporadic form, the tumor usually presents in middle or late life and is often unilateral in its location. In the familial form, the tumor usually becomes manifest within the first three decades of life and is usually bilateral in location. The familial form of the disease is thought to be inherited as a dominant autosomal trait and this familial form of medullary thyroid carcinoma can be part of a multiple endocrine adenomatosis (Steiner *et al.*, 1968; Sipple, 1961). The two most common associated findings are pheochromocytomas and hyperparathyroidism, often due to parathyroid hyperplasia. Although distant metastases can occur and the disease can be rapidly fatal, the growth of medullary thyroid carcinoma is often slow and indolent. In fact, in one recent study, an unusual degree of longevity has been demonstrated in a family affected by this tumor (MacIntyre, personal communication). The manifestations of the tumor itself are, therefore, often local (Melvin *et al.*, 1972).

Other neuroectodermal features occur in association with medullary thyroid carcinoma. The most striking of these are small polypoid neuromas of the eyelids, lips, and tongue, usually with profuse thickening of the lips (Fig. 10). These features are so characteristic that the facial appearance of nonrelated subjects with this syndrome makes them appear to be consanguinous. The proliferation of nerves, which causes these neuromas, can also occur throughout the intestine and sometimes may involve the bronchial tree and the bladder. Accompanying these multiple mucosal neuromas can be a Marfanoid habitus (Melvin *et al.*, 1972; Hill *et al.*, 1973).

There is a high incidence of hyperparathyroidism in patients with medullary thyroid carcinoma. This probably represents another expression of the genetic mechanism that is responsible for the familial pattern of this syndrome. Hyperplasia of the parathyroid glands, usually of the chief cell variety, is more common than adenoma (Steiner *et al.*, 1968; Melvin *et al.*, 1972; Hill *et al.*, 1973). It has been speculated that the hyperparathyroidism seen in these patients may represent a compensatory response to the high levels of calcitonin, presumably mediated by hypocalcemia due to the excessive concentrations of the hormone. How-

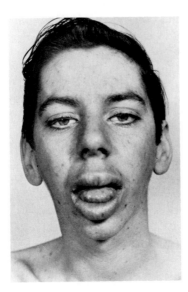

Fig. 10. Facial appearance of a patient with the familial syndrome involving multiple endocrine defects, including medullary thyroid carcinoma, and multiple neuromata of the eyelids, lips, and tongue. (From Melvin *et al.*, 1972.)

ever, in many patients, parathyroid hormone and calcium levels are normal despite the high levels of calcitonin. Additional support for an independent genetic mechanism for the hyperparathyroidism rather than a reactive disorder of the parathyroids also comes from the recent observation that some relatives of patients with medullary thyroid carcinoma have high circulating levels of parathyroid hormone prior to the development of medullary carcinoma. Furthermore, clinical hyperparathyroidism alone has been described in family members who do not have medullary thyroid carcinoma (Steiner *et al.*, 1968; Tashjian *et al.*, 1970; Melvin *et al.*, 1972; Beylin *et al.*, 1972; Hill *et al.*, 1973). However, recent observations suggest that there may be a functional as well as genetic relationship between the hyperparathyroidism and hypercalcitoninism seen in patients with this thyroid tumor (Deftos and Parthemore, 1974).

Despite these hormonal disorders, patients with medullary thyroid carcinoma have no readily recognizable abnormality of skeletal or mineral metabolism. Most of the patients are normocalcemic. When hypocalcemia does occur it is usually related to the common occurrence of diarrhea. The diarrhea is thought to be due, in part, to the excessive amounts of prostaglandin that can be secreted by these tumors. Another contributing mechanism to the diarrhea may be the high incidence of

ganglioneuromatosis and diverticulosis of the intestinal tract that is seen
in these patients (Melvin *et al.*, 1972; Hill *et al.*, 1973). Phosphate and
magnesium concentrations are also normal. The skeletal system in most
patients with this tumor is essentially normal according to standard
radiological, morphological, and dynamic studies. However, more sophisticated methods have recently demonstrated that both bone formation and
bone resorption can be reduced in patients with this tumor (Rasmussen
and Bordier, 1973). It is of interest that these patients are resistant to the
skeletal but not the renal effects of exogenous calcitonin (Singer and
Krane, 1973).

Another associated endocrinological disturbance in patients with
medullary carcinoma of the thyroid is the occurrence of Cushing's disease. In fact, the features of Cushing's disease may be so striking that
they dominate the clinical picture. In these patients, the Cushing's disease
is due to the production by the medullary thyroid carcinoma of ACTH.
This results in bilateral adrenal hyperplasia and corticosteroid excess.
The hyperadrenalism can be treated by surgical removal of the thyroid
carcinoma. Other endocrinological disorders have also been described in
patients with medullary thyroid carcinoma (Melvin *et al.*, 1972; Hill *et al.*,
1973).

4. Diagnosis

The diagnosis of medullary thyroid carcinoma should be considered in
any patient with a thyroid tumor. It should be especially suspected in the
relatives of patients who have the disease and in patients who have
thyroid tumor with histology that is atypical and does not conform to the
features described for tumors of those thyroid cells responsible for iodine
metabolism. The possibility of ACTH-producing medullary thyroid carcinoma should be considered in patients with otherwise unexplained
Cushing's syndrome.

The most reliable (nonsurgical) method for establishing the diagnosis of
medullary thyroid carcinoma is the measurement of blood calcitonin. The
large majority of patients with medullary thyroid carcinoma have increased basal concentrations of plasma calcitonin (Fig. 11). In fact plasma
calcitonin may be increased before there is any clinical evidence of the
presence of the tumor. Therefore, especially in familial cases, the presence of high levels of calcitonin may be a very early clue to the presence
of this malignancy. In the initial immunoassay studies, all patients with
this tumor had basal concentrations of calcitonin that were greater than
1000 pg/ml, clearly distinguishable from normal, and, therefore, diagnostic of the presence of the tumor (Tashjian *et al.*, 1970). However, subsequent studies demonstrated that some patients with this tumor had

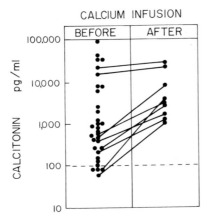

Fig. 11. Plasma calcitonin before and after calcium infusion in patients with medullary thyroid carcinoma. The majority of patients had basal levels of calcitonin that are clearly elevated above normal, represented by the dashed line. In some patients, however, it is only after calcium infusion that the plasma calcitonin is definitively diagnostic of the presence of this thyroid tumor.

basal levels of calcitonin that were lower than 1000 pg/ml and that, in some cases, could not be distinguished from normal; provocative tests of calcitonin secretion were necessary to establish the presence of tumor in these patients (Deftos and Potts, 1970; Potts *et al.*, 1971; Melvin *et al.*, 1972; Jackson *et al.*, 1973; Deftos, 1974). Furthermore, it is now apparent that in some of these patients basal plasma calcitonin may be intermittently elevated (Deftos, 1974). In these types of patients, provocative tests of calcitonin secretion may be useful in confirming the presence of this disease.

The most thoroughly evaluated provocative test for establishing the presence of medullary thyroid carcinoma in suspect patients without abnormally elevated basal levels of calcitonin is a 2–4-hour calcium infusion. Virtually all patients show a markedly increased level of plasma calcitonin following this procedure. Furthermore, in some patients with basal levels of the hormone that are not abnormal, the postinfusion values are diagnostic of the presence of tumor (Fig. 11). This provocative testing can lead to the diagnosis of the tumor in its earliest stages (Wolfe *et al.*, 1973). In some patients, a more convenient 10-minute infusion of calcium may establish the diagnosis (Parthemore *et al.*, 1974) (Fig. 12). This response to calcium indicates that the secretion of calcitonin by these malignant parafollicular cells is stimulated by the same ion that influences secretion of calcitonin by normal C cells (Potts and Deftos, 1974). In addition, EDTA-induced hypocalcemia suppresses the secretion of calcinonin by this tumor (Deftos

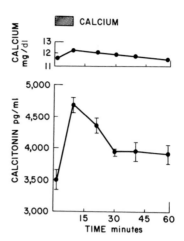

Fig. 12. Effect of a 150-mg calcium infusion on plasma calcium and calcitonin in a patient with medullary thyroid carcinoma. Even though plasma calcium increased less than 1 mg, there was still a significant increase in plasma calcitonin. (From Parthemore *et al.*, 1974.)

et al., 1971a). Therefore, medullary thyroid carcinoma is not autonomous in its secretory function but responds to the normal control mechanisms (Fig. 13).

Glucagon infusion can also stimulate the secretion of calcitonin in patients with medullary thyroid carcinoma, but, since it can release catecholamines, glucagon is potentially hazardous in patients who may have associated pheochromocytoma (Lawrence, 1967). In addition, its effects are not as consistent as those of calcium, and glucagon may, in fact, cause suppression of calcitonin release (Fig. 13). Therefore, despite its convenience of administration, glucagon is not as reliable an agent for the diagnosis of medullary carcinoma of the thyroid.

The effects of gastrin, a peptide that has been shown to stimulate the secretion of calcitonin in the porcine species and in some patients with hypocalcemia, has also been evaluated in patients with this tumor. This peptide, speculated to be a physiological stimulus for calcitonin secretion, has also been shown to be useful as a provocative agent for calcitonin secretion in patients with medullary thyroid carcinoma; in fact, one report describes gastrin infusion as a more reliable diagnostic procedure than calcium infusion (Hennessey *et al.*, 1974). The relative diagnostic value of calcium and gastrin awaits further comparative studies. The conflicting results that have been reported of the stimulatory effect of gastrin in medullary carcinoma of the thyroid (Melvin *et al.*, 1972; Hennessey *et al.*, 1973) may be due to its transient effect; calcitonin levels increase sharply

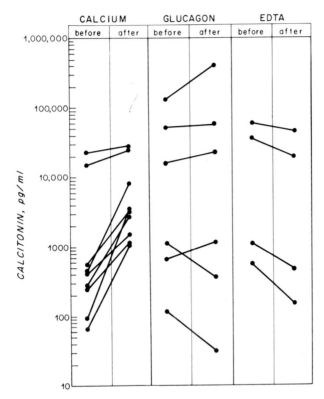

Fig. 13. Response of plasma calcitonin to functional tests of hormone secretion in a group of patients with medullary carcinoma of the thyroid. Calcium and EDTA, respectively, stimulate and suppress calcitonin. Glucagon has a variable effect.

immediately after gastrin infusion and can return to normal within several minutes (Hennessey *et al.*, 1973).

In summary, the measurement of calcitonin by radioimmunoassay thus offers a precise, reliable, and relatively simple test for establishing the diagnosis of medullary thyroid carcinoma (Clark *et al.*, 1969; Potts and Deftos, 1974). The use of provocative tests for calcitonin secretion, either calcium and/or gastrin infusion, are important ancillary procedures, which can lead to even earlier diagnosis. Since false-negative results can occur with either procedure, both should probably be used before excluding the diagnosis in the subject at risk because of family history. In many instances, plasma measurements of calcitonin can establish the presence of medullary carcinoma even before there is any clinical evidence of the disease. Total thyroidectomy, performed because of increased calcitonin detected in the blood prior to any sign or symptom or detectable thyroid abnormality, has lead to detection of microscopic foci of medullary carcinoma in the removed thyroid tissue (Melvin *et al.*, 1972). Recently, C-cell hyperplasia has been described as a histological precursor of this tumor (Wolfe *et al.*, 1973). Accordingly, calcitonin measurement is especially useful in relatives of these patients. Early diagnosis of the disease is important to effect a potential cure.

Several other bioactive substances have been identified (prostaglandins, serotonin, and histaminase) as secretory products of medullary carcinoma of the thyroid. Histaminase measurements may be especially helpful in identifying the presence of metastatic disease (Beylin *et al.*, 1972). However, the presence of these other substances does not seem to occur with enough consistency to make their measurement diagnostically useful. Prostaglandins, serotonin, and ACTH may be responsible for some of the signs and symptoms associated with the tumor, as previously discussed (Melvin *et al.*, 1972; Hill *et al.*, 1973).

5. *Treatment*

Suppression of tumor growth by thyroid hormone cannot be expected in these patients. The most effective treatment for patients with medullary thyroid carcinoma is surgical removal of the tumor (Melvin *et al.*, 1972; Hill *et al.*, 1973). In advanced cases, surgery is often palliative and directed at the symptoms due to local obstruction by the tumor of large veins or of the trachea. With the introduction of the immunoassay for calcitonin, however, the disease can be detected very early in some individuals from affected kindred; consequently, surgery in these cases may be curative.

Total thyroidectomy should be undertaken because of the multifocal distribution of the disease, especially in the familial form. Wide excision of lymph nodes is recommended, but radical neck dissection has not been fully evaluated. Surgical management is influenced by the presence of other associated endocrinopathies. For example, when pheochromocytomas are present, it may be expeditious to perform bilateral adrenalectomy first. This permits direct examination of the liver for the presence of metastases from the thyroid carcinoma. If such metastases are present, direct attack on the tumor may not be justified. Bilateral adrenalectomy may also be indicated in the patients with Cushing's disease due to the production of ACTH by a medullary thyroid tumor if the medullary carcinoma is already metastatic, and, therefore, cannot be removed. There is no extensive experience with radiotherapy or chemotherapy in the treatment of this disease (Hill *et al.*, 1973), although some case reports of adriamycin treatment have recently appeared (Gottlieb and Hill, 1974).

Whatever forms of therapy are used, the immunoassay for calcitonin can be used to monitor treatment (Goltzman *et al.*, 1974).

D. Measurement of Human Calcitonin

It has been emphasized in this chapter that the significance of calcitonin in human physiology is not well defined. A major impediment to the study of this hormone in humans has come from the conflicting results that have been reported about the measurement of this hormone in normal subjects. The first measurements of calcitonin in normal subjects were made by bioassay procedures in which basal concentrations of 200 to 1700 pg of calcitonin per ml of plasma were reported (Sturtridge and Kumar, 1968; Gudmundsson *et al.*, 1969). However, it became apparent that this method was subject to artifacts (Bell *et al.*, 1969). The first reported radioimmunoassay for human calcitonin was sufficiently sensitive only to record normal calcitonin levels as being less than 2000 pg/ml (Clark *et al.*, 1969). Using an immunoassay of improved sensitivity, Tashjian *et al.* (1970) reported that plasma calcitonin could be readily measured in the peripheral blood of normal adults and that its range was 20–400 pg/ml; there were not significant differences in calcitonin between normals and either chronic hypo- or hypercalcemic subjects. Using a similar method, Deftos (1971) reported that most normal subjects had undetectable (less than 100 pg/ml) basal values of plasma calcitonin. Some patients were found to have higher values, but artifacts were shown to operate in the radioimmunoassay for human calcitonin, which could have given spuriously high results. Although calcitonin gradients were demonstrated across the thyroid vein in some subjects, the possibility of an immunoassay artifact could not be definitely eliminated (Deftos *et al.*, 1971b). This finding was also observed in other laboratories (MacIntyre *et al.*, 1972). Subsequently, Melvin *et al.* (1971) and his colleagues reported in additional studies that basal calcitonin levels were less than 100 pg/ml (undetectable) in most normal subjects and never greater than 350–380 pg/ml (Melvin *et al.*, 1972; Baker *et al.*, 1973).

Several other laboratories have also reported conflicting results of basal calcitonin measurements. Beceiro *et al.* (1971) have reported normal ranges of 50–400 pg/ml and subsequently the same laboratory reported a mean ± S.D. of 270 ± 240 pg/ml (Samann *et al.*, 1973). Hesch *et al.* (1971) reported that most normals have values of 50–150 pg/ml but that approximately one-fourth of normals have values of less than 50 pg/ml (Hesch *et al.*, 1973). Using an immunometric assay, the same group reported normal calcitonin at 150 ± 140 pg/ml (Hesch *et al.*, 1973). The

Mayo Clinic has reported normal calcitonin values as 50–500 pg/ml with only 5% undetectable (Sizemore *et al.*, 1972), 65–393 pg/ml (Sizemore *et al.*, 1973a), and less than 500 pg/ml (Markey *et al.*, 1973); this group (Sizemore *et al.*, 1972) also reported a direct correlation between basal calcitonin and calcium, a result not confirmed by others (Silva *et al.*, 1974a; Heynen and Franchimont, 1974). Silva *et al.* (1973a,b) have reported a normal mean of 180 ± 97 pg/ml, and, in contrast to Tashjian *et al.* (1970), observed higher values in hypercalcemic subjects of 281 ± 91 and even a higher mean value of 510 pg/ml (110–2700 pg/ml) in a subsequent study (Silva *et al.*, 1974a). Silva *et al.* (1974a) also reported that normal women seemed to have lower basal concentrations than men, with 82% having values of <200 pg/ml and 24% having values <50 pg/ml in contrast to the male range of 63–450 pg/ml with only 4% <50 pg/ml.

Curiously, thyroidectomized patients had calcitonin concentrations of 63–110 pg/ml with a mean of 83 pg/ml whereas Melvin *et al.* (1972) reported that 22 of 25 thyroidectomized patients had undetectable plasma calcitonin. Patients with chronic renal failure had higher concentrations than normal with a mean of 690 ± 260 pg/ml and a range of 300–1200 pg/ml; dialysis and parathyroidectomy had no effect on plasma calcitonin (Silva *et al.*, 1974b). Heynen and Franchimont (1974) also found that patients with chronic renal failure had higher than normal plasma calcitonin, 500–3800 pg/ml (mean 1341) as compared to normals (10–580 pg/ml, mean 108) and even hypercalcemics (100–2000 pg/ml, mean 824). However, in contrast to Silva *et al.* (1974b), they noted a significant increase in calcitonin following dialysis. In addition, calcitonin was undetectable (<10 pg/ml) in 103 of 166 normal subjects. Furthermore, Heynen and Franchimont (1974) observed that higher than normal basal levels of calcitonin are seen in patients with Paget's disease (range 0–1200 pg/ml, mean ± S.E.M. 428 ± 151) and patients with pernicious anemia (range 0–1880 pg/ml, mean ± S.E.M. 787 ± 173 pg/ml). Beceiro *et al.* (1971) reported intermittently elevated levels of calcitonin in hypercalcemic states and Bieler *et al.* (1973) observed that normals have undetectable (less than 50 pg/ml) basal values of plasma calcitonin.

It has been suggested that calcitonin may be an important developmental hormone. There exist reports of increased plasma calcitonin over normal (270 ± S.D. 240 pg/ml) in umbilical cord blood (1890 ± S.D. 1000 pg/ml) and maternal plasma (660 ± S.D. 40 pg/ml) at term (Samaan *et al.*, 1973). This hypothesis is not supported by Baker's observation that calcitonin is undetectable (less than 100 pg/ml) in the majority of normal children of ages 5–10. In contrast to Silva *et al.* (1974a), there were no demonstrable sex differences in calcitonin levels in Baker's studies (Baker *et al.*, 1973).

Just as there is controversy about the measurement of basal levels of calcitonin in adults, considerable disagreement exists about measurement of the hormone during provocative tests of secretion. Calcium infusion has been the most reliable provocative test for calcitonin secretion in experimental animals and in humans with medullary carcinoma of the thyroid (Potts and Deftos, 1974). However, its effect in normal adults has not been well defined. Tashjian *et al.* (1970) reported that calcium infusion produced no detectable rise of calcitonin in 38% of normal adults; the remainder exhibited a mean calcitonin increase following calcium infusion of 100 pg/ml, and the increase in plasma calcitonin never exceeded either 550 (Melvin *et al.*, 1972) or 700 pg/ml (Jackson *et al.*, 1971). Heynen and Franchimont (1974) and Silva *et al.* (1974a) reported that approximately 80% of their subjects showed an increase in plasma calcitonin following calcium infusion with stimulated values similar to those reported by Melvin *et al.* (1972). Beceiro *et al.* (1971) reported that normal subjects exhibit a post-calcium infusion rise in calcitonin of up to 1000 pg/ml (Samaan *et al.*, 1973). Sizemore *et al.* (1972) reported that calcium infusion caused only a 20–30% increase in plasma calcitonin in normal adults but that oral calcium, even though it did not produce as great a rise in blood calcium as did calcium infusion, resulted in a 30–300% increase in plasma hormone concentration (Sizemore *et al.*, 1972). In contrast, Melvin *et al.* (1972) and Silva *et al.* (1973a,b) reported that oral calcium was less effective than calcium infusion in stimulating plasma calcitonin. The latter group observed an average maximal increase in plasma calcitonin of 230% following calcium infusion with a detectable rise occurring within 20 minutes of the start of the infusion; they also observed a 50% reduction in plasma calcitonin following EDTA-induced hypocalcemia (Silva *et al.*, 1973a,b, 1974a). Heynen and Franchimont (1974) do not give details about the increase they observed in calcitonin following oral calcium in two of five patients; in three or five patients, EDTA infusion decreased calcitonin. In our original studies (reviewed in Potts and Deftos, 1974), some normal subjects did exhibit an apparent increase in calcitonin following calcium infusion; however, assay artifacts were not conclusively ruled out (Deftos *et al.*, 1971b).

The most convincing evidence for calcitonin secretion in patients without medullary thyroid carcinoma using standard immunoassay procedures has come from studies of patients with hypocalcemic states following calcium infusion. In a group of patients with pseudohypoparathyroidism, idiopathic hypoparathyroidism, and osteomalacia, calcium infusion led to a marked rise in plasma calcitonin (Deftos *et al.*, 1972a,b, 1973a,b). The calcitonin levels found after calcium infusion in these patients approached the levels seen in some patients with medullary thyroid carcinoma. In some patients, the administration of pentagastrin also resulted in an increase in plasma calcitonin. It is likely that the hypocalcemia in these patients resulted in increased storage of calcitonin in the parafollicular cells and that the induced hypercalcemia resulted in the release of these increased calcitonin stores, producing a blood level that could be readily detected by existing assay systems. Recently, Baker *et al.* (1973) have also demonstrated intermittently elevated levels of calcitonin in pycnodysotosis.

There are several possible explanations for these discrepancies regarding the measurement of plasma calcitonin. Many of the reported measurements are made at or near the detection limits of the assay procedures. It is well known that artifacts are likely to operate under such conditions (Deftos, 1971; Deftos *et al.*, 1971b; MacIntyre *et al.*, 1972; Heynen and Franchimont, 1974). Attempts have been made in some studies to control for such artifacts by the use of adsorption or filtration procedures (Deftos *et al.*, 1971b; Samaan *et al.*, 1973; Baker *et al.*, 1973; Bieler *et al.*, 1973; Heynen and Franchimont, 1974). Although such procedures have been useful in demonstrating the operation of artifacts, they may introduce additional artifacts of their own (David *et al.*, 1973; Potts and Deftos, 1974).

Another potential explanation for these discrepancies in calcitonin measurements may result from the recently demonstrated immunochemical heterogeneity of plasma calcitonin (Singer and Habener, 1974) (Fig. 14). Since there are several immunological species of calcitonin in peripheral plasma, it may be that different antisera (in different laboratories) have varying affinities for the various circulating calcitonin species. As has been well documented with parathyroid hormone (Potts and Deftos, 1974), such a circumstance could result in varying estimations of calcitonin in the same plasma sample.

To further study the secretion of calcitonin, several laboratories have utilized immune concentration procedures to improve functional assay sensitivity (Parthemore and Deftos, 1974; Mohsen *et al.*, 1973; Tashjian and Voelkel, 1974). Preliminary reports from these laboratories indicated that basal levels of calcitonin in adults usually range from 0 to 100 pg/ml, but that some subjects do have higher levels (Fig. 15). The further application of extant and newer assays for calcitonin should help to define the importance of this hormone in humans.

1. Ectopic Calcitonin Production

Recent developments indicate that the calcitonin assay may be an important tool in the diagnosis of malignancy other than medullary thyroid carcinoma. Several laboratories have observed that other forms of cancer are also characterized by the increased production of calcitonin

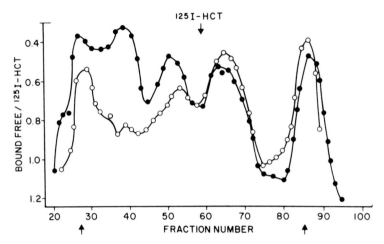

Fig. 14. Immunochemical heterogeneity of calcitonin in plasma. A plasma sample from a patient with medullary thyroid carcinoma was chromatographed on BioGel P-30. Each of the column fractions was immunoassayed with two different antisera for human calcitonin, represented by the opened and closed circles, respectively. Not only were there multiple peaks of immunoassayable calcitonin activity, but each of the two different antisera described different immunological peaks within the same plasma sample. Arrows at bottom represent the void and salt volumes of the column, respectively. The elution position of ^{125}I-labeled calcitonin is also shown.

(Milhaud *et al.*, 1972; Whitelaw and Cohen, 1973; Silva *et al.*, 1973a,b, 1974c; Deftos *et al.*, 1974a,b; Milhaud *et al.*, 1974; Coombes *et al.*, 1974). It was at first considered that the other forms of cancer derived from cells that were embryologically related to the C cells of the thyroid, which are neural crest in origin. However, such a wide variety of cancers has been associated with increased calcitonin production that such an hypothesis no longer seems tenable. Ectopic calcitonin production has been reported with a wide variety of nonthyroidal neoplasms, which include the following: intestinal, bronchial, and gastric carcinoids; pheochromocytoma; melanoma; carcinoma of the lung, especially oat cell; pancreatic carcinoma; maxillary carcinoma; prostatic carcinoma; uterine carcinoma; bladder carcinoma; breast carcinoma; leukemia. Thus, calcitonin may be a more general marker for the malignant transformation of cells, although neural crest cells may predominate in such calcitonin-producing tumors. The measurement of calcitonin may not only serve as a diagnostic marker for such tumors but may also be a guide to therapy (Fig. 16). Because of these observations, the detection of an elevated plasma level of calcitonin does not necessarily mean the presence of medullary thyroid carcinoma. The patient must now be evaluated for other malignant disorders. How-

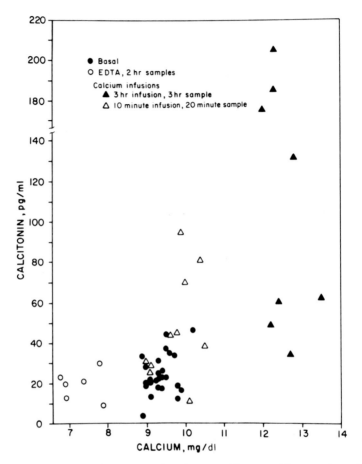

Fig. 15. Plasma calcitonin concentrations in normal human subjects as determined by immunoextraction of a 10-ml plasma sample and subsequent radioimmunoassay. Measurements were made in the basal state and during functional tests of hormone secretion. (From Parthemore and Deftos, 1974.)

ever, it may be possible by immunochemical means to determine if the abnormally elevated calcitonin is thyroidal or nonthyroidal in origin Deftos et al., 1974b).

These controversies notwithstanding, the aggregate of all studies suggests that this hormone does have a physiological role in human biology. Plasma calcitonin concentrations seem to respond to even minor perturbations of calcium and mineral homeostasis. Although not yet confirmed, age and sex differences in concentration have been reported and gastrointestinal control of calcitonin secretion has been postulated.

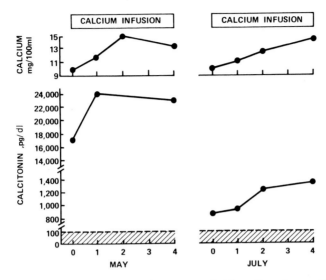

Fig. 16. Ectopic calcitonin production by a pancreatic islet cell carcinoma. Shown is the effect of calcium infusion on plasma calcitonin before (left) and after (right) streptozotocin therapy. Although there was an increase in plasma calcitonin during the induced hypercalcemia before and after treatment, the absolute level of calcitonin dropped markedly after streptozotocin therapy. (From Deftos *et al.*, 1974.)

In addition to the well-documented primary disorder of calcitonin secretion—medullary thyroid carcinoma—secondary disorders of hormone secretion may exist in certain calcium and skeletal diseases, renal diseases, gastrointestinal disorders, and a variety of other human diseases. Future studies using extant and newer assays for calcitonin should help to define further the physiological and pathophysiologic importance of calcitonin in humans.

IV. RECENT DEVELOPMENTS

Recent studies have begun to dispel doubts about the hormonal nature of calcitonin and about its physiological and pathophysiological significance in humans and other mammals (Deftos *et al.*, 1977). The regulation of calcitonin secretion (and/or metabolism) is becoming better defined with additional experimental, clinical, and *in vitro* studies (Deftos *et al.*, 1977). In addition to the growing list of calcitonin secretagogues, primary and/or secondary changes in hormone secretion have been demonstrated in several physiological states, such as alimentation, pregnancy, neonatal

TABLE I

Regulation of Calcitonin Secretion[a]

Calcium and related ions
Gastrointestinal factors
Age and sex
Calcitropic hormones[b]
Neuroendocrine factors
Iodine, T_4, and related factors
Other calcitonin secretagogues

---

[a]Adapted from Deftos, *et al.*, 1977
[b]Parathyroid hormone, Vitamin D metabolites, calcitonin

TABLE II

Conditions reported or postulated to be associated with abnormalities of calcitonin secretion and/or metabolism[a]

Condition	Possible mechanism
1. Medullary thyroid carcinoma	
a. C-cell hyperplasia	Genetic/function
b. Prehyperlasia	
2. Ectopic calcitonin production	Malignancy
3. Hypocalcemia	Calcium
4. Hypercalcemia/hypercalciuria	Calcium/gastrin
5. Hyperparathyroidism	Calcium/PTH/GI hormones
6. Malignancy	Possible factors
	calcium
	bone resorption
	prostaglandins
	CT secretagogues
7. Pancreatitis	Glucagon/nonthyroidal calcitonin
8. Pregnancy	Calcium/bone resorption
9. Neonatal hypocalcemia	Calcium/bone resorption
10. Renal disease	Metabolism/bone resorption/vitamin D
11. Bone disease	Bone resorption/CT secretagogues
a. Hyperostotic states	
Pycnodysostosis	
Engleman's disease	
Osteopetrosis	
b. Hyperesorptive States	
Osteitis fibrosa cystica	
Osteoporosis	
Renal osteodystrophy	

[a]Adapted from Deftos, *et al.*, 1977

hypocalcemia, lactation, and changes of serum calcium within the physiological range (Deftos *et al.*, 1977; Samaan *et al.*, 1973; Roos *et al.*, 1977; Dirksen and Anast, 1976; Anast, 1977; Toverud, 1977; Parthemore, 1977). Even more important is the demonstration of primary and secondary abnormalities of calcitonin secretion in a variety of disease states in addition to those previously discussed (Table II). Abnormalities of calcitonin secretion (and/or metabolism) have been implicated by preliminary studies in the pathogenesis of renal osteodystrophy (Lee *et al.*, 1977b; Deftos *et al.*, 1977; Kanis *et al.*, 1977). Less convincing at this time is a possible role for calcitonin in the hypocalcemia of pancreatitis (Canale and Donabedian, 1975; Robertson *et al.*, 1976). It is intriguing to speculate that the pancreas or adjacent gastrointestinal cells may be a source of calcitoninlike activity (Takaoka *et al.*, 1969; Sowa *et al.*, 1977). An increase in calcitonin secretion, presumably compensatory, can occur in chronic hypercalcemic states such as malignancy and primary hyperparathyroidism (Deftos *et al.*, 1977; Lee *et al.*, 1977a; Parthemore *et al.*, 1977; Parthemore and Deftos, 1977). Calcitonin abnormalities have been demonstrated in one hyperostatic state, pycnodysostosis, and may occur in others (Deftos *et al.*, 1977; Baker *et al.*, 1973). Decreased calcitonin reserve in females may play a role in the severity of osteitis fibrosa cystica occurring in primary hyperparathyroidism and in the pathogenesis of osteoporosis (Parthemore and Deftos, 1977; Milhaud, 1974). Preliminary studies in Paget's disease also suggest the presence of decreased calcitonin reserve (Deftos *et al.*, 1977). Finally, the recent discovery of calcitonin in the pituitary gland provides novel implications about the significance of this hormone (Deftos *et al.*, 1978). Thus, there is a growing body of clinical and experimental data which is elucidating the role of calcitonin in physiology and pathophysiology (Deftos *et al.*, 1977).

ACKNOWLEDGMENTS

The author is indebted to Susan Murphy for her expert secretarial assistance.

This research was supported by the Veterans Administration, the National Institutes of Health (AM15888), and the American Cancer Society.

REFERENCES

Adams, P. H., Jowsey, J., Kelly, P. J., Riggs, B. L., Kinney, V. R., and Jones, J. F. (1967). *Q. J. Med.* **36,** 1.

Anast, C. S.: Premature Infant Hypocalcemia, in Talmage, R. V. and Copp, H. D. (eds.), Proceedings of the 6th Parathyroid Conference (Amsterdam: Excerpta Medica, 1977).

Askanazy, M., and Rutishauser, E. (1933). *Virchows Arch. Pathol. Anat. Physiol.* **291,** 653.

Aub, J. C., Bauer, W., Heath, C., and Ropes, M. (1929). *J. Clin. Invest.* **7,** 97.

Baker, R. K., Wallach, S., and Tashjian, A. H. T., Jr. (1973). *J. Clin. Endocrinol. Metab.* **37,** 46.

Bateson, E. M., and Chander, S. (1965). *Br. J. Radiol.* **38,** 581.

Baume, L. J., Becks, H., and Evans, H. M. (1954). *J. Dent. Res.* **33,** 104.

Baxter, J. D., and Bondy, P. K. (1966). *Ann. Intern. Med.* **65,** 429.

Beceiro, J., Quais, S., Hill, C. S., Jr., and Samaan, N. A. (1971). *Clin. Res.* **19,** 367.

Bell, P. H., Dziobkowski, C., Barg, W. F., and Snedeker, E. H. (1969). *Lancet* **1,** 433.

Benoit, F. L., and Watten, R. H. (1968). *Metab. Clin. Exp.* **17,** 20.

Beylin, S. B., Beaven, M. A., Buga, L. M., and Keiser, H. R. (1972). *Am. J. Med.* **53,** 723.

Bieler, E. U., van Rooyen, R. J., deBruin, E. J. P., and Hoog, J. M. C. (1973). *Horm. Metab. Res.* **5,** 231.

Bijvoet, O. L. M., van der Sluys Veer, J., Greven, H. M., and Schellekens, A. P. M. (1972). *In* "Calcium, Parathyroid Hormone and the Calcitonins" (R. V. Talmage and P. L. Munson, eds.), Int. Congr. Ser. No. 243, p. 284. Excerpta Med. Found., Amsterdam.

Bouillon, R., and DeMoor, P. (1974). *J. Clin. Endocrinol. Metab.* **38,** 999.

Breuer, R. I., and McPherson, H. T. (1966). *Arch. Intern. Med.* **118,** 310.

Bussolati, G., and Pearse, A. G. E. (1967). *J. Endocrinol.* **37,** 205.

Canale, D. D. and Donabedian, R. K.: Hypercalcitoninemia in acute pancreatitis, Journal of Clinical Endocrinology and Metabolism 40:738, 1975.

Clark, M. B., Byfield, P. G. H., Boyd, G. W., and Foster, G. V. (1969). *Lancet* **2,** 74.

Coombes, R. C., Hillyard, C., Greenberg, P. B., and MacIntyre, I. (1974). *Lancet* **2,** 1080.

Copp, D. H., Cameron, E. C., Chaney, B. A., Davidson, A. G. F., and Henze, K. G. (1962). *Endocrinology* **70,** 638.

Copp, D. H., Cockcroft, D. W., and Keuh, Y. (1967). *Science* **158,** 924.

Cunliff, W. J., Black, M. M., Hall, R., Johnston, I. D. A., Hudgson, P., Shuster, S., Gudmundsson, T. V., Joplin, G. F., Williams, E. D., Woodhouse, N. J. Y., Galante, L., and MacIntyre, I. (1968). *Lancet* **2,** 63.

David, L., Erfling, W., Winnacker, J., and Anast, C. (1973). *Proc. 55th Annu. Meet. Am. Endocr. Soci.* Abstract No. 322.

Deftos, L. J. (1971). *Metab. Clin. Exp.* **20,** 1122.

Deftos, L. J. (1973). *In* "Clinical Aspects of Metabolic Bone Disease" (B. Frame, A.M. Parfitt, and H. Duncun, eds.), Int. Congr. Serv. No. 270, p. 178. Excerpta Med. Found., Amsterdam.

Deftos, L. J. (1974). *J. Am. Med. Assoc.* **227,** 403.

Deftos, L. J., and Parthemore, J. G. (1974). *J. Clin. Invest.* **54,** 416.

Deftos, L. J., and Potts, J. R., Jr. (1970). *Clin. Res.* **18,** 673.

Deftos, L. J., Goodman, A. D., Engelman, K., and Potts, J. T., Jr. (1971a). *Metab. Clin. Exp.* **20,** 428.

Deftos, L. J., Bury, A. E., Habener, J. F., Singer, F. R., and Potts, J. T., Jr. (1971b). *Metab. Clin. Exp.* **20,** 1129.

Deftos, L. J., Murray, T. M., Powell, D. A., Habener, J. F., Singer, F. R., Mayer, G. P., and Potts, J. T., Jr. (1972a). *In* "Calcium, Parathyroid Hormone and the Calcitonins" (R. V. Talmage and P. L. Munson, eds.), Int. Congr. Ser. No. 243, p. 140. Excerpta Med. Found., Amsterdam.

Deftos, L. J., Swenson, K., Bode, H., Hayak, A., Neer, R., and Potts, J. T., Jr. (1972b). *Clin. Res.* **20,** 217.

Deftos, L. J., Powell, D., Parthemore, J. G., and Potts, J. T., Jr. (1973a). *J. Clin. Invest.* **52,** 3109.

Deftos, L. J., Bury, A. E., Mayer, G. P., Habener, J. F., Singer, F. R., Powell, D., Krook, L., Watts, E. G., and Potts, J. T., Jr. (1973b). *Proc. Third Int. Symp. Endocrinol., 4th, 1972* p. 89.

Deftos, L. J., Rosen, S. W., and Sartiano, G. P. (1974a). *Clin. Res.* **22,** 486.

Deftos, L. J., McMillan, P. J., Sartiano, G. P., Robinson, A. G., Abuid, J., and Alberts, D. (1974b). (1976) Metabolism. 25, 543. *Copenhagen*.

Deftos, L. J., Roos, B. A., Knecht, G. L., Lee, J. C., Pavlinac, D., Bone, H. G., and Parthemore, J. G. Calcitonin Secretion, in Talmage, R. V. and Copp, H. D. (eds.), Proceedings of the 6th Parathyroid Conference (Amsterdam: Excerpta Medica, 1977).

Deftos, L. J., Burton, D., Bone, H. G., Catherwood, B. D., Parthemore, J. G., Moore, R. Y., Minick, S. and Guilleman, R. (1978). Life Sciences, in press.

Dirksen, M. C. and Anast, C. S.: Interrelationship of serum immunoreactive calcitonin and serum calcium in newborn infants. Pediatric Research 10:408, 1976.

Engfeldt, B., and Hertquist, S. O. (1954). *Acta Endocrinol.* **15,** 109.

Epstein, F. H., Freedman, L. R., and Levitin, H. (1958). *N. Engl. J. Med.* **259,** 782.

Fell, H. B., and Mellanby, E. (1956). *J. Physiol. (London)* **133,** 89.

Fisher, D. A. (1971). *In* "The Thyroid" (S. C. Werner and S. H. Ingbar, eds.), 3rd Ed. pp. 292 and 807.

Foster, G. V. (1964). *Nature (London)* **203,** 1029.

Fraser, S. A., Anderson, J. B., Smith, D. A. and Wilson, G. M. (1971). *Lancet* **1,** 981.

Freedberg, I. M. (1971). *In* "The Thyroid" (S. C. Werner and S. H. Ingbar, eds.), 3rd ed., pp. 515. Harper and Row

Friedlander, J. A., Williams, G. A., Bowser, E. N., Handerson, W. J., and Hoffens, E. (1965). *Proc. Soc. Exp. Biol. Med.* **120,** 20.

Galante, L., Gudmundsson, T. V., Mathews, E. W., Tse, A., Williams, E. D., Woodhouse, N. J. Y., and MacIntyre, I. (1968). *Lancet* **2,** 537.

Gimlett, T. M. D. (1964). *In* "The Thyroid Gland" (R. Pitt-Rivers and W. R. Trotter, eds.), Vol. 2, p. 198, Butterworth, London.

Gittes, R. F., and Irvin, G. L. (1966). *Endocrinology* **79,** 1033.

Goltzman, D., Potts, J. R., Jr., Ridgway, E. C., and Maloof, F. (1974). *J. Clin. Endocrinol. Metab.* **290,** 1036.

Gottlieb, J. A., and Hill, C. S., Jr. (1974). *N. Engl. J. Med.* **290,** 193.

Gudmundsson, T. V., Woodhouse, N. J. Y., and Osafo, T. D. (1969). *Lancet* **1,** 443.

Haddad, J., Birge, S., Couranz, S., and Avioli, L. V. (1969). *Clin. Res.* **17,** 285.

Harden, R. M., Harrison, M. T., Alexander, W. D., and Nordin, B. E. C. (1964). *J. Endocrinol.* **28,** 281.

Harrison, M. T., Harden, R. M., and Alexander, W. D. (1964). *J. Clin. Endocrinol. Metab.* **24,** 214.

Hazard, J. B., Hawk, W. A., and Crile, G. (1959). *J. Clin. Endocrinol. Metab.* **19,** 152.

Hennessey, J. F., Gray, T. K., Cooper, C. W., and Ontjes, D. A. (1973). *J. Clin. Endocrinol. Metab.* **36,** 200.

Hennessey, J. F., Wells, S. A., Ontjes, D. A., and Cooper, C. W. (1974). *J. Clin. Endocrinol. Metab.* **39,** 487.

Hesch, R. D., Hufner, M., and Hausenhager, R. (1971). *Horm. Metab. Res.* **3,** 140.

Hesch, R. D., Woodhead, S., Hufner, M., and Wolfe, H. (1973). *Horm. Metab. Res.* **5,** 235.

Heynen, G., and Franchimont, P. (1974). *Eur. J. Clin. Invest.* **4,** 213.

Hill, C. S., Jr., Ibañez, M. L., Samaan, N. A., Ahearn, M. J., and Clark, R. L. (1973). *Medicine (Baltimore)* **52,** 141.

Hirsch, P. F., and Munson, P. L. (1969). *Physiol. Rev.* **49,** 548.

Hirsch, P. F., Garthier, G. F., and Munson, P. L. (1963). *Endocrinology.* **73,** 244.

Horn, R. C. (1951). *Cancer* **4**, 697.

Jackson, C. E., Tashjian, A. H. T., Jr., and Block, M. A. (1971). *J. Lab. Clin. Med.* **78**, 817.

Jackson, C. E., Tashjian, A. H. T., Jr., and Block, M. A. (1973). *Ann. Intern. Med.* **78**, 845.

Jenkins, G. N. (1966). *In* "The Physiology of the Mouth," p. 199. Davis, Philadelphia, Pennsylvania.

Kanis, J. A., Earnshaw, M., Heynen, G., Ledingham, J. C. C., Oliver, D. O., Russell, G. G., Woods, C. G., Franchimont, P., and Gaspar, S.: Changes in histologic and biochemical indexes of bone turnover after bilateral nephrectomy in patients on hemodialysis, New England Journal of Medicine 296:1073, 1977.

Karnofsky, D., and Crinkhite, E. P. (1939). *Proc. Soc. Exp. Biol. Med.* **40**, 568.

Kennedy, J. W., and Talmage, R. V. (1972). *In* "Calcium, Parathyroid Hormone, and the Calcitonins" (R. V. Talmage and P. L. Munson, eds.), Int. Congr. Ser. No. 243, p. 407. Excerpta Med. Found., Amsterdam.

Kivirikko, K. I. (1971). *Int. Rev. Connect. Tissue Res.* **5**, 93.

Kivirikko, K. I., Koivulsalo, M., Laitinen, O., and Liesmaa, M. (1963). *Acta Physiol. Scand.* **57**, 462.

Kivirikko, K. I., Laitinen, O., and Lamberg, B. A. (1965). *J. Clin. Endocrinol. Metab.* **25**, 1347.

Krane, S. M. (1971a). *In* "The Thyroid" (S. C. Werner and S. H. Ingbar, eds.), 3rd ed., pp. 598 Harper & Row

Krane, S. M. (1971b). *In* "The Thyroid" (S. C. Werner and S. H. Ingbar, eds.), 3rd ed. 763 Harper & Row

Krane, S. M., Brownell, G. L., Stanbury, J. B., and Corrigan, H. (1956). *J. Clin. Invest.* **35**, 874.

Krane, S. M., Harris, E. D., Singer, F. R., and Potts, J. T., Jr. (1973). *Metab. Clin. Exp.* **22**, 51.

Krawitt, E. L. (1967). *Proc. Soc. Exp. Biol. Med.* **125**, 417.

Laake, H. (1955). *Acta Med. Scand.* **15**, 229.

Lawrence, A. M. (1967). *Ann. Intern. Med.* **66**, 1091.

Le Douarin, N., and Le Lievre, C. (1970). *C. R. Hebd. Seances Acad. Sci., Ser. D* **270**, 2857.

Lee, J. C., Catanzaro, A., Parthemore, J. G., Roach, B., and Deftos, L. J.: Hypercalcemia is disseminated coccidioidomycosis, New England Journal of Medicine, 297:431, 1977

Lee, J. C., Parthemore, J. G., and Deftos, L. J.: Calcitonin secretion in renal disease. Calc. Tiss. Res. 225:154, 1977

Lewin, I., and Samackson, J. (1972). *J. Lab. Clin. Med.* **76**, 1016.

Lowery, G. H., Aster, R. H., Carr, E. A., Ramon, G., Beierwaltes, W. H., and Spafford, N. R. (1958). *AMA J. Dis. Child.* **96**, 131.

MacIntyre, I., Foster, G. V., Woodhouse, N. J. Y., Bordier, P., Gudmundsson, T. V., and Joplin, G. F. (1972). *In* "Calcium, Parathyroid Hormone and the Calcitonins" (R. V. Talmage and P. L. Munson, eds.), Int. Congr. Ser. No. 243, p. 83. Excerpta Med. Found., Amsterdam.

McMillan, P. J., Hooker, W. M., and Deftos, L. J. (1974). *Am. J. Anat.* **140**, 73.

Malamos, B., Sfikakis, P., and Pandos, P. (1969). *J. Endocrinol.* **45**, 269.

Markey, W. S., Ryan, W. G., Economou, S. G., Sizemore, G. W., and Arnaud, C. D. (1973). *Ann. Intern. Med.* **78**, 898.

Marx, S. J., Woodward, C., Aurbach, G. D., Glossman, H., and Keutmann, H. T. (1973). *J. Biol. Chem.* **248**, 4797.

Melvin, K. E. W., and Tashjian, A. H. T., Jr. (1968). *Proc. Natl. Acad. Sci. U.S.A.* **59**, 1216.

Melvin, K. E. W., Miller, H. H., and Tashjian, A. H. T., Jr. (1971). *N. Engl. J. Med.* **285,** 1115.

Melvin, K. E. W., Tashjian, A. H. T., Jr., and Miller, H. H. (1972). *Recent Prog. Horm. Res.* **28,** 399.

Meyer, J. S., and Abdel-Bari, W. (1968). *N. Engl. J. Med.* **278,** 523.

Milhaud, G., Tubiana, M., Parmentier, C., and Coutris, G. (1968). *C. R. Hebd. Seances Acad. Sci.* **266,** 608.

Milhaud, G., Calmettes, C., Julienne, A., Thauaud, D., Bloch-Michel, H., Cavaillon, J. P., Colin, R., and Moukhtar, M. S. (1972). *In* "Calcium, Parathyroid Hormone and the Calcitonins" (R. V. Talmage and P. L. Munson, eds.), Int. Congr. Ser. No. 243, p. 56. Excerpta Med. Found., Amsterdam.

Milhaud, G., Calmettes, C., Taboulet, J., Julienne, A., and Moukhtar, M. S. (1974). *Lancet* **2,** 462.

Milhaud, G., Talbot, J. N., and Coutris, G.: Interet de l'analyse en composantes principales (A.C.P.) pour l'etude d'agents therapeutiques. Application au traitement au long cours de l'osteoporose par la calcitonine a faible dose, Therapie 29:611, 1974.

Mohsen, S., Moukhtar, A. J., Tharaud, D., Taboulet, J., and Milhaud, G. (1973). *C. R. Hebd. Seances Acad. Sci., Ser. D.,* 276:3445.

Munson, P. L. (1974). *Endocrinol. Proc. Int. Symp., 2nd, 1973* p.

Mutt, V. (1974). *Endocrinol. Proc. Int. Symp., 2nd, 1973* p.

Olsen, E. B., Jr., DeLuca, H. F., and Potts, J. T., Jr. (1972). *In* "Calcium, Parathyroid Hormone and the Calcitonins" (R. V. Talmage and P. L. Munson, eds.), Int. Congr. Ser. No. 243, p. 240. Amsterdam.

Parfitt, A. M., and Dent, L. E. (1970). *Found. J. Med.* **39,** 171.

Parsons, V., and Anderson, J. (1964). *Clin. Sci.* **27,** 313.

Parthemore, J. G., and Deftos, L. J. (1974). *Proc. 56th Annu. Meet., Am. Endocr. Soc.,* Abstract No. 300, p. 205.

Parthemore, J. G., Bronzert, D., Roberts, G., and Deftos, L. J. (1974). *J. Clin. Endocrinol. Metab.* **39,** 108.

Parthemore, J. G., Moriguchi, M., and Deftos, L. J.: Secondary hypercalcitoninism in primary hyperparathyroidism, Clinical Research 25:498A, 1977.

Parthemore, J. G., and Deftos, L. J.: Calcitonin secretion in primary hyperparathyroidism, Journal of Clinical Investigation, in press.

Parthemore, J. G., Knecht, G. L., and Deftos, L. J.: Calcitonin secretion in normal human subjects, Journal of Clinical Endocrinology and Metabolism, in press.

Pearse, A. G. E. (1968). *Proc. R. Soc. Med.* **170,** 71.

Pickering, D. E., and Fisher, D. A. (1958). *J. Chronic Dis.* **7,** 242.

Potts, J. T., Jr., and Deftos, L. J. (1974). *In* "Duncan's Diseases of Metabolism" (P. K. Bondy, ed.), 7th ed., p. 1225. Saunders, Philadelphia, Pennsylvania.

Potts, J. T., Jr., Niall, H. D., Keutmann, H. T., Deftos, L. J., and Parsons, J. A. (1970). *Calcitonin, Proc. Int. Symp, 2nd, 1960* p. 56.

Potts, J. T., Jr., Niall, H. D., and Deftos, L. J. (1971). *Curr. Top. Exp. Endocrinol.* **1,** 151.

Rasmussen, H., and Bordier, P. (1973). *N. Engl. J. Med.* **289,** 25.

Riekstniece, E., and Asling, C. W. (1966). *Proc. Soc. Exp. Biol. Med.* **123,** 258.

Robertson, G. M., Jr., Moore, E. W., Switz, D. M., Sizemore, G. W., and Estep, H. L.: Inadequate parathyroid response in acute pancreatitis, New England Journal of Medicine 294:512, 1976.

Roos, B. A., Bergeron, G., Guggenheim, K., and Deftos, L. J.: Maturational increases in plasma calcitonin related to gastrointestinal function. Clinical Research 25:398A, 1977.

Samaan, N. A., Hill, C. S., Beceiro, J. R., and Schultz, P. N. (1973). *J. Lab. Clin. Med.* **81,** 671.

Sataline, L. R., Powell, C., and Hamwi, G. J. (1962). *N. Engl. J. Med.* **267,** 646.

Silberberg, M., and Silberberg, R. (1943). *Arch. Pathol.* **36,** 512.

Silberberg, M., and Silberberg, R. (1947). *Anat. Rec.* **98,** 181.

Silva, O. L., Becker, K. C., Primack, A., Doppman, J., and Snider, R. H. (1973a). *Lancet* **2,** 443.

Silva, O. L., Snider, R. H., and Becker, K. L. (1973b). *Proc. 55th Annu. Meet., Am. Endocr. Soc.,* Abstract No. 184, p. 272.

Silva, O. L., Snider, R. H., and Becker, K. D. (1974a). *Clin. Chem.* **20,** 337.

Silva, O. L., Becker, K. C., Selawry, H. P., Snider, R. H., Moore, C. F., Bivins, L. E., and Shalhoub, R. J. (1974b). *Lancet* **1,** 1055.

Silva, O. L., Becker, K. C., Primack, A., Doppman, J., and Snider, R. H. (1974c). *N. Engl. J. Med.* **290,** 1122.

Singer, F. R., and Habener, J. F. (1974). *Clin. Res.* **22,** 167A.

Singer, F. R., and Krane, S. M. (1973). *Proc. 55th Annu. Meet. Am. Endocr. Soc.* Abstract No. 271.

Singer, O. L., Snider, R. H., and Becker, K. C. (1974a). *Clin. Chem.* **20,** 337.

Sipple, J. H. (1961). *Am. J. Med.* **31,** 163.

Sizemore, G. W., Leffler, J., Fisher, J., Oldham, S., Goldsmith, R., and Arnaud, D. (1972). *Clin. Res.* **20,** 441.

Sizemore, G. W., Go, V. L. W., Kaplan, E. L., Sanzenbacher, L. J., Holtermuller, K. H., and Arnaud, C. (1973a). *N. Engl. J. Med.* **288,** 641.

Sizemore, G. W., Holtermuller, K. H., and Go, V. L. W. (1973b). *Clin. Res.* **21,** 828.

Smith, D. A., Fraser, S. A., and Wilson, G. M. (1973). *Clin. Endocrinol. Metab.* **2,** 333.

Sowa, M., Appert, H. E., and Howard, J. M.: Hypocalcemic activity of pancreatic tissue homogenate in dog, Surgical Gynecology and Obstetrics 144:365, 1977.

Steiner, A. G., Goodman, A. D., and Powers, R. A. (1968). *Medicine (Baltimore)* **47,** 371.

Sturtridge, W. C., and Kumar, M. A. (1968). *Lancet* **1,** 725.

Takaoka, Y., Takamori, M., Ichinose, M., Shikaya, T., Igawa, N., Kikutani, M., and Yamamoto, Y.: Hypocalcemic action of a pancreatic factor and its clinical significance on the myasthenic patients, Acta Medica Nagasaki 13:28, 1969.

Talbot, N. B. (1939). *Endocrinology* **24,** 872.

Talmage, R. V., Anderson, J. J. B., and Kennedy, J. W. (1973). *Endocrinology* **94,** 413.

Tapp, E. (1966). *J. Bone Joint Surg., Br. Vol.* **48,** 526.

Tashjian, A. H. T., Jr., and Voelkel, E. F. (1974). *In* "Methods of Hormone Radioimmunoassay (B. M. Jaffe and H. R. Behrman, eds.), pp. 199–213.

Tashjian, A. H. T., Jr., Howland, B. G., Melvin, K. E. W., and Hill, C. S., Jr. (1970). *N. Engl. J. Med.* **283,** 890.

Toverud, S. V.: Hormonal Control of Calcium Metabolism in Lactation, in Talmage, R. V. and Copp, H. D. (eds.), Proceedings of the 6th Parathyroid Conference (Amsterdam: Excerpta Medica, 1977).

von Recklinghausen, F. (1891). *Festschr. Rudolf Virchow* Reimer, Berlin p. 1.

Walker, D. G. (1957). *Bull. Johns Hopkins Hosp.* **101,** 101.

Whedon, G. E., Neumann, W. F., and Jenkins, D. W. (1966). *In* "Progress in the Development of Methods in Bone Densitometry," March 25–27, 1965, Washington D. C. Sponsored by NIAMD and the American Institute of Biological Sciences. Published by Scientific and Technical Information Division of NASA.

Whitelaw, A. G. L., and Cohen, S. L. (1973). *Lancet* **2,** 443.

Wilkins, L. W. (1955). *Ann. N. Y. Acad. Sci.* **60,** 763.

Wilkins, L. W. (1962). *In* "The Diagnosis and Treatment of Endocrine Disorders in Childhood and Adolescence." Blizzard, R. M., and Migeon, C. J. (ed.), p. 93. Thomas, Springfield, Illinois.

Williams, E. D. (1967). *J. Clin. Pathol.* **20,** Suppl., 395.
Williams, G. A., Bowser, E. N., and Henderson, W. J. (1967). *Isr. J. Med. Sci.* **3,** 639.
Wolfe, H. J., Melvin, K. E. W., Cervi-Skinner, S. J., Al Saadi, A. A., Juliar, J. F., Jackson, C. E., Jackson, C. E., and Tashjian, A. H. T., Jr. (1973). *N. Engl. J. Med.* **289,** 437.

5

Paget's Disease of Bone

FREDERICK R. SINGER, ALAN L. SCHILLER,
ELEANOR B. PYLE, AND STEPHEN M. KRANE

I.	Introduction	490
II.	Historical Aspects	490
III.	Incidence and Epidemiology	490
IV.	Histopathology	494
	A. Pertinent Aspects of Differential Diagnosis	504
V.	Focal Manifestations	505
	A. Pain	506
	B. The Skull	506
	C. The Jaws	509
	D. The Spine	509
	E. The Pelvis and Extremities	513
VI.	Complications	518
	A. Fractures	518
	B. Associated Neoplasia	522
VII.	Metabolic Aspects of Paget's Disease	530
	A. Mineral Metabolism	530
	B. Collagen Metabolism	533
	C. Acute Effects of Calcitonin	540
	D. Citrate Metabolism	542
	E. Serum Alkaline Phosphatase	543
	F. Other Phosphatases	545
VIII.	Systemic Complications and Associated Diseases	545
	A. Hypercalciuria, Renal Calculi, and Hypercalcemia	545
	B. Hyperuricemia and Gout	546
	C. Calcific Periarthritis and Chondrocalcinosis	547
	D. Cardiovascular Complications	548
	E. Pseudoxanthoma Elasticum, Angioid Streaks, and Skin Changes	549
	F. Malabsorption Syndrome	550
IX.	Drug Treatment	551

Copyright © 1978 by Academic Press, Inc.
All rights of reproduction in any form reserved
ISBN 0-12-068702-X

A. Indications 551
B. Miscellaneous Drugs 552
C. Sodium Fluoride 552
D. Phosphate 553
E. Mithramycin 553
F. Diphosphonates 555
G. Glucagon 558
H. Calcitonin 558
X. Etiology 564
References 567

I. INTRODUCTION

Paget's disease of bone is a focal disorder of unknown etiology characterized initially by excessive resorption and subsequently by excessive formation of bone, culminating in a "mosaic" pattern of lamellar bone associated with extensive local vascularity and increased fibrous tissue in adjacent marrow. In the strict sense this is not a metabolic bone disease, since some portion of the skeleton is spared, no matter how widespread the disease process may be. It is the extraordinary extent of the abnormal remodeling seen in some cases and its metabolic consequences that make necessary a detailed consideration of the disorder in this volume.

II. HISTORICAL ASPECTS

Sir James Paget in 1876 described the clinical and pathological aspects of a disease resulting in focal enlargement and deformity of the skeleton (Fig. 1). His subsequent papers (Paget, 1877, 1882a,b) provided further details. It was his opinion that the pathological basis for the disease was a chronic inflammation of bone, hence the term osteitis deformans.

Descriptions of the disorder had been published earlier: Rullier (1812), Wrany (1867), Wilks (1869), and Czerny (1873) all reported single cases which resembled those of Paget. Nagant de Deuxchaisnes and Krane (1964) have summarized evidence that the disease may have existed in prehistoric times. A detailed historical review of Paget's disease can be found in *Paget's Disease of Bone* by Barry (1969).

III. INCIDENCE AND EPIDEMIOLOGY

The incidence of Paget's disease in a given population is extremely difficult to estimate because a substantial number of affected individuals

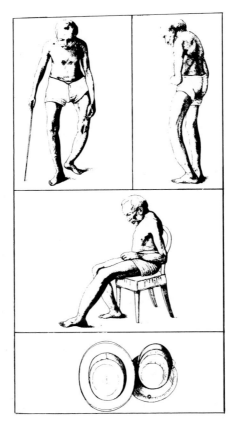

Fig. 1. The original patient of Sir James Paget showing marked skeletal deformities including enlargement of the skull, represented here by change in hat size.

are asymptomatic (Monroe, 1951). The types of studies that have been undertaken to obtain data are autopsies of unselected persons, review of roentgenograms, and review of hospital admissions. The first major study was that of Schmorl (1932) in Dresden who found at autopsy that 3% of 4614 patients over 40 years had Paget's disease. Collins (1956) in England found an incidence of 3.7% in 650 autopsies. These figures were confirmed by the radiological survey of Pyggot (1957) who found an incidence of 3.5% in London in 9775 patients over 45 years of age. The incidence in hospitalized patients, however, is less than 1%. Newman (1946) reported 82 cases out of 127,000 admissions (1 in 1548) at the Hospital of the University of Pennsylvania. Rosenkrantz and colleagues (1952) found 111 cases out of 94,112 patients (1 in 848) admitted to the New York Veterans Administration Hospital. Barry (1969) reviewed admissions to the main teaching hospitals of Australia and found 2630 cases out of 1,769,664 admissions (1 in 673).

The most striking aspect of the epidemiology of Paget's disease is the great variation in incidence throughout the world (Barry, 1969). It occurs most frequently in Great Britain, Australia, New Zealand, Germany, and perhaps France. The high incidence of the disease in Australia and New Zealand is accounted for entirely by people who migrated from the United Kingdom during World War II. The disorder is rare in India, China, Japan, the Middle East, Africa, and Scandinavia. Although accurate data are not available, in North and South America, Central Europe, the Mediterranean countries, and Russia the incidence appears to be intermediate in comparison to that found in the other two groups of countries. There can also be great variations within a country as evidenced by the report of Rosenbaum and Hanson (1969) who found a 15-fold greater incidence in Providence, Rhode Island, than in Lexington, Kentucky.

Characteristically Paget's disease is found in middle-aged or elderly patients. The incidence rises with increasing age so that by the ninth decade it has been reported to be 5-11%. The youngest patients described are over 20 years. The rare syndrome in children of congenital hyperphosphatasia characterized by fragile and deformed bones, which has also been called "juvenile Paget's disease" (Choremis *et al.*, 1958; Woodhouse *et al.*, 1972), does not have the morphologic characteristics of Paget's disease (Section IV,A). In the large series that have been reported, men are affected more frequently than women. For example, of the 2630 patients reported by Barry (1969), 1420 were men, a ratio of seven men to six women.

Paget's disease may occur in more than one member of a family. Evens and Bartter (1968) have reported a family with definite Paget's disease in seven members and probable disease in two others. Singer (1977a) has reported the disease to affect five brothers and two of their cousins, brother and sister, in one family. Jones and Reed (1967) described six cases in one family. We have found a family history of Paget's disease in 16% of 55 pagetic patients, including one family with six females involved. Despite the ample evidence of multiple cases of the disease occurring in families, Martin and Melick (1975) have found only five reported cases in identical twins. They felt that this lessened the possibility that genetic factors were critical in the pathogenesis of the disease. Montagu (1949) has postulated that the pattern may be sex-linked recessive, whereas McKusick (1972) thought it a simple autosomal Mendelian-dominant.

In an attempt to find a possible genetic marker for the disease we have determined the frequency of HLA antigens in 34 patients with Paget's disease. The results are presented in Table I. To determine whether the patient population differed significantly from the control, chi-square values were computed, and the resultant p values were multiplied by 21, the number of specificities tested. Although HLA-5 was about threefold greater in frequency in the patients, the p value did not reach significant levels (0.2). In two other small series of patients, no significant correlation was discovered (Seignalet, 1975; Roux et al., 1975). It may be that further testing in a larger population of patients would confirm a specific pattern of HLA antigens, which would allow identification of the potential pagetic subject, as has been accomplished for ankylosing spondylitis (Brewerton et al., 1973; Caffrey and James, 1973; Schlosstein et al., 1973) (Section V,D).

TABLE I

Phenotype Frequencies of HLA Specificities in Patients with Paget's Disease[a]

Antigen	Controls (64)[b] (%)	Paget's disease (34) (%)
HLA-1	38	26.5
HLA-2	44.6	44.1
HLA-3	21.5	29.4
HLA-9	17	17.6
HLA-10	18.5	20.6
HLA-11	4.6	5.9
W19	0	0
W28	7.7	5.9
HLA-5	7.7	23.5
HLA-7	18.5	26.5
HLA-8	24.6	5.9
HLA-12	17.0	26.5
HLA-13	3	0
W5	21.5	47.1
W10	18.5	35.3
W14	6	8.8
W15	6	0
W17	12.3	2.9
W18	4.6	2.9
W22	1.5	5.9
W27	4.6	8.8

[a] Data provided by Drs. R. Patel and D. W. Zschaeck.
[b] Controls were nonpagetic adults from Peter Bent Brigham Hospital, Boston, Massachusetts.

IV. HISTOPATHOLOGY

There is general agreement that the pathology of Paget's disease of bone may be divided into three phases. In the first, the osteolytic or "hot" phase, there is intense resorption of existing bone. This is soon accompanied by accelerated deposition of spicules of lamellar bone in a disorganized fashion (the mixed phase). In the final phase, the osteoblastic or "cold" phase, bone formation is dominant, and the irregularly shaped trabeculae are characterized by the "mosaic" pattern of cement lines, which appear haphazardly between fragments of lamellar bone. Any single bone may have separate foci, each of a different phase of the disease process, or various bones may be in different phases. It is possible for all three phases of the disorder to be found in the same focus in a single bone.

Since Paget's disease has as its diagnostic feature abnormal architecture of lamellar bone, a brief description of the histology of bone is necessary, although the reader is also referred to Chapter 4, Volume I, for additional information. Normal lamellar bone may be defined as bone with a parallel arrangement of collagen fibers (best visualized by polarized light), relatively few osteocytes per unit area of matrix, and a uniformity in size and shape of the osteocytes, which are generally small cells with dark nuclei. There are a number of types of lamellar bone in the cortex. The outer and inner circumferential lamellae are those on the periosteal and endosteal surfaces, respectively. These surround the osteones or Haversian systems, which are composed of concentric lamellae. The interstitial lamellae found between osteones are the remnants of previously formed and partially resorbed circumferential lamellae. The trabeculae of the medulla are also normally composed of lamellar bone but do not contain osteones.

Woven bone, which is almost never found under normal conditions after the epiphyses close, except in areas of the most rapid remodeling, is the type of bone most frequently seen in response to a stress, e.g., fracture or tumor. It may be defined as bone with a chaotic, unorganized pattern of collagen fibers, large numbers of osteocytes per unit area of matrix, and large variations in size and shape of the osteocytes. This type of bone is frequently seen in foci of Paget's disease, but the pattern of its deposition should be distinguished from the diagnostic "mosaic" pattern of pagetic lamellar bone. Although woven bone may occasionally be the predominant finding in an active phase of Paget's disease, it is not a diagnostic feature.

The major changes seen in the osteolytic phase of the disease are due to the osteoclast. These large multinucleated cells are often found in great

profusion adjacent to any bone surface and are derived from the pluripo-
tential mesenchymal bone marrow (Fig. 2). They may assume bizarre
shapes and contain as many as 100 nuclei (Rubenstein *et al.*, 1953; Bélanger *et al.*, 1968; Rasmussen and Bordier, 1974). Osteoclasts of this type
are rarely seen in other forms of nonneoplastic bone disorders such as
hyperparathyroidism. Such observations prompted Rasmussen and Bordier (1974) to suggest that Paget's disease is really a slow growing, benign,
hormonally responsive tumor.

The osteoclastic resorption occurs before there is luxuriant fibrous
tissue replacement of adjacent normal fatty or hematopoietic bone marrow. Noteworthy at this stage of the disease is the early development of
vascular hypertrophy, hyperplasia and venous ectasia in the marrow
spaces, and the influx of undifferentiated mesenchymal cells adjacent to
the osteoclastic foci. As resorption continues there is an increase in
fibrous tissue and the vascularity becomes extremely prominent. The
blood flow in this region may be 20 times that of normal, due mostly to
arteriolar hyperplasia and hypertrophy rather than arteriovenous shunts

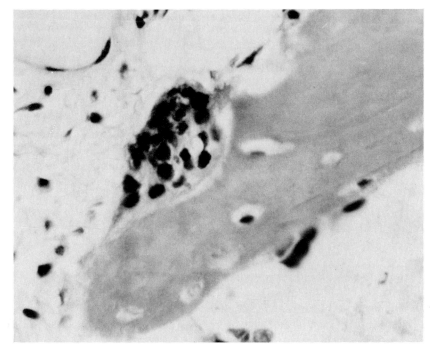

Fig. 2. A large multinucleated osteoclast resorbing a spicule of lamellar bone. Note the
loose fibrous marrow that has replaced the fatty marrow. H & E; ×790.

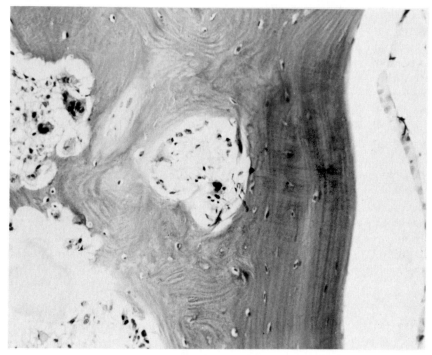

Fig. 3. Osteoclastic resorption of the cortex at the endosteal surface and within an osteone. The outer circumferential lamellae are still intact. H & E; ×190.

(Jaffe, 1972; Demmler, 1974). In the cortex the osteoclasts widen the osteones centrifugally until they become confluent with other osteones or Volkmann's canals. This process may continue until resorption extends to the endosteal and periosteal surfaces (Fig. 3). In some cases the outer circumferential lamellae will remain intact. If there is penetration of the outer circumferential lamellae, periosteal new bone formation occurs, often as woven bone that is deposited similarly to fracture callus. If the disease continues, this new bone will also be resorbed and eventually replaced by pagetic lamellar bone with its characteristic "mosaic" pattern.

Despite the fact that the osteoclast is the principal cell of interest in the lytic phase, foci of intense osteoblastic activity may also be seen. These osteoblasts usually lay down lamellar bone, often adjacent to areas of irregular resorption (Fig. 4). However, woven bone is also sometimes seen in these areas as if there were not enough time to make lamellar bone. Some evidence that this may be the case was provided by using tetracycline-labeled tissue to demonstrate that such newly formed bone is

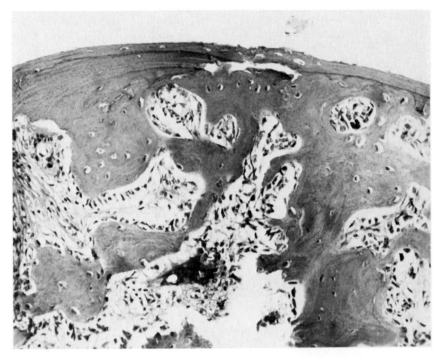

Fig. 4. Resorption of the cortex is almost complete, although a thin rim of outer cir-cumferential lamellae is still intact. Note the presence of osteoblasts laying down woven bone in response to the osteoclastic activity. H & E; ×190.

resorbed soon after it is manufactured (Lee, 1967). Occasionally an uncal-cified osteoid seam is the dominant histological finding.

Similar changes are seen in the cancellous bone of the medulla. This trabecular bone is rapidly attacked by numerous osteoclasts. Thin bands of new bone of either lamellar or woven type may also be found in the marrow cavity adjacent to areas of resorption. Occasionally, hemorrhagic cysts surrounded by fibrous marrow and hemosiderin-laden macrophages are found in the medulla. Such cysts may persist into the third phase of the disease. These defects develop from microinfarcts of trabecular bone and marrow secondary to rupture of the numerous thin-walled dilated vessels (Jaffe, 1972).

The mixed phase of the disease occurs when the osteoclasts become less numerous, their activity begins to wane, and osteoblasts become more numerous. New lamellar bone formation occurs with lines of easily recognized plump osteoblasts closely applied to bone. The appearance of classic pagetic bone with a "mosaic" arrangement of the cement lines becomes prominent. This diagnostic histological feature of Paget's disease is characterized by irregular, jigsaw-shaped pieces of lamellar bone with an erratic arrangement of cement lines (Fig. 5). The scalloped appearance of these cement lines represents sites of prior osteoclastic resorption. No osteone is completely intact and often no single unit of lamellar bone can be traced for any distance (Fig. 6). Bone lamellae haphazardly faceted together are readily observed using polarized light microscopy (Fig. 7). The interfaces between these units of bone are represented by the cement lines seen with light microscopy. Each new wave of osteolysis will leave a resorption line, which subsequently remains as a cement line when new lamellar bone is deposited. Thus pagetic bone represents the repeated pattern of resorption and deposition of lamellar bone waxing and waning in the same area. The marrow contiguous with areas of osteoblastic and osteoclastic activity is replaced by fibrovascular connective tissue (Fig. 8).

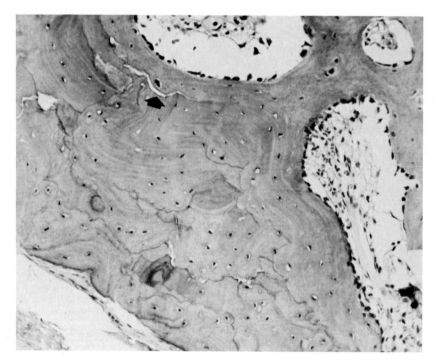

Fig. 5. The mixed phase, with prominent rows of osteoblasts lining lamellar bone, which is arranged in the typical "mosaic" pattern. Note the replacement of fatty marrow by loose fibrovascular marrow. The crack (arrow), which is an artifact, separates two units of lamellar bone and is usually seen as a blue cement line. H & E; ×190.

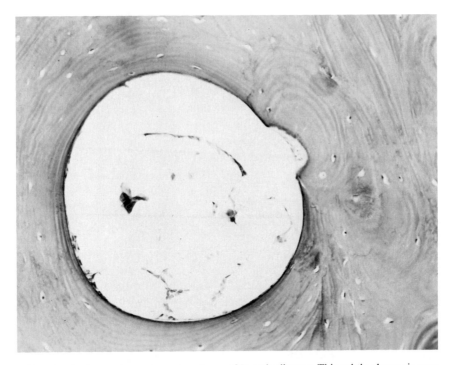

Fig. 6.   An incomplete osteone in a focus of Paget's disease. This subtle change is very common and often overlooked. H & E; ×190.

The osteoblastic phase of the disease features dense irregular masses of pagetic bone with relatively little cellular activity (Fig. 9). The marrow is mostly fibrous tissue entrapping scattered telangectatic vessels, with osteoblasts lined up along bone surfaces. There may be scattered chronic inflammatory cells present. Periodic acid-Schiff positive droplets are found in the marrow adjacent to some osteoblasts. The pagetic bone in the sclerotic phase has no tendency to orient around vascular canals or to form osteones and is therefore relatively avascular and grossly hard to cut. It has been found by Bélanger et al. (1968) using microradiography that the thin metachromatic cement lines of the early phases have formed into high density bands of calcification. Lee (1967) studied several patients using microradiography and tetracycline labeling and found that bone formation, defined as the percent volume of new bone added to the total bone volume per day, was increased 10 times that of normal bone. However, the rate of bone deposition on preexisting bone surfaces was only slightly above the normal rate of about 1 μm per day. He concluded that the overall increased formation rate was accounted for by increased

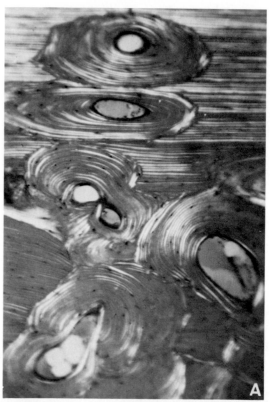

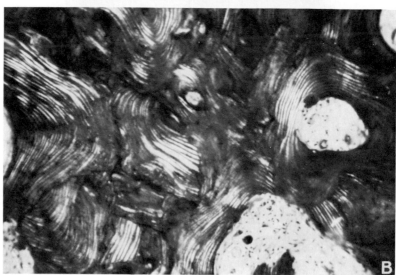

Fig. 7. Polarized views of lamellar bone. (A) Normal cortex with circumferential and concentric lamellar bone. H & E; ×150. (B) Lamellar bone in Paget's disease with its classic "mosaic" pattern. H & E; ×190.

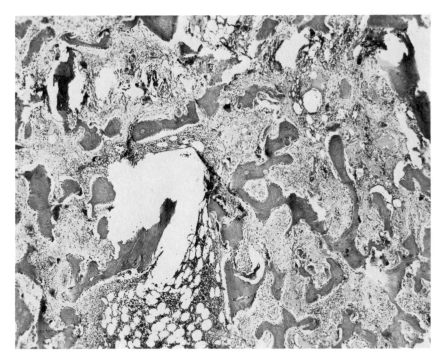

Fig. 8. A cross-sectional view of a rib showing the mixed phase of Paget's disease. Most of the cortex has been replaced by irregular spicules of pagetic bone and loose fibrovascular marrow. The remnants of medulla and hematopoietic marrow are seen in the lower center. H & E; ×44.

bone formation surfaces and therefore the osteoblast in Paget's disease is a normally functioning cell. Meunier (1977) has quantitated the calcification rate in patients with Paget's disease utilizing double labeling with tetracycline and found the rate to be twice that of normal bone.

It has been proposed by Bélanger *et al*. (1968) that the first morphologic event in Paget's disease is the resorption of surrounding lamellar bone by osteocytes (osteocytic osteolysis). Microradiographs of lamellar bone in a focus of Paget's disease close to the junction of normal bone have widened osteocyte lacunae with irregularly bosselated or etched borders. Bélanger *et al*. (1968) suggest that these lacunae continue to become resorbed by osteocytes until there is communication with a Haversian system or Volkmann's canal. Adjacent to these widened lacunae, periodic acid-Schiff and metachromatic stains are strongly positive, implying that resorption has indeed been occurring (Bélanger, 1969). The osteocytes in these lacunae may be either normal or pyknotic. Many lacunae may be empty, a hallmark of osteocytic death. Such a process was studied by

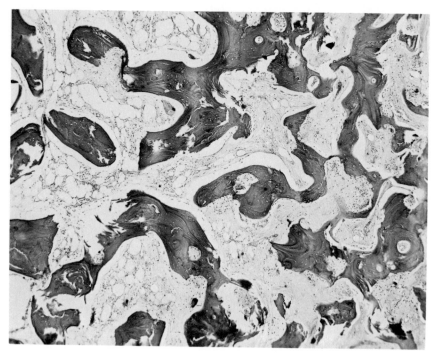

Fig. 9. The osteoblastic phase with thickened irregular spicules of pagetic bone and a loose fibrous marrow. There is very little cellular activity. H & E; ×44.

serially sectioning epon-embedded bone tissue so that each osteocyte lacuna was measured. Technical restrictions preclude a critical evaluation on our part regarding the validity of such a sequence of biological events. However, occasional osteocyte lacunae do appear scalloped and enlarged on random light microscopy sections (Fig. 10).

Bélanger *et al.* (1968) have speculated further that as resorption becomes accelerated and the disease progresses, resorption outpaces the maturation of the osteocytes so that there is a condensation of perilacunar

Fig. 10. Possible osteocytic osteolysis. (A) An enlarged scalloped osteocyte lacuna, which may represent osteocytic osteolysis. H & E; ×790. (B) Electron micrograph of demineralized bone from a different patient with Paget's disease illustrating an osteocyte with apparent resorptive activity. The osteocyte has a large lobulated nucleus and clumped chromatin. Note the large number of peripherally located dense bodies in the cytoplasm with the appearance of lysosomes. There are also vacuoles and dilated cisternae of the rough endoplasmic reticulum. The edge of the cell has numerous filapodia extending into the lacunar space, which contains amorphous material and loose collagen fibrils. The perilacunar wall is frayed and the osmiophilic lamina is lost. The collagenous structure of the bone is disorganized and there are no distinct lamellae. ×6840. (Courtesy of Dr. Barbara Mills.)

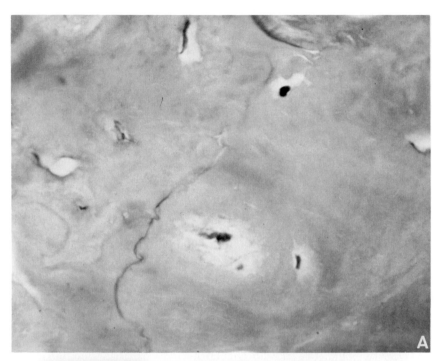

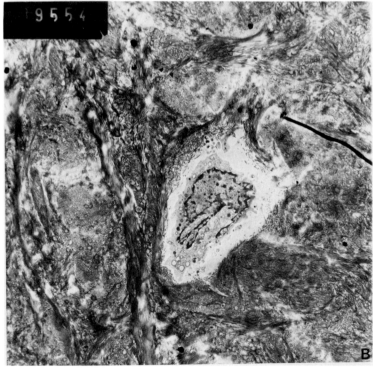

metachromatic substances about the immature osteocyte, contributing to the cement lines. These lines are seen on routine hematoxylin and eosin stains as a blue line at the interfaces between circumferential lamellae and osteones, between interstitial lamellae and osteones, or in trabecular bone when a new unit of bone is added to preexisting bone. Cement lines, therefore, are at the interface between units of bone, even between woven and lamellar bone. The later accumulation of these cement lines in lamellar bone creates the diagnostic "mosaic" pattern seen in Paget's disease. Both alpha radiography and microradiography demonstrate concurrent perilacunar mineral and matrix loss. Eventually, the poorly mineralized bone cannot undergo further osteocytic osteolysis and, by unknown mechanisms, osteoclastic activity is stimulated.

Although there may be more bone per unit volume in Paget's disease, it is architecturally unsound and weak. Grossly, the bone in the osteolytic phase may be soft enough to be cut with a knife if resorption and lack of calcification are severe enough. In the osteoblastic phase the macerated bone often crumbles like a pumice stone. This occurs presumably because the collagen fibers are not aligned along stress lines in each spicule or plate of bone. Although each spicule of bone is arranged according to stress lines, each one is weaker than a comparable normal spicule of lamellar bone and will readily break.

A. Pertinent Aspects of Differential Diagnosis

There are a few entities that may mimic histologically the pattern of pagetic bone, although none has the striking "mosaic" pattern of Paget's disease. In hyperparathyroidism irregular fragments of lamellar bone surrounded by a fibrous marrow adjacent to brown tumors or cysts are seen. However, there is no great profusion of cement lines, and dissecting osteitis, not seen in Paget's disease, is usually present. Similarly, periosteal reactions in syphilis or fracture callus may include spicules of lamellar bone with many cement lines, but one can usually still see a complete osteone and the cement lines are rarely in such chaotic profusion as in Paget's disease. Slowly formed reactive lamellar bone, such as that about a Schmorl's nodule in the spine, a Brodie's abscess in a long bone, or endosteal callus, may also be confused with Paget's disease. These lesions often have large trabeculae of lamellar bone, irregularly shaped, but cement lines are not very numerous. Accessory scaphoid bones, especially those subjected to constant pressure, also have a confusing histological picture, but again cement lines are not numerous (Jaffe, 1972). Osteoblastic metastases may stimulate formation of lamellar bone spicules, which are embedded in a sea of fibrous tissue. However, numerous cement lines are lacking in this new bone and metastatic tumor is often found trapped in the marrow.

In fibrous dysplasia, the trabeculae are irregularly shaped and consist of woven bone with numerous cement lines surrounded by dense fibrovascular connective tissue. However, prominent osteoblasts on the surface of bone trabeculae, a characteristic feature of Paget's disease, are not seen in fibrous dysplasia. Moreover, abnormal *lamellar* bone, diagnostic of Paget's disease, is absent in fibrous dysplasia.

Last, in the few cases of so-called congenital hyperphosphatasia studied microscopically (Eyring and Eisenberg, 1968; Thompson *et al.*, 1969; Woodhouse *et al.*, 1972), there are numerous irregular trabeculae of woven bone instead of a compact normal cortex with osteone formation. This rare, autosomal recessive disease, which occurs in children and has been called juvenile Paget's disease, osteoclasia, osteochalasia, and hyperostosis corticalis deformans juvenilis, is characterized by rapid turnover of subperiosteal bone and may share certain clinical and biochemical features of Paget's disease, e.g., multiple bone involvement, skull deformities, elevated urinary hydroxyproline excretion and serum alkaline phosphatase, and even the presence of angioid streaks. Histologically, however, the skeletal lesions can easily be differentiated since hyperphosphatasia represents a lack of normal cortical remodeling; hence the classic "mosaic" pattern of faceted units of *lamellar* bone is absent. We have recently had the opportunity to review the tumorous left radius in one of the three cases reported by Thompson *et al.* (1969). The mass had numerous misshapen spicules of mineralized woven bone surrounded by a dense fibrovascular marrow, similar to a focus of fibrous dysplasia. The pattern of Paget's disease was not present, and we feel that the term juvenile Paget's disease is not warranted.

V. FOCAL MANIFESTATIONS

The clinical presentation of a patient with Paget's disease depends on the extent and site of skeletal involvement. The disease may be monostotic or polyostotic, with or without symptoms. When polyostotic, the disease may lead to crippling deformities. Symptoms arise from fractures, enlargement, and excessive vascularity of bone, as well as from compression of neural structures. Joints may undergo degenerative changes due to abnormal stresses resulting from structurally altered, deformed bones. It is our impression that the patient with very severe, extensive disease may be withdrawn or somnolent, or complain of fatigue and weakness, even in the absence of specific involvement as described below. This is especially true in those patients with severe skull involvement. On the basis of angiographic studies it has been postulated that in some of these patients there may be a shunting of blood through the external carotid system to the detriment of the brain, a so-called "pagetic steal" (vol pagetique; Blotman et al., 1974).

A. Pain

Although the majority of pagetic lesions encountered are not painful (Vignon, 1974), pain may be prominent in patients with Paget's disease. It may result from the primary pagetic process or from complications that arise because of the abnormal bone. The pain associated with an uncomplicated pagetic lesion is dull and boring but may occasionally be sharp and radiating. Weight bearing may increase the severity of pain in lesions in the vertebrae, pelvis, and lower extremities, but nocturnal pain is also common in these areas. Khairi et al. (1973) have found that pagetic lesions which are detected by ^{18}NaF bone scan but not seen on roentgenograms are generally painful.

It is uncertain how the abnormal structure of the bone accounts for the development of pain. Steindler (1959) postulated that stretching of the periosteum as the bone enlarges and hyperemia of the marrow cavity may stimulate somatic sensory nerve endings in these areas. It is likely that microfractures are a significant cause of pain in weight-bearing areas. The overgrowth of bone encroaching on nervous tissue may result in severe pain syndromes; since associated neurological signs are frequently absent, it may prove difficult to determine the source of pain.

Frequently pain may be due to joint involvement by other disease processes distinct from Paget's disease such as degenerative arthritis, gouty arthritis, calcific periarthritis, or rheumatoid arthritis and its variants (Franck et al., 1974). It is of great importance to appreciate the variety of factors that can account for such pain in order to be able to institute the appropriate mode of therapy.

B. The Skull

Paget's disease involves the skull in two major patterns, although both may be present at the same time or one may develop into the other. Presumably the earliest lesion and one of the patterns seen in the skull that is usually asymptomatic has been termed osteoporosis circumscripta (Schüller, 1926; Kasabach and Gutman, 1937) (Fig. 11). Histologically the inner and outer tables are resorbed and replaced by fibrovascular tissue

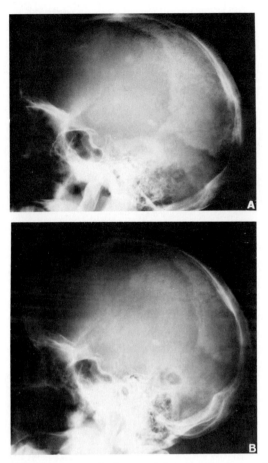

Fig. 11. Progression of osteoporosis circumscripta in Paget's disease. (A) The skull of a 52-year-old man, which shows a focal irregular osteoporotic area. (B) The same patient, 1 year later, now with almost total skull involvement.

(Jaffe, 1972). Therefore, grossly the involved area is red-violet because of the marrow shining through the absent tables. These circumscribed radiolucent areas in the calvarium may persist for years before new bone is deposited in a patchy fashion (Fig. 12). A second pattern, which may represent a later stage of osteoporosis circumscripta, is that where the skull may become markedly enlarged, usually greatest in the occipital and frontal regions. The circumference of the skull may increase by as much as 15 cm. This cortical thickening is primarily the result of deposition of pagetic bone on the outer table. As the process continues, however, the diploe is also replaced so that grossly the whole affected calvarium is

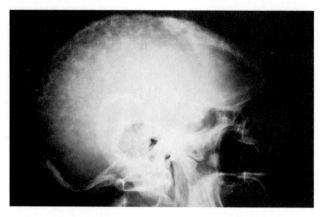

Fig. 12. An 83-year-old woman with a "honeycomb" skull produced by patchy deposition of new bone in a focus of osteoporosis circumscripta.

coarsely thickened yet still vascular. Roentgenograms at this stage may show the classic "cotton wool" appearance (Fig. 13).

The patient with an enlarged cranium may be asymptomatic or have a variety of problems. Rarely, the increased weight of the skull can make it difficult for the patient to hold his head erect, leading to spasm in the muscles of the neck. A potentially more serious complication caused by

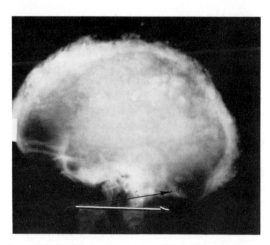

Fig. 13. An enlarged skull with the "cotton wool" pattern of diffuse cortical thickening and platybasia. Chamberlain's line (black arrow), which extends from the posterior end of the hard palate to the dorsal rim of the foramen magnum, is well below the tip of the dens. McGregor's line (white arrow), which extends from the posterior surface of the hard palate to the most caudal point of the occipital curve, is below the dens by more than 4 mm. Both of these measurements aid in defining platybasia.

pagetic remodeling of the base of the skull is the weakening of this area and its subsequent slow collapse onto the cervical spine. The degree of such basilar invagination or platybasia may be measured radiographically as an increase in the angle between the basisphenoid and the basilar portion of the occiput (Fig. 13). Although platybasia is not uncommon in Paget's disease, neurological abnormalities resulting from compression of structures in the posterior fossa (Wycis, 1944) or less commonly from cerebellar tonsillar herniation (Epstein and Epstein, 1969) are rare complications. Laminectomy of upper cervical vertebrae and suboccipital craniectomy have been successfully performed to relieve pressure on the structures of the posterior fossa (Wycis, 1944).

Difficulties in hearing and maintaining balance may arise when Paget's disease involves the temporal bone. This may be due to direct involvement of the ossicles, the labyrinth, or the external auditory canal by the pagetic process. Sensorineural loss from cochlear involvement or from impingement on the eighth cranial nerve by pagetic bone narrowing the auditory foramen may also decrease hearing (Waltner, 1965; Sparrow and Duvall, 1967; Davies, 1968).

Disturbance of function of other cranial nerves is highly unusual. Optic atrophy has been reported as a complication of Paget's disease, but Mackie (1956) found little evidence that pagetic bone compressed the optic nerve.

C. The Jaws

The jaws and bones of the face are uncommonly involved with Paget's disease. The maxilla is most often affected (Stafne and Austin, 1938). Leontiasis ossea, more typically seen in fibrous dysplasia, is a rare complication of Paget's disease which occurs when all the facial bones are involved.

Paget's disease involving the bone of the alveolar socket may produce serious dental problems (Cooke, 1956). All phases of the disease may involve the bone adjacent to the tooth, although the enamel and dentine are not affected. Particularly prominent is hyperplasia of the cementum surrounding the teeth, partial loss of the lamina dura, and severe displacement of the teeth (Barry, 1969) (Figs. 14 and 15).

D. The Spine

The spine, particularly in the lumbar and sacral regions, is one of the commonest sites in which Paget's disease is found. Although Paget's disease of the spine is most often asymptomatic, pain may be present. The

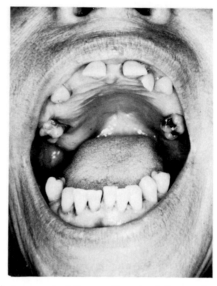

Fig. 14. Severe displacement of the maxillary teeth in a patient with Paget's disease.

early vertebral lesion may be indistinguishable from osteoporosis, especially when the entire body is involved. Radiologically the vertebral bodies most often appear enlarged with thickening at the margins and central coarse vertical striations (Fig. 16). Multiple vertebrae may be affected but often the disease skips vertebrae. The vertical height of a vertebra may be decreased due to weakness of the bone or a compression fracture may

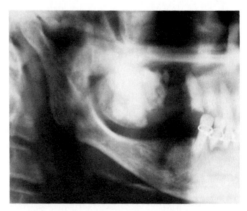

Fig. 15. A Panovex view of the mouth showing a marked hypercementosis appearing as a bosselated radiodense mass. Such a lesion could easily be confused with a dental tumor were it not for the associated pagetic changes in the adjacent bone. (Courtesy of Dr. W. Guralnick.)

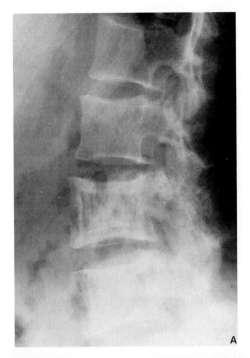

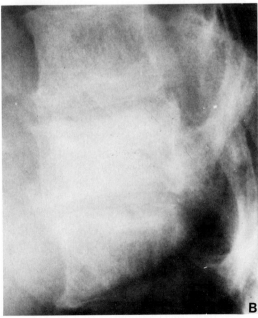

Fig. 16. Paget's disease of the spine in a 60-year-old man. (A) Enlarged vertebral bodies with thickened margins and coarse central vertical striations, the so-called "framed" vertebrae. (B) A higher power view.

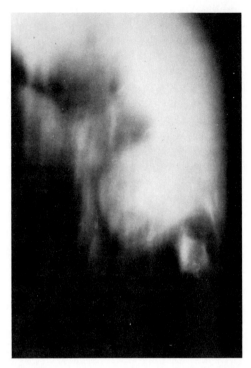

Fig. 17. A tomogram of a 61-year-old man with severe generalized Paget's disease and a rapidly growing paraspinal mass arising from several thoracic vertebrae.

develop. In extreme instances a vertebral body may even seem to disappear and be represented as a thin transverse osseous rod.

Compression of the spinal cord or nerve roots may result from enlarging vertebral bodies, pedicles, and laminae involved by Paget's disease (Wyllie, 1923; Hartman and Dohn, 1966). This is more common in the thoracic area. The symptoms resulting from these lesions include back pain, numbness and paresthesias of the feet, difficulty in walking, and progressive paresis of the legs. If untreated the patient may develop spastic paraparesis with abnormal bladder and bowel function and an upper thoracic sensory loss. Myelography performed in the lumbar and suboccipital regions reveals the inferior and superior limits of the compression, which often extends over multiple adjacent thoracic segments (Siegelman et al., 1968). The treatment of choice is decompressive laminectomy as spontaneous recovery does not occur. An uncommon feature found in some patients is the development of a discrete paraspinal mass, which represents partially calcified osteoid tissue that infiltrates the epidural region by direct extension from the vertebral periosteum and paraosseous connective tissue (Siegelman *et al.*, 1968). We have observed one such lesion in a 61-year-old man with extremely severe, generalized Paget's disease (urinary hydroxyproline 1200 mg per 24 hour), which appeared, over a period of months, on roentgenograms of the chest as a rapidly enlarging mass (Fig. 17). An exploratory thoracotomy performed to rule out a pleural tumor or malignant degeneration of the Paget's disease revealed a large oval mass arising from several thoracic vertebrae and consisting of a central marrow cavity and a peripheral capsule of pagetic bone. The significance of this extramedullary hematopoietic lesion is unclear since the patient was not anemic.

An association of ankylosing spondylitis and Paget's disease was reported by Bitar (1961) and Layani and colleagues (1961) in a total of six patients. Recently we have evaluated another six patients with Paget's disease who also had physical findings that suggested ankylosing spondylitis (Franck *et al.*, 1974). Limitation of chest expansion was present in each patient. Spinal flexion was impaired in four patients and four had peripheral joint disease. Apparent ossification of spinal ligaments was present in two patients and extensive osteophytosis in the other four. Sacroiliac joint obliteration occurred in four patients and squaring of the vertebral bodies in two. Syndesmophytes were not seen. Paget's disease was present in the pelvis of five patients and in the lumbosacral spine of four. Fatigue, stiffness, and back pain were common complaints. The clinical findings in this group of patients were strongly suggestive of ankylosing spondylitis but it is conceivable that pagetic involvement adjacent to certain joints might mimic spondylitis. From 88 to 96% of patients with ankylosing spondylitis have the HLA antigen W27 as compared to 8% or less of control populations (Brewerton *et al.*, 1973; Caffrey and James, 1973; Schlosstein *et al.*, 1973). We therefore compared the incidence of W27 in four of our six patients and none had the W27 HLA antigen. Such preliminary data support the possibility that small joints of the spine and the costovertebral joints may be affected secondarily by Paget's disease in adjacent bone.

E. The Pelvis and Extremities

In the extremities the femur and tibia are most commonly involved with Paget's disease. It is not unusual to find a monostotic focus in either of these bones (Fig. 18). When these bones are involved, clinical manifestations such as pain, deformity, and increase in skin temperature are usually present. The deformity associated with Paget's disease of the femur is an outward bowing combined with a coxa vara deformity causing external

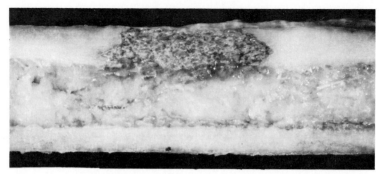

Fig. 18. An osteolytic focus of Paget's disease in the cortex of the tibia. Note the coarsely trabeculated pattern of bone spicules and the extremely rich vascular marrow within this focus. [From *The New England Journal of Medicine* (1963), **269**, 813.]

rotation of the lower leg. The tibia is usually bowed anteriorly and laterally (Fig. 19). The upper extremities are less frequently affected by Paget's disease and are often asymptomatic (Figs. 20 and 21). However, involvement of the ulna may lead to bowing of the arm. Rarely the disease may appear in the hands; it is usually in a single bone and is almost always asymptomatic (Fig. 22).

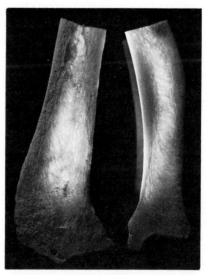

Fig. 19. A transillumination of a macerated hemisected tibia with Paget's disease showing the thickened cortex and densely packed, coarsely thickened trabeculae, as well as typical bowing deformity.

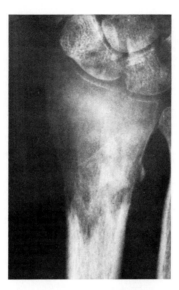

Fig. 20. An osteolytic monostotic focus of Paget's disease in the radius of a patient who presented with wrist pain. Note the classic flame shape or sawtooth pattern produced by the advancing edge of osteoclastic activity which distinguishes this lesion from a malignant tumor. (Courtesy of Dr. K. Proppe.)

The major clinical problem that may develop after years of involvement of the pelvis and upper femur is degenerative joint disease of the hip, which may cause considerable morbidity from pain and decreased mobility (Machtey *et al.*, 1966). Although Barry (1969) feels that the incidence of this problem is low, we have found this to be a common source of discomfort in the majority of our pagetic patients (Franck *et al.*, 1974). Involvement of the hip joint could result from Paget's disease of subchondral bone or from altered mechanics at the hip due to deformity of the entire bone. Roper (1971) suggested that if the narrowing of the hip joint space in patients with Paget's disease was predominantly superior in the zone of maximal weight bearing, this implied coincidental, unrelated degenerative joint disease. He concluded that if the joint space narrowing was medial and accompanied by protrusio acetabuli, the Paget's disease was the cause of the symptoms. In our study of 41 patients with disease involving 76 hips, we have found that pagetic involvement of the proximal femur in the absence of acetabular involvement is rare, whereas acetabular disease without femoral involvement is common (Franck *et al.*, 1974) (Fig. 23). Most of the latter patients have narrowing of the superior joint margin, usually without protrusio acetabuli, and are less symptomatic. The most severe disease occurs in patients with both

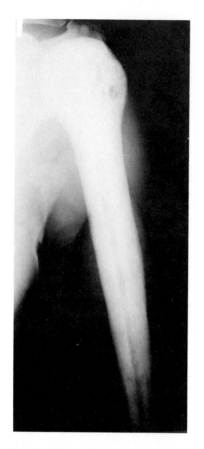 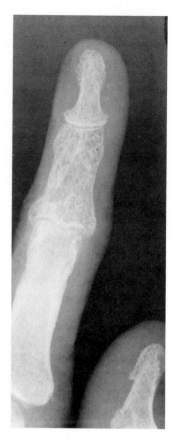

Fig. 21. Paget's disease of the humerus. Note the cyst in the humoral head representing cystic degeneration, which may occur in a focus of Paget's disease. The cortices are markedly thickened by coarse trabeculae.

Fig. 22. A 78-year-old man with severe generalized Paget's disease including asymptomatic involvement of the fingers. Note the thickened cortex of the proximal phalanx and the coarsely thickened trabeculae of the middle phalanx.

acetabular and proximal femoral disease (Fig. 24). Protrusio acetabuli is usually associated with both superior and medial joint space narrowing (Fig. 25). In these patients the abnormal remodeling of pagetic bone permits the forces of weight bearing to drive the femoral head both superiorly and medially. Some symptomatic relief from the pain of hip disease is obtained by the use of orthopedic devices, salicylates, or indomethacin, but in others total hip replacement is required for adequate relief of pain (Stauffer and Sim, 1976).

Knee pain is quite common in patients with Paget's disease of the femur

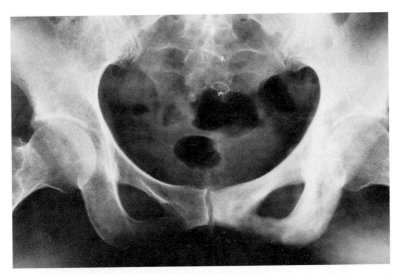

Fig. 23. Early involvement of the left half of the pelvis characterized by a dense rim of pagetic bone surrounding the acetabulum. This is a frequent early finding in the pelvis.

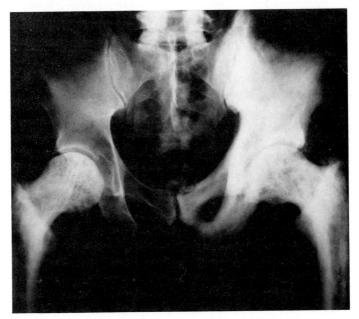

Fig. 24. More severe involvement of the left pelvis and femur by Paget's disease. Note that the left portion of the sacrum is also involved.

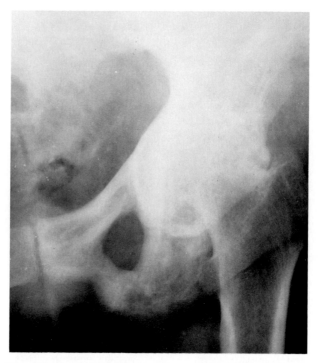

Fig. 25. Protrusio acetabuli in Paget's disease involving the proximal femur and acetabulum.

and tibia (Franck *et al.*, 1974) and is more likely to be present if the disease is adjacent to the joint. Severe joint space narrowing is common in these patients and almost always accompanied by pain, although the severity of the pain and impaired mobility of these patients is usually less than that of patients with hip disease. Paget's disease may involve the patella, which may become enlarged and warm to the touch. The focality of the disease is illustrated by the fact that such pagetic involvement may occur in the absence of any other involvement of the particular extremity and is not necessarily associated with Paget's disease of the femur or tibia (Fig. 26).

VI. COMPLICATIONS

A. Fractures

Fractures are the most common complication of Paget's disease (Collins, 1966). They are characteristically transverse whether complete or

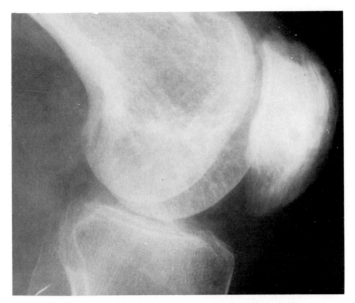

Fig. 26. Paget's disease of the patella. There is marked exaggeration of the cortical and medullary bone produced by the pagetic bone, following normal stress lines.

incomplete, and lie perpendicular to the cortex. The incomplete fissure fracture, or infraction, seen in the long bones is infrequently a precursor to complete transverse fractures (Allen and John, 1937) and need not result from external trauma. Femoral fractures are twice as common as fractures of the tibia (Jaffe, 1972); the main femoral site is just below the lesser trochanter, whereas the tibia is most frequently fractured in the upper third of the shaft (Harris and Krane, 1968). The small cortical incomplete fractures often occur at multiple sites on a single long bone, primarily along the periosteal edge of the convex surface of the curved bone and penetrating to various depths through the cortex. Roentgenograms have narrow slit-like radiolucent transverse lines (Fig. 27).* Repeated occurrence and remodeling of incomplete fractures is partly responsible for the increase in total degree of curvature in diseased tubular bone. The majority of incomplete fractures occur during the osteolytic

---

*It is possible that these transverse radiolucencies, particularly on the convex aspect of the femur, do not initially represent fractures but are enlarged vascular channels. Roentgenograms obtained at different degrees of rotation have shown that the radiolucencies, in some patients at least, do not penetrate to the outer cortex at any point as would be expected with fractures (B. Maldague, unpublished). These regions could still be weak relative to the rest of the bone and therefore be the site of initiation of fractures.

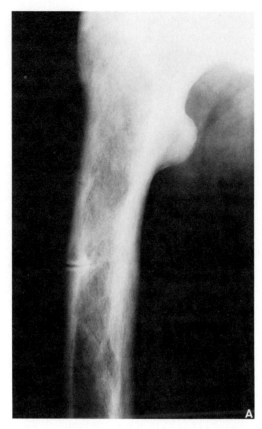

Fig. 27. Fractures in Paget's disease. (A) Two fissure fractures of a femur involved by Paget's disease. (B) One month later a complete "chalk stick" fracture occurred at the site of the distal fissure fracture. Note that the proximal fissure fracture is still present. (C) A month after the fracture was pinned, it began to heal. (D) Two years later a complete "chalk stick" fracture occurred at the site of the proximal fissure fracture.   *(Continued)*

phase, while complete fractures tend to be more common in the osteoblastic phase. This would be anticipated, since the energy required for the propagation of the fracture is dissipated by the numerous separate trabeculae of the bone of the lytic phase.

Fractures in pagetic bone can heal as efficiently as in normal bone while the callus underlying the break itself undergoes the bony changes of Paget's disease. In complete fractures, which are usually transverse as if the bone were snapped like a piece of chalk, the periosteum will be torn with a wide separation of fragments. There is a bias (over 30%) for

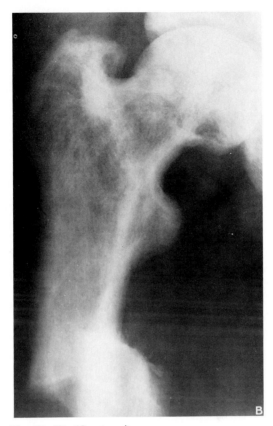

Fig. 27. (B) *(Continued)*

complete shaft fractures just below the lesser trochanter, with flexion ab-
duction deformity of the proximal fragment. This subtrochanteric site contrasts vividly with the bias toward femoral neck fracture found in older
persons without Paget's disease. Since incomplete fractures are most
common at the subtrochanteric level, this area would be the site of the
most extensive femoral remodeling and proliferation of abnormal bone in
Paget's disease. Accordingly, a combination of internal expansion and
remote compression trauma might be sufficient to elicit complete fracture.
Tibial fractures follow the femoral pattern. Sometimes the fibula, which is
not ordinarily diseased, can be fractured as a sequel to tibial breaks.
Pelvic fracture is usually through one or both pubic or ischial rami. It is
often difficult to determine whether vertebral body deformity is a result of
pagetic resorption or represents authentic fracture.

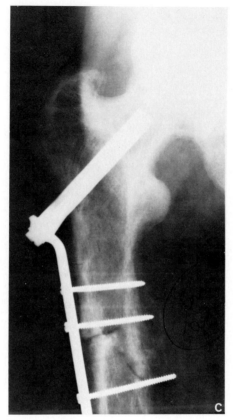

Fig. 27. (**C**) *(Continued)*

It has been noted by Barry (1969) that spontaneous fracture may occur through an osteolytic lesion of Paget's disease and result in rapid local spread of the pagetic osteolytic process. This can be confused radiographically with a malignant change (Grainger and Laws, 1957; Barry, 1961).

B. Associated Neoplasia

The exact incidence of malignant change in Paget's disease is unknown. Although there have been estimates as high as 10% in generalized, severe disease (Jaffe, 1972), an incidence well below 1% probably reflects a more accurate picture if all cases are taken into account (Collins, 1966; Barry,

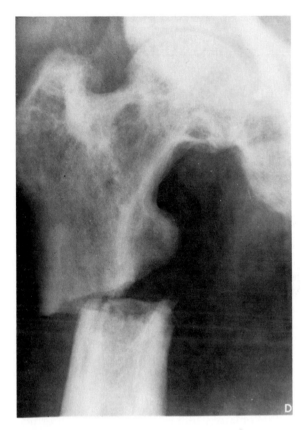

Fig. 27. (D) *(Continued)*

1969). Of all patients over the age of 40 with bone sarcoma, however, about one-fifth will have Paget's disease (McKenna *et al.*, 1964). In Barry's series (1969) of 116 sarcomas arising in Paget's disease, men were affected twice as often as women. Malignant change was rare below the age of 50. The most common symptoms were pain and swelling, which may have predated radiographic findings by a period of months. Pain may be absent with skull involvement. In some cases the neoplasm, as a soft tissue tumor, may be the presenting sign (Jaffe, 1972). Some correlation has been thought to exist between the fracture site and the site of sarcomatous change, but it is unsubstantiated since a neoplasm has rarely been histologically demonstrated at a fracture site, even though both occur in the same bone (Barry, 1969). Furthermore, in one survey no predisposition to malignancy was found following fracture (McKenna *et al.*, 1964). Therefore, local injury or excessive trauma, so often invoked as causally related to malignant transformation, is more likely to be the event that draws attention to the previously undetected tumor.

Sarcomas in pagetic patients occur most frequently in the femur, humerus, skull, face, and pelvis but are uncommon in vertebrae (Barry, 1969). This is in sharp contrast to the distribution of Paget's disease itself, which usually affects the vertebrae, skull, pelvis, femur, and tibia and less commonly the humerus. The reasons why sarcomatous change favors the humerus (Poretta *et al.*, 1957; Barry, 1969) are obscure. Such malignant change always takes place within a focus of Paget's disease. Therefore, only in cases of advanced and extensive polyostotic disease are multifocal sarcomas found (Grainger and Laws, 1957; Hilker, 1959; Boutouras and Goodsit, 1963; Schajowicz and Slullitel, 1966; Jaffe, 1972) and when they do occur, the skull is most commonly the site (Barry, 1969). Jaffe (1972) has described cases where only one bone was involved with Paget's disease in which sarcoma developed. In studies by Collins (1966) Paget's disease was polyostotic in two-thirds of the patients with sarcoma. Autopsy data also suggested that each sarcoma is of independent origin and not metastatic. Multiple scalp tumors were seen in 24 cases in Barry's series (1969) of 116 sarcomas. Such lesions were often associated with lysis of the underlying calvarium and invasion directly into the brain. Death ensued within 6 months after diagnosis.

The sarcomas vary widely in cell composition (Barry, 1969; Jaffe, 1972), reflecting the pluripotentiality of the mesenchymal elements of the bone marrow. Sarcomatous tumors have a spectrum of histological patterns, which include the following: (1) cell-poor, collagen-rich fibrosarcomas (Fig. 28); (2) poorly differentiated fibrosarcomas with abundant giant cells; (3) anaplastic sarcomas with giant cells, spindle cells with plump nuclei, and osteoclast-like giant cells resembling so-called malignant giant cell tumors of bone; (4) rare chondrosarcomas, nine of which were reviewed by Barry (1969); (5) conventional giant cell tumors found mostly in the skull, but with occasional spinal, innominate, or femoral involvement; (6) sarcomatous stroma that may contain osteoid and may be classified as osteosarcoma; (7) reticulum cell sarcoma (Lauchlan and Walsh, 1963); and (8) multiple myeloma (Riffat, 1968). This histological spectrum appears to be a continuum from benign to malignant since benign but bizarre cellular changes in fibrous bone marrow remote from

---

Fig. 28. A spindle cell sarcoma. (A) The tumor consists almost wholly of fibroblasts swirling around fragments of pagetic bone. H & E; ×190. (B) Atypical mitoses are easily seen in the spindle sarcoma cells. H & E; ×750.

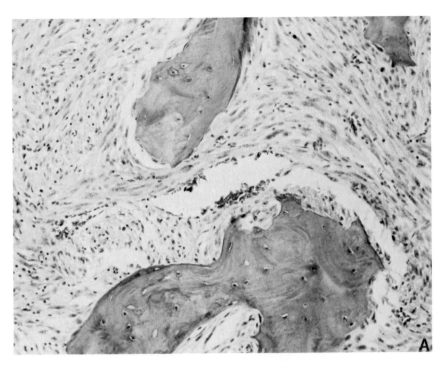

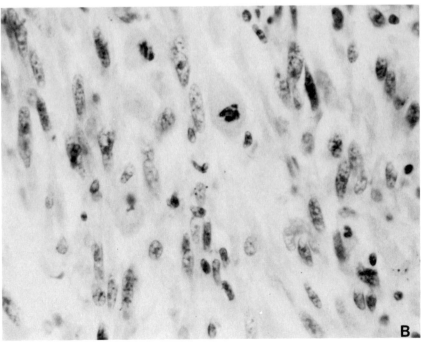

the tumor site may be seen (von Albertini, 1928; Jaffe, 1972). Thus there is a danger in interpreting a biopsy taken from one portion of a tumor, since different histological patterns may be found in different parts of the neoplasm, and for this reason we prefer the broadly descriptive term sarcoma. As Jaffe (1972) concluded: "It would seem that the connective tissue from which they (sarcomas) arise may reveal, even within the same tumor, manifold potentialities for differentiation and dedifferentiation along mesenchymal lines."

Radiographically sarcomas usually appear as small, irregular radiolucent foci with mottled or speckled areas of calcification superimposed on the background of Paget's disease (Fig. 29). The dense areas of tumor

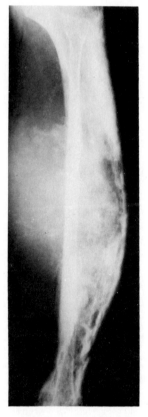

Fig. 29. An 82-year-old man with osteosarcoma arising in a tibia afflicted with Paget's disease. The tumor has extended into the soft tissue and has multiple radiodense areas, some of which have the trabecular pattern of bone formation. Note the underlying changes of Paget's disease extensively involving the tibia.

bone or the sunburst pattern characteristic of osteosarcoma of the young are not usually seen in sarcoma associated with Paget's disease. In addition, the tumors associated with Paget's disease are not confined to the ends of the bones but occur anywhere along the shaft. For example, in Barry's series (1969) of 24 tumors involving the femur, 10 were in the proximal third of the shaft, 5 in the mid-third, and 9 in the distal third. Most tibial tumors were in the proximal portion of the shaft. Sarcomas appear to originate in the medulla (Barry, 1969; Jaffe, 1972), as manifested by the radiographic signs of early subcortical medullary bone lysis. This progresses to cortical bone loss and the eventual development of a soft tissue mass. A pathological fracture may be seen as a terminal event of this biological sequence (Barry, 1969).

The prognosis for sarcomas arising in Paget's disease is dismal (Barry, 1969; Jaffe, 1972). Most patients die within 2 years after the diagnosis is established. In Barry's series of 116 tumors (1969) no patient survived longer than 5 years with the average duration of survival being 12 months from diagnosis. Those cases with multiple sarcomas died within 6 months with pulmonary metastases (Jaffe, 1972). At present, radiotherapy is only palliative and the treatment of choice appears to be amputation if the tumor is painful or disfiguring. The role of adriamycin, methotrexate with citrovorum factor and other chemotherapeutic agents, alone and in combination in osteosarcoma patients, is under intense investigation (Jaffe and Watts, 1976).

A peculiar neoplasm deserving special mention here is the giant cell tumor associated with Paget's disease. These are uncommon sarcomas and almost always involve some portion of the calvarium or facial bones. In Barry's review (1969) of 15 such tumors (5 in the calvarium, 2 each in the maxilla and mandible, and 1 in the humerus, ilium, tibia, and ethmoid) a spectrum ranging from classic benign giant cell tumors to malignant sarcomas with giant cells was seen. Similar cases have been reported under the broad term of giant cell tumor. Therefore, the prognosis varies with each case report. However, survival rates appear to be much better than for other sarcomas (Jaffe, 1972). Jaffe (1972) has described an astounding case where, over an 8-year period, 12 such tumors appeared successively in the frontal, parietal, temporal, occipital, and facial bones. We had under our care a man with extensive polyostotic Paget's disease known since age 35 (serum alkaline phosphatase levels as high as 114 Bodansky Units) who at age 46 was discovered to have a tumor containing giant cells in the mandible. He was treated with currettage and radiation but the tumor recurred on several occasions over several years. Eleven years after the mandibular lesion was identified he developed a right iliac bone tumor with iliac vein obstruction, which was identical histologically to the lesion in the jaw (Fig. 30). The pelvic lesion did not respond to radiation therapy but became smaller with calcitonin administration. At the time of the patient's death from coronary heart disease, 19 years after the jaw lesion was discovered, there was no evidence of metastases.

Microscopically these tumors consisted of benign spindle cells with plump fusiform nuclei and clumped chromatin or nucleoli. Mitoses were rare. Scattered among these cells were osteoclast-type giant cells not randomly dispersed, but congregated about foci of hemorrhage or scar and often associated with hemosiderin-laden macrophages. Some of the giant cells had phagocytized erythrocytes. Small scattered fragments of

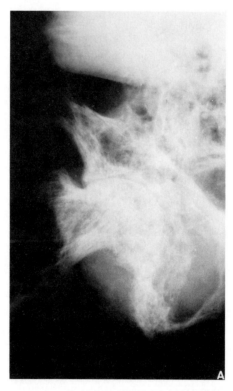

Fig. 30. A giant cell tumor in the right iliac bone of a 57-year-old man with extensive Paget's disease of most bones. (A) The tumor is represented as a large cystic defect in the ilium. There is severe Paget's disease of the pelvis and femur. Histologically the tumor was similar to a giant cell reparative granuloma of the jaw in the same individual. (B) The jaw and iliac lesions were composed of benign spindle cells with plump fusiform nuclei and prominent nucleoli. The many osteoclast-type giant cells were generally arranged about areas of hemorrhage. H & E; ×270. (C) Such giant cells often engulfed large aggregates of erythrocytes. H & E; ×700.

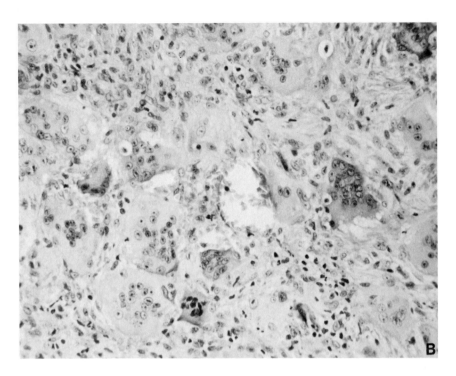

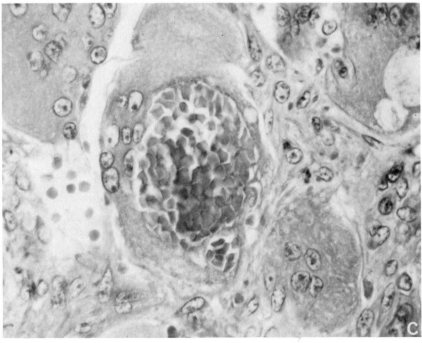

pagetic bone were adjacent to some tumor cells in addition to reactive woven bone spicules, which were generally peripherally disposed. Fibrous marrow adjacent to these tumors had similar gradations of cellular atypicality such that the tumors merged subtly with the nearby fibrous marrow. We felt these lesions to be an atypical proliferative process similar to the giant cell reparative granuloma of the jaw. This case illustrates the most benign form of the giant cell lesions seen associated with Paget's disease.

Attempts have been made to correlate the skeletal distribution of Paget's disease with that of metastatic cancer, but the correlation would hold only for the axial skeleton, which is among the most favored sites for metastases of many types of cancer. The ribs are a preferential site for metastases but are nearly exempt from Paget's disease. On the other hand the tibia, which is among the most favored sites of Paget's disease, is an infrequent location for metastatic cancer (Barry, 1969). A correlation would seem to depend on the degree of abnormal bone vascularization. The few examples of the coexistence of multiple myeloma and Paget's disease, two diseases that commonly affect the axial skeleton of the elderly, appear to be coincidence (Riffat, 1968).

VII. METABOLIC ASPECTS OF PAGET'S DISEASE

A. Mineral Metabolism

Clinical and histopathological evidence suggests that the primary defect in Paget's disease is excessive resorption of bone in a focal area. Characteristically this excessive resorption is soon accompanied by an increase in bone formation which may continue on after the resorption has slowed down. Despite the focal nature of the disorder and its limited extent in some patients, the increased remodeling is readily detected and involves both the mineral and organic phases of bone.

As bone is resorbed, mineral ions are released into the extracellular fluid. If excessive resorption occurs in one part of the skeleton, the increased concentration of mineral ions in the extracellular fluid would, because of the hypercalcemia, decrease secretion of parathyroid hormone and increase renal clearance of calcium. However, in patients with Paget's disease, concentrations of calcium and phosphorus in plasma are usually normal,* parathyroid hormone concentrations by radioim-

---

*For example, in our series of 29 patients with Paget's disease of varying extent and severity (F. R. Singer and S. M. Krane, unpublished), the mean (±S.E.) fasting serum calcium was 9.35 ± 0.08 and phosphorus 3.7 ± 0.08 mg per dl, all within the normal range for this laboratory (Castleman and McNeely, 1970).

munoassay are within the normal range (Riggs *et al.*, 1971; Singer *et al.*, 1972b; Burckhardt *et al.*, 1973), and urinary calcium excretion is not characteristically increased in the absence of fractures of bone or immobilization of patients in bed (Nagant de Deuxchaisnes and Krane, 1964). This implies that the increased release of mineral ions that results from increased bone resorption must be accompanied by closely geared reutilization locally of such ions for the formation of new mineral phase. Therefore, the external calcium balance in Paget's disease, which reflects *differences* in bone formation and resorption, does not usually give any indication of the *rates* of these processes. Analysis of the disappearance from the plasma of tracer doses of mineral ions does indicate how greatly accelerated turnover of these ions may be, even though the process may be confined to a limited region of the skeleton.

The results of studies of several authors using [47]Ca (Avioli and Henneman, 1964), [45]Ca, [85]Sr (Nagant de Deuxchaisnes and Krane, 1964; Coutris *et al.*, 1975; Lauffenburger *et al.*, 1977; Schiano and Eisenger, 1977), and [25]Mg (Avioli and Berman, 1968), although not strictly comparable quantitatively, have all shown that the rates of both bone formation and resorption are greatly increased in patients with polyostotic Paget's disease. The pattern of disappearance of injected [47]Ca from the serum of a patient with extensive Paget's disease is shown in Fig. 31. From data of this sort it is possible to calculate the size of the exchangeable calcium pool and rates of entrance into (v_{0-}) and exit from (v_{0+}) this pool (Aubert

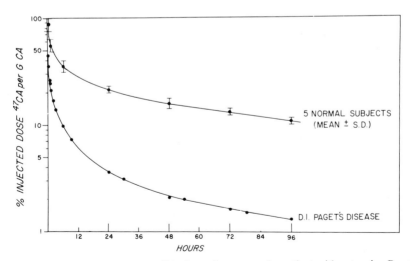

Fig. 31. The pattern of loss of [47]Ca from the serum of a patient with extensive Paget's disease as compared to that from five normal subjects. (From Nagant de Deuxchaisnes and Krane (1964). By permission from the publisher, the Williams and Wilkins Co.).

and Milhaud, 1960; Aubert *et al.*, 1963). Although there is disagreement as to the significance of such calculations and their physiological meaning, it is possible to use the numbers derived to compare different subjects to each other and to normals. The increased values for v_{0+} and v_{0-} calculated in patients with Paget's disease are *mean* rates for the whole skeleton. It should be emphasized that some areas would be remodeling at rates manyfold that of others. Calculations of the kinetic parameters in patients such as those listed in Table IV (Section VII,B) probably overestimate rates of calcium resorption, v_{0-} (as well as calcium deposition, v_{0+}). However, in comparison with the rates calculated for normal subjects, both formation and resorption may be increased occasionally more than 20-fold. Although the physical properties of ^{32}P have precluded its widespread use to study phosphorus kinetics in man, it is likely that an abnormality similar to that observed with the tracer cations would be seen. Fluoride ions can be incorporated into the hydroxyapatite crystal lattice and evidence of increased retention of absorbed fluoride has also been found in patients with Paget's disease (Nagant de Deuxchaisnes and Krane, 1964).

Although the whole body turnover of mineral ions is increased in pagetic subjects, results obtained by external scanning following administration of the radioactive isotopes ^{47}Ca, ^{85}Sr, ^{18}F, and diphosphonate coupled to ^{99m}Tc (Pendergrass *et al.*, 1973) indicate that the tracer is localized mainly to diseased areas of the skeleton. It was found that pagetic bone initially took up more ^{47}Ca than normal bone and retained the isotope for longer periods of time (Nagant de Deuxchaisnes and Krane, 1964). This increased uptake is not due entirely to rapid exchange processes, since the high level of activity persists in the involved bones even when the plasma activity has reached low levels. Whether such retention is the result of the formation of new mineral phase or some long-term exchange process (Lee *et al.*, 1965; Harris and Heaney, 1970) is not yet known. However, the intensity of the remodeling in diseased bone may clear tracer ions so rapidly from the blood that little is available for uptake by normal bone. Uptake over an *uninvolved* tibia at an arbitrary interval following injection of ^{47}Ca is less in patients with Paget's disease than in normal subjects. The kinetic data obtained in patients with Paget's disease imply that, despite enormous increases in both bone resorption and formation, the rates of the two processes are very similar.

We have speculated in the past (Nagant de Deuxchaisnes and Krane, 1964) that the increase in bone formation is the homeostatic response of the organism to maintain the concentration of calcium in the plasma constant despite the great egress of calcium from bone to extracellular fluid. It is possible that it is this homeostatic requirement for bone formation that accounts for the irregular deposition of new bone which characterizes Paget's disease. The delicate equilibrium between formation and resorption is easily upset by such events as fractures or immobilization of the patient and would be reflected in alterations in calcium balance or in elevation of serum calcium level.

B. Collagen Metabolism

1. Pagetic Bone Collagen

When bone is resorbed, not only is there release of mineral ions from the inorganic phase but there is resorption of the organic phase as well. As discussed in Chapter 1, Volume I, the organic phase of bone consists mainly of collagen in addition to a variety of noncollagenous proteins.

That the arrangement of the lamellae of collagen fibers in pagetic bone is abnormal is easily seen with polarized light microscopy. There is little information on other aspects of the structure of collagen in the abnormal bone. The amino acid composition of some samples of pagetic bone analyzed after demineralization in EDTA is indistinguishable from normal bone (Table II) (Krane *et al.*, 1977). The relative amounts of the glycosylated hydroxylysines are also comparable. In only one sample of pagetic bone was there an increase in the amount of glucosylgalactosylhydroxylysine relative to galactosylhydroxylysine. Since in Paget's disease the normal fatty or hematopoietic marrow may be replaced by fibrous tissue, it is possible that the relative increase in diglycosylated hydroxylysine in the one sample reflects the contribution of the immature woven pagetic bone or the fibrous tissue, which may have chemical characteristics more closely resembling those of skin than of bone collagen. Other analytical techniques (e.g., determination of amino acid sequence or type of inter- and intramolecular cross-links) may uncover other differences in collagen structure to account for the characteristic histological appearances that distinguish pagetic from normal bone. Misra (1975) has reported the relative increase of a minor cross-link, hydroxylysinonorleucine, in pagetic bone. The significance of this observation remains to be determined. In preliminary studies by A. H. Kang (unpublished), the distribution pattern of the peptides obtained by cleavage of insoluble demineralized pagetic bone with cyanogen bromide was similar to normal bone, suggesting no major alteration of primary structure.

2. Collagenolysis

In order to resorb bone it is first necessary to remove the inorganic mineral phase so that the collagen and other components of the organic

TABLE II

Chemical Composition of Pagetic Bone[a]

	Pagetic bone					
	1	2	3	4	5	
Amino acid			(residues/1000 residues)			Control
4-Hydroxyproline	102	113	109	100	108	$100.5^b \pm 5.9$
Aspartic acid	52	51	48	52	53	48.5 ± 0.9
Threonine	21	21	19	21	21	18.0 ± 0.9
Serine	37	38	36	39	38	36.2 ± 0.8
Glutamic acid	85	84	80	86	85	80.7 ± 1.7
Proline	122	129	124	128	125	120.7 ± 2.8
Glycine	290	277	307	281	282	311.0 ± 3.8
Alanine	104	109	110	111	110	111.2 ± 1.8
½ Cystine	1.4	0.6	0	0.5	0.9	0.3 ± 0.1
Valine	26	25	23	20	26	24.2 ± 1.7
Methionine	6.2	7.3	3.0	11.4	7.7	5.6 ± 0.6
Isoleucine	11	11	10	11	12	10.2 ± 0.8
Leucine	28	27	26	24	28	25.9 ± 1.0
Tyrosine	6	4.8	2.5	5.5	5.3	4.0 ± 0.2
Phenylalanine	15	15	13	18	16	13.6 ± 1.0
Hydroxylysine	5.4	5.0	3.8	6.7	4.2	4.2 ± 0.7
Lysine	28	24	28	28	20	29.0 ± 2.8
Histidine	6.4	2.0	4.2	1.5	1.8	5.6 ± 0.3
Arginine	52	55	51	55	56	48.5 ± 2.4
Total hydroxylysine glycosides (%)	27	33	33	27	56	30^c
Glucosylgalactosyl-hydroxylysine galactosylhydroxylysine	0.422	0.743	0.396	0.464	0.390	0.474^c

[a] From Krane et al. (1977) using methods of Pinnell *et al.* (1972).
[b] Mean ± S.D. from Pinnell *et al.* (1972).
[c] Pinnell *et al.* (1971).

matrix can be attacked by collagenolytic (Eisen *et al.*, 1970) and other enzymes (Vaes, 1968) released from bone-resorbing cells (Stern *et al.*, 1963; Kaufman *et al.*, 1965; Fullmer and Lazarus, 1967; Shimizu *et al.*, 1969; Sakamoto *et al.*, 1972, 1973). The resorption of bone collagen in Paget's disease is probably mediated by the same factors that are involved in normal skeletal remodeling, as shown by studies in which biopsy specimens of bone from patients with Paget's disease incubated *in vitro* release significantly greater label from collagen gels than do specimens of normal bones (Gardner *et al.*, 1970). Whether this enhanced collagenolysis is due to increased numbers of bone-resorbing cells or enhanced activity of each cell is not known.

3. Hydroxyproline and Hydroxylysine Excretion

In normal animals and man, the free hydroxylysine (Sinex and Van Slyke, 1955) and hydroxyproline (Stetten, 1949) released from collagen-derived peptides are not reutilized for collagen synthesis and are degraded to small carbon fragments (Adams, 1970; Kivirikko, 1970). However, oligopeptide-bound hydroxyproline (Kivirikko, 1970) and hydroxylysine (Dubovsky et al., 1964; Nagant de Deuxchaisnes and Krane, 1967; Krane et al., 1977) and glycosylated hydroxylysine (Segrest and Cunningham, 1970; Askenasi, 1973; Askenasi et al., 1976; Krane et al., 1977) are excreted in the urine, the rate of excretion roughly reflecting the rate of collagen degradation. The finding of increased urinary excretion of peptides containing hydroxyproline and other collagen markers in patients with Paget's disease provides a useful tool for the study of collagen turnover in man.

The excretion of hydroxyproline-containing peptides is greater than normal in almost all patients with Paget's disease, even in those with monostotic involvement (Dull and Henneman, 1963; Kivirikko, 1970). In general, the amount of hydroxyproline excreted is directly correlated with the extent of the Paget's disease (Khairi et al., 1973; Franck et al., 1974) as well as with the degree of disease activity as determined, for example, by ^{47}Ca kinetics (Nagant de Deuxchaisnes and Krane, 1964). The fact that the concentrations of oligopeptide hydroxyproline in the plasma are also increased (Bijvoet et al., 1968), despite rapid clearance by the kidney (Benoit and Walton, 1968), indicates that the increased urinary excretion is not due simply to increased renal clearance. Although the evidence is indirect, it is likely that the excessive urinary excretion of hydroxyproline in pagetic subjects has its source in bone. The evidence is as follows: (1) The level of excretion of hydroxyproline is directly related to the extent and the degree of the activity of the Paget's disease. (2) As will be discussed in detail later in this chapter (Section IX), treatment of Paget's disease with agents that have their major effects on bone (e.g., calcitonin) results in decreased hydroxyproline excretion. (3) There is no histopathologic evidence that collagens in tissues other than bone, such as the dermis, are involved to a degree sufficient to explain the increased collagen degradation, although minor morphologic changes in appearance of the dermis in pagetic subjects have been observed. (4) The total urinary excretion of hydroxylysine as well as hydroxyproline is increased in Paget's disease and the pattern of glycosylated hydroxylysines excreted in the urine of several patients studied resembles that of bone collagen (Askenasi et al., 1976; Krane et al., 1977). The ratio of glucosylgalac-tosylhydroxylysine:galactosylhydroxylysine in five patients with exten-sive Paget's disease ranged from 0.40 to 0.74, closer to that of bone collagen (0.47) than to that of skin (2.06) or other collagens (>2.0). The urinary ratios are distinctly lower than the mean of 1.49 in nonpagetic subjects (Askenasi, 1973).

4. Other Collagen Peptides

Dialyzable oligopeptides containing hydroxyproline comprise over 90% of the total urinary hydroxyproline (Meilman *et al.*, 1963; Kivirikko, 1970). These consist primarily of the dipeptide prolylhydroxyproline and its diketopiperazine and the tripeptide glycylprolylhydroxyproline. The sequence of the peptide components is consistent with that in mammalian collagens in which glycine occurs every third residue and 4-hydroxyproline only in the residue preceding glycine, never in the position following glycine.

One might expect that other peptides of the collagen sequence, such as glycylproline, would be excreted in the urine in excess when collagen degradation is increased. Scriver (1964) identified glycylproline in the urine of patients with rickets and found that the rate of its excretion diminished with healing of the rickets. More recently Alderman *et al.* (1969) observed marked increases in urinary excretion of glycylproline in patients with a familial skeletal disorder characterized by thickened cortices of long bones, bow deformities, and fractures. They were also able to detect glycylproline in the urine of some subjects with rickets and osteogenesis imperfecta but were unable to find the peptide in the urine of patients with other bone diseases including Paget's disease, although data on hydroxyproline excretion in these patients were not given. In preliminary studies S. R. Pinnell and S. M. Krane (unpublished) found the excretion of glycylproline to range from 1.04 to 1.47 μmoles per mg creatinine in four samples of urine from a patient with severe Paget's disease and total urinary hydroxyproline excretion averaging 1300 μg per mg creatinine (normal adults usually excrete <40 μg hydroxyproline per mg creatinine). The level of excretion of glycylproline in this subject was in the range of that reported by Alderman *et al.* (1969) for their patients. However, the hydroxyproline excretion in the pagetic subject was six times greater and is consistent with the observations of Alderman *et al.* (1969) that the excretions of glycylproline and hydroxyproline are not directly proportional.

5. Nondialyzable Urinary Hydroxyproline

The nondialyzable fraction of urinary hydroxyproline consists of a number of heterogeneous polypeptides of approximately similar molecular weight, averaging about 5000 (Krane *et al.*, 1967, 1970; Haddad *et al.*, 1970b). These polypeptides obtained from the urine of patients with

Paget's disease share several characteristics with the collagen chains including the typical amino acid composition, susceptibility to proteolytic cleavage with purified clostridial collagenase, and a negative optical rotation in solution which increases on cooling. The amino acid composition of the polypeptides partially purified from the urine of three pagetic subjects (Krane *et al.*, 1967, 1970) is shown in Table III. Some features that distinguish several of these peptides from bone collagens are the high ratio of 4-hydroxyproline to proline, the absence of 3-hydroxyproline, and the high ratio of lysine relative to arginine. It seems likely, however, that these polypeptides are derived from bone for reasons similar to those considered above which suggest that the major source of total urinary

TABLE III

Amino Acid Composition of Selected Urinary Polypeptides from Patients with Paget's Disease Compared to Human Bone Collagen[a,b]

Amino acid	D.I.[c]	Sa[c]	Ma 6[d]	Ma 9[d]	Human bone collagen
3-Hydroxyproline	—	—	—	—	0.5
4-Hydroxyproline	114	106	111	134	98
Aspartic acid	90	98	94	78	48
Threonine	29	39	28	31	21
Serine	50	51	34	56	39
Glutamic acid	89	83	83	90	74
Proline	77	93	104	74	116
Glycine	323	285	312	317	317
Alanine	113	114	135	95	112
½ Cystine	0	0	3	0	0
Valine	25	23	20	27	23
Methionine	—	—	—	—	4
Isoleucine	4	6	5	0	10
Leucine	6	13	9	2	26
Tyrosine	2	3	2	2	4
Phenylalanine	3	6	3	2	14
Hydroxylysine	5	7	6	8	5
Lysine	44	38	34	68	30
Histidine	4	8	4	2	7
Arginine	21	26	12	14	51

[a] From Krane *et al.* (1970).
[b] Values are residues per 1000 residues.
[c] Purified by DEAE cellulose chromatography.
[d] Peak fractions numbered 6 and 9 from column of phosphocellulose measured by absorption at 230 nm.

hydroxyproline in Paget's disease is bone. However, the pattern of distribution of the glycosylated hydroxylysines in the urinary polypeptide fraction is different from that of whole bone or whole urine from pagetic subjects, with a ratio of glucosylgalactosylhydroxylysine:galactosylhydroxylysine of about 1.7 (Krane *et al.*, 1977).

The results of studies using tracer doses of ^{14}C-proline in three patients with Paget's disease were similar and suggested that these nondialyzable urinary polypeptides are related to collagen synthesis. Within hours following oral administration of the ^{14}C-proline, ^{14}C-hydroxyproline was detected in the urinary polypeptide fraction. At the peak of labeling, the specific activity in the polypeptide fraction was several-fold greater than that in the oligopeptide fraction (Fig. 32). After chromatography on phosphocellulose of one of these polypeptide peaks the specific activity of the ^{14}C-hydroxyproline was higher in every fraction isolated than in the total dialyzable small peptide fraction. Polypeptides similar to these were also found in the urine of patients with other skeletal disorders including severe fibrous dysplasia of bone, hyperphosphatasia, and hyperparathyroidism with osteitis fibrosa, all conditions characterized by high skeletal turnover (Krane *et al.*, 1970). A similar portion of the hydroxyproline in the urine of normal subjects is also nondialyzable, although the chemical composition of the normal polypeptides has not been determined.

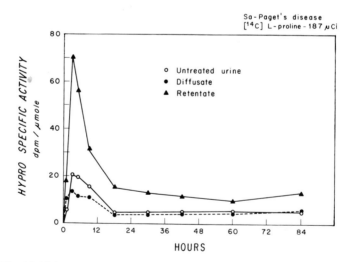

Fig. 32. Multiple specific activities of ^{14}C-hydroxyproline (hypro) in urine and its fractions after dialysis as a function of time after administration of ^{14}C-proline to a patient with Paget's disease. (From Krane *et al.*, 1967 *Science* **157,** 713.) Copyright 1967 by the American Association for the Advancement of Science.

It is likely that the collagen-like polypeptides excreted in the urine in large amounts by patients with Paget's disease, representing about 10% of the total hydroxyproline, are somehow related to collagen synthesis. Current evidence suggests that the chains of collagen are synthesized as a continuous polypeptide starting as a precursor form with extra amino acids at the amino-terminal end (procollagen); the data are not compatible with an assembly of subunits of the chain (Vuust and Piez, 1970, 1972; Grant and Prockop, 1972). Amino acid analyses of the amino-terminal polypeptide fragments of procollagen chains (Bornstein *et al.*, 1972) obtained from chick calvaria in culture show no resemblance to the polypeptides isolated from the urine of pagetic subjects, although data on the extra peptide portion of procollagens from other species are so far incomplete. Whatever the position on the collagen chains of the urinary polypeptides, the evidence is most consistent with the idea that there is some selective removal either of newly synthesized chains or portions of chains in bone and that this material contributes to the urinary polypeptides.

Taubman and colleagues (1976) have reported elevated concentrations of "procollagen" in sera of patients with Paget's disease. They utilized a radioimmunoassay developed specifically for the nonhelical portions of procollagen, probably towards one carboxyterminus. The serum levels correlated reasonably well with urinary hydroxyproline excretion and alkaline phosphatase activity, and returned towards normal with treatment with disodium etridronate.

The pattern of alteration in the metabolism of mineral ions and matrix components in patients with Paget's disease is thus consistent with the high rate of skeletal turnover inferred from radiological and histological observations in the course of the disorder. We noted that the mineral ion kinetics probably overestimate the mean rate of bone calcium deposition and resorption and that the total urinary hydroxyproline excretion reflects both (bone) collagen synthesis and degradation. The urinary hydroxyproline contained in low molecular weight fractions largely reflects collagen breakdown. However, an unknown portion of these peptides has been cleaved to yield free hydroxyproline which, in turn, has been further degraded in the liver (Kivirikko, 1970). Therefore, the calculation of collagen degradation based on the excretion of hydroxyproline peptides alone gives too low an estimate. Determination of the glycosylated hydroxylysines (Segrest and Cunningham, 1970; Askenasi, 1973; Askenasi *et al.*, 1976; Krane *et al.*, 1977) may provide a more accurate index of collagen degradation, since their further metabolism is relatively limited. In view of these limitations, we have estimated the amount of bone resorbed in a number of pagetic patients based on ^{47}Ca kinetics and compared these with others based on total hydroxyproline excretion as shown in Table IV. Since the level of hydroxyproline excretion was high in these subjects, sources of collagen other than bone would be expected to contribute little to total excretion and the figure based on matrix resorption would be a minimum one. Therefore, the magnitude of the turnover determined by ^{47}Ca kinetics is not unreasonable.

C. Acute Effects of Calcitonin

The use of the calcitonins in treatment of Paget's disease will be discussed subsequently (Section IX,H). However, the acute effects of calcitonin are so striking in pagetic subjects that it is appropriate to discuss them as they relate to bone turnover. Bijvoet *et al.* (1968) were the first to demonstrate that a decrease in serum calcium and phosphorus concentrations was readily produced by injection of porcine calcitonin in pagetic patients, whereas no such response was detected in normal subjects. The fall in serum calcium was accompanied by a marked decrease in plasma levels and urinary excretion of hydroxyproline peptides. These results were confirmed and extended to include the effects of salmon calcitonin by Singer *et al.* (1972b) and Krane *et al.* (1973). The major decrease in hydroxyproline excretion occurs in the oligopeptide fraction. Observations that, in response to calcitonin administration, the ratio of glucosylgalactosylhydroxylysine:galactosylhydroxylysine rises (from the low values of bone) as the total hydroxylysine and hydroxyproline fall are consistent with a decrease in degradation of *bone* collagen rather than

TABLE IV

Calcium Resorption and Hydroxyproline Excretion in Paget's Disease[a]

Patient	Calcium resorption rate (v_{0-}) (1) (g/24 hour)	Hydroxyproline excretion (2) (g/24 hour)	Bone resorption (g/24 hour) based on	
			(1)	(2)
1	14.2	0.590	50.7	17.5
2	6.9	0.497	24.6	14.8
3	4.9	0.238	17.5	7.1
4	4.1	0.114	14.6	3.4
5	3.6	0.147	12.9	4.4
6	3.5	0.223	12.5	6.6
7	2.3	0.078	8.2	2.3
Normal values	<0.670	<0.040	<2.4	<1.2

[a] Calculated from Nagant de Deuxchaisnes and Krane (1964).

collagen from some other source (Krane *et al.*, 1977). The decrease in bone resorption induced by calcitonin appears to be due to an inhibition of osteoclastic activity. Within 30 minutes after administration of calcitonin to pagetic patients, the osteoclasts become less adherent to bone, lose their ruffled borders, and begin to fragment (Fig. 33; Singer *et al.*, 976).

It seems reasonable to conclude, since the calcitonins have been shown to have their major action on decreasing bone resorption, that the pagetic subject in whom bone turnover is markedly accelerated would show the greatest serum calcium response to a decrease in bone resorption. Krane *et al.* (1973) demonstrated that normal subjects respond to calcitonin by decreasing total urinary hydroxyproline excretion without significantly changing serum calcium levels. The fall in total urinary hydroxyproline excretion was similar in percentage to that seen in patients with Paget's disease, although the absolute decrease was orders of magnitude less. As in the patients with Paget's disease, the decrease in excretion of polypeptide hydroxyproline was not as marked as that of the oligopeptide hydroxyproline and the ratio of polypeptide/oligopeptide excreted rose at the nadir of the calcitonin response. We have proposed that the decrease in plasma and urinary hydroxyproline is greater than the

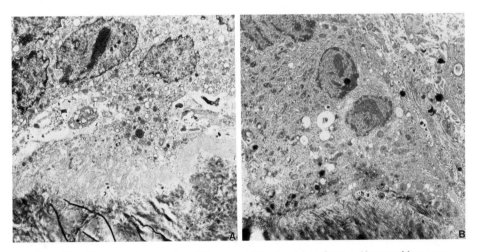

Fig. 33. Electron micrographs of iliac crest biopsies taken from a 60-year-old woman with Paget's disease (A) prior to and (B) 30 minutes following 20 μg salmon calcitonin IV. (A) Edge of active osteoclast showing wide ruffled border containing collagen fibrils and bone mineral. Note numerous as well as large vacuoles immediately adjacent to the ruffled border. ×4200. (B) Osteoclast displaying reduction in activity shown by the loss of the ruffled border and relatively smooth appearance of the cytoplasmic membrane bordering bone. Note the reduction in numbers of vacuoles but an increase in autophagic vacuoles compared to the initial biopsy. ×7800. Courtesy of Dr. Barabara G. Mills).

decrease seen in plasma calcium because the size of the exchangeable calcium pool is large relative to rates of entry into this pool, even in Paget's disease where the amount of calcium entering and leaving the pool is much greater than normal. In contrast, the pool of small peptides containing hydroxyproline is small relative to rates of entry into this pool from degradation of collagen. Therefore, a given decrease in resorption would more profoundly affect the oligopeptide hydroxyproline pool than the calcium pool. The results of this study also suggest that an acute decrease in bone matrix formation (as shown by decrease in excretion of polypeptide hydroxyproline) accompanies the fall in bone resorption. Whether this response is mediated by parathyroid hormone or by a fall in plasma phosphorus is not known.

D. Citrate Metabolism

A large fraction of total body citrate is present in bone, where it is bound to calcium ions on the surface of the inorganic Ca-P crystals. When bone is resorbed the release of calcium ions is accompanied in many systems by release of citrate (Neuman and Neuman, 1958; Kenny, 1961). Parathyroid hormone inhibits citrate oxidation and release in bone and other tissues (Nisbet, et al., 1970; Costello et al., 1971) and increases plasma citrate levels. Hypocitremia follows parathyroidectomy and the citrate levels can be restored by administration of parathyroid hormone (Costello et al., 1971). Calcitonin decreases the effects of parathyroid hormone on citrate accumulation by bone in culture (Nisbet et al., 1970) and decreases plasma citrate when administered to rats (Costello et al., 1971).

In human diseases associated with decreased bone resorption, such as hypoparathyroidism, reduced concentrations of serum citrate are found. In hypercalcemic states such as hyperparathyroidism with osteitis fibrosa (Watson, 1959), citrate levels are usually increased (Harrison, 1956). Urinary citrate levels parallel those of calcium in patients with renal stone disease, with and without hyperparathyroidism (Hodgkinson, 1963) and the administration of parathyroid extract increases the urinary citrate excretion in hypoparathyroidism (Shorr et al., 1942).

In Paget's disease the serum citrate levels may be elevated in patients with high alkaline phosphatase levels even though the serum calcium levels are normal (Kissin and Kreeger, 1954). This is consistent with other evidence of increased bone resorption. We have measured urinary citrate excretion by the method of Natelson et al. (1948) in a few patients with extensive Paget's disease. Basal levels of excretion in two patients with severe disease were 600 and 1390 μg per mg creatinine and total hydroxyproline excretion was 610 and 1300 μg per mg creatinine, respectively. Although the range of citrate excretion in normal subjects is broad (Brodwall *et al.*, 1972) and there is some diurnal variation in the excretion pattern, it is probable that the citrate excretion in the more severely affected subject was increased. However, in both patients citrate excretion increased strikingly following calcitonin injection. In the subject whose data are shown in Fig. 34 serum citrate levels prior to calcitonin infusion were elevated to 4.9 mg per dl, well above the upper limit of normal of 3.6 mg per dl (Watson, 1959). At the peak of the response to calcitonin, citrate levels fell to 4.1 mg per dl and citrate clearance increased from 13.9 to 37.0 ml per minute. It is probable that the initial fall in serum citrate resulted from calcitonin suppression of bone resorption but that the increased urinary citrate excretion and clearance was due to an increase in secretion of parathyroid hormone.

E. Serum Alkaline Phosphatase

The role of alkaline phosphatase in bone and its pattern of variation in disease in general has been discussed in detail in Chapter 3, Volume I.

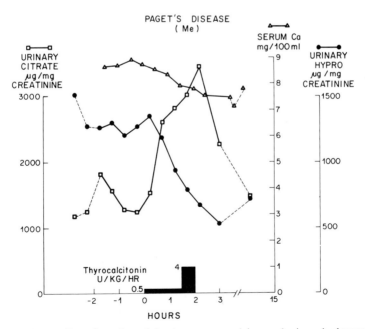

Fig. 34. Acute effect of porcine calcitonin on serum calcium and urinary hydroxyproline and citrate excretion in a 69-year-old woman with Paget's disease.

Elevation of the level of the enzyme in serum is characteristically seen in patients with Paget's disease, an observation made first by Kay (1929). Indeed, the highest recorded values for alkaline phosphatase are found in patients with Paget's disease. The level correlates with the extent as well as the activity of the disease, as does the level of urinary hydroxyproline excretion. Serum alkaline phosphatase and urinary hydroxyproline excretion also correlate with each other (Khairi *et al.*, 1973; Franck *et al.*, 1974) (Fig. 35). It is distinctly unusual to see markedly elevated levels in patients with isolated involvement of a small bone such as a vertebral body. However, isolated involvement of larger bones is associated with a broad range of phosphatase levels. In our experience, involvement of the skull alone is often associated with levels of phosphatase high in proportion to percentage of skeleton involved; the converse is true for pelvic involvement (Franck *et al.*, 1974). When the disorder enters the osteoblastic phase and cellular activity decreases, even extensive involvement may be associated with limited elevations.

In patients followed over years the levels of phosphatase tend to show a long-term upward trend with a tendency to plateau in a range characteristic for that individual (Woodard, 1959). Some patients show cyclic fluctuations about this more or less constant baseline. Occasionally, if osteosarcoma develops on the background of Paget's disease, a sudden elevation in serum phosphatase may be observed (Woodard, 1959), whereas in other patients no such striking increase takes place and even normal

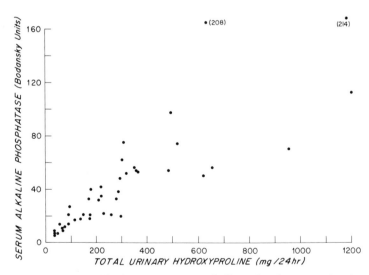

Fig. 35. The relationship between serum alkaline phosphatase and urinary hydroxyproline excretion in 42 patients with Paget's disease. (From Franck *et al.*, 1974.)

levels may be present (Porretta *et al.*, 1957). In almost all studies the alkaline phosphatase in patients with Paget's disease is indistinguishable from that normally present in bone and circulating in the plasma of patients with other skeletal disorders (see Chapter 3, Volume I).

F. Other Phosphatases

In patients with Paget's disease and moderately elevated alkaline phosphatase levels, the activity of 5'-nucleotidase is usually normal. Modest elevations in 5'-nucleotidase may be seen, however, in serum from patients with very high alkaline phosphatase levels (Hill and Sammons, 1967). The level of acid phosphatase is usually normal in patients with Paget's disease, although in subjects with widespread, advanced lesions and very high alkaline phosphatase, mild elevations of acid phosphatase levels may be found (Sullivan *et al.*, 1942). Using monophenyl phosphate as substrate, it was found that 18% of 96 patients with Paget's disease had levels between 3.0 and 4.9 units and only 3% between 5.0 and 9.9 units (normal values <3.0 units). However, with β-glycerophosphate as substrate, in only 1 pagetic patient out of more than 100 was an elevation of acid phosphatase noted (Woodard, 1952, 1959).

VIII. SYSTEMIC COMPLICATIONS AND ASSOCIATED DISEASES

A. Hypercalciuria, Renal Calculi, and Hypercalcemia

Urinary calcium excretion in patients with Paget's disease may be high, low, or normal (O'Reilly and Race, 1932) because the amount excreted appears to be dependent on the rates of bone resorption and formation relative to each other (Nagant de Deuxchaisnes and Krane, 1964), as well as upon a variety of influences including parathyroid hormone. In those patients with bone resorption greater than formation, hypercalciuria is more likely to occur. The majority of patients with Paget's disease have similar rates of resorption and formation, however, and therefore urinary calcium excretion is usually normal. Hypercalciuria may also occur when there are fractures or when patients are immobilized.

In an individual patient hypercalciuria may predispose to the formation of renal calculi (see Chapter 7, Volume I). This does not appear to be a common complication of Paget's disease, although in one series 15.6% of patients had urinary calculi (Moehlig and Adler, 1937). Nagant de Deuxchaisnes and Krane (1964), after reviewing the literature on this subject, found an overall incidence of 5% among 1382 pagetic patients. They felt that two factors other than the Paget's disease accounted for such an association. Since patients with urinary calculi frequently have roentgenograms of the abdomen and pelvis, asymptomatic and presumably incidental Paget's disease in these areas would be detected more readily. Also prostatic hypertrophy, which is quite common in elderly males, often leads to urinary tract obstruction, infection, and calculi. Ridlon (1962) found that more than half of 22 pagetic patients with urinary calculi had prostatic hypertrophy.

Hypercalcemia is a distinctly uncommon occurrence in patients with Paget's disease. Nagant de Deuxchaisnes and Krane (1964) were able to find in the literature only 17 patients with a serum calcium greater than 12 mg per dl after excluding those patients with hyperparathyroidism and multiple myeloma. Reifenstein and Albright (1944) originally reported that it was the immobilized patient who had hypercalcemia. It was also noted that patients who sustained fractures developed hypercalcemia, but it was difficult to separate the general effects of immobilization of the patient from the local effects of the fracture in such patients.

Hypercalcemia in patients with Paget's disease may also develop as a result of coincidental hyperparathyroidism or malignancy. Rarely hyperparathyroidism may be misdiagnosed as Paget's disease because of radiological similarities in pelvic lesions (Gutman and Parsons, 1938; Ellis and Hochstim, 1960). A complete skeletal survey and, if necessary, measurement of serum parathyroid hormone concentration should distinguish the two disorders.

B. Hyperuricemia and Gout

The association of Paget's disease and gout may be found in some of the early descriptions of Paget's disease (Paget, 1882b). Despite further reports of such an association between these two diseases (Feiring, 1946; Serre and Mirowze, 1952; Weiss and Segaloff, 1959; Wright, 1966), there has been little evidence to indicate that patients with Paget's disease have an increased incidence of hyperuricemia or gout.

Recent studies of the concentration of serum uric acid and the incidence of gout in 47 patients with Paget's disease have provided new evidence that implicates the pagetic process as an etiological factor in the development of gout (Franck et al., 1974). In this study of 28 men and 18 women, 19 patients (40.4%), 16 of whom were men, were found to be hyperuricemic. Serum uric acid concentrations in the group correlated with both the extent and the activity of the bone disease as defined by the percent of bone involved radiologically, the serum alkaline phosphatase, and the total urinary hydroxyproline excretion. Seven of the male patients had clinical episodes of gouty arthritis. Urinary uric acid excretion was measured in six patients. Three were hyperuricosuric and three were hypouricosuric. The one patient who had a family history of gout had the most severe form of the disease (Fig. 36). It seems reasonable to speculate that the turnover of nucleic acid in the active cells of pagetic bone might increase the urate pool and result in secondary hyperuricemia.

C. Calcific Periarthritis and Chondrocalcinosis

Franck and colleagues (1974) reviewed the roentgenograms of multiple joints from 55 patients with Paget's disease and found a 36% incidence of periarticular calcifications. The association, although striking, may be coincidental. The shoulder was most commonly involved but the elbow, wrist, hip, knee, metacarpophalangeal, and interphalangeal joints also were involved. Acute inflammatory episodes occurred in relation to these deposits. In general the calcifications were not adjacent to areas of Paget's disease and there was no correlation between the extent of the Paget's disease and the calcifications.

Radi and colleagues (1970) have reported that 6 of 14 patients with Paget's disease had chondrocalcinosis on roentgenograms of wrists and

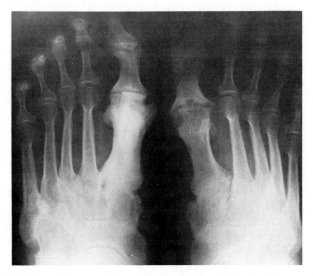

Fig. 36. A 59-year-old man with gout and generalized Paget's disease who has both diseases involving the left first metatarsal. The pagetic bone is radiodense and widened. The associated scalloped destruction of the metatarsal head is due to gouty arthritis. (From Franck *et al.*, 1974.)

knees. In contrast to this report, Franck and colleagues (1974) found only 2 instances of chondrocalcinosis in 54 patients who had wrist and knee films. The main difference between the two series of patients was that the latter group had a mean serum alkaline phosphatase seven times greater than the group with chondrocalcinosis. It is conceivable that the high concentration of alkaline phosphatase, which probably acts as a pyrophosphate at neutral pH, might protect against the development of chondrocalcinosis.

D. Cardiovascular Complications

In the osteolytic and mixed phases of Paget's disease there is a marked increase in blood flow through involved extremities, manifested often by elevated skin temperature over the affected bones (Edholm et al., 1945). That this increased blood flow is not due to anatomic arteriovenous anastomoses but rather to increased perfusion of pagetic bone was shown by Rutishauser et al. (1954), who injected the vessels of such bone at autopsy, and by Rhodes et al. (1972), who showed there were no such channels greater than 15 μm in diameter through the injection of microspheres. Others have concluded that there is associated vascular hyperplasia and ectasia in pagetic bone (Demmler, 1974).

Recently it has been shown that most if not all of the increased blood flow to pagetic extremities can be accounted for by increased cutaneous flow, as measured with water plethysmographs and by demonstrating that epinephrine iontophoresis reduces blood flow of an affected extremity almost to normal (Heistad et al., 1975). In addition, local heating of the extremity failed to increase the blood flow in the pagetic limb as in a normal limb. Thus reflex cutaneous dilatation must be the explanation for the cutaneous hyperthermia and the elevated pO_2 in the venous blood of an involved extremity. How much bone vascularity increases the blood flow remains unknown.

Increased cardiac output may be found in patients with generalized disease involving at least 30% of the skeleton (Edholm et al., 1945; Howarth, 1953; Lequime and Denolin, 1955), although we have observed increased cardiac output in a patient with Paget's disease limited to the skull. This increased cardiac output in the elderly patient with Paget's disease may give rise to congestive heart failure but is generally responsive to the usual modes of treatment.

Intracardiac calcification has been reported in association with Paget's disease. Harrison and Lennox (1948) concluded that calcification of the cardiac tissues was five times more common in patients with generalized Paget's disease than in control subjects. Such calcification may involve the interventricular septum and the aortic and mitral valves. Heart block may develop as a result of septal calcification; however, the valvular calcifications are generally not of clinical significance. King *et al.* (1969) reported one patient with calcification of the interventricular septum, aortic and mitral valves, and complete heart block who required a permanent transvenous pacemaker.

Arterial calcifications are a common finding in patients with Paget's disease. O'Reilly and Race (1932) found an incidence of 43% in their patients. The calcifications are particularly common in limb arteries and were visible by radiographic examination in 50% of patients studied by Acar and colleagues (1968). Such calcifications are generally of the Mönckeberg type (medial involvement and preservation of the lumen) and are usually of no clinical importance.

E. Pseudoxanthoma Elasticum, Angioid Streaks, and Skin Changes

The association of pseudoxanthoma elasticum and Paget's disease (Larmande and Margaillan, 1957; Shaffer *et al.*, 1957; Moretti *et al.*, 1962) has provoked speculation that Paget's disease may be a widespread disorder of connective tissue rather than a disease limited to the skeleton. Characteristics common to these two diseases include angioid streaks, vascular calcification, and skin calcification (Paton, 1972). Although this concept is interesting, it is incompatible with the fact that the vast majority of patients with Paget's disease have normal skin and no excessive mobility of the joints.

We have examined skin biopsies from six patients with Paget's disease, in which four had abnormal patterns of elastic fibers. The histological changes included a decrease in the number of the superficial fine elastic fibers with fragmentation and clumping of fibers as seen with elastic tissue stains. In the reticular layer the coarse fibers were sparse and the few remaining ones were greatly fragmented so that few interconnecting bundles were present. Such changes were also noted by Paton (1972), but he felt that after treatment with various connective tissue stains and digestion with β-glucuronidase there was no evidence of any abnormality in the collagen or elastic fibers. Paton (1972) explained his findings on the basis of the great variation of the cutaneous elastic fibers found normally in various parts of the skin or various portions of the body. We have not been able to refute this valid point, since the normal variations of cutaneous elastic fibers have not been well documented. Therefore, although the changes in the skin may be purely specious, we have recorded our findings so that future investigators may deal with this problem.

Although angioid streaks are found in 8 to 15% of advanced cases of Paget's disease (Paton, 1972), comparatively little has been written about such lesions in Paget's disease (Fig. 37). The changes described for the angioid streaks seen in Paget's disease are histologically identical to those of pseudoxanthoma elasticum. These changes are basophilia and cracking of Bruch's membrane and proliferation of fibrovascular tissue through the defects. It is felt that since calcification may occur at the site of elastic fibers in the skin of patients with Paget's disease, the same event may occur in Bruch's membrane (Paton, 1972).

Preliminary evidence that supports the concept of a generalized connective tissue abnormality in patients with Paget's disease has been reported by Francis and Smith (1974). These investigators examined the nature of skin collagen in 11 patients and control subjects. They found a decreased amount and stability of a polymeric collagen fraction in the pagetic patients and speculated that a progressive failure of glycoprotein and collagen cross-linking reactions could account for the observed abnormalities.

F. Malabsorption Syndrome

Somayaji (1968) described eight patients with Paget's disease who had a variable pattern of gastrointestinal malabsorption. Diarrhea, steatorrhea,

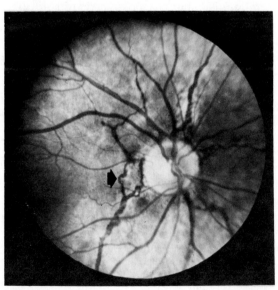

Fig. 37.   Multiple angioid streaks in Paget's disease (arrow indicates most extensive one).

xylose malabsorption, and folate deficiency were prominent features in these patients. It was postulated that secondary folate deficiency or relative ischemia of the bowel secondary to increased bone blood flow might be responsible for the observations. No confirmatory reports have been published.

IX. DRUG TREATMENT

A. Indications

Most patients with Paget's disease require no treatment, since the disorder is usually asymptomatic and it produces little or no morbidity. The advanced age of many affected individuals would also preclude the use of potentially toxic drugs. However, there are several criteria that we propose for considering patients with Paget's disease as potential candidates for specific therapy. These have been grouped under definite and possible indications in Table V.

Various modes of treatment affect certain manifestations of Paget's disease. Bone pain is decreased by a variety of drugs, and elevated cardiac output is diminished as a result of suppression of the activity of the disease. There have been no formal studies on the use of drugs in the control of hypercalcemia, hypercalciuria, or gout in the pagetic patient,

TABLE V

Indications for Drug Treatment of Paget's Disease

Definite
  1. Severe bone pain corresponding to areas of pagetic involvement as demonstrated by roentgenograms and/or isotope scanning procedures
  2. Cardiac failure associated with a high output state
  3. Hypercalcemia due to the Paget's disease
  4. Recurrent renal calculi due to hypercalciuria

Possible
  1. Multiple fractures in pagetic bone
  2. Scheduled orthopedic surgery of an extensive nature involving pagetic bone or associated with prolonged immobilization
  3. Skeletal compression of nerve tissue
  4. Early onset of Paget's disease in an area where disabling deformity is to be anticipated
  5. Prevention of osteogenic sarcoma
  6. Otherwise unexplained disabling weakness and fatigue in a patient with severe, extensive Paget's disease

---

although on theoretical grounds there is a strong likelihood that suppression of the disease would help correct these complications. Much more clinical investigation will be required to determine the effect of treatment in prevention of pathological fractures or osteogenic sarcoma, in the preoperative preparation of a patient about to undergo an osteotomy or other orthopedic procedure, and in the patient with neurological deficit. If it can be shown that drug treatment not only can suppress existing disease but also prevent the appearance of lesions in other bones, it would be important to treat younger patients with mild Paget's disease in order to prevent the onset of disabling disease. There are some patients with widespread Paget's disease who have disabling weakness and lassitude. If such clinical problems cannot be explained by other disease mechanisms, then treatment of the Paget's disease may be considered.

B. Miscellaneous Drugs

Many drugs have been used to treat Paget's disease, including arsenic (O'Reilly and Race, 1932), magnesium carbonate (Gill and Stein, 1936), aluminum acetate (Ghormley and Hinchey, 1944; Helfet, 1952), anabolic steroids (Kolb, 1959; McGavack et al., 1961), folic acid (Rosenkrantz et al., 1952), phenylbutazone (Nagant de Deuxchaisnes and Krane, 1964), acetylsalicylic acid (Maurice et al., 1962; Henneman et al., 1963; Avioli and Henneman, 1964; Nagant de Deuxchaisnes and Krane, 1964, 1974; Galmiche and Levy, 1967) and adrenocorticosteroids or ACTH (Berman, 1936; Watson, 1939; Charvat and Belohradsky, 1952; Neugebauer, 1953; Albright and Henneman, 1955; Rapaport et al., 1957; Henneman et al., 1963). Some of these drugs were evaluated at a time when only subjective criteria were used to assess efficacy. Others, particularly acetylsalicylic acid and adrenocorticosteroids, have produced significant suppression of the disease but this was transient, and intolerable side effects or toxicity developed with continued use. At present none of these drugs is widely used. However, we have found antiinflammatory drugs such as acetylsalicylic acid and indomethacin of use in controlling symptoms associated with degenerative joint disease, especially of the hips.

During the last 10 years another group of drugs has been introduced for treatment of Paget's disease. Although there is much to be learned about the clinical pharmacology of these drugs, several have proved to be effective in treatment.

C. Sodium Fluoride

This agent has been evaluated in the management of both osteoporosis and Paget's disease. Fluoride ion is incorporated into the crystal lattice of hydroxyapatite by substitution for hydroxyl ions. It increases the crystallinity of poorly crystalline hydroxyapatite. Excessive intake of fluoride results in overgrowth of abnormally dense bones. The mechanism by which this occurs is unknown, although fluoride in high concentrations inhibits the action of many enzymes.

Chronic administration of fluoride to patients with Paget's disease has been reported to induce calcium retention and relieve bone pain (Purves, 1962; Bernstein *et al.*, 1963; Rich *et al.*, 1964). Avioli and Berman (1968) reported that fluoride decreased exchangeable magnesium and magnesium turnover rate in one patient and lowered urinary hydroxyproline excretion and serum alkaline phosphatase levels in four patients. The serum alkaline phosphatase increased with short-term therapy and decreased with long-term therapy. Other studies of shorter duration have not produced such impressive results (Nagant de Deuxchaisnes and Krane, 1964; Higgins *et al.*, 1965; Lukert *et al.*, 1967). The different conclusions reached in these studies might be explained by (1) the small numbers of patients studied in all but one of the reports, (2) failure of the measurements made to reflect accurately the activity of the disease, and (3) the wide variation in the duration of the studies (Riggs and Jowsey, 1972). Clearly, more extensive studies are needed to define the safety and efficacy of this potent bone-seeking ion in the treatment of Paget's disease.

D. Phosphate

Oral phosphate supplementation has been used with varying degrees of success in the treatment of hypophosphatemic rickets, hypercalcemia, hypercalciuria, and osteoporosis. Goldsmith (1972) has studied the effects of administering the equivalent of 1 to 2 g of elemental phosphorus as phosphate daily to three patients with Paget's disease. He reported improvement of bone pain, decreased cardiac output, decreased urinary calcium excretion, and a more positive calcium balance in all three patients. One patient had a significant decrease in serum alkaline phosphatase concentration. In two of the patients the hemodynamic and metabolic effects did not persist. Phosphate supplementation may be useful in controlling hypercalcemia or hypercalciuria associated with Paget's disease (Nagant de Deuxchaisnes and Krane, 1964), but whether the disease process is altered with this agent still remains conjectural.

E. Mithramycin

Mithramycin is an antibiotic that has proved to be an effective antitumor drug in the treatment of embryonal tumors of the testis. The drug also has a potent cytotoxic effect on bone cells, which has made it an effective agent in the control of hypercalcemia. Ryan and his colleagues (1969, 1970, 1972) have used mithramycin in the treatment of 50 patients with Paget's disease. The drug was administered by intravenous infusion, usually for 10 days, at a dose of 15–25 μg/kg/day. Urinary hydroxyproline excretion was measured in 17 patients before and after treatment. The mean pretreatment level was 267 mg per 24 hour; this fell to a mean level of 44 mg per 24 hour after treatment. Serum alkaline phosphatase fell from a mean pretreatment level of 30.5 to 11.7 Bessey-Lowry-Brock Units in the 50 patients (Fig. 38). The investigators reported that bone pain was relieved in most patients within 4 days. Biopsies of bone in four patients before and after treatment showed a marked decrease in the number of osteoclasts and osteoblasts. One patient demonstrated apparent improvement in bone structure as evidenced by filling in of a cystic area noted radiologically, although no biopsy was taken to confirm that normal

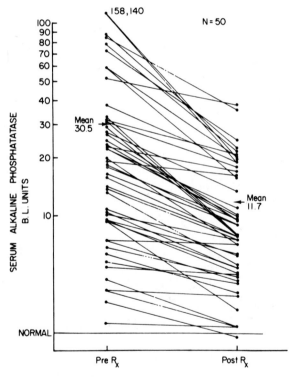

Fig. 38. The effect of mithramycin therapy on serum alkaline phosphatase (Bessey-Lowry-Brock Units) in 50 patients with Paget's disease. (From Ryan *et al.*, 1972.)

bone had indeed filled in the defect. All patients had a transient rise in serum levels of hepatic enzymes and three patients had a transient increase in blood urea nitrogen levels. Many patients had prolonged relief of symptoms after the 10-day course of therapy. Serum alkaline phosphatase remained suppressed in some of these for almost 1 year after the initial treatment. Condon and colleagues (1971) have also reported suppression of Paget's disease in three patients treated with mithramycin; one of the patients experienced a transient rise in blood urea concentration. Epstein (1974) found no evidence of hepatic or renal toxicity in six patients treated with 15 μg/kg. Mithramycin induces an acute hypocalcemic response which stimulates parathyroid hormone secretion (Ajlouni and Theil, 1975). The hypocalcemia may persist for days (Elias and Evans, 1972). Lebbin et al. (1974) treated 13 patients with mithramycin, on an outpatient basis; they concluded that the drug was both effective and safe to use in active Paget's disease and that signs of its potential toxicity were transient and controllable. Use of mithramycin was associated with improved bone scans in 11 of 11 patients reported by Russell, Lentle, and colleagues (Russell and Lentle, 1974; Lentle et al., 1976).

Mithramycin and other cytotoxic drugs, such as actinomycin D, have been shown to suppress the activity of Paget's disease (Jesserer et al., 1967; Fennelly and Groarke, 1971) by suppressing increased bone turnover. However, the use of potentially lethal drugs to treat a chronic disorder like Paget's disease must be undertaken with extreme caution. Until extensive studies with smaller doses of the drug provide data that are reassuring in terms of toxicity and efficacy, the widespread use of such drugs seems unwarranted.

F. Diphosphonates

Diphosphonates are bone-seeking compounds that have P–C–P bonds and produce effects similar to those of pyrophosphate. They retard precipitation of calcium phosphate from solution and slow the growth and dissolution of hydroxyapatite crystals. One such compound is disodium etidronate (disodium ethane-1-hydroxyl-1,1-diphosphonate). The drug can be administered orally, although gastrointestinal absorption is variable.

Disodium etidronate produced biochemical remissions in 9 of 10 patients with Paget's disease treated with 20 mg per kg daily for up to 29 weeks (Smith et al., 1973). The fall in urinary hydroxyproline excretion and plasma alkaline phosphatase levels persisted for at least 3 months after discontinuing the drug (Fig. 39). Symptomatic improvement was

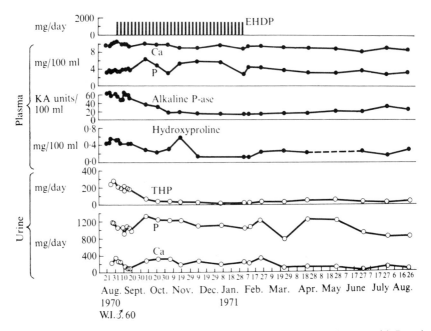

Fig. 39. The effects of disodium etidronate (EHDP) on a 60-year-old man with Paget's disease. Note the continued low levels of plasma and urinary hydroxyproline (THP) and plasma alkaline phosphatase after stopping the drug. (From Smith *et al.*, 1973.)

noted in three of the patients. Bone biopsies were obtained in six patients after treatment and two before treatment. The two main histological features of the biopsies were a reduction in the number of osteoclasts and osteoblasts and an irregular increase in the thickness of osteoid that covered all bone surfaces. The deposition of thick layers of osteoid occurred in both pagetic and uninvolved, normal bone. The appearance of osteoid in the bone supports the view that this drug acts to impair matrix mineralization. It is possible that such an increase in osteoid may be the mechanism by which bone resorption is decreased. Smith and colleagues (1973) measured urinary nondialyzable hydroxyproline in four patients treated with disodium etidronate and found that the absolute amount decreased in each patient, but in two patients the ratio of nondialyzable to total hydroxyproline increased significantly. This observation is compatible with the observed increase in osteoid. More extensive studies by these investigators in 47 patients with Paget's disease have confirmed the initial observations (Russell *et al.*, 1974). They found a dose-related suppression of the raised alkaline phosphatase in plasma and total hydroxyproline in urine and that a single course of treatment could maintain a biochemical remission for up to 2 years after stopping treatment. Histological evaluation of bone biopsies revealed suppression of the Paget's disease, and at a dose of 20 mg/kg there was an increase in unmineralized osteoid. A similar observation was made by Gunčaga and colleagues (1974), who found a broadening of osteoid seams and defective tetracycline uptake of pagetic bone in eight patients treated with 20 mg/kg of disodium etidronate. De-Vries and Bijvoet (1974) found an increase in unmineralized osteoid with as little as 7.5 mg/kg in some patients. Another unexplained observation in patients treated with the drug is the development of hyperphosphatemia (Smith et al., 1973; Gunčaga et al., 1974; Russell et al., 1974). Altman and colleagues (1973) have carried out a double-blind study on 47 patients and have found disodium etidronate to be more effective than a placebo in the treatment of the disease. Bone biopsies were not reported in this preliminary communication. It is difficult to evaluate the symptomatic improvement noted in a later paper by this same group (Khairi et al., 1974), because the placebo effect is marked.

These early studies indicated that disodium etridronate might prove to be highly effective in the treatment of Paget's disease; except for inconstant hyperphosphatemia, no systemic toxicity was observed during its administration.

However, we observed that six of twelve patients treated with high doses of this drug (20 mg/kg/day) developed severe pain over the sites of pagetic involvement within four to six weeks (Kantrowitz et al., 1975). In several, pain necessitated discontinuation of therapy. These six had significantly more severe disease, judging by levels of serum alkaline phosphatase and by hydroxyproline excretion. In addition, of 29 patients treated, seven (all treated with 10–20 mg/kg/day) developed ten fractures, mostly at the sites of increased radiolucency in long bones. Nine of these fractures were considered pathologic. Histologic examination showed encasement of pagetic trabeculae by hypomineralized nonpagetic lamellar bone. Subsequent studies have confirmed these observations of pathological fractures and/or impaired mineralization on high doses of disodium etidronate (Meunier et al., 1975; Reiner et al., 1975; Caniggia et al., 1976; Finerman et al., 1976; Jung et al., 1976; Canfield et al., 1977; Khairi et al., 1977; Stein et al., 1977). The results of two studies do indicate that 5 mg/kg dosage can produce beneficial clinical effects in the absence of impaired mineralization and fractures (Alexandre and Meunier, 1977; Canfield et al., 1977). Hosking and colleagues (1976) utilized human calcitonin, 0.5 mg daily, in combination with disodium etidronate, 7.5 mg/kg, to achieve marked biochemical suppression without impairing mineralization in nine patients. Parathyroid function appears to remain stable during treatment with disodium etidronate but after discontinuing treatment with

20 mg/kg, plasma calcium falls and serum immunoreactive parathyroid hormone concentration and urinary cyclic AMP excretion rise (David *et al.*, 1976). This apparently arises from the increased need of the skeleton for calcium to remineralize the excess osteoid.

Disodium etidronate therapy has not been reported to produce radiological improvement, but bone scans have been observed to return toward normal (Goldman *et al.*, 1975; Finerman *et al.*, 1976; Stein *et al.*, 1977; Wellman *et al.*, 1977). Disodium etidronate at a low dose (7.5 mg/kg) in combination with human calcitonin proved quite effective in decreasing the uptake of [99]technetium -disodium etidronate by pagetic lesions (Vellenga *et al.*, 1976).

G. Glucagon

Care and colleagues (1970) reported that glucagon stimulated the porcine thyroid gland to release calcitonin. This observation led Condon (1971) to study the effects of glucagon infusions in four patients with Paget's disease. The hormone was infused in doses ranging from 0.2 to 0.8 mg/hour for two to eighteen days. The maximum daily dose was 20 mg. In each patient there was a prompt decrease in urinary hydroxyproline excretion and/or alkaline phosphatase concentration. Bone pain which was present in two patients was relieved by this treatment. Calcitonin was not detectable in the plasma of two patients before or after four hours of glucagon infusion.

We have studied the effect of glucagon in two patients with Paget's disease and have not been able to demonstrate suppression of the disease with the hormone. The results of the treatment are summarized in Table VI. The side effects in both patients included nausea, and one patient had diarrhea during treatment.

H. Calcitonin

Calcitonin is a peptide hormone, the main pharmacological effect of which is to retard bone resorption. It accomplishes this, at least in part, through an early, rapid inhibition of osteoclast function and by decreasing the number of osteoclasts.

Milhaud and colleagues (1968) suggested and Bijvoet and colleagues (1968; Bijvoet and Jansen, 1967) and Canniggia and Gennari (1968) first demonstrated that calcitonin produces an early, dramatic hypocalcemic effect in patients with Paget's disease. Bijvoet *et al.* (1968) noted a striking, acute decrease in urinary hydroxyproline excretion in such patients, and a transient decrease of 90% in one pagetic patient was subsequently reported by Singer *et al.* (1972b).

TABLE VI

Glucagon Treatment of Paget's Disease

Patient	Alkaline phosphatase (Bessey-Lowry-Brock Units)	Urinary hydroxyproline (mg/24 hour)
A.O.		
Before treatment	5.8	62
After 1 mg daily (7 days) and 5 mg daily (14 days)	6.5	58
J.P.		
Before treatment	46	1052
After 5 mg daily (6 days) and 10 mg daily (2 days)	51	1057

Porcine calcitonin was used in the initial studies of the chronic effects of calcitonin in patients with Paget's disease (Bell *et al.*, 1970; Bijvoet *et al.*, 1970; Bomparu and Ceccato, 1970; Courvoisier *et al.*, 1970; Gavazzoli *et al.*, 1970; Haddad *et al.*, 1970a; Neer *et al.*, 1970; Rapado *et al.*, 1971; Reig *et al.*, 1971; Shai *et al.*, 1971; Dubé *et al.*, 1972; Milhaud *et al.*, 1972; Renier *et al.*, 1974; Eisman *et al.*, 1974; Lesh *et al.*, 1974; Moffatt *et al.*, 1974; Kanis *et al.*, 1975; Renier *et al.*, 1975; Melick *et al.*, 1976; Martin *et al.*, 1977; Nicolle *et al.*, 1977). When it was shown that salmon calcitonin was more potent in acutely lowering plasma calcium in man (Singer *et al.*, 1972b; Galante *et al.*, 1973), this form of the hormone was introduced into clinical trials (DeRose *et al.*, 1972, 1974; Goldfield *et al.*, 1972; Haddad and Caldwell, 1972; Singer *et al.*, 1972b, 1974, 1976, 1977; Schuhmacher *et al.*, 1973; Avramides *et al.*, 1974, 1975, 1976; Hamilton, 1974; Kanis *et al.*, 1974; Lesh *et al.*, 1974; Chapuy *et al.*, 1975; Crosbie *et al.*, 1975; Grimaldi *et al.*, 1975; Staehelin, 1975; Wallach *et al.*, 1975; Woodhouse *et al.*, 1975; Bouvet, 1977; Evans and Slee, 1977; Oreopoulos *et al.*, 1977; Singer and Ahrne-Collier, 1977; Woodhouse *et al.*, 1977). Human calcitonin has also been available, in limited amounts, for treatment of patients with Paget's disease (Woodhouse *et al.*, 1971, 1972; Singer *et al.*, 1972a, 1974, 1977; Greenberg *et al.*, 1974; Rojanasathit *et al.*, 1974; Menzies *et al.*, 1975; Burckhardt *et al.*, 1977; Evans, 1977; Haddad and Rojanasathit, 1977; Haymovits *et al.*, 1977; Singer and Ahrne-Collier, 1977; Ziegler *et al.*, 1977).

The clinical experience with all three forms of calcitonin has, in general, been similar. The exceptions to this will be discussed. The hormone has been administered by subcutaneous or intramuscular injection, usually on a daily basis. With few exceptions the patients have responded with a fall in urinary hydroxyproline within days and a fall in serum alkaline phosphatase levels within weeks. Calcium balance has become more positive during the initial 1–4 months of treatment (Bijvoet *et al.*, 1970; Shai *et al.*, 1971; Woodhouse *et al.*, 1971; Avramides *et al.*, 1974; Haymovits *et al.*, 1977). More prolonged treatment (9 to 19 months) is not associated with any change in calcium balance (Oreopoulos *et al.*, 1977). In 10 patients treated 6 to 23 months, total body calcium as assessed by neutron activation actually fell by 4% (Wallach *et al.*, 1975). ^{45}Ca uptake by bone has decreased (Woodhouse *et al.*, 1971) and clinical improvement has been documented (loss of bone pain, decreased cardiac output, decreased skin temperature, and improved neurological function). With few exceptions, hearing has not been observed to improve in patients with hearing deficits, although it has been suggested that treatment may prevent further hearing loss (Shai *et al.*, 1971; Moffatt *et al.*, 1974; Grimaldi *et al.*, 1975; Menzies *et al.*, 1975; Solomon *et al.*, 1977). Of particular interest is the radiological improvement reported by Doyle and colleagues (1974). In some patients they observed the formation of a more normal cortex in long bones, restoration of the corticomedullary junction, and a reduction in the total diameter of the shaft of expanded bones. The disease process did not appear to progress radiologically during the treatment period in patients treated with 1 mg of human calcitonin daily. Improvement in bone scans during long-term calcitonin therapy has also been reported (Lavender *et al.*, 1977; Waxman *et al.*, 1977).

As the number of patients treated and the duration of treatment have increased, several patterns of response to calcitonin are apparent. Some patients have complete biochemical and clinical remissions (Woodhouse *et al.*, 1971; Hamilton, 1974; Singer *et al.*, 1974) (Fig. 40). A larger group exhibits an initial decrease in parameters of bone turnover, but normalization of bone turnover does not occur as treatment continues (Fig. 41). These patients maintain clinical improvement as they continue to have signs of decreased bone turnover (DeRose *et al.*, 1972, 1974; Singer *et al.*, 1972b, 1974; Greenberg *et al.*, 1974; Hamilton, 1974). This pattern has been termed a plateau response. A third group of patients responds initially as the others, but as treatment continues, biochemical and clinical parameters return to pretreatment status (Fig. 42) (DeRose *et al.*, 1972, 1974; Haddad and Caldwell, 1972; Singer *et al.*, 1972a, b, 1974, 1977b; Rojanasathit *et al.*, 1974; Haddad and Rojanasathit, 1977; Singer and Ahrne-Collier, 1977).

The plateau response has been observed in patients treated with each type of calcitonin (DeRose *et al.*, 1972; Greenberg *et al.*, 1974; Singer *et al.*, 1974). In an attempt to exclude inadequate dosage of hormone as a factor in the plateau response, Singer and colleagues (1972b) increased the dose of salmon calcitonin up to 10-fold in four patients but found no

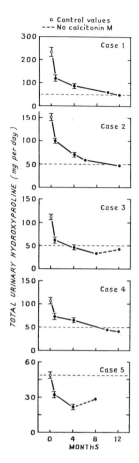

Fig. 40. The effect of human calcitonin (calcitonin M) on urinary hydroxyproline excretion in five patients with Paget's disease. Upper limit of normal is indicated by dashed line. (From Woodhouse *et al.*, 1971.)

significant further decreases in the biochemical indices of disease activity.

Resistance to the effects of calcitonin has been found in some patients treated with porcine and salmon calcitonin. In most instances this has been associated with the presence of high titers of neutralizing antibodies to these species of calcitonin (Haddad and Caldwell, 1972; Singer *et al.*, 1972a, 1974, 1977b, c; Rojanasathit *et al.*, 1974; Haddad and Rojanasathit, 1977; Woodhouse *et al.*, 1977). The precise incidence of this treatment complication is in dispute. In three studies the conclusion was reached that antibodies seldom interfered with the hormone's therapeutic effectiveness (DeRose *et al.*, 1974; Martin *et al.*, 1977; Woodhouse *et al.*,

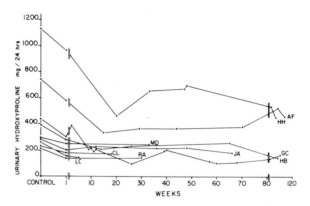

Fig. 41. The effect of salmon calcitonin on urinary hydroxyproline excretion in nine patients with Paget's disease. Upper limit of normal is 40 mg/24 hour. Note the "plateau response." (From Singer *et al.*, 1974).

1977). However, Haddad and Caldwell (1972) studied 15 patients treated with porcine and/or salmon calcitonin and found that 66% of those treated with the porcine hormone and 40% of those treated with salmon calcitonin developed high antibody titers and resistance. In the largest series reported thus far, 21% of 70 patients treated with salmon calcitonin became resistant (Singer and Ahrne-Collier, 1977). In 13 of the 15 resistant patients in this series, high antibody titers were found. The development of resistance in two patients with no detectable antibodies remains unexplained. Previous studies have reported apparent calcitonin resistance in

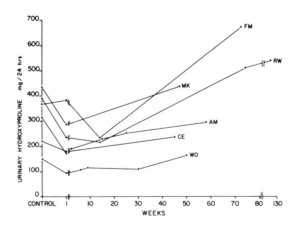

Fig. 42. The effect of salmon calcitonin on urinary hydroxyproline excretion in six patients with Paget's disease. Note the initial decrease and return to control or higher levels. (From Singer *et al.*, 1974).

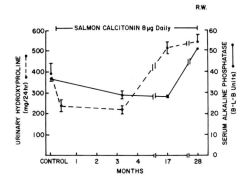

Fig. 43. Response of a 62-year-old woman treated for twenty-eight months with salmon calcitonin. After an initial decrease of bone turnover, she became resistant to continuing treatment. Antibodies to salmon calcitonin were present in her serum at a titer of 1:8000 at twenty-eight months. (From Singer *et al.*, 1977).

the absence of significant antibody titers (Dubé *et al.*, 1973; DeRose *et al.*, 1974). In patients treated with human calcitonin significant antibody titers have not been found (Burckhardt *et al.*, 1977; Dietrich and Fischer, 1977; Evans, 1977; Haymovits *et al.*, 1977; Singer *et al.*, 1977). Human calcitonin has proven effective in treating patients resistant to salmon or porcine calcitonin (Singer *et al.*, 1972a, 1974, 1977; Rojanasathit *et al.*, 1974; Haddad and Rojanasathit, 1977; Singer and Ahrne-Collier, 1977). An example of this is illustrated in Figs. 43 and 44.

Another factor that might alter the clinical response of patients treated with calcitonin is the known stimulation of parathyroid hormone secretion

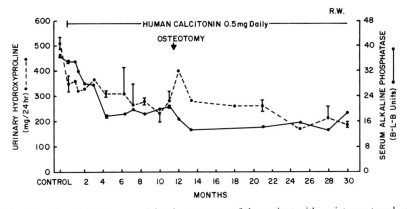

Fig. 44. Results of human calcitonin treatment of the patient with resistance to salmon calcitonin illustrated in Fig. 43. Note the continuing response after thirty months. (From Singer *et al.*, 1977).

by calcitonin-induced hypocalcemia (Riggs *et al.,* 1971; Singer *et al.,* 1972b; Chapuy *et al.,* 1975). Dubé and colleagues (1972) found a slight elevation of serum immunoreactive parathyroid hormone in five patients treated with porcine calcitonin and felt that the development of secondary hyperparathyroidism could account for resistance to calcitonin. Burckhardt and colleagues (1973) studied the parathyroid hormone response to calcitonin-induced hypocalcemia in 12 patients before and during treatment with salmon calcitonin and found no evidence of hypersecretion after treatment. Other investigators also found no evidence of hyperparathyroidism in their patients (DeRose *et al.,* 1974; Greenberg *et al.,* 1974; Burckhardt *et al.,* 1977; Evans *et al.,* 1977; Oreopoulos *et al.,* 1977; Ziegler *et al.,* 1977). The possibility remains, however, that the daily increase in parathyroid hormone secretion, which occurs in patients until bone turnover is returned to normal, may interfere with their clinical response. Conclusive evidence for such an occurrence would be provided if these patients showed the histological changes of hyperparathyroidism in bone uninvolved with Paget's disease. There is a suggestion that this may occur in one study (Ziegler *et al.,* 1977).

In one study (R. A. Evans, 1977), the stimulation of endogenous calcitonin was attempted in nine pagetic patients by treating with a high calcium intake, a low phosphorus diet, aluminum hydroxide gel and methychlothiazide. A fall in plasma alkaline phosphatase and relief of bone pain were noted. Plasma calcitonin determinations were not done.

After seven years of clinical trials with calcitonin in Paget's disease there is no question that the hormone can effectively and safely suppress elevated bone turnover. Although side effects of nausea and facial flushing may be troublesome in certain patients, there has been no significant toxicity reported in any patient (Lesh *et al.,* 1974). Improvement in bone pain has usually been observed, including one double blind study (Bouvet, 1977). It should be stressed that joint pain and pain from nerve or spinal cord compression are unlikely to be improved by treatment. Future investigation should more adequately evaluate the indications for treatment and the appropriate dosage regimens for the several forms of calcitonin. Earlier studies suggest that relatively high doses may be needed to improve radiological features of the disease (Doyle *et al.,* 1974), whereas symptomatic and biochemical improvement may occur at low doses (Singer, 1977b).

X. ETIOLOGY

Speculation as to the cause of Paget's disease began with the initial paper of Paget (1877). His concept of the disease as a chronic inflammatory disorder has not gained widespread acceptance, in large part because there are few inflammatory cells in pagetic lesions. Interest in this idea was revived by the reports of Albright and Henneman (1955) and Maurice and colleagues (1962) in which the antiinflammatory drugs ACTH, cortisone, and aspirin were shown to suppress Paget's disease. Since cortisone and related steroids in high doses may inhibit protein synthesis, their effect on Paget's disease may represent interference with the function and/or differentiation of osteoclasts and osteoblasts rather than an "antiinflammatory effect." Similarly, the effect of acetylsalicylic acid on Paget's disease may be to alter prostaglandin synthesis in bone cells rather than to suppress inflammation in a nonspecific manner.

Abnormalities of hormone secretion have been proposed as an etiological factor in the development of Paget's disease (DaCosta et al., 1915). The pituitary gland (Moehlig and Adler, 1937) and the parathyroid glands (Ballin, 1933) have been implicated. A deficit or excess secretion of any known pituitary hormone has not been reported in patients with Paget's disease and lesions compatible with the disease do not occur in hypopituitarism or in any known syndrome of pituitary hormone excess. As previously discussed, hyperparathyroidism may mimic to some extent and may coexist with Paget's disease, but it is clearly not an etiological factor. The role of calcitonin in the etiology of Paget's disease deserves close scrutiny since this hormone has such a potent effect upon osteoclasts and may suppress the disease. The lack of a thyroid gland in mammals, including humans, does not result in skeletal lesions despite the absence of calcitonin. Further evidence against the role of calcitonin in the pathogenesis of Paget's disease is provided by the reports of normal concentrations of calcitonin in the circulation of pagetic patients (Heynen and Franchimont, 1974; Singer, 1977a).

The possibility that Paget's disease is a tumor of bone has been stressed by Rasmussen and Bordier (1974), who point out that the large numbers of nuclei in osteoclasts and the bizarre forms of osteoblasts that are seen may represent neoplastic phenomena.

The remarkable increase in the vasculature of involved bone has led to speculation that the disease is primarily vascular in origin (Cone, 1922; Moore, 1951). However, it is still not resolved whether the hypervascularity seen is primary or secondary to the bone disease.

McKusick (1972) has suggested that, based on family studies, the presence of angioid streaks, and an association with pseudoxanthoma elasticum, Paget's disease may be a genetically determined, generalized disorder of connective tissue. This implies that an inborn error of metabolism of connective tissue may exist in patients with Paget's disease. We have found that the amino acid content and other compositional characteristics of skin and bone are normal in several patients, but other defects, such as abnormal cross-linking of bone collagen could be present (Francis and Smith, 1974, Misra, 1975).

Another possibility, and one amenable to investigation with modern techniques, is that Paget's disease could result from viral infection years before the disorder becomes clinically manifest. Consistent with this theory are the following observations: (1) The very nature of this disease, which is characterized by the processes of bone destruction, bone formation, and associated fibrosis with minimal inflammation, is suggestive of a subacute, ongoing process, which could be a response to chronic infection. Bacteria have not been isolated from these lesions, but the possibility of viral infection still exists. (2) The presence in pagetic lesions of giant osteoclasts with large numbers of nuclei, although not specific, is reminiscent of multinucleated syncytial giant cells, which are a feature of viral lesions. Indeed, multinucleated cells can be produced at will *in vitro* in the presence of and as a direct result of virus infection of cultured cells (Harris *et al.*, 1966). (3) Paget's disease characteristically is detected in individuals after the age of 40, consistent with an infection of long latency. (4) The distribution of the disease in the population is spotty, common in some regions, sparing others. (5) Multiple cases are seen in families where

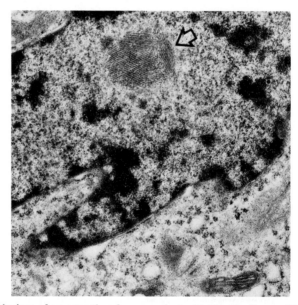

Fig. 45. Nucleus of an osteoclast from a patient with Paget's disease. The arrow indicates the characteristic nuclear inclusion in longitudinal section. Each microfilament measures approximately 150 Å in diameter. Decalcified; ×20,250. (From Singer *et al.*, 1976). Permission from Blackwell Scientific Publications, Ltd.

it has not been proven that the clustering is genetic in origin. (6) Intranuclear formations of a filamentous character (Fig. 45) have been observed in the nuclei of osteoclasts in biopsies of 41 patients (Rebel *et al.*, 1974, 1975, 1976; Mills and Singer, 1976). They resemble intranuclear inclusions found in the brain cells of patients with subacute sclerosing panencephalitis, a disorder which is caused by a measles-like paramyxovirus (Oyanagi *et al.*, 1971).

After more than 100 years we finally may be nearing an understanding of the disorder which Paget was the first to suggest was of an inflammatory nature.

REFERENCES

Acar, J., Delbarre, F., and Waynberger, M. (1968). *Arch. Mal. Coeur Vaiss.* **61,** 849.

Adams, E. (1970). *Int. Rev. Connect. Tissue Res.* **5,** 1.

Ajlouni, K., and Theil, G. B. (1975). *Am. J. Med. Sci.* **13,** 18.

Albright, F., and Henneman, P. H. (1955). *Trans. Assoc. Am. Physicians* **68,** 238.

Alderman, M. H., Frimpter, G. W., Isaacs, M., and Scheiner, E. (1969). *Metab., Clin. Exp.* **18,** 692.

Alexandre, C., and Meunier, P. (1977). "Le Traitement de la Maladie Osseuse de Paget par L'Ethane-1 Hydroxy-1, 1 Diphosphonate (EHDP)." Effets cliniques, biologiques et histologiques chez 69 malades. Association Corporative des Etudiants en Médecine de Lyon, Lyon.

Allen, M. L., and John, R. L. (1937). *Am. J. Roentgenol. Radium Ther.* [N. S.] **38,** 109.

Altman, R. D., Johnston, C. C., Khairi, M. R. A., Wellman, H., Serafini, A. N., and Sankey, R. R. (1973). *N. Engl. J. Med.* **289,** 1379.

Askenasi, R. (1973). *Biochim. Biophys. Acta* **304,** 375.

Askenasi, R., DeBacker, M., and Devos, A. (1976). *Calcif. Tissue Res.* **22,** 35.

Aubert, J. P., Bronner, F., and Richelle, L. J. (1963). *J. Clin. Invest.* **42,** 885.

Aubert, J. P., and Milhaud, G. (1960). *Biochim. Biophys. Acta* **39,** 122.

Avioli, L. V., and Berman, M. (1968). *J. Clin. Endocrinol. Metab.* **28,** 700.

Avioli, L. V., and Henneman, P. H. (1964). *In* "Dynamic Studies of Metabolic Bone Disease" (O. H. Pearson and G. F. Joplin, eds.), pp. 185–197. Blackwell, Oxford.

Avramides, A., Baker, R. K., and Wallach, S. (1974). *Metab., Clin. Exp.* **23,** 1037.

Avramides, A., Flores, A., DeRose, J., and Wallach, S. (1975). *Br. Med. J.* **3,** 632.

Avramides, A., Flores, A., DeRose, J., and Wallach, S. (1976). *J. Clin. Endocrinol. Metab.* **42,** 459.

Ballin, M. (1933). *J. Bone Joint Surg.* **15,** 120.

Barry, H. C. (1961). *J. Bone Joint Surg., Am. Vol.* **43,** 1122.

Barry, H. C. (1969). "Paget's Disease of Bone." Williams & Wilkins, Baltimore, Maryland.

Bélanger, L. F. (1969). *Calcif. Tissue Res.* **4,** 1.

Bélanger, L. F., Jarry, L., and Uhthoff, H. K. (1968). *Rev. Can. Biol.* **27,** 37.

Bell, N. H., Avery, S., and Johnston, C. C., Jr. (1970). *J. Clin. Endocrinol. Metab.* **31,** 283.

Benoit, F. L., and Walton, R. H. (1968). *Metab., Clin. Exp.* **17,** 20.

Berman, L. (1936). *Endocrinology* **20,** 226.

Bernstein, D. S., Guri, C., Cohen, P., Collins, J. J., and Tamvakopoulos, S. (1963). *J. Clin. Invest.* **42,** 916.

Bijvoet, O. L. M., and Jansen, A. P. (1967). *Lancet* **2,** 471.

Bijvoet, O. L. M., van der Sluys Veer, J., and Jansen, A. P. (1968). *Lancet* **1,** 876.
Bijvoet, O. L. M., van der Sluys Veer, J., and Smeenk, D. (1970). *In* "Calcitonin 1969, Proc. 2nd Int. Symp." (S. Taylor and G. Foster, eds.) pp. 531–539. Heinemann, London.
Bitar, E. (1961). *Rev. Med. Moyen-Orient* **18,** 477.
Blotman, F., Suquet, P., Labauge, R., and Simon, L. (1974). *In* "La Maladie de Paget. Symposium International" (D. J. Hioco, ed.), pp. 79–87. Laboratoire Armour Montagu, Paris.
Bomparu, R., and Ceccato, S. (1970). *G. Gerontol.* **18,** 720.
Bordier, P., Rasmussen, H., and Dorfman, H. (1974). *Am. J. Med.* **56,** 850.
Bornstein, P., von der Mark, K., Wyke, A. W., Ehrlich, H. P., and Monson, J. M. (1972). *J. Biol. Chem.* **247,** 2808.
Boutouras, G. D., and Goodsit, E., (1963). *J. Int. Coll. Surg.* **40,** 380.
Bouvet, J.-P. (1977). *Nouv. Presse Med.* 6, 1447.
Brewerton, D. A., Hart, F. D., Nicholls, A., Caffrey, M., James, D. C. O., and Sturrock, R. D. (1973). *Lancet* **1,** 904.
Brodwall, E. K., Wertlie, L., and Myhre, E. (1972). *Acta Med. Scand.* **192,** 137.
Burckhardt, P. M., Singer, F. R., and Potts, J. T., Jr. (1973). *Clin. Endocrinol.* **2,** 15.
Burckhardt, P., Ducommun, J., and Hessler, C. (1977). *In* "Human Calcitonin and Paget's Disease" (I. MacIntyre, ed.), pp. 155–166, H. Huber, Bern, Switzerland.
Caffrey, M. F. P., and James, D. C. O. (1973). *Nature (London)* **242,** 121.
Canfield, R., Rosner, W., Skinner, J., McWhorter, S., Resnick, L., Feldman, F., Kammerman, S., Ryan, K., Kunigonis, M., and Bohne, W. (1977). *J. Clin. Endocrinol. Metab.* **44,** 96.
Canniggia, A., and Gennari, C. (1968). *Minerva Med.* **59,** 279.
Canniggia, A., Gennari, C., Guideri, R., Vattimo, A., and Nardi, P. (1976). *Minerva Med.* **67,** 1.
Care, A. D., Bates, R. F. L., and Gitelman, H. J. (1970). *J. Endocrinol.* **48,** 1.
Castleman, B., and McNeely, B. U. (1970). *N. Engl. J. Med.* **283,** 1276.
Cautris, G., Cayla, J., Rondier, J., Talbot, J.-N., Bonvarlet, J.-P., and Milhaud, G. (1975). *Rev. Rhum. Mal. Osteo-Articulaires* **42,** 759.
Chapuy, M.-C., Meunier, P., Terrier, M., David, L., and Vignon, G. (1975). *Path. Biol.* 23, 349.
Charvat, J., and Belohradsky, K. (1952). *Cas. Lek. Cesk.* **91,** 45.
Choremis, C., Yannakos, D., Papadatos, C., and Baroutsou, E. (1958). *Helv. Paediatr. Acta* **13,** 185.
Collins, D. H. (1956). *Lancet* **2,** 51.
Collins, D. H. (1966). "Pathology of Bone." Butterworth, London.
Condon, J. R. (1971). *Br. Med. J.* **4,** 719.
Condon, J. R., Reith, S. B. M., Nassim, J. R., Millard, F. J. C., Hilb, A., and Stainthorpe, E. M. (1971). *Br. Med. J.* **1,** 421.
Cone, S. M. (1922). *J. Bone Joint Surg.* **4,** 751.
Cooke, B. E. D. (1956). *Ann. R. Coll. Surg. Engl.* **19,** 223.
Costello, L. C., Stacey, R., and Stevens, R. (1971). *Horm. Metab. Res.* **3,** 120.
Courvoisier, B., DeBarros, Q., Jacot, C., and Zender, R. (1970). *Schweiz. Med. Wochenschr.* **100,** 26.
Crosbie, W. A., Mohamedally, S. M., and Woodhouse, N. J. Y. (1975). *Clin. Sci. Mol. Med.* **48,** 537.
Czerny, V. (1873). *Wien. Med. Wochenschr.* **23,** 985.
DaCosta, J. C., Funk, E. H., Bergeim, O., and Hawk, P. B. (1915). *Publ. Lab. Jefferson Med. Coll. Hosp.* **6,** 1.

David, L., Chapuy, M. C., Meunier, P. (1976). *In* Phosphate Metabolism, Kidney and Bone (L. Avioli, P. Bordier, H. Fleish, S. Massry, and E. Slatopolsky, eds.) pp. 345–358, Armour Montagu, Paris.

Davies, D. G. (1968). *Acta Oto-Laryngol., Suppl.* **242.**

Demmler, K. (1974). *Dsch. Med. Wochenschr.* **99,** 91.

DeRose, J., Avramides, A., Baker, R. K., and Wallach, S. (1972). *Semin. Drug Treat.* **2,** 51.

DeRose, J., Singer, F. R., Avramides, A., Flores, A., Dziadiw, R., Baker, R. K., and Wallach, S. (1974). *Am. J. Med.* **56,** 858.

DeVries, H. R., and Bijvoet, O. L. M. (1974). *Neth. J. Med.* **17,** 281.

Dietrich, F. M., and Fischer, J. A. (1977). *In* "Human Calcitonin and Paget's Disease" (I. MacIntyre, ed.), pp. 179–194, H. Huber, Bern, Switzerland.

Doyle, F. H., Pennock, J., Greenberg, P. B., Joplin, G. F., and MacIntyre, I. (1974). *Br. J. Radiol.* **47,** 1.

Doyle, F. H. (1977). *In* "Human Calcitonin and Paget's Disease" (I. MacIntyre, ed.), pp. 124–137, H. Huber, Bern, Switzerland.

Dubé, W. J., Goldsmith, R. S., Arnaud, S. B., and Arnaud, C. D. (1972). *In* "Calcium, Parathyroid Hormone and the Calcitonins" (R. V. Talmage and P. L. Munson, eds.), Int. Congr. Ser. No. 243, pp. 113–115. Excerpta Med. Found., Amsterdam.

Dubé, W. J., Goldsmith, R. S., Arnaud, S. B., and Arnaud, C. D. (1973). *Mayo Clin. Proc.* **48,** 43.

Dubovsky, J. F., Formankova, J., and Dubovska, E. (1964). *Cas. Lek. Cesk.* **103,** 187.

Dull, T. A., and Henneman, P. H. (1963). *N. Engl. J. Med.* **268,** 132.

Edholm, O. G., Howarth, S., and McMichael, J. (1945). *Clin. Sci.* **5,** 249.

Eisen, A. Z., Bauer, E. A., and Jeffrey, J. J. (1970). *J. Invest. Dermatol.* **55,** 359.

Eisman, J. A., Xipell, J. M., Sloman, J. G., Jerums, G., and Martin, T. J. (1974) *Med. J. Aust.* **1,** 564.

Ellis, K., and Hochstim, R. J. (1960). *Am. J. Roentgenol., Radium Ther. Nucl. Med.* [N. S.] **83,** 732.

Epstein, B. S., and Epstein, J. A. (1969). *Am. J. Roentgenol., Radium Ther. Nucl. Med.* [N. S.] **107,** 535.

Epstein, S. (1974). *S. Afr. Med. J.* **48,** 1328.

Evans, G. A., and Slee, G. C. (1977) *Br. Med. J.* **1,** 357.

Evans, I. M. A. (1977). *In* "Human Calcitonin and Paget's Disease" (I. MacIntyre, ed.), pp. 111–123, H. Huber, Bern, Switzerland.

Evans, R. A. (1977). *Aust. N. Z. J. Med.* **7,** 259.

Evens, R. G., and Bartter, F. C. (1968). *J. Am. Med. Assoc.* **205,** 900.

Eyring, E. J., and Eisenberg, E. (1968). *J. Bone Joint Surg., Am. Vol.* **50,** 1099.

Feiring, W. (1946). *N. Engl. J. Med.* **46,** 631.

Fennelly, J. J., and Groarke, J. F. (1971). *Br. Med. J.* **1,** 423.

Finerman, G. A. M., Gonick, H. C., Smith, R. K., and Mayfield, J. M. (1976). *Clin. Orthop. Related Res.* **20,** 115.

Francis, M. J. O., and Smith, R. (1974). *Lancet* **1,** 841.

Franck, W. A., Bress, N. M., Singer, F. R., and Krane, S. M. (1974). *Am. J. Med.* **56,** 592.

Fullmer, H. M., and Lazarus, G. (1967). *Isr. J. Med. Sci.* **3,** 758.

Galante, L., Joplin, G. F., MacIntyre, I., and Woodhouse, N. J. Y. (1973). *Clin. Sci.* **44,** 605.

Galmiche, P., and Levy, P. (1967). *Rev. Rhum. Mal. Osteo-Articulaires* **34,** 185.

Gardner, B., Gray, H., and Hedayati, H. (1970). *Surg. Forum* **21,** 467.

Gavazolli, L., Coscelli, C., Gnudi, A., and Passeri, N. (1970). *G. Gerontol.* **18,** 347.

Ghormley, R. K., and Hinchey, J. J. (1944). *J. Bone Joint Surg.* **26,** 811.

Gill, A. B., and Stein, I. (1936). *J. Bone Joint Surg.* **18,** 941.

Goldfield, E. B., Braiker, B. M., Prendergast, J. J., and Kolb, F. O. (1972). *J. Am. Med. Assoc.* **221**, 1127.

Goldman, A. M., Braunstein, P., Wilkinson, D., and Kammerman, S. (1975). *Radiology* **117**, 365.

Goldsmith, R. S. (1972). *Semin. Drug Treat.* **2**, 69.

Grainger, R. G., and Laws, J. W. (1957). *Br. J. Radiol.* **30**, 120.

Grant, M. E., and Prockop, D. J. (1972). *N. Engl. J. Med.* **286**, 194, 242, 291.

Greenberg, P. B., Doyle, F. H., Fisher, M. T., Hillyard, C. J., Joplin, G. F., Pennock, J., and MacIntyre, I. (1974). *Am. J. Med.* **56**, 867.

Grimaldi, P. M. G. B., Mohamedally, S. M., and Woodhouse, N. J. Y. (1975). *Br. Med. J.* **2**, 726.

Gunčaga, J., Lauffenburger, T., Lentner, C., Dambacher, M. A., Haas, H. G., Fleisch, H., and Olah, A. J. (1974). *Horm. Metab. Res.* **6**, 62.

Gutman, A. B., and Parsons, W. B. (1938). *Ann. Intern. Med.* **12**, 13.

Haddad, J. G., Jr., and Caldwell, J. G. (1972). *J. Clin. Invest.* **51**, 3133.

Haddad, J. G., Jr., Birge, S. J., and Avioli, L. V. (1970a). *N. Engl. J. Med.* **283**, 549.

Haddad, J. G., Jr., Couranz, S., and Avioli, L. V. (1970b). *J. Clin. Endocrinol. Metab.* **30**, 282.

Haddad, J. G., Jr. and Rojanasathit, S. (1977). *In* "Human Calcitonin and Paget's Disease" (I. MacIntyre, ed.), pp. 195–206, H. Huber, Bern, Switzerland.

Hamilton, C. R., Jr., (1974). *Am. J. Med.* **56**, 315.

Harris, E. D., Jr., and Krane, S. M. (1968). *Bull. Rheum. Dis.* **18**, 506.

Harris, H., Watkins, J. F., Ford, C. E., and Schoefl, G. I. (1966). *J. Cell Sci.* **1**, 1.

Harris, W. H., and Heaney, R. P. (1970). "Skeletal Renewal and Metabolic Bone Disease." Little, Brown, Boston, Massachusetts.

Harrison, C. V., and Lennox, B. (1948). *Br. Heart J.* **10**, 167.

Harrison, H. E. (1956). *Am. J. Med.* **20**, 1.

Hartman, J. T., and Dohn, D. F. (1966). *J. Bone Joint Surg., Am. Vol.* **48**, 1079.

Haymovits, A., Zluizek, V., Ling, A. S. C., Hobitz, H., and Fotino, M. (1977). *In* "Human Calcitonin and Paget's Disease" (I. MacIntyre, ed.), pp. 138–154, H. Huber, Bern, Switzerland.

Heistad, D. D., Abboud, F. M., Schmid, P. G., Mark, A. L., and Wilson, W. R. (1975). *J. Clin. Invest.* **55**, 69.

Helfet, A. J. (1952). *S. Afr. Med. J.* **26**, 703.

Henneman, P. H., Dull, T. A., Avioli, L. V., Bastomsky, C. H., and Lynch, T. N. (1963). *Trans. & Stud. Coll. Physicians Philadelphia* **31**, 10.

Heynen, G. and Franchimont, P. (1974). *Europ. J. Clin. Invest.* **4**, 213.

Higgins, B. A., Nassim, J. R., Alexander, R., and Hilb, A. (1965). *Br. Med. J.* **1**, 1159.

Hilker, R. (1959). *Lancet* **1**, 527.

Hill, P. G., and Sammons, H. G. (1967). *Q. J. Med.* **36**, 457.

Hodgkinson, A. (1963). *Clin. Sci.* **24**, 167.

Hosking, D. J., Bijvoet, O. L. M., Van Aken, J., and Will, E. J. (1976). *Lancet* **1**, 615.

Howarth, S. (1953). *Clin. Sci.* **12**, 271.

Jaffe, H. L. (1972). "Metabolic, Degenerative, and Inflammatory Diseases of Bones and Joints." Lea & Febiger, Philadelphia, Pennsylvania.

Jaffe, N., and Watts, H. G. (1976). *J. Bone Joint Surg., Am. Vol.* **58**, 634.

Jesserer, H., Chlud, K., and Wondner, G. (1967). *Wien. Klin. Wochenschr.* **79**, 137.

Jones, J. V., and Reed, M. F. (1967). *Br. Med. J.* **4**, 90.

Kanis, J. A., Horn, D. B., Scott, R. D. M., and Strong, J. A. (1974). *Br. Med. J.* **3**, 727.

Kanis, J. A., Fitzpatrick, K., and Strong, J. A. (1975). *Quart. J. Med.*, (N. S.) **44**, 399.

Kantrowitz, F. G., Byrne, M. H., Schiller, A. L., and Krane, S. M. (1975). *Arthritis Rheum.* **18,** 407.

Kasabach, H. H., and Gutman, A. B. (1937). *Am. J. Roentgenol. Radium Ther.* [N. S.] **37,** 577.

Kaufman, E. J., Glimcher, M. J., Mechanic, G. L., and Goldhaber, P. (1965). *Proc. Soc. Exp. Biol. Med.* **120,** 632.

Kay, H. D. (1929). *Br. J. Exp. Pathol.* **10,** 253.

Kenny, A. D. (1961). *In* "The Parathyroids" (R. O. Greep and R. V. Talmage, eds.), pp. 275–291. Thomas, Springfield, Illinois.

Khairi, M. R. A., Wellman, H. N., Robb, J. A., and Johnston, C. C., Jr. (1973). *Ann. Intern. Med.* **79,** 348.

Khairi, M. R. A., Johnston, C. C., Jr., Altman, R. D., Wellman, H. N., Serafini, A. N., and Sankey, R. R. (1974). *J. Am. Med. Assoc.* **230,** 562.

Khairi, M. R. A., Meunier, P., Edouard, C., Courpron, P., Bernard, J., Derosa, G. P., and Johnston, C. C., Jr. (1977). *Calcif. Tissue Res.* **22,** (Suppl.), 355.

King, M., Huang, J., and Glassman, E. (1969). *Am. J. Med.* **46,** 302.

Kissin, B., and Kreeger, N. (1954). *Am. J. Med. Sci.* **228,** 301.

Kivirikko, K. I. (1970). *Int. Rev. Connect. Tissue Res.* **5,** 93.

Kolb, F. O. (1959). *Calif. Med.* **91,** 245.

Krane, S. M., Muñoz, A. J., and Harris, E. D., Jr. (1967). *Science* **157,** 713.

Krane, S. M., Muñoz, A. J., and Harris, E. D., Jr. (1970). *J. Clin. Invest.* **49,** 716.

Krane, S. M., Harris, E. D., Jr., Singer, F. R., and Potts, J. T., Jr. (1973). *Metab., Clin. Exp.* **22,** 51.

Krane, S. M., Kantrowitz, F. G., Byrne, M., Pinnell, S. R., and Singer, F. R. (1977) *J. Clin. Invest.* **59,** 819.

Larmande, A., and Margaillan, A. (1957). *Bull. Soc. Ophtalmol. Fr.* **70,** 206.

Lauchlan, S. C., and Walsh, M. J. (1963). *Can. Med. Assoc. J.* **88,** 891.

Lauffenburger, T., Olah, A. J., Dambacher, M. A., Guncaga, J., Lentner, C., and Haas, H. G. (1977). *Metab. Clin. Exp.* **26,** 589.

Lavender, J. P., Evans, I. M. A., Arnot, R., Bowring, S., Doyle, F. H., Joplin, G. F., and MacIntyre, I. (1977). *Br. J. Radiol.* **50,** 243.

Layani, F., Françon, J., and Wattebled, R. (1961). *Sem. Hop.* **37,** 1037.

Lebbin, D., Ryan, W. G., and Schwartz, T. B. (1974). *Ann. Intern. Med.* **81,** 635.

Lee, W., Marshall, J. H., and Sissons, H. A. (1965). *J. Bone Joint Surg., Br. Vol.* **47,** 157.

Lee, W. R. (1967). *J. Bone Joint Surg., Br. Vol.* **49,** 146.

Lentle, B. C., Russell, A. S., Heslip, P. G., and Percy, J. S. (1976). *Clin. Radiol.* **27,** 129.

Lequime, J., and Denolin, H. (1955). *Circulation* **12,** 215.

Lesh, J. B., Aldred, J. P., Bastian, J. W., and Kleszynski, R. R. (1974). *In* "Endocrinology 1973, Proc. Int. Symp., 4th, 1973 p. 409–424.

Lukert, B. P., Bolinger, R. E., and Meeks, J. C. (1967). *J. Clin. Endocrinol. Metab.* **27,** 828.

McGavack, T. H., Seegers, W., and Reifenstein, E. C., Jr. (1961). *J. Am. Geriatr. Soc.* **9,** 533.

Machtey, I., Rodnan, G. P., and Benedek, T. G. (1966). *Am. J. Med. Sci.* **251,** 524.

McKenna, R. J., Schwinn, C. P., Soong, K. Y., and Higinbotham, N. L. (1964). *Cancer* **17,** 42.

Mackie, E. G. (1956). *Trans. Ophthalmol. Soc. U. K.* **76,** 267.

McKusick, V. (1972). "Heritable Disorders of Connective Tissue." Mosby, St. Louis, Missouri.

Martin, T. J., Jerums, G., Melick, R. A., Xipell, J. M., and Arnott, R. (1977). *Aust. N. Z. J. Med.* **7,** 36.

Maurice, P. F., Lynch, T. N., Bastomsky, C. H., Dull, T. A., Avioli, L. V., and Henneman, P. H. (1962). *Trans. Assoc. Am. Physicians* **75**, 208.

Meilman, E., Urivetsky, M. M., and Rapoport, C. M. (1963). *J. Clin. Invest.* **42**, 40.

Melick, R. A., Ebeling, P., and Hjorth, R. J. (1976). *Br. Med. J.* **1**, 627.

Melick, R. A., and Martin, T. J. (1975). *Aust. N. Z. J. Med.* **5**, 564.

Menzies, M. A., Greenberg, P. B., and Joplen, G. F. (1975). *Acta Oto-Laryngol.* **79**, 378.

Meunier, P. (1977). *In* "Human Calcitonin and Paget's Disease" (I. MacIntyre, ed.), pp. 78–92, H. Huber, Bern, Switzerland.

Meunier, P., Chapuy, M. C., Courpron, P., Vignon, E., Edouard, C., and Bernard, J. (1976). *Rev. Rhum. Mal. Osteo-Articulaires* **42**, 699.

Milhaud, G., Tsien-Ming, L., Nesralla, H., Moukhtar, M. S., and Perault-Staub, A. (1968). *Calcitonin, Proc. Thyrocalcitonin C Cells, 1967* pp. 347–360.

Milhaud, G., Calmettes, C., Julienne, A., Tharaud, D., Bloch-Michel, H., Cavaillon, J. P., Colin, R., and Moukhtar, M. S. (1972). *In* "Calcium, Parathyroid Hormone and the Calcitonins" (R. V. Talmage and P. L. Munson, eds.), Int. Congr. Ser. No. 243, pp. 56–70, Excerpta Med. Found. Amsterdam.

Mills, B. G., and Singer, F. R. (1976). *Science* **194**, 201.

Misra, D. P. (1975). *J. Clin. Pathol.* **28**, 305.

Moehlig, R. C., and Adler, S. (1937). *Surg., Gynecol. Obstet.* **64**, 747.

Moffatt, W. H., Morrow, J. D., and Simpson, N. (1974). *Br. Med. J.* **4**, 203.

Monroe, R. T. (1951). "Diseases of Old Age." Harvard Univ. Press, Cambridge, Massachusetts.

Montagu, M. F. A. (1949). *Am. J. Hum. Genet.* **1**, 44.

Moore, S. (1951). *J. Bone Joint Surg., Am. Vol.* **33**, 421.

Moretti, G. F., Texier, L., and Staffen, J. (1962). *Sem. Hop.* **38**, 3813.

Nagant de Deuxchaisnes, C., and Krane, S. M. (1964). *Medicine (Baltimore)* **43**, 233.

Nagant de Deuxchaisnes, C., and Krane, S. M. (1967). *Am. J. Med.* **43**, 508.

Nagant de Deuxchaisnes, C., and Krane, S. M. (1974). *In* "La Maladie de Paget. Symposium International" (D. J. Hioco, ed.), pp. 196–213. Laboratoire Armour Montagu, Paris.

Natelson, S., Pincus, J. B., and Lugovoy, J. K. (1948). *J. Biol. Chem.* **175**, 745.

Neer, R. M., Parsons, J. A., Krane, S. M., Deftos, L. J., Shields, C. L., and Potts, J. T., Jr. (1970). *Calcitonin, Proc. Int. Symp., 2nd, 1969* pp. 547–554.

Neugebauer, R. (1953). *Wien. Med. Wochenschr.* **103**, 827.

Neuman, W. F., and Neuman, M. W. (1958). "The Chemical Dynamics of Bone Mineral." University of Chicago Press, Chicago, Illinois.

Newman, F. W. (1946). *J. Bone Joint Surg.* **28**, 798.

Nicolle, M.-H., Grondard, E., Francois, N., and Maury, M. (1977). *Nouv. Presse Med.* **6**, 1567.

Nisbet, J. A., Helliwell, S., and Nordin, B. E. C. (1970). *Clin. Orthop.* **70**, 220.

O'Reilly, T. J., and Race, J. (1932). *Q. J. Med.* **25**, 471.

Oreopoulos, D. G., Husdan, H., Harrison, J., Meema, H. E., McNeil, K. G., Murray, T. M., Oglivie, R., and Rapaport, A. (1977). *Canad. Med. Assoc. J.* **23**, 851.

Oyanagi, S., ter Meulen, V., Katz, M., and Kaprowski, H. (1971). *J. Virol.* **7**, 176.

Paget, J. (1877). *Med.-Chir. Trans.* **60**, 37.

Paget, J. (1882a). *Br. Med. J.* **2**, 1189.

Paget, J. (1882b). *Med.-Chir. Trans.* **65**, 225.

Paton, D. (1972). "The Relation of Angioid Streaks to Systemic Disease." Thomas, Springfield, Illinois.

Pendergrass, H. P., Potsaid, M. S., and Castronovo, F. P., Jr. (1973). *Radiology* **107**, 557.

Pinnell, S. R., Fox, R., and Krane, S. M. (1971). *Biochim. Biophys. Acta* **229**, 119.

Pinnell, S. R., Krane, S. M., Kenzora, J. E., and Glimcher, M. J. (1972). *N. Engl. J. Med.* **286**, 1013.

Porretta, C. A., Dahlin, D. C., and Janes, J. M. (1957). *J. Bone Joint Surg., Am. Vol.* **39**, 1313.

Purves, M. J. (1962). *Lancet* **2**, 1188.

Pyggot, F. (1957). *Lancet* **1**, 1170.

Radi, I., Epiney, J., and Reiner, M. (1970). *Rev. Rhum. Mal. Osteo-Articularies* **37**, 385.

Rapado, A., Hawkins, F. G., Torres, J. A., and Traba, M. L. (1971). *Rev. Clin. Esp.* **122**, 387.

Rapaport, E., Kuida, H., Dexter, L., Henneman, P. H., and Albright, F. (1957). *Am. J. Med.* **22**, 252.

Rasmussen, H., and Bordier, P. (1974). "The Physiological and Cellular Basis of Metabolic Bone Disease." Williams & Wilkins, Baltimore, Maryland.

Rebel, A., Malkani, K., and Basle, M. (1974). *Nouv. Presse Med.* **3**, 1299.

Rebel, A., Bregeon, C., Basle, M., and Malkani, K. (1976). *Rev. Rhum. Mal. Osteo-Articulaires* **42**, 637.

Rebel, A., Malkani, K., Basle, M., and Bregeon, C. (1976). *Calcif. Tissue Res.* **20**, 187.

Reifenstein, E. C., Jr., and Albright, F. (1944). *N. Engl. J. Med.* **231**, 343.

Reig, A. A., Madaria, E. Z., Justiniano, E. H., Rubio, J. M. R., San Millan, M. G., and Merchante, S. C. (1971). *Rev. Clin. Esp.* **122**, 395.

Reiner, M., Jung, A., Seiler, A., Schenk, R., and Fleisch, H. (1975). *Schweiz. Med. Wschr.* **105**, 1701.

Renier, J. C., Boasson, M., Jallet, P., and Bernat, M. (1974). *Rev. Rhum. Mal. Osteo-Articulaires* **40**, 557.

Renier, J.-C., Bernat, M., Brégeon, C., Gallois, Y., Rebel, A., Basle, M., Auvinet, B., and Pitoes, M. (1975). *Rev. Rhum. Mal. Osteo-Articulaires* **42**, 731.

Rhodes, B. A., Greyson, N. D., Hamilton, C. R., Jr., White, R. I., Jr., Giargiana, F. A., Jr., and Wagner, H. N., Jr. (1972). *N. Engl. J. Med.* **287**, 686.

Rich, C., Ensinck, J., and Ivanovich, P. (1964). *J. Clin. Invest.* **43**, 545.

Ridlon, H. C. (1962). *J. Urol.* **87**, 499.

Riffat, M. G. (1968). *J. Lyon Med.* **219**, 1035.

Riggs, B. L., and Jowsey, J. (1972). *Semin. Drug Treat.* **2**, 65.

Riggs, B. L., Arnaud, C. D., Goldsmith, R. S., Taylor, W. F., McCall, J. T., and Sessler, A. D. (1971). *J. Clin. Endocrinol. Metab.* **33**, 115.

Rojanasathit, S., Rosenberg, E., and Haddad, J. G., Jr. (1974). *Lancet* **2**, 1412.

Roper, B. A. (1971). *Clin. Orthop. Relat. Res.* **80**, 33.

Rosenbaum, H. D., and Hanson, D. J. (1969). *Radiology* **92**, 959.

Rosenkrantz, J. A., Wolf, J., and Kaicher, J. J. (1952). *Arch. Intern. Med.* **90**, 610.

Roux, H., Mercier, P., Maestracci, D., Eisinger, J., and Recordier, A. M. (1975). *Rev. Rhum. Mal. Osteo-Articulaires* **42**, 661.

Rubinstein, M. A., Smelin, A., and Freedman, A. L. (1953). *Arch. Intern. Med.* **92**, 684.

Rullier, P. R. (1812). *Bull. Fac. Med. Paris* **2**, 94.

Russell, A. S., and Lentle, B. C. (1974). *Can. Med. Assoc. J.* **110**, 397.

Russell, R. G. G., Smith, R., Preston, C., Walton, R. J., and Woods, C. G. (1974). *Lancet* **1**, 894.

Rutishauser, E., Veyrat, R., and Rouiller, C. (1954). *Presse Med.* **62**, 654.

Ryan, W. G., Schwartz, T. B., and Perlia, C. P. (1969). *Ann. Intern. Med.* **70**, 549.

Ryan, W. G., Schwartz, T. B., and Northrup, G. J. (1970). *J. Am. Med. Assoc.* **213**, 1153.

Ryan, W. G., Schwartz, T. B., and Northrup, G. (1972). *Semin. Drug Treat.* **2**, 57.

Sakamoto, S., Goldhaber, P., and Glimcher, M. J. (1972). *Calcif. Tissue Res.* **10**, 142.

Sakamoto, S., Goldhaber, P., and Glimcher, M. J. (1973). *Calcif. Tissue Res.* **12**, 247.

Schajowicz, F., and Slullitel, I. (1966). *J. Bone Joint Surg., Am. Vol.* **48,** 1340.
Schiano, A., and Eisenger, J. (1977). *Sem. Hôp. Paris.* **20,** 1131.
Schlosstein, L., Terasaki, P. I., Bluestone, R., and Pearson, C. M. (1973). *N. Engl. J. Med.* **288,** 705.
Schmorl, G. (1932). *Virchows Arch. Pathol. Anat. Physiol.* **283,** 694.
Schuhmacher, C. A., Scurry, M. T., and Deiss, W. P., Jr. (1973). *Arch. Intern. Med.* **131,** 722.
Schüller, A. (1926). *Br. J. Radiol.* **31,** 156.
Scriver, C. R. (1964). *Can. J. Physiol. Pharmacol.* **42,** 357.
Segrest, J. P., and Cunningham, L. W., (1970). *J. Clin. Invest.* **49,** 1497.
Seignalet, J. (1975). *Lyon Medit. Med.* **11,** 222.
Serre, H., and Mirowze, J. (1952). *Presse Med.* **60,** 595.
Shaffer, B., Copelan, H. W., and Beerman, H. (1957). *AMA Arch. Dermatol.* **76,** 622.
Shai, F., Baker, R. K., and Wallach, S. (1971). *J. Clin. Invest.* **50,** 1927.
Shimizu, M., Glimcher, M. J., Travis, D., and Goldhaber, P. (1969). *Proc. Soc. Exp. Biol. Med.* **130,** 1175.
Shorr, E., Almy, T. P., Sloan, M. H., Taussky, H., and Toscani, V. (1942). *Science* **96,** 587.
Siegelman, S. S., Levine, S. A., and Walpin, L. (1968). *Clin. Radiol.* **19,** 421.
Sinex, F. M., and Van Slyke, D. D. (1955). *J. Biol. Chem.* **216,** 245.
Singer, F. R., Aldred, J. P., Neer, R. M., Krane, S. M., Potts, J. T., Jr., and Bloch, K. J. (1972a). *J. Clin. Invest.* **51,** 2331.
Singer, F. R., Keutmann, H. T., Neer, R. M., Potts, J. T., Jr., and Krane, S. M. (1972b). *In* "Calcium, Parathyroid Hormone and the Calcitonins" (R. V. Talmage and P. L. Munson, eds.), Int. Congr. Ser. No. 243, pp. 89–96. Excerpta Med. Found., Amsterdam.
Singer, F. R., Neer, R. M., Goltzman, D., Krane, S. M., and Potts, J. T., Jr. (1974). *Endocrinol. Proc. Int. Symp., 4th, 1973* pp. 397–408.
Singer, F. R. (1977a). "Paget's Disease of Bone." Plenum, New York, New York.
Singer, F. R. (1977b). *Clin. Orthop. Rel. Res.* **127,** 86.
Singer, F. R., and Ahrne-Collier, J. (1977). *In* "Endocrinology, 1977. Proceedings of the Sixth International Symposium" (I. MacIntyre, ed.), in press. Elsevier/North Holland, Amsterdam.
Singer, F. R., Melvin, K. E. W., and Mills, B. G. (1976). *Clin. Endocrinol.* **5,** 333s.
Singer, F. R., Rude, R. K. and Mills, B. G. (1977). *In* "Human Calcitonin and Paget's Disease" (I. MacIntyre, ed.), pp. 93–110, H. Huber, Bern, Switzerland.
Smith, R., Russell, R. G. G., Bishop, M. C., Woods, C. G., and Bishop, M. (1973). *Q. J. Med.* **42,** 235.
Solomon, L. R., Evanson, J. M., Canty, D. P., and Gill, N. W. (1977). *Br. Med. J.* **2,** 485.
Somayaji, B. N. (1968). *Br. Med. J.* **4,** 278.
Sparrow, N. L., and Duvall, A. J., III. (1967). *J. Laryngol. Otol.* **81,** 601.
Staehelin, A. (1975). *Schweiz. Med. Wschr.* **105,** 1704.
Stafne, E. C., and Austin, L. T. (1938). *J. Am. Dent. Assoc.* **25,** 1202.
Stauffer, R. N., and Sem, F. H. (1976). *J. Bone Joint Surg., Am. Vol.* **58,** 476.
Stein, I., Shapiro, B., Ostrum, B., and Beller, M. L. (1977). *Clin. Orthop. Related Res.* **122,** 347.
Steindler, A. (1959). "Lectures on the Interpretation of Pain in Orthopedic Practice." Thomas, Springfield, Illinois.
Stern, B. D., Mechanic, G. L., Glimcher, M. J., and Goldhaber, P. (1963). *Biochem. Biophys. Res. Commun.* **13,** 137.
Stetten, M. R. (1949). *J. Biol. Chem.* **181,** 31.
Sullivan, T. J., Gutman, E. B., and Gutman, A. B. (1942). *J. Urol.* **48,** 426.

Taubman, M. B., Kammerman, S., and Goldberg, B. (1976). *Proc. Soc. Exp. Biol. Med.* **152,** 284.

Thompson, R. C., Jr., Gaull, G. E., Horwitz, S. J., and Schenk, R. K. (1969). *Am. J. Med.* **47,** 209.

Vaes, G. (1968). *J. Cell Biol.* **39,** 676.

Vellenga, C. J. L. R., Pauwels, E. K. J., Bijvoet, O. L. M., and Hosking, D. J. (1976). *Radiologia Clin.* **45,** 292.

Vignon, G. (1974). *In* "La Maladie de Paget. Symposium International" (D. J. Hioco, ed.), pp. 17–26. Laboratoire Armour Montagu, Paris.

von Albertini, A. (1928). *Virchows Arch. Pathol. Anat. Physiol.* **268,** 259.

Vuust, J., and Piez, K. A. (1970). *J. Biol. Chem.* **245,** 6201.

Vuust, J., and Piez, K. A. (1972). *J. Biol. Chem.* **247,** 856.

Wallach, S., Avramides, A., Flores, A., Bellavia, J., and Cohn, S. (1975). *Metab. Clin. Exp.* **24,** 745.

Waltner, J. G. (1965). *Arch. Otolaryngol.* **82,** 355.

Watson, E. M. (1939). *Can. Med. Assoc. J.* **41,** 561.

Watson, L. (1959). *Proc. R. Soc. Med.* **52,** 349.

Waxman, A. D., Ducker, S., McKee, D., Siemsen, J. K., and Singer, F. R. (1977). *Radiology,* **125,** 761.

Weiss, T. E., and Segaloff, A. (1959). "Gouty Arthritis and Gout." Thomas, Springfield, Illinois.

Wellman, H. N., Shanwrecker, D., Robb, J. A., Khairi, M. R., and Johnston, C. C. (1977). *Clin. Orthop. Rel. Res.* **127,** 55.

Wilks, S. (1869). *Trans Pathol. Soc. London* **20,** 273.

Woodard, H. Q. (1952). *Cancer* **5,** 236.

Woodard, H. Q. (1959). *Am. J. Med.* **27,** 902.

Woodhouse, N. J. Y., Bordier, P., Fisher, M., Joplin, G. F., Reiner, M., Kalu, D. N., Foster, G. V., and MacIntyre, I. (1971). *Lancet* **1,** 1139.

Woodhouse, N. J. Y., Fisher, M. T., Sigurdsson, G., Joplin, G. F., and MacIntyre, I. (1972). *Br. Med. J.* **4,** 267.

Woodhouse, N. J. Y., Crosbie, W. A., and Mohamedally, S. M. (1975). *Br. Med. J.* **4,** 686.

Woodhouse, N. J. Y., Mohamedally, S. M., Sald-Nehad, F., and Martin, T. J. (1977). *Br. Med. J.* **2,** 927.

Wrany, —— (1867). *Vierteijahresschr. Prakt. Heilkd.* **93,** 79.

Wright, J. T. (1966). *Australas. Radiol.* **10,** 365.

Wycis, H. T. (1944). *J. Neurosurg.* **1,** 299.

Wyllie, W. G. (1923). *Brain* **46,** 336.

Ziegler, R., Holz, G., Raue, F., Minne, H., and Delling, G. (1977). In "Human Calcitonin and Paget's Disease" (I. MacIntyre, ed.), pp. 167–178, H. Huber, Bern, Switzerland.

6

Disorders of Mineral Metabolism in Malignancy

JOHN S. RODMAN AND LOUIS M. SHERWOOD

I. Introduction 578
II. Effects of Hypercalcemia 578
    A. Neurologic 578
    B. Gastrointestinal 580
    C. Cardiovascular 582
    D. Renal 584
III. Clinical Occurrence 585
    A. Breast Cancer 587
    B. Myeloma, Leukemia, and Lymphoma 589
    C. Lung Tumors and Others Associated with Hypercalcemia .. 590
IV. Pathogenesis of Tumor-Associated Hypercalcemia 590
    A. Calcium Balance Considerations 590
    B. Mechanisms of Tumor-Associated Hypercalcemia 591
    C. Ectopic Parathyroid Hormone Production 595
    D. New Hypercalcemic Syndrome 604
    E. Differential Diagnosis 605
    F. Other Calcium Disorders Associated with Tumors 608
        1. Hypophosphatemic Osteomalacia 608
        2. Hypocalcemia 609
V. Treatment of Hypercalcemia 610
    A. Hydration and Electrolyte Replacement 611
    B. Mobilization 615
    C. Dietary Control 615
    D. Specific Therapy 616
    E. Nonspecific Therapy 617
    F. Comparison of Available Modalities 621
References 622

577

Copyright © 1978 by Academic Press, Inc.
All rights of reproduction in any form reserved
ISBN 0-12-068702-X

I. INTRODUCTION

Hypercalcemia is a common and serious complication of malignant disease. This review discusses its frequency, the mechanisms underlying its appearance, and its effects on various organ systems. The presenting clinical features of tumors associated with hypercalcemia and the management of acute and chronic hypercalcemic states are described. Attention is also given to certain aspects of other disorders of calcium metabolism associated with cancer.

II. EFFECTS OF HYPERCALCEMIA

The maintenance of a normal calcium concentration is critical for normal bone formation, blood coagulation, cardiac contractility, and exocrine and endocrine secretion as well as autonomic, central, and peripheral nervous system function. Calcium is known to stabilize biological membranes and to decrease their permeability to monovalent cations. Furthermore, it serves as an inhibitor of membrane-bound adenyl cyclase, an enzyme known to be crucial in the activation of various neuromuscular and secretory functions. In other cellular and subcellular reactions, calcium may act as an enzyme cofactor or as a direct participant in a metal–enzyme complex. When hyper- or hypocalcemia ensues, the effects can be manifested in many different organ systems and may mimic many of the protean effects of the malignancy they complicate. It is not uncommon for hypercalcemia to be misdiagnosed as cerebral metastases, gastroenteritis, or even malingering.

A. Neurologic

In general, the extent of the central nervous system symptomatology is related to the degree of elevation of the serum calcium, but in the individual patient the chronicity of the calcium abnormality and the rapidity of its change may be important modulating factors in its expression. Usually, the earliest central nervous system signs are drowsiness and lethargy. As the serum calcium rises, the patient becomes progressively confused, disoriented, and eventually stuporous and comatose. There is generalized muscle weakness with hypotonic or absent deep tendon reflexes. Headache is occasionally a prominent feature. While this nonspecific picture of mental and physical dulling associated with depression of neuron function is the general rule, it is by no means the only way that hypercalcemia can affect the nervous system.

Fitz and Hallman (1952) described a patient with a florid paranoid reaction and hallucinations, which was corrected by removal of a parathyroid adenoma. Another patient developed delusions of threats on her life, which cleared after partial parathyroidectomy (Delay *et al.*, 1970). Other mental disturbances attributed to hypercalcemia in a review article by Karpati and Frame (1964) included aggressive bickering behavior, childlike whining actions, and acute depressive reactions. All symptoms were reversed when the calcium returned to normal. Petersen (1968) reported that more than half of 54 patients with hyperparathyroidism demonstrated some form of psychopathology and he specifically excluded those patients referred primarily for psychiatric disorders. Mild changes were reflected in a neurasthenic personality, characterized by disturbances in affect and drive, and occasionally by impairment of memory. In more severe cases, acute organic psychosis developed. The emotional changes were correlated directly with the degree of elevation of the serum calcium rather than the concentration of parathyroid hormone. When peritoneal dialysis reduced the serum calcium in one patient, an acute organic psychosis was terminated.

Although localizing neurological signs are not usually associated with hypercalcemia, there are several reports of their occurrence. Herishami *et al.* (1970) described a woman with inoperable breast cancer who developed left-sided Jacksonian seizures after testosterone therapy elevated the serum calcium. When her calcium concentration was controlled, the seizures and the abnormality in the right hemisphere on her electroencephalogram (EEG) disappeared. Of course, one must wonder whether the hormonal manipulation had not affected the growth of a small cerebral metastasis, thereby creating an epileptogenic focus. Streeto (1969) reported a hypoparathyroid patient receiving vitamin D who developed ataxia and visual scotomata. She was felt to have basilar artery insufficiency until a calcium of 16.4 mg/100 ml was discovered and her symptoms were reversed when normocalcemia was restored. Simpson (1954) described four patients with nerve deafness associated with hyperparathyroidism, three of whom showed improvement in hearing after parathyroid surgery.

An increased cerebrospinal fluid protein of 145–170 mg/100 ml was reported in a fatal case of hyperparathyroidism (Edwards and Daum, 1959). In a review of the literature, these authors found 24 cases of hypercalcemia of diverse etiologies in which the spinal fluid protein was reported. Three of the patients, despite lack of evidence of primary neurological disease, had protein levels greater than 60 mg/100 ml.

The electroencephalogram in the hypercalcemic patient, while nonspecific, does show characteristic changes. There is progressive slow-ing of the record as the calcium rises. Paroxysms of frontal dominant, moderately high voltage, 2 to 4 cycles per second (cps) activity last for 1 to 2 seconds and recur every 4 to 10 seconds. Restoration of normocalcemia usually produces reversion to a normal record, but unlike hypoglycemia where conversion of the abnormality produces an instant response, there may be a time lag of several days or weeks after appropriate treatment (Moure, 1967; Allen *et al.*, 1970). Similarly, Evaldson *et al.* (1969) found that a lower index (mean of the cps frequency distribution), was likely to be associated with a higher serum calcium, but emphasized that a normal record can exist despite a value greater than 15 mg/100 ml. The hypercalcemic EEG has been misinterpreted as indicating diffuse cerebral metastases (Smith *et al.*, 1968); Strickland *et al.*, 1967).

Because the central nervous system manifestations of hypercalcemia are so diverse, the serum calcium should be determined on every patient who presents with confusion, neurologic or unexpected psychiatric problems. One of us (L.M.S.) has observed three elderly women whose hyperparathyroidism was first manifested by changing sensorium after they were put on bed rest for traumatic hip fractures. Lehrer and Levitt (1960) reported three patients with hypercalcemia who were initially diagnosed incorrectly as having primary neurologic disease. One was subjected to a pneumoencephalogram and a left carotid anteriogram before a serum calcium was drawn. Patten *et al.* (1974) recently showed evidence for atrophy of types I and II muscle fibers and altered motor unit potentials, presumably due to neuropathic changes, in a number of patients with primary hyperparathyroidism.

B. Gastrointestinal

The depressive action of hypercalcemia on autonomic nervous tissue probably accounts for much of the gastrointestinal symptomatology it produces. Constipation, often bordering on obstipation, is the rule, although diarrhea may sometimes occur. Anorexia followed by uncontrolled vomiting often ensues as the serum calcium rises. Repeated emesis will in turn cause hypokalemic alkalosis, which aggravates the toxic effects of hypercalcemia. Atony may produce increased gastric residual volume (Mavligit, 1970) and, in the peptic ulcer patient, can masquerade as pyloric obstruction (Sataline, 1962).

The relationship between serum calcium concentration and peptic ulcer disease involves both neural and hormonal mechanisms, which have only been partially clarified. When the calcium is low, as in infantile tetany, gastric secretion is depressed (Babbott *et al.*, 1923). In one adult patient with idiopathic hypoparathyroidism, gastric free acid was absent whenever the serum calcium was less than 7.0 mg/100 ml. When the calcium concentration was raised from a nadir of 5.6 mg/100 to 12.7 mg/100 ml, there was a progressive increase in free acid and a fall in pH. In addition, both pepsin concentration and total pepsin output increased (Donegan and Spiro, 1960, Spiro, 1970). When normal patients are given calcium infusions, the basal acid level may increase by more than fourfold to as much as 52% of the Histalog-stimulated value. Hypercalcemia, however, does not increase the gastric secretory response to Histalog (Barreras and Donaldson, 1967a). These same authors (1967b) described a patient with three parathyroid adenomas, severe peptic ulcer disease, and elevated basal acid secretion. When a normal serum calcium was restored by removal of the adenomas, basal gastric acid secretion fell from an average of 19.5 mEq/hour to 2.1 ± 1.3 mEq/hour. In the year following surgery, when the serum calcium was in the normal range, calcium infusion reproduced the gastric hypersecretion noted preoperatively. On the other hand, Donegan and Spiro (1960) reported that only one of five hyperparathyroid patients showed a fall in gastric acid production after successful surgical treatment of their disease. When the serum calcium concentration exceeds 18 mg/100 ml, metastatic gastric calcification occurs and achlorhydria may result (Spiro, 1960).

Both atropine and pentolinium block the hyperacidity induced by calcium infusions. Administration of magnesium has an effect opposite to that of calcium and interferes with the characteristic augmentation of gastric secretion produced by hypercalcemia (Barreras and Donaldson, 1967a,b). As calcium is well known to facilitate, and magnesium to inhibit, acetylcholine release, these data suggest that the effect of calcium on gastric mucosal secretion may be mediated by neural mechanisms.

The development of a satisfactory assay for serum gastrin has permitted studies that shed a different light on the relationship between hypercalcemia and peptic ulcer disease. Trudeau and McGuigan (1969) studied a patient with hyperparathyroidism 12 years after total gastrectomy had been performed for the Zollinger-Ellison syndrome. Before a neck exploration was undertaken, the serum calcium was 12 mg/100 ml and the serum gastrin 12,000 pg/ml. When parathyroidectomy reduced the calcium to 7 mg/100 ml, the gastrin level fell more than 20-fold to 550 pg/ml. Subsequent infusions of calcium again raised the gastrin level, but administration of parathyroid extract did not. It appears that the stimulation of gastric acid secretion by hypercalcemia is mediated, in part, by the polypeptide hormone gastrin (McGuigan, 1970).

In 1957, Cope et al., first described the relationship between hyperparathyroidism and pancreatitis. At least three different mechanisms have been proposed to explain this association (Turchi et al., 1962). Coffey et *al.* (1959) suggested that precipitation of calcium carbonate and phosphate in alkaline pancreatic juice causes obstruction of pancreatic ducts. Dreiling (1961) showed that high doses of parathyroid hormone injected into mice produce necrosis of pancreatic tissue. Although calcium by itself does not activate typsinogen, rising calcium concentrations do enhance its conversion to trypsin (Haverbeck *et al.,* 1960).

In an interesting series of experiments, Kelly (1968) thyroparathyroidectomized a group of rats and then transplanted varying amounts of parathyroid tissue into prepared pouches in their back muscles. No pancreatic necrosis or calcifications were found, but the degree of edema of the pancreas was directly proportional to the amount of parathyroid tissue transplanted. Pancreatic juice calcium and trypsin, but not anylase, were increased whenever the serum calcium was elevated. Those data lend support to the mechanism proposed by Haverbeck *et al.* (1960) that calcium induces typsinogen activation.

Calcium is also a cofactor in the activation of enzymes in the clotting casade. Baer and Neu (1966) found microthrombi in the kidneys and pancreas of an elderly woman with hyperparathyroidism and pancreatitis. They hypothesized that abnormalities of intravascular coagulation might account for the pancreatic disease. There have been other reports suggesting that hypercalcemia, especially when associated with malignancy, may result in a hypercoagulable state (Hilgard, 1970).

C. Cardiovascular

During their investigations with a calcium infusion test, Moore and Smith (1963) found that 9 of 19 patients showed at least a 30-mm increase in systolic blood pressure. In one patient, the blood pressure rose from 130/80 to 230/140. After the infusion was stopped, no other cause for paroxysmal hypertension was found. Earl *et al.* (1966) described a postthyroidectomy, hypoparathyroid man who developed a blood pressure of 224/160 while being treated with vitamin D and calcium lactate. When therapy was withheld and the calcium normalized, the blood pressure fell to 150/90. In a group of 57 patients receiving intravenous calcium infusions, Weidmann *et al.* (1972) found a significant correlation between the changes in both systolic and diastolic blood pressure and the increment in the serum calcium. The hypertensive response was more common in patients with advanced renal failure (serum creatinine greater than 4 mg/100 ml) but bore no relation to the presence or absence of preexisting hypertension. Some patients with primary hyperparathyroidism and hypertension have elevated plasma renin activity (Brinton *et al.,* 1975).

Hypocalcemia will apparently lower the blood pressure, under certain conditions. Intravenous phosphates, discussed in Section V, E, 5, can produce abrupt falls in the serum calcium and concomitant hypotension (Shackney and Hasson, 1967). When hypocalcemia is induced by EDTA infusion, significant orthostatic hypotension sometimes occurs (Soffer *et al.*, 1960). On the other hand, hyperparathyroid patients, and especially those with bone disease, may sustain a major decrease in their serum calcium levels after successful neck explorations. Tetany is common under these circumstances, but hypotension is not.

The physiologic effects of calcium on vascular smooth muscle tone are complex and affected by variations in many factors. In the dog forelimb and kidney vessels, combinations of hypercalcemia, hypokalemia, alkalosis, and hypomagnesemia produce greater vasoconstriction than does any single factor (Haddy *et al.*, 1963). Physiologic salt solutions containing 120 mM Na inhibit the contractile response to calcium present in sodium-free media (Sitrin and Bohr, 1971). With other factors constant, rising calcium concentrations produce progressive vasoconstriction and, at levels up to 2 mM, potentiate the contractile response to nonrepinephrine (Hiraoka *et al.*, 1968). Calcium depletion causes dilatation of small blood vessels (Overbeck *et al.*, 1961) and blunts the vasoconstrictive effect of epinephrine (Waugh, 1962).

Hypercalcemia increases myocardial contractility and shortens ventricular systole. With high enough calcium concentrations, cardiac arrest in systole may occur. Characteristic alterations of the electrocardiogram include shortening of the Q-T interval primarily by an effect on the length of the ST segment, which is inversely proportional to the level of the serum calcium up to about 20 mg/100 ml (Bronsky *et al.*, 1961). There may be coving of the ST segment with loss of the isoelectric portion and broadening of the T wave (Muggia and Heinemann, 1970). Reversible first degree heart block and the Wenckebach phenomenon (Crum and Till, 1960) have been described. Although bradycardia has been reported (Hoff *et al.*, 1939), nonspecific tachycardia is frequently present in these patients with systemic disease.

The deaths of two patients on digitalis who had received small amounts of intravenous calcium (Bower and Mengle, 1936) heightened the concern of clinicians about the known synergistic effect of calcium and digitalis on the myocardium. Like rising calcium concentrations, digitalis preparations increase myocardial contractility and shorten systolic ejection time. EDTA infused into normal young men antagonizes the effects of deslanoside on these parameters (Cohen *et al.*, 1965). Doses of digitalis that induce contracture also induce a net uptake of calcium by the myocardial cell. At lower levels of glycoside, the calcium influx is elevated, but it is difficult to demonstrate an increase in total intracellular calcium (Langer, 1972).

Individually, calcium and digitalis may each cause ventricular irritability and fibrillation. Sustained lowering of the serum calcium doubles the doses of acetyl strophanthidin required to produce ventricular arrhythmias. Digitalis, in turn, prevents the pump failure and hypotension induced by profound hypocalcemia (Lown *et al.*, 1960). However, when dogs who had received 90% of the ventricular tachycardia-inducing dose of ouabain had their serum calcium concentrations raised as high as 46.2 mg/100 ml, no digitalis arrhythmias were present (Lown *et al.*, 1960). Although these experiments were short-term studies, they do raise important questions concerning the clinical importance of the interaction between hypercalcemia and digitalis.

D. Renal

The most characteristic alteration of renal function seen in hypercalcemic states is an inability to concentrate the urine. Hyposthenuria is manifested at low urine flows and during mannitol diuresis (Epstein *et al.*, 1959). In 28 of 50 patients with documented hyperparathyroidism, the urinary specific gravity was never greater than 1.014. Nine additional patients had their highest value between 1.014 and 1.017 (Hellström, 1954). The reduction in concentrating capacity occurs out of proportion to the general derangement of renal function. Epstein *et al.* (1958) gave a series of 18 rats, 200,000 units or more of vitamin D_2 subcutaneously daily for 4 days and found an average urine osmolarity of 1625 mOs/liter in contrast to 2630 mOs/liter in the controls. The BUN was elevated in only 5 of the 18 animals and phenol red excretion dropped an average of only 5% (67 to 62%) from pretreatment values. Petersen and Edelman (1964) demonstrated an inhibitory effect of calcium on the action of vasopressin on the toad bladder.

High concentrations of calcium injected directly into the renal tubule decrease the permeability of the distal tubule to water but not the proximal tubule (Lassiter *et al.*, 1967). Sodium efflux from both the proximal and distal tubules is inhibited in the rat (Gutman and Gottschalk, 1966), but patients with hypercalcemia of various etiologies are still able to conserve sodium on a diet of 9 mEq per day (Gill and Bartter, 1961). In hypercalcemia, medullary sodium content is reduced (Manitius *et al.*, 1960) probably because of a direct and immediate effect on sodium transport by the thick ascending limb of Henle's loop (Suki *et al.*, 1969). This, rather than the collecting tubule, is probably the site where the concentrating defect is generated (Bennett, 1970; Epstein, 1971). That hyposthenuria is not a function of changes in glomerular filtration rate has been demonstrated (Zeffren and Heinemann, 1962; Suki *et al.*, 1969).

Hypercalcemia has been reported to stimulate the secretion of acid into the urine (Richet *et al.*, 1963) and, paradoxically, to impair ammonia excretion in some patients (Heinemann, 1963). Metabolic alkalosis is common in patients with nonparathyroid induced hypercalcemia, and acidosis usually occurs only when azotemia supervenes. In a series of 20 patients with hypercalcemia secondary to neoplasia, metabolic alkalosis, defined by an elevated arterial blood pH with normal or high serum bicarbonate levels, was present in all but one patient (Heinemann, 1963). Balance studies failed to demonstrate hydrogen ion loss, potassium depletion, chloride deficiency, or contraction of the extracellular volume. It was proposed that increased bone destruction or turnover increased the availability of the buffering capacity of the skeleton. With hypercalcemia due to hyperparathyroidism, on the other hand, a mild hyperchloremic acidosis is common, probably as a result of the effect of parathyroid hormone in increasing bicarbonate clearance (Barzel, 1971; Morris, 1969; Wills and McGowan, 1964). In hypercalcemia, Tm_{PAH} is usually depressed, more than is inulin clearance, suggesting that tubular function is disturbed more than glomerular filtration. Proteinuria is usually slight unless there is accompanying hypertension or congestive heart failure. Small molecular weight proteins including lysozyme may appear in the urine (Hayslett et al., 1968).

In the kidney, as elsewhere in the body, calcium precipitates in dead or dying tissue, or in areas where there is a local increase in pH (anterior corneal surface, gastric mucosa, alveolar lining, pancreas, synovium). After mercury poisoning, for example, the calcium is deposited in the cortex, chiefly in the proximal tubules. In hypercalcemic states, on the other hand, the deposits occur in the medullary tissue. The earliest changes occur in the cells of the collecting ducts and ascending loop of Henle, the areas of the tubules known to be involved in concentrating the urine. Distal tubular calcifications occur later while the proximal tubules are surprisingly spared (Manitius et al., 1960; Steck et al., 1937; Epstein, 1971).

Acute hypercalcemia produces rather minimal histologic changes as would be expected in view of the rapidity with which the clinical manifestations may be reversed. Chronic hypercalcemia tends to produce interstitial calcium deposits, infiltration with chronic inflammatory cell and fibrous tissue (Anderson, 1939), and, of course, renal stones (see Chapter 7, Volume I).

III. CLINICAL OCCURRENCE

In reviewing the 5-year experience at Memorial Hospital between 1954 and 1958, Myers (1960) reported 430 cases of tumor-related hypercalcemia (Table I). Of those, more than half were due to mammary car-

TABLE I

Diagnoses in 430 Patients Having Hypercalcemia Associated with Malignancy[a]

Primary site	Number	Maximum serum calcium (mg/100 ml)												Roentgenograms of the skeleton		
		11	12	13	14	15	16	17	18	19	20	21	22	Pos.	Neg.	Not done
Breast	225	54	37	35	23	17	15	16	16	5	3	3	4	209	14	2
Lung	29	6	4	4	5	3	3	1	2	2	1			21	5	3
Kidney	18	1	3	2	1	3	3	3	2					14	3	1
Cervix	12	1	4	1	2	2	1			1				4	4	4
Myeloma	11	1	2	1		3	1				1			11	0	0
Lymphoma	33	7	5	4	4	5	3	1	3		1			16	10	7
Leukemia	13	9	3		1									2	5	6
Miscellaneous[b]	89	15	20	13	15	10	4	4	2	4	1			57	15	17

[a] Modified after Myers (1960).

[b] Miscellaneous includes 11 prostate; 9 neuroblastoma; 8 melanoma; 8 rhabdomyosarcoma; 7 thyroid; 4 larynx; 3 each vagina, tonsil, tongue; 2 each ovary, uterus, floor of the mouth, nasopharynx, stomach, adrenal, salivary gland; 1 each urethra, esophagus, pancreas, fibromyxoliposarcoma, osteogenic sarcoma, liver, Ewing's sarcoma, hemangiopericytoma, leiomyosarcoma, malignant thymoma, and 9 metastatic tumors of undetermined primary site.

cinoma, reflecting, at least in part, the physician's familiarity with abnormalities of the serum calcium in that disease and its more frequent determination. Malignancies of kidney, lung, cervix, and the leukemia-lymphoma group accounted for 116 patients, or 27%. Despite the prevalence of gastrointestinal tumors in the general population, only two gastric and no colonic malignancies were included in that series. The most obvious explanation would appear to be that the latter neoplasms ordinarily metastasize to the liver first and rarely invade bone. However, as will be discussed below, tumor-associated hypercalcemia may occur even in the absence of demonstrable malignant involvement of bone.

A. Breast Cancer

This deserves special discussion, not only because it is the malignancy most often associated with hypercalcemia, but also because it is the only tumor, with the possible exception of prostate cancer, in which the hypercalcemia may be iatrogenic. Of 145 patients with breast cancer reported by Jessiman *et al.* (1963), 33 developed hypercalcemia on one or more occasions for a total of 59 episodes. Spontaneous elevations occurred 41 times (69%), while hormone therapy appeared to be responsible on 11 occasions. One patient developed hypercalcemia after oophorectomy. The remaining six episodes were ascribed to disturbances in water balance, presumably due to dehydration. Other authors (Graham *et al.,* 1963) reported that between 10 and 33% of patients with breast cancer will become hypercalcemic at some time in their course.

Galasko (1969) and Galasko and Burn (1971) reported some abnormality of calcium metabolism in 69% of a series of 127 mammary cancer patients. Roughly one-third had hypercalciuria with normocalcemia, one-third had asymptomatic elevations of the serum calcium, and the rest had progressive hypercalcemia. Spontaneous hypercalcemia tends to be associated with more advanced metastatic disease and a graver prognosis than does the hormone-induced abnormality (Mannheimer, 1965).

There are no adequate guidelines for predicting the consequences of hormonal manipulation on the serum calcium in breast cancer patients. Occasionally, in a premenopausal woman, hypercalcemia may be cyclic with the menses. In such patients, ablative therapy offers a good prospect for control of the tumor as well as the serum calcium. Pearson *et al.* (1954) reported three patients in whom oophorectomy caused tumor regression. Administration of estrogens to those patients was followed by recurrence of bone pain and return of serum and urinary calcium to the elevated precastration levels.

In postmenopausal women with breast carcinoma, estrogens have often been the hormonal therapy of first choice. The physician, however, must be aware of possible paradoxical responses to treatment. One 72-year-old woman, many years postmenopausal, developed an increased urinary calcium when treated with estrogens. She later benefited from castration (Baker, 1956). Another example of an unpredictable response was a patient discussed by Kennedy *et al.* (1953). A 63-year-old woman 5 years post-radical mastectomy had multiple metastases including a large supraorbital tumor mass displacing the globe downward. The patient was normocalcemic. By the fourth day of diethylstilbesterol therapy, the serum calcium had risen to 13.4 mg/100 ml. Despite disorientation associated with a calcium as high as 16.7, estrogen treatment was continued. The ocular mass regressed, the back pain diminished, pulmonary lesions disappeared, and the patient entered positive calcium balance with evident bone healing. If the hypercalcemia merely represents an "estrogen flare" to be followed by tumor regression as was demonstrated in this case, then one may carry the patient over the critical period with appropriate fluid and corticosteroid therapy. On the other hand, if the estrogen therapy appears to provide impetus for tumor growth, it should be stopped and other therapeutic measures substituted. Beckett (1969) discussed 36 postmenopausal breast cancer patients of whom 7 displayed hypercalcemia. Those seven, with an average age of 46, tended to be younger and to have more rapidly progressive disease than patients without hypercalcemia. The author suggests that this type of patient not be continued on estrogens but rather be considered for ablative or cytotoxic therapy.

Researchers have also implicated androgens (Myers *et al.*, 1956) and progestational agents (Kaufman *et al.*, 1964) in hypercalcemia. Those investigators suggested that testosterone-induced blood calcium elevation was due to hepatic conversion of the androgen to an estrogenic substance. Jessiman *et al.*, (1963) have proposed a similar mechanism. However, there have been numerous reports of favorable responses to testosterone after estrogen failure and even of hypercalcemia induced by testosterone after initial successful therapy with the hormone (Muirhead, 1967; Kennedy *et al.*, 1953). There is no evidence that progesterones are interconverted to estrogenic substances. With recent advances in combination chemotherapy for breast cancer and its institution at earlier phases in the disease, hormone-induced hypercalcemia should be seen less frequently.

When hypercalcemia occurs in a breast cancer patient receiving hormonal therapy, it is often advisable to change to a different form of treatment or perform an ablative procedure. Prednisone (30–60 mg/

day) is often effective in controlling the hypercalcemia either by a direct effect on the tumor itself or on bone, or because of unknown factors created by the new hormonal environment. In rare cases (Muirhead, 1967) estrogen therapy may succeed where corticosteroids have failed.

B. Myeloma, Leukemia, and Lymphoma

Osteolytic lesions of multiple myeloma associated with extensive bone destruction are responsible for the elevation of either the serum or urinary calcium at some time in the course of almost all patients with this disease. A new mechanism for the production of hypercalcemia in multiple myeloma has been proposed (Luben *et al.*, 1974) vide infra.

In Myers' (1960) series, patients with myeloma, leukemia, and lymphoma accounted for 13% of the total number of patients. This relatively high frequency may have been due to the nature of the patients referred to Memorial Hospital. Nevertheless, the osteolytic lesions of multiple myeloma and extensive bone destruction are associated with elevation of either the serum or urinary calcium at some time in the course of almost all patients with this disease. Hypercalcemia may be accentuated by immobilization due to pathologic fractures that often occur (Chapter 6, Volume I). Furthermore, the effects of hypercalcemia on renal function may further compromise kidneys that are already damaged by deposits of myeloma proteins, amyloid, or uric acid.

Less often appreciated is the occasional association of hypercalcemia with leukemia. It has been described with acute, subacute, and chronic leukemias of both lymphatic and myelogenous types (Mawdsley and Holman, 1957; Kronfield and Reynold, 1964; Knisley, 1964; Benvenisti *et al.*, 1969; Ballard and Marcus, 1970; Buer, 1970; Haskell *et al.*, 1971; Stein, 1971). Hypercalcemia may be a premonitory sign in blastic transformation of the chronic leukemias (Steinberg *et al.*, 1971; Steinberg, 1972) or a presenting symptom in acute leukemia. Since the diagnosis of malignancy may be missed on examination of the peripheral smear, some patients presenting with hypercalcemia have undergone parathyroidectomy before the appropriate bone marrow examination was made (Jordan, 1966). A recent report (Zidar *et al.*, 1976) suggests that leukemic cells may occasionally produce parathyroid hormone.

Elevated calcium concentrations have been described with reticulum cell sarcoma, lymphosarcoma, cutaneous lymphosarcoma, and Hodgkin's disease (Krabakow *et al.*, 1957; Moses and Spencer, 1963; Dube *et al.*, 1968; Anonymous, 1970; Canellos, 1974) and is, in general, associated with destructive lesions of bone, although ectopic production of parathyroid hormone has been reported (Sherwood *et al.*, 1967).

C. Lung Tumors and Others Associated with Hypercalcemia.

In addition to breast cancer, tumors of the bronchus, kidney, prostate, thyroid and cervix are the ones that metastasize most frequently to bone. In the male, carcinoma of the lung is the most frequent cause of cancer-associated hypercalcemia. In a study of 200 patients with untreated bronchogenic carcinoma, Bender and Hansen (1974) reported a frequency of hypercalcemia of 12.5%. Twenty-three percent of patients with epidermoid, 12.7% with anaplastic, 2.5% with adeno, and none with small cell carcinoma had hypercalcemia. Fifty-six percent with hypercalcemia did not have osseous metastases, and small cell carcinoma which most commonly metastasized to bone was not associated with an increased calcium.

IV. PATHOGENESIS OF TUMOR-ASSOCIATED HYPERCALCEMIA

A. Calcium Balance Considerations

As noted in Chapter 1, Volume I, the concentration of calcium in the plasma reflects a dynamic equilibrium between calcium and phosphate ions in the extracellular fluid (which exist in saturated or near saturated solution) and the corresponding ions in the labile mineral pool of bone. Superimposed on this basic physical-chemical equilibrium is the negative feedback control for serum calcium produced by the parathyroid glands. Contributing to the overall dynamic state are oral intake of calcium, urinary and fecal losses, vitamin D and its metabolites and varying rates of skeletal turnover. Parathyroid hormone and vitamin D work in concert to maintain the normal mobilization of calcium and phosphate from bone, while vitamin D, in addition, enhances intestinal transport of calcium. Through its effects on the renal tubular handling of calcium, phosphate and bicarbonate, parathyroid hormone further modulates calcium homeostasis. Although calcitonin has been shown to have an effect antagonistic to that of parathyroid hormone in that it blocks the exit of mineral from bone, it is probably not a major factor in calcium homeostasis in adult man (Sherwood, 1967; Schneider and Sherwood, 1974; Chapter 8).

Based on the above considerations, hypercalcemia would occur under the following circumstances: (1) where there is an excess of parathyroid hormone due to primary hyperparathyroidism or to a tumor that produces parathyroid hormone or another calcium-mobilizing substance, thereby disrupting the normal negative feedback mechanisms; (2) excessive quantities or sensitivity to vitamin D, thereby causing enhanced mobilization of calcium from bone and transport of calcium across the gastrointestinal mucosa; and (3) increases in skeletal turnover caused by the presence of abnormal tumor tissue or increased metabolic activity of bone such as in hyperthyroidism or immobilization. When the kidneys are unable to excrete all of the additional calcium added to the extracellular fluid by excessive intestinal absorption or increased bone breakdown, hypercalciuria is soon followed by hypercalcemia. In patients with excessive quantities of parathyroid hormone, hypercalcemia is present at lower levels of urinary calcium because the effect of the hormone is to increase tubular levels of urinary calcium (see Chapter 2, Volume I, and Chapter 1, this volume).

Myers (1962) stressed the difference between "equilibrium" and "balance." Calcium balance refers to the net change in total body calcium, which amounts to the net traffic in skeletal calcium, since 99% of body calcium is in the bones. The typical cancer patient with osteolytic metastasis, for example, might be hypercalcemic and in negative calcium balance. Adequate hydration which restored normocalcemia would still leave the patient in negative balance. Accelerated resorption of bone is also reflected in increased excretion of the hydroxyproline in the urine (Bonadonna et al., 1966). Furthermore, studies of patients on metabolic units (Pearson, 1964; Myers, 1972) have shown that when skeletal metastasis has occurred, both bone accretion and breakdown rates are increased over their normal values of 400–500 mg/day. Even in the normocalcemic patient in neutral calcium balance, the miscible calcium pool may be increased as a new equilibrium point is established (see Table II).

B. Mechanisms of Tumor-Associated Hypercalcemia

Most tumors produce hypercalcemia by direct invasion of bone. Osteolytic lesions may be demonstrable by routine radiologic studies but the lesion must be greater than 1 cm in size to be seen and, in one series, only 50% of the histologically demonstrable lesions were found by routine radiographs (Bachman and Sproule, 1955). With the new nuclear medicine techniques of radioactive scanning, accuracy has been improved considerably. Bone marrow biopsy may also be helpful in establishing the presence of skeletal metastasis (Hyman, 1955), but negative findings obviously do not rule out malignant invasion of bone. Often the presence of bony metastasis is established only after painstaking postmortem study.

TABLE II

Calcium Homeostasis in Normal and Pathologic States

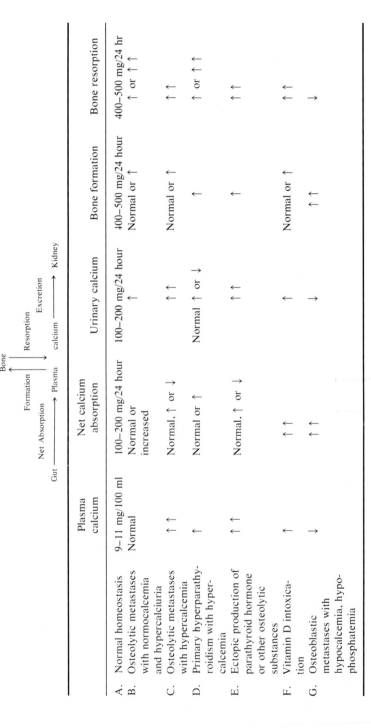

Gut ——Net Absorption——→ Plasma · Bone (Formation ←— / Resorption —→) · calcium ——Excretion——→ Kidney

	Plasma calcium	Net calcium absorption	Urinary calcium	Bone formation	Bone resorption
A. Normal homeostasis	9–11 mg/100 ml	100–200 mg/24 hour	100–200 mg/24 hour	400–500 mg/24 hour	400–500 mg/24 hr
B. Osteolytic metastases with normocalcemia and hypercalciuria	Normal	Normal or increased	↑	Normal or ↑	↑ or ↑↑
C. Osteolytic metastases with hypercalcemia	↑↑	Normal, ↑ or ↓	↑↑	Normal or ↑	↑↑
D. Primary hyperparathyroidism with hypercalcemia	↑	Normal or ↑	Normal, ↑ or ↓	↑	↑ or ↑↑
E. Ectopic production of parathyroid hormone or other osteolytic substances	↑↑	Normal, ↑ or ↓	↑↑	↑	↑↑
F. Vitamin D intoxication	↑	↑↑	↑	Normal or ↑	↑↑
G. Osteoblastic metastases with hypocalcemia, hypophosphatemia	↓	↑↑	↓	↑↑	↓

Primary hyperparathyroidism is occasionally present with back pain and vertebral fractures. This does not necessarily imply the presence of a metastatic neoplasm (Dauphine *et al.*, 1975).

Von Recklinghausen's original description (1891) of the progress of skeletal metastases is probably still valid today: (1) they are blood-borne; (2) they appear first in the marrow cavity; (3) subperiosteal extensions develop chiefly where main foramina traverse the cortical bone; (4) bones affected in order of frequency are vertebrae, proximal femurs, pelvis, ribs, sternum, proximal humerus, and the skull.

In addition to direct invasion of bone, a variety of other mechanisms have been proposed as the basis for cancer-related hypercalcemia. Although there have been reports of increased tubular reabsorption of calcium in cancer patients, thought not to have ectopic parathyroid hormone production (Nordin and Peacock, 1969), it is unlikely that the kidney plays any significant direct role. It has been suggested that increased protein binding might account for some elevation of the total serum calcium, but studies by Walser (1962) have dispelled this idea. A possible exception occurs in a rare multiple myeloma patient. In one recently reported case of multiple myeloma, the ionized calcium was normal while the total serum calcium was as high as 7.2 mEq/liter (Lindegarde and Zettervall, 1973). Although hypercitricemia has been reported with some tumors (Rottino *et al.*, 1952; Lemon and Kotob, 1961), there is no evidence to date that this chemical abnormality accounts for the hypercalcemia. Conceivably, malignant tumors could in some way interfere with the action of calcitonin on bone, thus promoting skeletal breakdown. In adult man, however, complete absence of this recently recognized hormone leads to no difficulties in skeletal or calcium homeostasis (Schneider and Sherwood, 1974).

Implants of breast and lung cancer placed against the rat calvarium produce intense osteolysis whereas normal breast and lung tissue do not (Gordan *et al.*, 1962). Since some breast cancers contain esters of stigmasterol and 7-dehydrositosterol, lipids that possess osteolytic activity in parathyroidectomized rats, it has been suggested that those substances might be responsible for hypercalcemia (Gordan *et al.*, 1966, 1967). However, since those sterols also occur in animal tumors not associated with hypercalcemia and are components of the normal diet, there is some question as to what role, if any, they may play in the production of abnormal calcium metabolism (Rice, 1969; Rice *et al.*, 1971). Haddad *et al.* (1970) have shown, in fact, that the levels of phytosterols in serum and breast tissue did not differ among normal females, lactating mothers, and patients with breast cancer.

The idea that malignant tumors might produce a substance that would induce parathyroid hyperplasia was first advanced by Klemperer (1923). Stone *et al.* (1961) revived interest in that theory and suggested that subtotal parathyroidectomy might be indicated in certain patients with cancer. There have been many reports of parathyroid hyperplasia or adenomas accompanying malignant tumors (Dent and Watson, 1964; Huvos *et al.*, 1969; Katz *et al.*, 1970), but there seems to be no reason for invoking the presence of a parathyrotropic hormone or to ascribe any more than a coincidental association in these instances (Anderson *et al.*, 1962; Kohout, 1966; Grimes *et al.*, 1967; Rothschild *et al.*, 1964). Myers (1972) described a woman with cancer of the cervix associated with hypercalcemia and hypophosphatemia. Because the possibility of a coexistenting parathyroid adenoma was considered, the patient underwent neck exploration. Although four normal glands were found, total parathyroidectomy was performed in an unsuccessful effort to control the serum calcium. In that instance, the parathyroid glands were clearly not involved in the production of the hypercalcemia.

Homotransplants of rabbit VX2 carcinoma regularly induce hypercalcemia without demonstrable bone metastases. In this interesting animal model, it was found that thyroparathyroidectomy did not affect the ability of the tumor to induce and maintain hypercalcemia. These data tend to contradict the notion that a parathyrotropic substance is involved and instead support the concept that some malignant tumors may elaborate osteolytic substances that act directly on bone (Vogel *et al.*, 1967) (vide infra).

Rice (1969) has described an interesting testicular tumor in rodents that produces hypercalcemia in response to gonadotropin administration. The tumor did not contain parathyroid hormone and presumably produced an osteolytic substance responsible for the elevation of the serum calcium.

More recently, Tashjian *et al.* (1972) reported that a transplantable mouse fibrosarcoma, which enhanced the resorption of bone in tissue culture, was synthesizing and secreting large quantities of a bone resorption-stimulating prostaglandin E_2. Voelkel *et al.* (1975) recently demonstrated that rabbits bearing the VX2 carcinoma also produce the prostaglandin. Evidence to support the etiology of hypercalcemia from prostaglandins in the two animal models is as follows (Tashjian 1974, 1975): (1) hypercalcemia is associated with animal tumors that do not usually metastasize to bone; (2) there is a high content of bone-resorbing activity and PGE_2 in tumor tissue extracts; (3) tumor cells in cloned-tissue culture release large amounts of bone-resorbing activity and PGE_2; (4) decreases in production of PGE_2 are found in cell culture and in animals with indomethacin, an inhibitor of prostaglandin synthesis; (5) parallel decreases in calcium and PGE_2 occur when indomethacin is administered to tumor-bearing animals that are hypercalcemic; (6) there are increased concentrations of PGE_2 in the venous drainage from the tumor; (7) infusion of PGE_2 into rats under certain experimental conditions will produce hypercalcemia (Franklin and Tashjian, 1975). Raisz *et al.* (1975) have recently noted that some of the components of complement will stimulate the synthesis of PGE_2 locally, providing an additional mechanism for stimulating bone resorption. Bennet *et al* (1975) have speculated that prostaglandin production by malignant breast tumors may facilitate metastasis to bone.

Luben *et al.* (1974) reported a new bone-resorbing factor from human lymphocytes that they named osteoclast-activating factor (OAF). It is a soluble mediator of bone resorption identified in the supernatant fluid from human peripheral leukocytes cultured in the presence of antigen or phytomitogen. In organ culture, OAF has been a potent stimulator of osteoclastic resorption of fetal bone. It appears to be a low molecular weight protein (less than 25,000 daltons), but it has not yet been purified to homogenous form. OAF activity has been found in the supernatant fluid from cultured lymphoid cell lines from patients with multiple myeloma, Burkitt's lymphoma, and malignant lymphoma, but not in cell lines from normal subjects or patients with other neoplasms (Mundy *et al.*, 1974, 1975). Bone-resorbing activity could be distinguished from PGE_2, parathyroid hormone, and vitamin D-like compounds on the basis of dose–response curves. OAF activity also appears to be sensitive to inhibition by glucocorticoids, and it can cause prolonged resorption of fetal rat bone after brief exposure (Raisz *et al.*, 1975). There may be both large and small molecular weight forms of OAF.

C. Ectopic Parathyroid Hormone Production

There is considerable evidence that some malignant cells are able to produce hormones (Table III). Thus, it is believed that specific genetic repressors, instituted at some indeterminate time in development, are apparently removed and the genetic information usually available for transcription only to specialized endocrine cells is utilized by cells originating from other tissues (Gellhorn, 1958, 1969). Roof *et al.* (1971) have raised objections to the depressor-deletion theory on two grounds. Their objection that ectopic parathyroid hormone production is specific for only certain tumors is not a valid objection since the theory does not imply an all-or-none concept. Furthermore, there are recent reports (Mavligit *et al.,* 1971; Melick *et al.,* 1972) of the production of parathyroid hormone by breast cancer, cited by Roof *et al.* (1971) as an example of a nonproducer of parathyroid hormone. Their second point, that cancer-associated hormones appear to have characteristics different from the native hormone, is discussed below.

TABLE III

Nonparathyroid Tumors Believed to Be Associated with Ectopic Production of Parathyroid Hormone or Other Osteolytic Substance[a]

I. Lung
  A. Squamous cell carcinoma
    Conner et al. (1956)
    Case Records (1957)
    Gold and Shnider (1959)
    Carey (1962)
    Fry (1962)
    Meador et al. (1962)
    Lafferty and Pearson (1963)
    Case Records (1964)
    Gault and Kinsella (1965)
    Horeau et al. (1965)
    Taylor and Siemsen (1965)
    Berson and Yaww (1966)[b]
    Turkington et al. (1966)
    Daughtry et al. (1967)
    Sherwood et al. (1967)[b]
    Omenn et al. (1969)[b]
    Sherwood (1971)
    Bender and Hansen (1974)
    Benson et al. (1974)[b]
    Palmieri et al. (1974)[b]
    Seyberth et al. (1975)[c]
  B. Other
    Bender and Hansen (1974)
    Gutman et al. (1936)
    Myers (1962)
    Tashjian et al. (1964)
    Sherwood et al. (1967)[b]
    Robertson et al. (1976)[c]
    Seyberth et al. (1975)[c]
II. Genitourinary and adrenal
  A. Renal cell carcinoma
    Case Records (1941)
    Plimpton and Gellhorn (1956)
    Alanis and Flanagan (1959)
    Borm (1961)
    Case Records (1961a)
    Case Records (1961b)
    David et al. (1962)
    Pinals and Krane (1962)
    Goldberg et al. (1964)[b]
    Lamberg et al. (1964)
    Tashjian et al. (1964)
    Tremblay and Ansell (1964)
    Lytton et al. (1965)[b]
    Thomas and Karat (1966)
    O'Grady et al. (1965)[b]

    Omenn et al. (1969)[b]
    Buckle et al. (1970)[b]
    Blair et al. (1973)[b]
    Benson et al. (1974)[b]
    Brereton et al. (1974)[c]
    Robertson et al. (1975)[c]
    Ito et al. (1975)[c]
    Robertson et al. (1976)[c]
  B. Renal pelvis
    1. Transitional cell
      Bourne et al. (1964)
    2. Squamous cell
      Dean et al. (1969)
  C. Bladder
    Cope et al. (1961)
    Loebel and Walkoff (1962)
    Svane (1964)
  D. Testes
    1. Anaplastic
      Omenn (1971)
    2. Seminoma
      King et al. (1972)
  E. Penis—squamous cell
    Anderson and Glenn (1965)
    Rudd (1972)
  F. Adrenal
    Sherwood et al. (1967)[b]
  G. Ovary
    1. Undifferentiated carcinoma
      Omenn et al. (1969)
    2. Papillary cystadenoma
      Plimpton and Gellhorn (1956)
      Noeninckx and Van Laethem (1962)
      Seifert and Seeman (1967)
      McGahey and Raker (as cited in
        Omenn et al., 1969)
    3. Hypernephroid carcinoma
      Abouav et al. (1959)
    4. Malignant dysgerminoma
      Breidal and Ritchie (1962)
    5. Mesonephroma
      Ross and Shelley (1968)
      Smith et al (1968)
      Ferenczy et al. (1971)
  H. Uterus
    1. Stromal cell carcinoma
      Orlando and Macanic (1972)
    2. Endometrial carcinoma

596

(Continued)

TABLE III *(Continued)*

Plimpton and Gellhorn (1956)
Horeau *et al*. (1965)
3. Leiomyosarcoma
    Seftel and Gusberg (1965)
I. Cervix
    Stone *et al*. (1961)
J. Vulva—squamous cell sarcoma
    Schatten *et al*. (1968)
    Omenn *et al*. (1969)
III. Breast
    Mavligit *et al*. (1971)[b]
    Melick *et al*. (1972)[b]
IV. Lymphoma and leukemia
    A. Acute leukemia
        Neiman and Li (1972)
        Zidar *et al*. (1976)
    B. Lymphoma
        1. Hodgkin's disease
            Plimpton and Gellhorn (1956)
        2. Lymphosarcoma
            Myers (1956a)
            Plimpton and Gellhorn (1956)
        3. Reticulum cell sarcoma
            Sherwood *et al*. (1967)[b]
        4. Burkitt's lymphoma
            Mundy *et al*. (1974)[d]
    C. Multiple Myeloma
        Mundy *et al*. (1974, 1975)[d]
V. Gastrointestinal
    A. Colon
        Case Records (1963)[b]
        Omenn *et al*. (1969)
        Benson *et al*. (1974)[b]
    B. Esophagus and Stomach
        Snedecor and Baker (1964)
        Deftos *et al*. (1976)[b]
        Robertson *et al*. (1976)[c]

C. Pancreatic carcinoma
    Lucas (1960)
    Magnenat and Perret (1961)
    Snedecor and Baker (1964)
    Tashjian *et al*. (1964)
    Albert *et al*. (1969)
    Omenn *et al*. (1969)[b]
    Palmieri *et al*. (1974) (islet cell)
    Seyberth *et al*. (1975)[c]
    Deftos *et al*. (1976)[b]
D. Liver and biliary
    1. Hepatoma
        Keller *et al*. (1966)
        Knill-Jones *et al*. (1970)[b]
    2. Hepatoblastoma
        Tashjian (1969)[b]
    3. Hemangiosarcoma
        Case Records (1953)
        Case Records (1967)
    4. Cholangiocarcinoma
        Samuelsson and Werner (1963)
        Anonymous (1967)
        Naide *et al*. (1968)
        Palmieri *et al*. (1974)[b]
VI. Other
    A. Parotid (anaplastic)
        Sherwood *et al*. (1967)[b]
        Robertson *et al*. (1976)[c]
    B. Melanoma
        Menguy (1969)
    C. Retroperitoneal sarcoma
        Melick *et al*. (1972)[b]
    D. Epidermoid
        1. Floor of mouth
            Deconti (1971)
        2. Alveolar ridge
            Omenn *et al*. (1969)

[a] The above table includes several groups of tumors.

[b] In one group immunochemical identification of a parathyroid hormone-like material in serum or tumor has been provided. In others, this has not been tested and the diagnosis of ectopic parathyroid hormone production has been suggested on clinical grounds. It is likely that some of these cases would fall into the category of patients recently suggested by Powell *et al*. (1973) in which a calcium-mobilizing substance other than parathyroid hormone (but as yet unidentified) is present. The 11 patients described by Powell *et al*. include 4 with carcinoma of the lung, 2 with renal cell carcinoma, 2 with ovarian carcinoma, and 1 each with pancreatic carcinoma, reticulum cell sarcoma, and mammary dysplasia with intraductal papillomatosis. In retrospect these may contain a prostaglandin that mobilized calcium.

[c] Indicates confirmation of prostaglandin in serum or tumor.

[d] Indicates presence of osteoclast activating factor.

The first description of the ectopic hormone syndrome was that of an oat cell carcinoma of the lung with features of Cushing's syndrome (Brown, 1928). Since then, numerous reviews on the subject have appeared (Lipsett *et al.*, 1964; Lipsett, 1968; Hobbs, 1968; Myers *et al.*, 1956; Bower and Gordon, 1965; Wyss *et al.*, 1971; DiLollo *et al.*, 1969; Pietrek, 1969; Leprat, 1969; Lista, 1966; Sherwood, 1976). Production of a humoral substance has been implicated in neoplasms associated with inappropriate antidiuresis, hypoglycemia, hyperadrenocorticism, hyperparathyroidism, precocious puberty, erythrocytosis, hyperthyroidism and other syndromes. The initial metabolic error for each of those disorders might be explained by the actions of a single polypeptide. None of the nonprotein hormones have been identified in neoplasms of tissues other than those in which the hormones are normally produced. Thus, Cushing's syndrome occurring with nonadrenal tumors results from *de novo* production of ACTH rather than from synthesis of corticosteroids. It is not illogical to propose that *de novo* synthesis of a polypeptide in any metabolically active cell already geared for protein synthesis is more likely, since it would require only a small adjustment in messenger RNA synthesis. On the other hand, for a nonsteroid-producing cell to initiate the production of a steroid molecule would require the mobilization of a vast synthetic machinery involving a complex brigade of enzymes.

In 1941, Albright discussed a now famous patient, a 51-year-old male with a renal cell carcinoma associated with hypercalcemia and hypophosphatemia. Three normal parathyroid glands were found during neck exploration. When a large osteolytic lesion in the ilium was irradiated, the serum calcium returned to normal and the phosporous rose. Although the crude bioassay available at that time was negative, Albright hypothesized that the tumor might have produced its metabolic effects by elaborating a parathyroid hormone-like substance.

Five years earlier, in a patient with bronchial carcinoma, Gutman *et al.* (1936) had described a patient with cancer and hypercalcemia, but without skeletal metastases. Plimpton and Gellhorn (1956) added 10 more patients, including 4 patients with hypernephroma, in which there were similar findings. In three of their patients, surgical resection of the tumors resulted in return of the serum calcium to normal. Similar results were described by Connor *et al.* (1956) in two patients with lung cancer. In one patient regrowth of the tumor 4 months after surgery was associated with recurrent hypercalcemia. Just before death, the serum calcium fell, and at postmortem examination, the tumor was necrotic. In the experimental model described above, rabbits receiving transplants of VX2 carcinoma developed hypercalcemia and hypophosphatemia in the absence of roentgenographic evidence of skeletal metastases. If the tumor was rejected, the abnormalities of calcium and phosphorus metabolism were reversed. When the bones were examined at postmortem, parathyroid-hormone-like bone resorption without evidence of tumor invasion was found (Wilson *et al.*, 1961). It is now known that osteolysis was due to prostaglandins, not parathyroid hormone (Voelkel, 1975).

The first firm evidence for the ectopic production of a parathyroid hormone-like substance was provided by Goldberg *et al.* (1964), who reported a positive parathyroid hormone assay in the primacy tumor and a metastasis of a renal adenocarcinoma. The same group of investigators (Tashjian *et al.*, 1964; Munson *et al.*, 1965) later obtained positive immunologic assays for parathyroid hormone in pancreas, lung, and colpn cancers. These studies, however, were based on complement fixation inhibition rather than direct assay. Sherwood *et al.* (1967), using a radioimmunoassay, were first able to measure a parathyroid hormone-like substance quantitatively in four lung cancers, an anaplastic parotid tumor, an adrenal adenocarcinoma, and a reticulum cell sarcoma (Figs. 1 and 2).

It has been suggested that malignant tumors might have an avidity for certain hormones, acting thereby as hormone "sponges" (Unger and Lochner, 1964). To maintain that such a trapping mechanism exists is to suppose that a tumor can extract the hormone from blood so efficiently as to concentrate it to more than a thousand times the plasma level. Furthermore, evidence to dispute that theory was provided in a case reported by Knill-Jones *et al.* (1970). An arteriovenous gradient of parathyroid hormone across a carcinoma of the intrahepatic bile ducts was demonstrated in a patient whose calcium and phosphorus blood levels of 17.6 and 1.4 mg/100 ml, respectively, returned to normal following resection and liver transplant. Similarly, circulating concentrations of immunoassayable parathyroid hormone were elevated before surgery and fell to normal after the transplant. Blood samples taken in the operating room showed a significant rise in the hormone concentration from the hepatic artery and portal vein to the hepatic vein.

Clinical observations that have supported the concept that parathyroid hormone may be produced in tumors of hypercalcemic patients include the following (Table III): (1) absence of skeletal metastases; (2) hypophosphatemia; (3) normal parathyroid glands found during surgery or at postmortem examination; (4) return to normocalcemia with surgical extirpation or radiation therapy of the tumor; (5) recurrence of hypercalcemia with renewed tumor growth; (6) immunoassay.

Gellhorn (1969) suggested that firmer support for the concept would be supplied by (1) isolation of sufficient material in purified form to permit amino acid sequence analysis so that identity with native parathyroid hormone could be established and (2) demonstration of net synthesis of

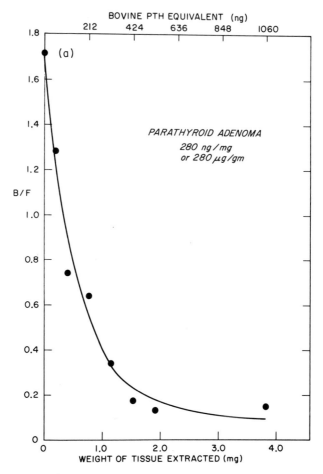

Fig. 1. Comparison of radioimmunoassay curves for extract of parathyroid adenoma (a) and adrenal carcinoma (b) from patients with hypercalcemia. The ordinate indicates the ratio of labeled parathyroid hormone bound and free (B/F) in radioimmunoassay and displacement by increasing quantities of tissue extract.

the hormone in tissue culture. The latter has been reported by Tashjian (1969) who established a clonal line from free floating cells in the ascitic fluid of a patient with a hepatoblastoma. Those cells secreted immunoassayable parathyroid hormone for several months *in vitro*. With serial propagation, however, the cells lost their parathyroid hormone-secreting ability. Gellhorn's first requirement, the establishment of identity with native parathyroid hormone, has never been satisfied. In the studies of Sherwood *et al.* (1967), the protein extracted from the tumors was identi-

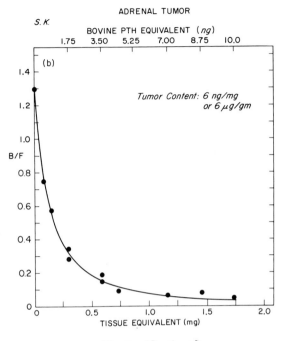

Fig. 1.   (*Continued*)

cal in immunologic activity and molecular weight to native parathyroid hormone (Figs. 1–3).

In the reviews of ectopic parathyroid hormone production (or pseudohyperparathyroidism) by Lafferty (1966) and Omenn *et al.* (1969), hypernephroma and bronchogenic carcinoma together accounted for well over half of the neoplasms reported (Table III). Lung cancer was the most common of the ectopic hormone-producing tumors. A greater number and variety of hormones have been produced by pulmonary neoplasms than by any other single tumor.

In an unselected series of 185 patients with histologically confirmed bronchial carcinoma, 16 were found to have associated endocrine disturbances. Eleven patients were hypercalcemic, three showed inappropriate antidiuresis, three had hypertrophic osteoarthropathy, one had Cushing's syndrome, and one showed gynecomastia (Azzopardi *et al.*, 1970). Sixteen percent of their patients coming to necropsy had hypercalcemia in the absence of skeletal metastases (Azzopardi and Whittaker, 1969). Berson and Yalow (1966) found higher than normal concentrations of parathyroid hormone in a significant number of patients with bronchogenic carcinoma even when they were not hypercalcemic. Amatruda

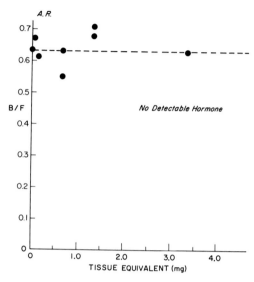

Fig. 2. Radioimmunoassay study of tumor extract from a patient with carcinoma of the lung and hypercalcemia due to metastasis to bone. No parathyroid hormone-like material was present.

(1969) and others (Omenn *et al.*, 1969; Raymond, 1968; Sperber, 1969; Turkington *et al.*, 1966) have emphasized an association between squamous cell tumors and hypercalcemia, on the one hand, and oat cell carcinoma and hyperadrenocorticism and inappropriate antidiuresis, on the other. Recent studies (Gewirtz and Yalow, 1974) have suggested that ACTH may be present radioimmunoassay in a much wider variety of lung tumors than previously shown. Azzopardi and Whittaker (1969) suggested that surgical material might be biased in favor of squamous cell tumors because of their greater resectability. The highly malignant nature of oat cell tumors makes them more likely to be associated with widespread metastases. Nevertheless, there does appear to be an empiric correlation between the squamous cell and possibly large cell type of lung cancer and ectopic hypercalcemia (Bender and Hansen, 1974). Other reports of hyperparathyroid-like states with bronchogenic tumors include those of Carey (1966), Taylor and Siemsen (1965), Cragg (1971), and Case Records (1957, 1970).

Table III includes the list of tumors other than lung and kidney in which a hyperparathyroid-like or hypercalcemic state has been reported.

The problem of distinguishing between primary hyperparathyroidism and ectopic production of the hormone arises when a patient presents with hypercalcemia and a lower than normal serum inorganic phosphorus. According to Lafferty (1966), cancer, rather than disease of the

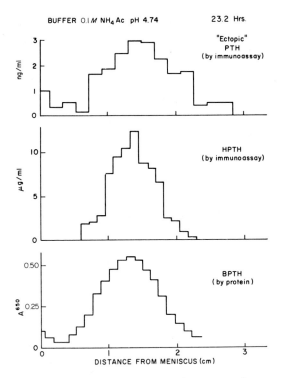

Fig. 3. Sedimentation rates for ectopic parathyroid hormone in tumor extract ("Ectopic" PTH), extract of human parathyroid adenoma (HPTH), and purified bovine hormone (BPTH) in sucrose density gradient in preparative ultracentrifuge. Sedimentation was performed in an SW-65 swinging bucket rotor at 65,000 rpm for 23.2 hours in ammonium acetate buffer (Sherwood *et al.*, 1967).

parathyroid glands, is the more likely diagnosis if (1) anemia is present, (2) the serum chloride level is less than 102 mEq/liter in a patient who is not vomiting and does not have respiratory acidosis, (3) the serum calcium is greater than 14 mg/100 ml, (4) the patient is male, (5) renal calculi are not present, and (6) the alkaline phosphatase is more than 20 King-Armstrong units, as this probably reflects liver rather than bone disease. Osteitis fibrosa cystica was present in only 2 of the 35 cases reviewed by this author. The differences in the frequency of bone changes in ectopic and primary hyperparathyroidism are most likely related to the duration of the disease (see Chapter 1). Patients with malignant tumors probably succumb to complications of their cancer before the diffuse skeletal reabsorption characteristic of parathyroid excess can develop. However, several patients with typical hyperparathyroid bone changes have been reported (Albert *et al.*, 1969; Azzopardi and Whittaker, 1969; Lamberg *et al.*, 1964). In one patient with Hodgkins disease and ectopic production of

parathyroid hormone, both recurrent renal calculi and typical subperiosteal bone resorption were manifest (Scholz et al., 1973).

The situation is complicated by the more than occasional coexistence of
primary hyperparathyroidism and a malignant tumor. Of the 50 patients
with primary hyperparathyroidism seen at Memorial Hospital, there were
12 with coexistenting neoplasms (Fahey and Myers, 1972). This series was
heavily skewed by the nature of the patients referred to the hospital.
Myers (1972) reports that hypophosphatemia occurs more frequently with
lung or kidney cancers than with lymphomas, myeloma, or breast carcinoma. He suggests, therefore, that a low serum phosphorus in a patient
with one of the latter diseases should cause the physician to consider
coexistenting primary hyperparathyroidism. In a series of 388 patients with
breast cancer, hypophosphatemia was found in only 3, all of whom had
coexistenting parathyroid adenomas (Gordan et al., 1962). In addition,
calcium ion has an effect on renal phosphate clearance independent of
hormones (Eisenberg, 1965; Schussler et al., 1972).

D. New Hypercalcemic Syndrome

One of us (Sherwood, 1971) discussed a case of squamous cell carcinoma of the lung associated with hypercalcemia at a clinicopathologic
conference. Despite the presence of hypophosphatemia and the absence
of skeletal metastases at both roentgenographic and postmortem examinations, no immunoassayable parathyroid hormone was detected in the
tumor or the peripheral blood. Subsequently, Powell et al. (1972a) reported five patients with tumors associated with hypercalcemia and
hypophosphatemia in the absence of demonstrable bone metastases. In all
patients, surgical treatment, radiation, or chemotherapeutic ablation reversed the biochemical abnormalities. Bone resorption was demonstrated
by tumor extracts from three patients in an in vitro mouse calvarium
bioassay. Despite these findings, radioimmunoassay for parathyroid hormone was negative in tumor extracts and the peripheral blood from all five
patients, one of whom has recently been described in detail (Singer et al.,
1973). It appears that some other humoral substance, distinct from
parathyroid hormone (and possibly a prostaglandin) was generated by
these tumors. The series of such patients was increased to 11 (Powell et
al., 1973), but the biologically active factor was not identified.

There is now evidence that some patients who have ectopic hypercalcemia without evidence for excessive parathyroid hormone are producing
prostaglandin in their tumor tissue. The first clinical evidence was provided by Brereton et al. (1974), who described a patient with renal cell
carcinoma and hypercalcemia which responded to treatment with indomethacin. High concentrations of prostaglandin E- and F-like materials

were found in liver metastases from the tumor. In a second report by Robertson *et al.* (1975), a patient with renal cell carcinoma and hypercalcemia had elevated levels of immunoreactive PGE in the plasma and low levels of parathyroid hormone. A third patient (Ito *et al.*, 1975) with renal cell carcinoma had decreasing serum calcium concentrations with indomethacin therapy, but no prostaglandin measurements were made. The most extensive report was by Seyberth *et al.* (1975) who studied 29 patients with solid tumors, 14 of whom had hypercalcemia. Their control group included 6 patients with hyperparathyroidism and 6 with hypercalcemia and malignant hematologic disorders. There were significant elevations of PGE-M, a metabolite of prostaglandins E_1 and E_2, in the urine of 12 of 14 hypercalcemic patients and only modest elevations in 7 of the 15 tumor patients with a normal serum calcium. Normal levels of the metabolite were found in the control subjects. Undetectable levels of parathyroid hormone were found in the blood of patients with hypercalcemia. Treatment with indomethacin or aspirin resulted in a decrease in PGE-M excretion but a variable decrease in serum calcium. Although these observations did not establish whether the tumor or some other tissue was the source of the prostaglandin, they established more firmly the relationship between tumor hypercalcemia and prostaglandins. Robertson *et al.* (1976), reported elevated immunoreactive PGE in 4 of 11 hypercalcemic cancer patients who also had low parathyroid (PTH) values. Further studies of prostaglandins and other tumor osteolytic substances are necessary to clarify their frequency in states of malignancy and hypercalcemia. It is possible that production of PGE or other calcium-mobilizing substances may be more common than parathyroid hormone as a cause of ectopic hyperplasia.

E. Differential Diagnosis

In the patient with severe hypercalcemia, the difficulties in differential diagnosis usually center around the question of primary hyperparathyroidism or hypercalcemia in association with malignancy (with or without metastases). Other disorders such as sarcoidosis, vitamin D intoxication, hyperthyroidism, and the milk alkali syndrome are usually readily excluded by history or simple laboratory tests. Although the radioimmunoassay for parathyroid hormone has become more widely available and better established as a diagnostic tool, persistent elevation of the serum calcium in the absence of other known causes remains the best diagnostic clue to the diagnosis of primary hyperparathyroidism. In differentiating primary disease of the parathyroid glands from malignancy, the following points should be considered:

1. *The degree of hypercalcemia.* The majority of patients with primary hyperparathyroidism have only mild elevations of the serum calcium (up to 12.5 mg/100 ml) unless they have very large adenomas or are subjected to immobilization or acute dehydration (see Chapter 1, Volume 1). Marked elevations of the serum calcium are more common in patients with ectopic hypercalcemia or with metastatic bone disease.

2. *The presences of hypophosphatemia.* Hypophosphatemia was present in 46% of 682 patients with primary hyperparathyroidism (Strott and Nugent, 1968). It is less common in patients with malignancy. But it has been well described in ectopic hypercalcemia states. The diagnostic value of the serum inorganic phosphorus is diminished in patients with renal failure and/or dehydration. Although the clearance of phosphate by the kidney is increased and the tubular reabsorption of phosphorus decreased in the classical patient with primary hyperparathyroidism, there is so much overlap with patients with nonparathyroid malignancy that these tests are of limited value.

3. *Elevation of the alkaline phosphatase.* In general, elevation of the serum alkaline phosphatase in patients with primary hyperparathyroidism is found only in those with radiographic evidence of bone disease. More often, elevation of the serum alkaline phosphatase in the hypercalcemic patient reflects an increase in the liver isoenzyme associated with hepatic metastases or other disease of the liver. In patients with carcinoma of the breast or prostate that is metastatic to bone, elevation of the alkaline phosphatase may indicate the activity of osteoblastic metastases. In 30 of 33 breast cancer patients, hypercalcemia was associated with a falling serum alkaline phosphatase (Griboff *et al.,* 1954). The enzyme level tends to rise during recovery from hypercalcemia (Lee and Lloyd, 1971). An additional consideration is the recently published evidence of production of an ectopic isoenzyme of alkaline phosphatase by 27 patients with lung, ovarian, colon, breast, lymphomatous, uterine, cervical, myelomatous, and other tumors (Stolbach, *et al.,* 1969). Alkaline phosphatase elevations ranged as high as 125 King-Armstrong Units, and the isoenzyme was heat stable and indistinguishable both biochemically and immunologically from placental alkaline phosphatase (see Chapter 3, Volume I).

4. *Radiographic or bone marrow biopsy evidence for skeletal metastases.* The presence of skeletal metastases does not rule out the possibility that the tumor is also producing parathyroid hormone or some other calcium-mobilizing substance. Only radioimmunoassays or bioassays for parathyroid hormone or other agents can document these syndromes (Sherwood *et al.,* 1967).

5. *General state of debilitation.* The presence of anemia, weight loss,

or other constitutional symptoms would support a malignant cause for the hypercalcemia.

6. *Electrolyte and acid–base considerations*. As noted in Chapters 2, Volume I, and 1 (this volume), parathyroid hormone is known to cause changes in tubular reabsorption of bicarbonate and to produce a tendency toward hyperchloremic acidosis. Barzel (1971), in fact, has measured arterial pH in patients with parathyroid disorders and has reported a significant decrease in pH in patients with hyperparathyroidism. In patients with hypercalcemia due to metastatic malignancy, on the other hand, a mild metabolic alkalosis is reported to be common (Heinemann, 1963). A strict differentiation of these disorders on the basis of acid–base balance is clouded by the frequent presence of nausea and vomiting that may accompany severe hypercalcemia and lead to hypochloremic metabolic alkalosis. This consideration may account for Lafferty's (1966) observation that patients with ectopic hyperparathyroidism did not have elevated serum chlorides. Furthermore, the presence of respiratory acidosis or of severe renal disease may further complicate the picture.

7. *Elevation of circulating parathyroid hormone*. An increase in immunoreactive parathyroid hormone in the peripheral blood documents the presence of hyperparathyroidism but does not necessarily indicate its source. Elevations of the hormone could be produced both by primary parathyroid disease or by the ectopic production of hormone by tumor. Recent studies by Riggs *et al.* (1971) suggest that the hormone produced by nonparathyroid tumors may be less immunoreactive (with an altered slope in the radioimmunoassay) than the hormone produced by the normal parathyroid gland. With their assay, they claim to be able to differentiate the two disorders but, no studies of the tumors or tumor extracts were done. The altered immunoreactivity of the circulating ectopic hormone could be due to (a) synthesis and secretion of an altered polypeptide; (b) secretion of a precursor or intermediate form of parathyroid hormone due to a lack of the enzyme necessary for conversion to the 84 amino acid polypeptide; (c) abnormal metabolism or breaddown of parathyroid hormone in the serum or tissues of patients with cancer; or (d) secretion of additional factor(s) by the tumor that affect the radioimmunoassay.

Additional studies of ectopic hyperparathyroidism by the same group (Benson *et al.*, 1974) involved the fractionation of serum on columns of BioGel P-150 and radioimmunoassay of immunoreactive parathyroid hormone (PTH). Smaller quantities of carboxyl-terminal fragments were found in plasma samples from these patients than in primary hyperparathyroidism, although the quantity of intact hormone was the same. It has recently been demonstrated that the carboxyl-terminal fragment is the dominant hormonal form of parathyroid hormone in plasma (Segre *et al.*, 1972). The authors concluded that the decreased quantity of immunoreactive carboxyl-terminal fragment in ectopic hyperparathyroidism probably accounted for the relatively low values of PTH (Riggs *et al.*, 1971), but that there was sufficient intact hormone to account for the production of hypercalcemia. They also raised the tantalizing possibility that a larger form of PTH than intact hormone might be present in the plasma of some patients with the ectopic syndrome.

Because of the complexities involved in the synthesis, secretion and metabolism of parathyroid hormone (see Chapter 1), careful studies of the hormone in tumor tissue and peripheral blood as well as studies incorporating radioactive amino acids into tumor hormone are required. In synthetic studies *in vitro* with a squamous cell tumor, Hamilton *et al.* (1977) showed production of a hormone similar to, but not necessarily identical with, the native molecule. At present, it is uncertain what percentage of the patients with ectopic hypercalcemia have production of parathyroid hormone, prostaglandin or other osteolytic substances (such as osteoclast activating factor) to account for their disorder. More definitive studies will involve the chemical analysis of large numbers of tumors and correlations with clinical data.

The recent development of sophisticated angiographic and venous catheterization techniques now makes possible localization of the source of the elevated circulating parathyroid hormone. In patients with primary hyperparathyroidism (Powell *et al.*, 1972b; Eisenberg *et al.*, 1974), selective sampling from neck and mediastinal veins has permitted precise preoperative localization of parathyroid tumors (see Chapter 1, Volume I). In the patient with hepatoblastoma reported by Knill-Jones *et al.* (1970) assay of hepatic vein blood documented the source of the elevated parathyroid hormone. A similar study of a renal cell carcinoma producing the hormone was reported by Blair *et al.* (1973). Heath *et al.* (1974) used selective catherization to prove the diagnosis of primary hyperparathyroidism in a patient with an associated malignancy. Arterial and venous sampling of tumors of the lung and kidney (the most common sites of ectopic production of parathyroid hormone) is readily performed.

F. Other Calcium Disorders Associated with Tumors

1. Hypophosphatemic Osteomalacia

An unusual disturbance of calcium metabolism, hypophosphatemic osteomalacia, has been associated with certain tumors. Salassa *et al.* (1970)

described two patients in whom removal of a sclerosing hemangioma was followed by an increase in serum inorganic phosphorus, relief of clinical symptoms and radiologic evidence of healing of the osteomalacia. In the one patient in whom parathyroid hormone was measured, removal of the tumor caused a rise in immunoassayable parathyroid hormone. In another report, removal of an ossifying mesenchymal tumor of the pharynx resulted in cure of vitamin D-resistant rickets (Olefsky et al., 1972).

Other reports have included patients with pleomorphic sarcomas, neurofibromas, and mesenchymal tumors (Stanbury, 1972). The etiology of the phosphaturia is uncertain, although a recent report suggests the possibility of decreased renal 1-α-hydroxylase activity (Orezner and Feinglos, 1977).

2. Hypocalcemia

Occasionally, a low rather than a high serum may complicate the course of a malignant tumor. Other causes of hypocalcemia usually include: (1) deficient calcium intake; (2) vitamin D deficiency (or resistance); (3) malabsorption; (4) acute or chronic pancreatitis; (5) renal disease; (6) hypoproteinemia; (7) hypoparathyroidism; (8) pseudohypoparathyroidism; and (9) Cushing's syndrome. Rarely, metastases to the parathyroid glands produce a hypoparathyroid state (Horwitz et al., 1972), but often mechanisms other than those listed above must be invoked to explain cancer hypocalcemia.

Osteoblastic metastases have been reported to lower the serum calcium (Ehrlich et al., 1963; Ludwig, 1962). Balance studies suggest that increased skeletal avidity for calcium accounts for the lowered serum concentration (Randall and Lireman, 1964). Normal subjects given 469 mg of calcium gluconate in a 4 hour intravenous infusion retain between 60 and 70%. Patients with lytic metastases, however, retain about 50% of the infused calcium, and the majority of those with blastic metastases retain more than 90% (Spencer et al., 1967). In the latter group, urinary calcium fell in some cases to levels below 10 mg/24 hours. Pearson (1964) did not observe tetany in his patients, but Hall et al. (1966), in contrast, reported three patients in whom a Chvostek sign was present. In two patients, symptoms of slurred speech, drowsiness, disorientation, and coma were reversed by calcium infusions. Positive calcium balance and hypocalcemia were reported in several patients who had rapid healing of breast and prostate cancers following modification of the hormonal environment (Ludwig, 1962; Hall et al., 1966).

Jaffe et al. (1972) reported 135 children with leukemia, 14 of whom had one or more hypocalcemic episodes. Five were associated with acute renal shut-down. In the remaining patients, a variety of gastrointestinal, hormonal, and chemotherapeutic factors were probably operative. All patients received transfusions, but the citrate in bank blood would lower primarily ionized calcium and not necessarily the total calcium. In two patients in whom hypomagnesemia and hypocalcemia were present, elevation of the serum calcium was achieved only after magnesium sulfate was given. Zusman *et al.* (1973) reported 4 children with acute lymphoblastic leukemia who developed hyperphosphatemia, hyperphosphturia and hypocalcemia, presumably due to increased endogenous phosphorus release from destruction of lymphocytes.

It is not uncommon on an oncology service to see hypocalcemic patients in whom the serum magnesium is also depressed from prolonged parenteral nutrition, severe vomiting, or diarrhea. A normal serum calcium may sometimes be restored by magnesium replacement alone (Muldowney *et al.*, 1970). Magnesium is an essential cofactor in many enzyme systems, and when magnesium concentration is low, parathyroid hormone release is depressed regardless of the calcium concentration. Thus, there is a good theoretical rationale to explain cancer-associated hypocalcemia in the presence of hypomagnesemia (Targovnik *et al.*, 1971; Sherwood and Abe, 1972; Schneider and Sherwood, 1974).

Calcitonin or another as yet undiscovered hypocalcemic hormone might be produced by tumors. However, even in medullary cancer of the thyroid gland, where large amounts of calcitonin are produced, hypocalcemia is not a usual feature of the disease. Silva *et al.* (1976) reported 16 patients with bronchogenic carcinoma who had elevated levels of calcitonin, particularly adeno and oat cell carcinoma. In some cases, the thyroid gland rather than the tumor was the source of calcitonin, but hypocalcemia was not observed. Simultaneous ectopic production of parathyroid hormone and calcitonin has been described in two patients (Deftos *et al.*, 1976).

V. TREATMENT OF HYPERCALCEMIA

The clinical picture of hypercalcemia varies greatly in its manifestations and severity. It is not at all unusual to see an asymptomatic patient with primary hyperparathyroidism whose serum calcium is 14 or 15 mg/100 ml, while another patient with disseminated cancer may be stuporous when the serum calcium is only 12 mg/100 ml. Factors such as the rapidity with which the serum calcium rises, accompanying renal failure and electrolyte disturbances, cardiovascular status, and the general state of debilitation will vary the clinical response to hypercalcemia. These factors and the state of consciousness, rather than the absolute level of the serum calcium, should determine the vigor and speed with which attempts are made to lower the calcium.

A. Hydration and Electrolyte Replacement

The most important measures in the treatment of acute hypercalcemia are the restoration of adequate hydration and an increase in calcium excretion (Table IV). This is best accomplished by normal saline infusions. Dextrose solutions, except when the patient is hypernatremic, are less effective partially because water tends to enter the intracellular compartment, but also because calcium excretion is linked to sodium excretion. Walser (1961) reported that plasma free calcium ion clearance remained equal to sodium clearance during diuresis with water, sodium chloride, sodium bicarbonate, mannitol, and glucose. The relationship was independent of variations in calcium or sodium intake, urinary flow, or urinary ionic strength. Kleeman et al. (1966) found that the change in calcium clearance in hypercalcemic dogs produced by acute reductions in glomerular filtration rate was primarily the consequence of simultaneous alterations in sodium excretion. Changing the diet of a normal man from one containing 25 mEq of sodium to one with 350 mEq of sodium can raise urinary calcium excretion from 180 mg to as much as 580 mg in 24 hours without any change in calcium intake (Kleeman et al., 1964). Since 99% of filtered calcium is normally reabsorbed by the renal tubule, a small change in tubular reabsorption can cause a marked increase in urinary calcium excretion.

1. Sodium Infusion

Initially, the fall in serum calcium with saline infusion is due chiefly to reduction in the protein-bound calcium. Ordinarily, only about one-half of the plasma calcium is protein bound. In the dehydrated patient with hemoconcentration, this fraction may be increased. Restoration of the extracellular fluid volume will not immediately change the ionized calcium concentration but will lower the total serum calcium concentration.

The amount of saline that should be given to each patient depends on the degree of dehydration and the tolerance of the patient's cardiovascular system to salt; thus more liberal fluid therapy would be given to younger patients with normal cardiac reserve. However, often the administration of only a liter or two of normal saline in 24 hours will be sufficient to break the vicious cycle of dehydration, vomiting, decreased urinary output, diminished calcium excretion, and rising serum calcium.

Other electrolyte abnormalities should be corrected as well. As a con-

TABLE IV

Evaluation of Methods for the Treatment of Acute Hypercalcemia[a]

Form of therapy	Dosage	Route of administration	Effects on urinary calcium	Mechanism of action	Potential complications	Limitations to use
Sodium chloride infusion	2–3 liters of 0.9% sodium chloride over 6 hours (1.45% saline may also be used)	Intravenous	Increased	Increased urinary excretion of calcium associated with natriuresis	Sodium overload; hypernatremia; hypokalemia; hypomagnesia	Hypertension; congestive heart failure; renal insufficiency
Furosemide	40–80 mg/hour	Intravenous	Increased	Increased urinary excretion of calcium	Hypokalemia: volume depletion; hypomagnesemia; calcium depletion	Renal failure with oliguria not responsive to furosemide and saline
Sodium sulfate infusion	3 liters of isotonic sodium sulfate over 9 hours	Intravenous	Increased	Increased urinary excretion of calcium	Sodium overload; hypernatremia; hypokalemia; hypomagnesemia	Hypertension; congestive heart failure; renal insufficiency
Phosphate	1–3 gm phosphorus per day	Oral	Decreased	Bony or extraskeletal deposition of calcium phosphate; prevention of bone resorption; increased bone formation?; binding of calcium in gastrointestinal tract	Hyperphosphatemia; hypotension and shock; extraskeletal calcification	Renal insufficiency; high normal or elevated serum phosphorus

TABLE IV (*Continued*)

Phosphate	50 mmoles over 6–8 hours	Intravenous	Decreased	As above, except for gastrointestinal binding	As above	As above, use only when all other methods are inadequate
Corticosteroids	30 mg prednisone (or equivalent) or more per day	Oral or parenteral	Variable	Antagonism to vitamin D effects on intestine; inhibition of bone mobilization of calcium (anti-OAF)	Hypercorticism or acute steroid complications	Delayed effect; generally not effective in hyperparathyroidism
Mithramycin	25 μg/kg of body weight	Intravenous	Not increased	?Antagonism to calcium mobilization from bone (interference with parathyroid hormone and/or vitamin D effect and physicochemical equilibrium) ? anti-tumor	Bleeding disorder; hepatic dysfunction; renal insufficiency	Bone marrow or liver failure

[a] Modified after Suki *et al.* (1969)

sequence of protracted vomiting, altered renal function, and contraction of the extracellular space, hypokalemic alkalosis frequently accompanies severe hypercalcemia. Furthermore, administration of large amounts of saline potentiates potassium loss by facilitating sodium–potassium exchange in the distal tubule. Prompt potassium replacement is of particular importance in the patient taking a digitalis preparation, as the effects of digitalis, hypercalcemia, and hypokalemia may be synergistic on the myocardium (*vide supra*). Hypomagnesemia can also enhance digitalis toxicity. Conversely, magnesium sulfate has an antiarrhthymic effect on digitalis-induced aberrations of cardiac rhythm (Seller, 1971). Since *in vitro* experiments have shown that magnesium depletion may stimulate parathyroid hormone release and, at least theoretically, potentiate the hypercalcemia, magnesium replacement is also essential (Targovnik *et al.*, 1971, Schneider and Sherwood, 1974). A paradoxical effect has been noted at extremely low concentrations of magnesium, however. Under these circumstances it appears that parathyroid hormone secretion is decreased rather than increased. It is conceivable that hypercalcemia might even be partially reversed in the patient with severe hypomagnesemia (Sherwood and Abe, 1972).

Isotonic sodium sulfate (0.12 M) has proved somewhat more effective than saline infusion in promoting calciuresis (Chakmakjian and Bethune, 1966). Unless hyperkalemia is present, 0.005 M potassium sulfate and 0.002 M magnesium sulfate should be added to prevent depletion of these cations. Each liter will lower the plasma calcium by about 1 mg/100 ml (Walser, 1970). In addition to promoting natriuresis, which obligates calcium excretion, the infusion provides sulfate ion that complexes calcium. Diminished protein binding as a result of the increase in plasma ionic strength may contribute to the effect of sodium sulfate, but is of lesser importance. In unanesthetized dogs, ionized calcium rose from a control value of 40–65% to 75–90% during sulfate infusion when the concentration of plasma sulfate reached 20 mmoles/liter. In another experiment, calcium clearance was increased from 10% of the glomerular filtration rate during saline, sodium bicarbonate, and sucrose diuresis to 16% during sulfate diuresis (Walser, 1958).

Hypernatremia has been reported as a complication of sulfate therapy (Hekhman and Walsh, 1967). Actually, since the concentration of sodium in isotonic sodium sulfate is 240 mEq/liter, hypernatremia is both expected and desirable. Benvenisti *et al.* (1969) raised the serum sodium concentration in one patient to as high as 168 mEq/liter without apparent side effects. Another complication of more concern is fluid overload, especially in the patient with compromised cardiac reserve.

2. Diuretics

In an effort to prevent congestive heart failure and to combine the calciuretic effects of sodium and certain diuretics, Suki *et al.* (1970) suggested a form of therapy, which has subsequently been successfully used by others (LeGall *et al.,* 1971). Furosemide (80–100 mg every 1–2 hours) is combined with saline infusion to replace urinary output. Considerable reduction in the serum calcium occurred in all of the patients studied. The patient's fluid balance must be monitored closely and urinary losses of potassium and magnesium, which are likely to be considerable, must be replaced.

The increased excretion of calcium induced by furosemide cannot be accounted for by a change in GFR and is probably due to a decrease in tubular reabsorption (Tambyak and Lim, 1969). Thiazides decrease renal excretion of calcium and should not be used in any hypercalcemic patient.

B. Mobilization

Prolonged immobilization is known to increase urinary calcium in normal man (Dietrich, 1948), and about 10% of such subjects will develop asymptomatic hypercalcemia (Walser, 1970, Chapter 6, Volume I). In normocalcemic patients with increased skeletal breakdown due to tumor, Paget's disease, or hyperparathyroidism, imposed bed rest for an independent reason may result in significant elevation of plasma calcium. It is not simply the lack of physical activity that results in increased osteolysis, since exercise on a tricycle ergometer in the lying position will not prevent the metabolic abnormalities in normal subjects. Neither is the use of a tilt table of any avail. Weight bearing is essential; simple quiet standing is sufficient to reverse the negative calcium balance (Issekutz *et al.,* 1966).

C. Dietary Control

It seems logical to reduce the calcium content of the diet in the hypercalcemic patient. However, except in conditions where gastrointestinal absorption of calcium is excessive (e.g., sarcoidosis and vitamin D intoxication), dietary limitations are not likely to be effective. Halving the dietary calcium in a normal man does not reduce urinary calcium by 50%. Instead, the percent calcium absorbed by the gut is augmented so that the amount of calcium excreted in the urine falls only slightly. In the rat, calcium deprivation causes the enhanced transport of the cation from mucosa to serosa (Kimberg, 1969; Deluca and Schnoes, 1976). The adaptive mechanism works in reverse so that gut absorption of calcium is greatly reduced in hypercalcemic states not characterized by vitamin D excess or increased sensitivity to calciferol.

As most foods that are high in calcium also contain a significant amount of phosphorus, dietary restrictions may have a paradoxical effect if oral phosphate supplements are not given. Furthermore, with significant hypercalcemia, nausea and emesis will prevent the patient from having significant intake. The patient should be given a diet containing no diary products and less than 200 mg calcium, but the physician should not be lulled into thinking that dietary control accomplishes much.

D. Specific Therapy

Primary consideration should be given to the underlying cause of the hypercalcemia. Often, this is easily treated and no ancillary measures need be employed. For example, the mild serum elevation that sometimes occurs in hyperthyroidism and Addisonian crisis need only be followed while appropriate specific therapy is given. Vitamin D intoxication and the milk–alkali syndrome may be treated by simply withholding the offending agents unless the hypercalcemia is severe. If primary hyperparathyroidism is diagnosed, the patient should be referred to a surgeon skilled in surgery of the parathyroid gland.

Specific therapy for tumor-associated hypercalcemia is a more difficult problem. The intricacies of manipulating the hormonal environment of breast cancer have already been discussed. Whenever possible, surgery should be considered as there have been numerous reports of restoration of normocalcemia following tumor excision (Myers, 1968; Plimpton and Gellhorn, 1956). Usually the fall in serum calcium occurs within the first 2 days postoperatively, if it will occur at all. Even if the entire tumor cannot be removed, surgery should be considered as a means of controlling the bulk of the tumor (Myers, 1972).

The use of radiation therapy to control hypercalcemia was first described by Albright and Reifenstein (1948). Radiation therapy may be aimed at osseous metastases as well as soft tissue tumor masses.

Chemotherapy is most likely to be effective in controlling hypercalcemia when it is caused by one of the lymphomas or leukemias. The hypercalcemia complicating a case of reticulum cell sarcoma and acute leukemia in a 58-year-old woman was initially controlled with a course of cytosine arabinoside (Benvenisti et al., 1969). Myers (1966) described a woman with lymphosarcoma in whom a serum calcium of 20.2 mg/100 ml was restored to normal by nitrogen mustard therapy, Intravenous methotrexate was successful in treating a patient with hypercalcemia associated with cutaneous lymphosarcoma (Dubé et al., 1968). By contrast, hypercalcemia accompanying solid tumors, with the exception of breast and prostate cancer, is less likely to be treated successfully with chemotherapy. Recent widespread use of combination chemotherapy may improve these results, however.

E. Nonspecific Therapy

1. EDTA

Ethylenediaminetetracetic acid is effective in reducing the ionized calcium in hypercalcemic patients (Spencer et al., 1956) but only for short periods of time. It acts by forming a stable chelate with calcium. If treatment with this compound is begun, methods that measure total serum calcium, such as atomic absorption spectrophotometry, cannot be used as there will be circulating Ca–EDTA complexes. Either a titrametric method or one that measures ionized calcium must be employed. EDTA has fallen into disfavor because the decrease in serum calcium it produces is short lived, pain at the site of intravenous infusion is often severe, and irreversible damage to the proximal convoluted tubules may occur (Dudley et al., 1955; Holland et al., 1953; Foreman et al., 1956).

2. Corticosteroids

The hypercalcemia of both sarcoidosis and vitamin D intoxication usually responds to corticosteroid administration. In these disease entities, steroids might actually be considered a form of specific therapy as they act in part by antagonizing the effects of calciferol on the gastrointestinal tract (Kimberb, 1969). In other situations, their mode of action is less clear. An elevated calcium concentration unexpectedly fell toward normal when cortisone was used to treat one patient with severe hyperthyroidism. When steroids were withheld, the calcium rose again (Sataline, 1962).

Although there have been scattered reports of the hypercalcemia of hyperparathyroidism responding to the administration of steroids, the vast majority do not (Walser, 1971; Gwinup and Sayle, 1961). Typically, when a response does occur, it is incomplete, as in the case reported by Hodges and Waterhouse (1967) where the calcium fell from 16.9 mg to 13.3 mg/100 ml.

Corticosteroids are often a mainstay of nonspecific medical treatment of the hypercalcemia of malignancy. They are most likely to be effective in treating breast cancer, multiple myeloma, and lymphosarcoma and are usually of little value with the nonlymphoid solid tumors (Myers, 1972). In 1958, Myers presented 11 patients with tumor-associated hypercalcemia treated with steroids. There were five positive responses (2 breast cancers, 2 lymphosarcomas, and 1 adenocarcinoma of unknown etiology) and two partial responses (1 breast and 1 myeloma). Two renal carcinomas, 1 rhabdomyosarcoma, and 1 breast cancer failed to respond. Thalassinos and Joplin (1970) found much less favorable results; only 1 of 13 random cancer patients, including myeloma cases, become normocalcemic with steroid therapy. Ashkar *et al.* (1971), however, in a series of 45 patients, reported that all of their myeloma patients and 90% of other tumors showed a diminution of the serum calcium.

The mechanism of action of steroids in multiple myeloma has been studied (Lazor and Rosenberg, 1964). These investigators showed that prednisone acted to decrease bone resorption rather than decreasing gut absorption or augmenting renal loss of calcium. Using radioactive calcium, Bentzel *et al.* (1964) found that miscible calcium pool size, bone formation rate, and bone resorption rate were increased in hypercalcemic myeloma patients and diminished by prednisone therapy. The serum calcium was reduced in all of the patients in whom it was elevated. The action of osteoclast activating factor, now implicated in the mechanism of myeloma-hypercalcemia, is inhibited by corticosteroids (Luben *et al.,* 1974, Mundy *et al.,* 1974).

3. Calcitonin

On a theoretical basis, the inhibitory effect of calcitonin on bone resorption makes it the ideal agent for treating hypercalcemia, but so far both the purified porcine hormone and synthetic human and salmon calcitonin have been clinically disappointing. Haas and Dumbacher (1968), in a group of hypercalcemic patients of diverse etiology, demonstrated a fall of about 2 mg/100 ml in the serum calcium by the end of a 3-hour infusion of 10–100 MRC units. Other studies have suggested limited effectiveness of calcitonin in short-term control of hypercalcemia (Kammerman and Canfield, 1970; West *et al.,* 1971). The hormone seems to have its greatest usefulness in the management of hypercalcemia associated with diffuse increase in bone resorption (Muckle *et al.,* 1969).

4. Mithramycin

Mithramycin is an antibiotic produced by the microorganism *Streptomyces plicatus*. Like actinomycin D, it is a potent inhibitor of DNA-induced RNA synthesis (Anonymous, 1971). The compound has been used in the chemotherapy of several neoplasms but the most favorable results have been achieved with embryonal cell testicular tumors (Kofman and Eisenstein, 1963; Kofman et al., 1964; Brown and Kennedy, 1956; Ream et al., 1968). During the experimental trials, the hypocalcemic properties of the drug were discovered.

The calcium-lowering dose of mithramycin is 25 μg/kg, which is about one-tenth of the antitumor dose. It is therefore unlikely that the drug acts by inhibiting neoplastic growth. Tritiated mithramycin does localize in areas of active bone resorption but concentrates to a greater degree in normal liver and kidney (Kennedy et al., 1967). Indirect evidence has suggested that the drug acts either by blocking the peripheral action of parathyroid hormone or by rendering the patient resistant to vitamin D (Baum, 1967, 1968; Haussler and McCain, 1977). High doses of vitamin D do not overcome the effect of mithramycin. There is no increase in hydroxyproline turnover, which usually accompanies bone healing (Parsons et al., 1967).

Mithramycin administered intravenously will lower the serum calcium in 24 to 48 hours in the majority of patients (Perlia, 1969; Perlia et al., 1970). The duration of effect is variable but may last up to a week as demonstrated by Muggia et al. (1968) in studying the related compound dactinomycin. Singer et al. (1970) used mithramycin to control the intractable hypercalcemia associated with parathyroid carcinoma.

The primary toxicity of mithramycin is dose-related bleeding associated with thrombocytopenia. As many of the patients in whom this therapy is entertained already have compromised marrow reserve, the drug may be contraindicated when it would be most helpful. However, Harrington et al. (1970) reported 43 consecutive patients with neoplasia-associated hypercalcemia treated with mithramycin who developed no toxicity more serious than nausea and occasional vomiting. Myers (1972) has suggested that dactinomycin may be preferable to mithramycin because of the platelet toxicity, but the latter has been more extensively studied.

5. Phosphates

Probably the first use of phosphates in the treatment of hypercalcemia was in the three patients reported by Bulger et al. (1930). Although the therapy was initially successful, extensive calcifications were found in the lungs, gastric mucosa, and kidneys at postmortem examination in one of the patients. After Albright et al. (1932) condemned the use of phosphates 2 years later, there were no significant reports of their use in treating hypercalcemia for 30 years. Then, in a patient with probable hyperparathyroidism who had had three negative neck explorations, Dent (1962) used oral phosphates in the long-term management of hypercalcemia and bone pain. It was not until 1966, however, when Goldsmith and Ingbar reintroduced phosphate therapy, that its use became widespread.

The effect of phosphates is independent of any action on the kidney (Hulley *et al.*, 1969). Phosphates, when given orally, may produce small elevations in fecal calcium. Whether given intravenously or by mouth, their chief actions are to decrease serum and urinary calcium by promoting uptake of the divalent cation from the circulation into bone and by decreasing active bone resorption. Eisenberg (1970) found that strontium and ^{47}Ca were actively removed from the circulation into a labile mineral pool from which they were released when the phosphate infusion was stopped. In bone culture, Raisz and Neiman (1969) showed that active resorption was progressively inhibited by increasing the phosphate concentration of the medium. Oral administration of phosphate will prevent the hypercalciuria, which occurs in healthy young men put to bed for prolonged periods (Hulley *et al.*, 1971). Such studies may have implications for astronauts exposed to extended periods of weightlessness and the attendant mineral loss from the skeleton (Chapter 6, Volume I).

Evidence presented by Massry *et al.* (1968) suggests that changes in the serum calcium induced by phosphate therapy are directly related to changes in the molar product of calcium and phosphate in the serum. In other words, there may be physiochemical precipitation of $CaHPO_4$ as its solubility product is exceeded (Herbert *et al.*, 1966). Several observations, however, suggest that this view may be oversimplified. Treatment with intravenous phosphates may result in levels of serum phosphorus that are lower than those obtained before therapy. Precipitation of $CaHPO_4$ could not account for a simultaneous fall in the serum calcium. In addition, the serum calcium often remains low for several days after a phosphate infusion is stopped, implying that the calcium is not removed to a crystal form that is in equilibrium with the circulation. Simultaneous effects of phosphate ion on stimulating bone formation (with utilization of both calcium and phosphate) may therefore be operative.

Since the initial report by Goldsmith and Ingbar (1966) there has been considerable controversy over the efficacy and safety of phosphate therapy. The principal fear is that extraskeletal calcifications will form and damage vital structures. In a group of rats made hypercalcemic with vitamin D, Spaulding and Walser (1970) found significantly higher tissue calcium levels in phosphate-treated animals compared with controls. The recent literature contains numerous reports of massive and pathological calcification of the myocardium, lungs, blood vessels, spleen, pancreas, and endocrine glands (Fierer *et al.*, 1970; Marti and Cox, 1970; Carey *et al.*, 1968). Acute renal failure and hypotension have also been reported as major complications of phosphate therapy (Breuer and LeBauer, 1967; Bernheim and Vischer, 1968; Barjon *et al.*, 1970).

Goldsmith and Ingbar (1967) maintain that the complications seen by others are the result of too rapid infusion of intravenous phosphate. They and others (Kahil *et al.,* 1967; Thalassinos and Joplin, 1968) have not found increased soft tissue calcification over that expected with the degree of hypercalcemia present.

While Walser (1970) concluded that the use of intravenous phosphates is to be deplored because other less hazardous methods of treatment are available, Fulmer *et al.* (1972) feel that phosphates are superior to sulfate in the treatment of tumor-associated hypercalcemia. They report that the fall in serum calcium can be predicted from the amount of phosphate infused: 25 mmoles phosphate produced an average decline of 1.1 mg%; 50 mmoles, 2.44 mg%; 75 mmoles, 4.13 mg%; and 100 mmoles, 6.08 mg% (Dimich *et al.,* 1969). The maximum dose recommended by Goldsmith and Ingbar was 50 mmoles of intravenous phosphate over 6 to 8 hours. Even the proponents of phosphate therapy, however, urge caution in its use when azotemia is present (Myers, 1972), although Goldsmith and Ingbar did report a fall in urea nitrogen in a few of the patients in their original paper.

While calcification along a vein at the site of a phosphate infusion has been reported (Goldsmith and Ingbar, 1966; Carey *et al.,* 1968), one of us (J.R.) has seen arterial calcification develop in a patient treated with intravenous phosphates.

6. Miscellaneous

Both hemodialysis (Eisenberg and Cotch, 1968; Raphael *et al.,* 1971) and calcium-free peritoneal dialysis (Nolph and Stoltz, 1971) have been used successfully in treating hypercalcemic crisis. Fluorides (Bierman *et al.,* 1969) and glucagon (Paloyan *et al.,* 1967) have been reported to reduce serum calcium in experimental animals. Anabolic steroids (Landau and Kappas, 1965), estrogens (Gallagher and Nordin, 1972; Sigurdsson *et al.,* 1973), and hexestrol, a synthetic estrogenic compound (Goepfert *et al.,* 1966), have been employed to treat hyperparathyroidism. None of these drugs has been used extensively enough to indicate its real clinical usefulness, and other agents are as or more useful in the treatment of hypercalcemia.

F. Comparison of Available Modalities

The various forms of therapy are compared in Table IV. When controversy exists over several forms of therapy, none of them is likely to be ideal. Nowhere is that maxim more true than in the treatment of hypercalcemia. Intravenous phosphates are undoubtedly the most effective in assuring a sustained fall in the serum calcium. However, their safety, as discussed above, is of concern. Oral phosphates and some of the other modalities discussed, while less dangerous, are also less reliable in lowering the serum calcium. Pechet *et al.* (1967) have suggested that thyrocalcitonin, which decreases bone resorption, and oral phosphates, which promote bone formation, should be combined in the therapy of hypercalcemia. Whatever form of nonspecific therapy chosen, the most important treatment is ultimately that directed at the underlying disorder. Vigorous hydration with intravenous saline and furosamide are often sufficient to resolve acute hypercalcemia (Schneider and Sherwood, 1974).

REFERENCES

Abouav, J., Berkowitz, S. B., and Kolb, F. O. (1959). *N. Engl. J. Med.* **260,** 1057.
Alanis, B. F., and Flanagan, J. F. (1959). *J. Am. Med. Assoc.* **171,** 2076.
Albert, D. J., Miller, M., Hubay, C. A., and Persky, L. (1969). *J. Urol.* **101,** 443.
Albright, F. (1941). *N. Engl. J. Med.* **225,** 789.
Albright, F., and Reifenstein, E. C. (1948). "The Parathyroid Glands and Metabolic Bone Disease," p. 92. Williams & Wilkins, Baltimore, Maryland.
Albright, F., Bauer, W., Claflin, D., and Cockrill, J. R. (1932). *J. Clin. Invest.* **11,** 411.
Allen, E. M., Singer, F. R., and Melamed, D. (1970). *Neurology* **20,** 15.
Amatruda, T. T., Jr. (1974). *In* "Duncan's Diseases of Metabolism." (P. K. Bondy and L. E. Rosenberg, eds.), 6th ed., Vol. 2, p. 1629. Saunders, Philadelphia, Pennsylvania.
Anderson, E. D., and Glenn, J. F. (1965). *J. Am. Med. Assoc.* **192,** 328.
Anderson, H. C., Rothschild, E. O., and Myers, W. P. L. (1962). *Clin. Res.* **10,** 328.
Anderson, W. A. D. (1939). *Arch. Pathol.* **27,** 753.
Anonymous. (1967). *Arch. Klin. Med.* **213,** 73.
Anonymous. (1970). *Am. J. Med.* **48,** 367.
Anonymous. (1971). *Clin. Pharmacol. Ther.* **12,** 310.
Ashkar, F. S., Miller, R., and Katims, R. B. (1971). *Lancet* **1,** 41.
Azzopardi, J. G., and Whittaker, R. S. (1969). *J. Clin. Pathol.* **22,** 718.
Azzopardi, J. G., Freeman, E., and Poole, G. (1970). *Br. Med. J.* **4,** 528.
Babbott, F. L., Jr., Johnston, J. A., and Haskins, C. H. (1923). *Am. J. Dis. Child.* **26,** 486.
Bachman, A. L., and Sproule, E. (1955). *Ann. N. Y. Acad. Sci.* **31,** 146.
Baer, L., and Neu, H. (1966). *Ann. Intern. Med.* **64,** 1062.
Ballard, H. S., and Marcus, A. J. (1970). *N. Engl. J. Med.* **282,** 663.
Baker, W. H. (1956). *Am. J. Med.* **21,** 714.
Barjon, P., Pages, A., and Barjon, A. C. (1970). *Presse Med.* **78,** 2333.
Barreras, R., and Donaldson, B. M., Jr. (1967a). *Gastroenterology* **52,** 670.
Barreras, R., and Donaldson, R. M., Jr. (1967b). *N. Engl. J. Med.* **276,** 1122.
Barzel, U. S. (1971). *Lancet* **1,** 1329.
Baum, M. (1967). *Lancet* **2,** 613.
Baum, M. (1968). *Br. J. Cancer* **22,** 176.
Beckett, V. L. (1969). *Cancer* **24,** 610.
Bender, R. A., and Hansen, H. (1974). *Ann. Int. Med.* **80,** 205.
Bennett, A., Simpson, J. S., McDonald, A. M., and Stamford, T. F. (1975). *Lancet* **1,** 1218.
Bennett, C. M. (1970). *J. Clin. Invest.* **49,** 1447.

Benson, R. C., Riggs, B. L., Pickard, B. M., and Arnaud, C. D. (1974). *J. Clin. Invest.* **54**, 175.
Bentzel, C. M., Carbone, P. P., and Rosenberg, L. (1964). *J. Clin. Invest.* **43**, 2132.
Benvenisti, D., Sherwood, L. M., and Heinemann, H. O. (1969). *Am. J. Med.* **46**, 976.
Bernheim, C., and Vischer, T. (1968). *Schweiz. Med. Wochenschr.* **98**, 641.
Berson, S. A., and Yalow, R. S. (1966). *Science* **154**, 907.
Bierman, H. R., Viner, M. L., Kovacs, E. T., and Bruner, J. A. (1969). *Ann. Intern. Med.* **70**, 1105.
Blair, J. A., Jr., Hawker, C. D., and Utiger, R. D. (1973). *Metab., Clin. Exp.* **22**, 147.
Bonadonna, G., Merlino, M. J., Myers, W. P. L., and Sonenberg, M. (1966). *N. Engl. J. Med.* **275**, 298.
Borm, D. (1961). *Endokrinologie* **41**, 291.
Bourne, H. H., Tremblay, R. E., and Ansell, J. S. (1964). *N. Engl. J. Med.* **21**, 1005.
Bower, B. F., and Gordan, G. S. (1965). *Annu. Rev. Med.* **16**, 83.
Bower, J. O., and Mengle, H. A. K. (1936). *J. Am. Med. Assoc.* **106**, 1151.
Breidal, H. D., and Ritchie, B. C. (1962). *Med. J. Aust.* **1**, 208.
Brereton, H. D., Halushka, P. V., Alexander, R. W., Mason, D. M., Keiser, H. R., and DeVita, V. T., Jr. (1974). *N. Engl. J. Med.* **291**, 83.
Breuer, R. I., and LeBauer, J. (1967). *J. Clin. Endocrinol. Metab.* **27**, 695.
Brinton, G. S., Jubiz, W., and LaGerguist, L. D. (1975). *J. Clin. Endocrin. Metab.* **41**, 1025.
Bronsky, D., Dubin, A., Kushner, D. S., and Walstein, S. S. (1961). *Am. J. Cardiol.* **7**, 840.
Brown, J. H., and Kennedy, B. J. (1965). *N. Engl. J. Med.* **272**, 111.
Brown, W. H. (1928). *Lancet* **2**, 1022.
Buckle, R. M., McMillan, M., and Mallinson, C. (1970). *Br. Med. J.* **4**, 724.
Buer, M. D. (1970). *South. Med. J.* **63**, 591.
Bulger, H. A., Dixon, H. H., and Barr, D. P. (1930). *J. Clin. Invest.* **9**, 143.
Canellos, G. P. *Ann. New York Acad. Sci.* **230**, 228, 1974.
Carey, R. W., Schmitt, G. W., Kopald, H. H., and Kantrowitz, P. A. (1968). *Arch. Intern. Med.* **122**, 150.
Carey, V. C. I. (1962). *Am. Rev. Respir. Dis.* **85**, 258.
Carey, V. C. I. (1966). *Am. Rev. Respir. Dis.* **93**, 584.
Case Records Massachusetts General Hospital. (1941). *N. Engl. J. Med.* **225**, 789.
Case Records Massachusetts General Hospital. (1953). *N. Engl. J. Med.* **248**, 248.
Case Records Massachusetts General Hospital. (1957). *N. Engl. J. Med.* **256**, 750.
Case Records Massachusetts General Hospital. (1961a). *N. Engl. J. Med.* **265**, 242.
Case Records Massachusetts General Hospital. (1961b). *N. Engl. J. Med.* **265**, 953.
Case Records Massachusetts General Hospital. (1963). *N. Engl. J. Med.* **269**, 801.
Case Records Massachusetts General Hospital. (1964). *N. Engl. J. Med.* **270**, 898.
Case Records Massachusetts General Hospital. (1967). *N. Engl. J. Med.* **276**, 629.
Case Records Massachusetts General Hospital. (1970). *N. Engl. J. Med.* **282**, 269.
Chakmakjian, Z. H., and Bethune, J. E. (1966). *N. Engl. J. Med.* **275**, 862.
Coffey, R. J., Canary, J. J., and Dumais, C. C. (1959). *Am. Surg.* **25**, 310.
Cohen, S., Weissler, A. M., and Schoenfield, C. D. (1965). *Am. Heart J.* **69**, 502.
Connor, T. B., Thomas, W. C., Jr., and Howard, J. E. (1956). *J. Clin. Invest.* **35**, 697.
Cope, O., Culver, P. J., Mixter, C. G., and Nardi, G. I. (1957). *Ann. Surg.* **145**, 857.
Cope, O., Barnes, B. A., Castleman, B., Mueller, G. C. E., and Roth, S. I. (1961). *Ann. Surg.* **154**, 491.
Cragg, J. (1971). *Br. Med. J.* **2**, 110.
Crum, W. D., and Till, H. J. (1960). *Am. J. Cardiol.* **6**, 838.
Daughtry, D. C., Chesney, J. G., Spear, H. C., Gentsch, T. O., and Larsen, P. B. (1967). *Dis. Chest* **52**, 632.

Dauphine, R. T., Riggs, B. L., and Scholz, D. A. (1975). *Ann. Int. Med.* **83,** 365.

David, N. J., Verner, J. V., and Engel, F. L. (1962). *Am. J. Med.* **33,** 88.

Dean, A. C., Lambie, A. T., and Shivas, A. A. (1969). *Br. J. Surg.* **56,** 375.

Deconti, R. C. (1971). *Conn. Med.* **35,** 275.

Deftos, L. J., McMillan, P. J., Sartiano, G. P., Abuid, J., and Robinson, A. G. (1976). *Metabolism* **25,** 543.

Delay, J., Lemperiere, T., and Feline, A. (1970). *Ann. Med. Intern.* **121,** 457.

Deluca, H. T., and Schnoes, H. K. (1976). *Ann. Rev. Biochem.* **45,** 631.

Dent, C. E. (1962). *Br. Med. J.* **2,** 1495.

Dent, C. E., and Watson, L. C. A. (1964). *Br. Med. J.* **2,** 218.

Dietrich, A. (1948). *Frank. Z. Pathol.* **59,** 398.

DiLollo, F., Fazzini, G., and Morini, P. L. (1969). *Osp. Ital. Chir.* **21,** 251.

Dimich, A. B., Rothschild, E. O., Fulmer, D. H., Freed, B. R., and Myers, W. P. L. (1969). *Clin. Res.* **17,** 588.

Donegan, W. L., and Spiro, H. M. (1960). *Gastroenterology* **38,** 750.

Dreiling, D. A. (1961). *J. Am. Med. Assoc.* **175,** 183.

Drezner, M. K., and Feinglos, M. N. (1977). *J. Clin. Invest.* **60,** 1046.

Dubé, W. J., Clerkin, E. P., and Oberfield, R. V. (1968). *J. Am. Med. Assoc.* **203,** 359.

Dudley, H. R., Ritchie, A. C., Schilling, A., and Baker, W. H. (1955). *N. Engl. J. Med.* **252,** 331.

Earl, J. M., Kurlzman, N. A., and Moses, R. H. (1966). *Ann. Intern. Med.* **64,** 378.

Edwards, G. A., and Daum, S. M. (1959). *Arch. Intern. Med.* **104,** 29.

Ehrlich, M., Goldstein, N., and Heinemann, H. O. *Metab. Clin. Exp.* **12,** 516.

Eisenberg, E. (1965). *J. Clin. Invest.* **44,** 942.

Eisenberg, E. (1970). *N. Engl. J. Med.* **282,** 889.

Eisenberg, E., and Gotch, F. A. (1968). *Arch. Intern. Med.* **122,** 258.

Eisenberg, H., Pallotta, J., and Sherwood, L. M. (1974). *Am. J. Med.* **56,** 810.

Epstein, F. H. (1971). *In* "Diseases of the Kidney" (M. B. Strauss and L. G. Welt, eds.), p. 908. Little, Brown, Boston, Massachusetts.

Epstein, F. H., Rivera, M. J., and Carone, F. A. (1958). *J. Clin. Invest.* **37,** 1702.

Epstein, F. H., Beck, D., Carone, F. A., Levitin, H., and Manitius, A. (1959). *J. Clin. Invest.* **38,** 1214.

Evaldsson, U., Ertekin, C., Ingvar, D. H., and Waldenström, J. G. (1969). *J. Chronic Dis.* **22,** 431.

Fahey, T., and Myers, W. P. L. (1972). As cited in Myers (1972).

Ferenczy, A., Okagaki, T., and Richart, R. M. (1971). *Cancer* **27,** 427.

Fierer, J. A., Wagner, B. M., and Strebel, R. F. (1970). *Am. J. Cardiol.* **26,** 423.

Fitz, T. E., and Hallman, B. L. (1952). *Arch. Intern. Med.* **89,** 547.

Foreman, H., Finnegan, C., and Lushbaugh, G. C. (1956). *J. Am. Med. Assoc.* **160,** 1042.

Franklin, R. B., and Tashjian, A. H., Jr. (1975). *Endocrinology* **97,** 240.

Fry, L. (1962). *Br. Med. J.* **1,** 301.

Fulmer, D. H., Dimich, A. B., Rothschild, E. O. (1972). *Arch. Intern. Med.* **129,** 923.

Galasko, C. S. (1969). *Proc. R. Soc. Med.* **62,** 487.

Galasko, C. S., and Burn, J. I. (1971). *Br. Med. J.* **3,** 573.

Gallagher, J. C., and Nordin, B. E. C. (1972). *Lancet* **1,** 503.

Gault, M. H., and Kinsella, (1965). *Can. Med. Assoc. J.* **92,** 317.

Gellhorn, A. (1958). *J. Chronic Dis.* **8,** 158.

Gellhorn, A. (1969). *Adv. Intern. Med.* **15,** 299.

Gewirtz, G., and Yalow, R. S. (1974). *J. Clin. Invest.* **53,** 1022.

Gill, J. R., and Bartter, F. C. (1961). *J. Clin. Invest.* **40,** 716.

Goepfert, H., Smart, C. R., and Rochlin, D. B. (1966). *Ann. Surg.* **164,** 917.

Gold, G. L., and Shnider, B. C. (1959). *Ann. Intern. Med.* **51,** 890.
Goldberg, M. F., Tashjian, A. J., Jr., Orcler, S. E., and Dammin, G. J. (1964). *Am. J. Msd.* **36,** 805.
Goldsmith, R. S., and Ingbar, S. H. (1966). *N. Engl. J. Med.* **274,** 1.
Goldsmith, R. S., and Ingbar, S. H. (1967). *Ann. Intern. Med.* **67,** 463.
Gordan, G. S., Eisenberg, E., Loken, H. F., Garder, B., and Nayashida, T. (1962). *Recent Prog. Horm. Res.* **18,** 297.
Gordan, G. S., Cantino, T. J., Erhardt, L., Hansen, J., and Lubich, W. (1966). *Science* **151,** 1226.
Gordan, G. S., Fitzpatrick, M. E., and Lubick, W. P. (1967). *Trans. Assoc. Am. Physicians* **80,** 183.
Graham, W. P., Gardner, B., Thomas, A. N., Gordan, G. S., Loken, H. F., and Goldman, L. (1963). *Surg., Gynecol. Obstet.* **117,** 709.
Griboff, S. I., Hernmann, J. B., Smelin, A., and Moss, J. (1954). *J. Clin. Endocrinol. Metab.* **14,** 378.
Grimes, B. J., Fisher, B., Finn, F., and Danowski, T. S. (1967). *Acta Endocrinol. (Copenhagen)* **56,** 510.
Gutman, A. B., Tyson, T. L., and Gutman, E. B. (1936). *Arch. Intern. Med.* **58,** 379.
Gutman, U., and Gottschalk, C. W. (1966). *Isr. J. Med. Sci.* **2,** 243.
Gwinup, G., and Sayle, B. (1961). *Ann. Intern. Med.* **55,** 1001.
Haas, H. G., and Dumbacher, M. A. (1968). *Helv. Med. Acta* **34,** 327.
Haddad, J. G., Jr., Couranz, S., and Avioli, L. V. (1970). *J. Clin. Endocrinol. Metab.* **30,** 174.
Haddy, F. J., Scott, J. B., Florio, M. A., Daugherty, R. M., Jr., and Huizenga, J. N. (1963). *Am. J. Physiol.* **204,** 202.
Hall, T. C., Griffiths, C. T., and Petranek, J. R. (1966). *N. Engl. J. Med.* **275,** 1474.
Harrington, G., Olson, K. B., Horton, J., Cunningham, T., and Wright, A. (1970). *N. Engl. J. Med.* **283,** 1172.
Hamilton, S. W., Hartman, C. R., and Cohn, D. V. (1977). *J. Clin. Endocrin. Metab.* **45,** 1023.
Haskell, C. M., Devita, V. T., and Canellos, G. P. (1971). *Cancer* **27,** 872.
Haussler, M. R., and McCain, T. A. (1977). *New Engl. J. Med.* **297,** 974.
Haverbeck, B. J., Dyce, B., Bundy, H., and Edmondson, H. A. (1960). *Am. J. Med.* **29,** 424.
Hayslett, J. P., Perillie, P. E., and Finch, S. C. (1968). *N. Engl. J. Med.* **279,** 506.
Heath, D. A., Shimkin, P. M., and Wolfe, D. R. (1974). *J. Clin. Endocrinol. Metab.* **38,** 618.
Heckman, B. A., and Walsh, J. H. (1967). *N. Engl. J. Med.* **276,** 1082.
Heinemann, H. O. (1963). *Metab. Clin. Exp.* **12,** 792.
Hellström, J. (1954). *Acta Endocrinol. (Copenhagen)* **16,** 30.
Herbert, L. E., Lemann, J., Jr., Petersen, J. R., and Lennon, E. J. (1966). *J. Clin. Invest.* **45,** 1886.
Herishami, Y., Abramsky, O., and Levy, S. (1970). *Eur. Neurol.* **4,** 283.
Hilgard, P. (1970). *N. Engl. J. Med.* **283,** 436.
Hiraoka, M., Yamagishi, S., and Sano, T. (1968). *Am. J. Physiol.* **214,** 1084.
Hobbs, C. B., and Miller, A. L. (1968). *J. Clin. Pathol.* **19,** 119.
Hodges, M., and Waterhouse, C. (1967). *Arch. Intern. Med.* **120,** 75.
Hoff, H. E., Smith, P. K., and Winkler, A. W. (1939). *Am. J. Physiol.* **125,** 162.
Holland, J. F., Danielson, E., and Sahagian-Edwards, A. (1953). *Proc. Soc. Exp. Biol. Med.* **84,** 359.
Hollander, W., Jr., and Blythe, W. B. (1971). *In* "Diseases of the Kidney" (M. B. Strauss and L. G. Welt, eds.), p. 933, Little, Brown, Boston.
Horeau, J., Guenel, J., Bureau, L., and Dubigeon, M. (1965). *Presse Med.* **73,** 3057.

Horwitz, C. A., Myers, W. P. L., and Foote, F. W. (1972). *Am. J. Med.* **52**, 797.

Hulley, S. B., Goldsmith, R. S., and Ingbar, S. H. (1969). *Am. J. Physiol.* **217**, 1570.

Hulley, S. B., Vogel, J. M., Donaldson, C. D., Bayers, J. H., Friedman, R. J., and Rosen, S. N. (1971). *J. Clin. Invest.* **50**, 2506.

Huvos, A., Muggia, F. M., and Markewitz, M. (1969). *N. Y. State J. Med.* **69**, 2042.

Hyman, G. A. (1955). *Cancer* **8**, 576.

Issekutz, B., Jr., Blizzard, J., Burkhead, N. C., and Rodhal, I. C. (1966). *J. Appl. Physiol.* **21**, 1013.

Ito, H., Sanada, T., and Katayama, T. (1975). *N. Engl. J. Med.* **293**, 558.

Jaffe, N., Kim, B. S., and Vawter, G. F. (1972). *Cancer* **29**, 392.

Jessiman, A. G., Emerson, K. J., Shan, R. C., and Moore, F. D. (1963). *Ann. Surg.* **157**, 377.

Jordan, G. W. (1966). *Am. J. Med.* **41**, 381.

Kahil, M., Orman, B., Gyorkey, F., and Brown, H. (1967). *J. Am. Med. Assoc.* **201**, 721.

Kammerman, S. F., and Canfield, R. C. (1970). *J. Clin. Endocrinol. Metab.* **31**, 70.

Karpati, G., and Frame, B. (1964). *Arch. Neurol. (Chicago)* **10**, 387.

Katz, A., Kaplan, L., Massry, S. G., Heller, R., Plotkin, D., and Knight, I. (1970). *Arch. Surg. (Chicago)* **101**, 582.

Kaufman, R. J., Rothschild, E. O., Escher, G. C., and Myers, W. P. L. (1964). *J. Clin. Endocrinol. Metab.* **24**, 1235.

Keller, R. T., Goldscheider, I., and Lafferty, F. W. (1966). *Medicine (Baltimore)* **45**, 247.

Kelly, T. R. (1968). *Arch. Surg. (Chicago)* **97**, 267.

Kennedy, B. J., Tibbetts, D. M., Nathason, I. T., and Aub, J. C. (1953). *Cancer Res.* **13**, 445.

Kennedy, B. J., Sandbert-Wolheim, M., Loken, M., and Yarbro, J. W. (1967). *Cancer Res.* **27**, 1534.

Kimberg, D. V. (1969). *N. Engl. J. Med.* **280**, 1396.

King, W. W., Cox, C. E., and Boyce, W. H. (1972). *J. Urol.* **107**, 809.

Kleeman, C. R., Bohannon, J., Bernstein, D., Ling, S., and Maxwell, M. H. (1964). *Proc. Soc. Exp. Biol. Med.* **115**, 29.

Kleeman, C. R., Ling, S., Bernstein, D., Maxwell, M. H., and Chapman, L. (1966). *J. Clin. Invest.* **45**, 1032.

Klemperer, P. (1923). *Surg., Gynecol. Obstet.* **36**, 11.

Knill-Jones, R. P., Buckle, R. M., Parsons, V., Calne, R. Y., and Williams, R. (1970). *N. Engl. J. Med.* **282**, 704.

Knisley, E. R. (1966). *Arch. Intern. Med.* **118**, 14.

Kofman, S., and Eisenstein, R. (1963). *Cancer Chemother. Rep.* **32**, 77.

Kofman, S., Medrek, R. J., and Alexander, R. W. (1964). *Cancer* **17**, 938.

Kohout, E. (1966). *Cancer* **19**, 925.

Krabakow, B., Miner, M. F., and King, F. H. (1957). *N. Engl. J. Med.* **256**, 59.

Kronfield, S. L., and Reynold, R. B. (1964). *N. Engl. J. Med.* **271**, 399.

Lafferty, F. W. (1966). *Medicine (Baltimore)* **45**, 24.

Lafferty, F. W., and Pearson, O. H. (1963). *J. Clin. Endocrinol. Metab.* **23**, 891.

Lamberg, P. A., Pekonen, R., and Frick, M. H. (1964). *Acta Med. Scand.* **176**, 187.

Landau, R. L., and Kappas, A. (1965). *Ann. Intern. Med.* **62**, 1223.

Langer, G. A. (1972). *Circulation* **46**, 180.

Lassiter, W. E., Frick, A., Rumrich, G., and Ullrich, K. J. (1967). *Pfluegers Arch. Gesamte Physiol.* **285**, 90.

Lazor, M. Z., and Rosenberg, L. E. (1964). *N. Engl. J. Med.* **270**, 749.

Lee, C. A., and Lloyd, H. M. (1971). *Cancer* **27**, 1099.

LeGall, J. R., Raphael, J. C., and Offenstadt, G. (1971). *Ann. Med. Interne* **122**, 613.

Lehrer, G. M., and Levitt, M. F. (1960). *J. Mt. Sinai Hosp., N. Y.* **27,** 10.

Lemon, H. M., and Kotob, N. (1961). *Cancer* **14,** 934.

Leprat, J. (1968). *Bruxelles-Med.* **48,** 5.

Lindegarde, F., and Zettervall, O. (1973). *Ann. Intern. Med.* **78,** 396.

Lipsett, M. B. (1968). *Adv. Metab. Dis.* **3,** 111.

Lipsett, M. B., Odell, W. D., Rosenberg, L. E., and Waldmann, T. A. (1964). *Ann. Intern. Med.* **61,** 733.

Lista, G. A. (1966). *Prensa Med. Argent.* **53,** 1260.

Loebel, A. S., and Walkoff, C. S. (1962). *N. Y. State J. Med.* **62,** 101.

Lown, B., Black, H., and Moore, F. D. (1960). *Am. J. Cardiol.* **6,** 309.

Luben, R. A., Mundy, G. R., Trummel, C. L., and Raisz, L. G. (1974). *J. Clin. Invest.* **53,** 1473.

Lucas, P. G. (1960). *Br. Med. J.* **1,** 1330.

Ludwig, G. D. (1962). *Ann. Intern. Med.* **56,** 676.

Lytton, B., Rosof, B., and Evans, J. S. (1965). *J. Urol.* **93,** 127.

McGuigan, J. E. (1970). *N. Engl. J. Med.* **283,** 137.

Magnenat, V. P., and Perret, C. (1961). *Gastroenterologia* **96,** 197.

Manitius, A., Levitan, H., Beck, D., and Epstein, F. H. (1960). *J. Clin. Invest.* **39,** 693.

Mannheimer, I. H. (1965). *Cancer* **18,** 679.

Marti, M. C., and Cox, J. N. (1970). *Schweiz. Med. Wochenschr.* **100,** 927.

Massry, S. G., Muellar, E., Silverman, A. G., and Kleeman, C. R. (1968). *Arch. Intern. Med.* **121,** 307.

Mavligit, G. (1970). *Lancet* **2,** 1188.

Mavligit, G. M., Cohen, J. L., and Sherwood, L. M. (1971). *N. Engl. J. Med.* **285,** 154.

Mawdsley, C., and Holman, R. L. (1957). *Lancet* **1,** 78.

Meador, C. K., Liddle, G. W., Island, D. P., Nicholson, W. E., Lucas, C. P., Nuckton, J. G., and Leutscher, J. A., (1962). *J. Clin. Endocrinol.* **22,** 693.

Melick, R. A., Martin, R. A., and Hicks, J. D. (1972). *Br. Med. J.* **2,** 204.

Menguy, R. (1969). *Surg. Clin. North Am.* **49,** 49.

Moore, W. T., and Smith, L. H., Jr. (1963). *Metab., Clin. Exp.* **12,** 447.

Morris, R. C. (1969). *N. Engl. J. Med.* **281,** 1405.

Moses, A. M., and Spencer, H. (1963). *Ann. Intern. Med.* **59,** 531.

Moure, J. M. B. (1967). *Arch. Neurol. (Chicago)* **17,** 34.

Muckle, R. M., Mason, A. M. S., and Middleton, J. E. (1969). *Lancet* **1,** 1128.

Muggia, F. M., and Heinemann, H. O. (1970). *Ann. Intern. Med.* **73,** 281.

Muggia, F. M., Heinemann, H. O., Bélanger, R., and Weinstein, I. B. (1968). *Clin. Res.* **16,** 558.

Muirhead, W. (1967). *Can. Med. Assoc. J.* **97,** 569.

Muldowney, F. P., McKenna, T. J., Kyle, L. H., Freaney, R., and Swan, M. (1970). *N. Engl. J. Med.* **282,** 61.

Mundy, G. R., Luben, R. A., Raisz, L. G., Oppenheim, J. J., and Buell, D. N. (1974). *N. Engl. J. Med.* **290,** 867.

Mundy, G. R., Raisz, L. G., Cooper, R. A., Schechter, G. P., and Salmon, S. E. (1974). *N. Engl. J. Med.* **291,** 1041.

Munson, P. L., Tashjian, A. J., Jr., and Levine, L. (1965). *Cancer Res.* **25,** 1062.

Myers, W. P. L. (1956a). *Cancer* **9,** 1135.

Myers, W. P. L. (1956b). *Med. Clin. North Am.* **40,** 871.

Myers, W. P. L. (1958). *Cancer* **11,** 83.

Myers, W. P. L. (1960). *Arch. Surg. (Chicago)* **80,** 308.

Myers, W. P. L. (1962). *Adv. Intern. Med.* **2,** 163.

Myers, W. P. L. (1966). *Med. Clin. North Am.* **50**, 763.

Myers, W. P. L. (1968). *In* "Lung Cancer" (W. L. Watson, ed.), p. 488. Mosby, St. Louis, Missouri.

Myers, W. P. L. (1972). *Proc. Clin. Conf., M. D. Anderson Hosp.*

Myers, W. P. L., West, C. D., Pearson, O. H., and Karnofsky, D. A. (1956). *J. Am. Med. Assoc.* **161**, 127.

Naide, W., Matz, R., and Spear, P. W. (1968). *Am. J. Dig. Dis.* **13**, 705.

Neiman, R. S., and Li, H. C. (1972). *Cancer* **30**, 942.

Noeninckx, F. R. S., and Van Laethem, L. (1962). *Acta Clin. Belg.* **14**, 406.

Nolph, K. D., and Stoltz, M. L. (1971). *Clin. Res.* **19**, 481.

Nordin, B. E. C., and Peacock, M. (1969). *Lancet* **2**, 1280.

O'Grady, A. S., Morse, L. J., and Lee, J. B. (1965). *Ann. Intern. Med.* **63**, 858.

Olefsky, J., Kempson, R., Jones, H., and Reaven, G. (1972). *N. Engl. J. Med.* **286**, 740.

Omenn, G. S. (1971). *Pediatrics* **47**, 613.

Omenn, G. S., Roth, S. I., and Baker, W. H. (1969). *Cancer* **24**, 1004.

Orlando, R. C., and Macanic, B. I. (1972). *J. Am. Med. Assoc.* **222**, 1183.

Overbeck, H. W., Molnar, J. I., and Haddy, F. J. (1961). *Am. J. Cardiol.* **8**, 533.

Palmieri, G. N. A., Nordquist, R. E., and Omenn, G. S. (1974). *J. Clin. Invest.* **53**, 1726.

Paloyan, E., Palozan, D., and Harper, P. V. (1967). *Metab., Clin. Exp.* **16**, 35.

Parsons, V., Baum, M., and Self, M. (1967). *Br. Med. J.* **1**, 474.

Patten, B. M., Bilezekian, J. P., Mallette, L. E., Prince, A., Engel, W. K., and Aurbach, G. D. (1974). *Ann. Int. Med.* **80**, 182.

Pearson, O. H. (1964). *Proc. Natl. Cancer Conf.* **5**, 445.

Pearson, O. H., West, C. D., Hollander, V. P., and Treves, N. E. (1954). *J. Am. Med. Assoc.* **154**, 234.

Pechet, M. M., Bobadilla, E., Carrol, E., and Hesse, R. H. (1967). *Am. J. Med.* **43**, 696.

Perlia, C. P. (1969). *Ann. Intern. Med.* **70**, 1103.

Perlia, C. P., Gubisch, N. J., Wolter, J., Edelberg, D., Dederick, M. M., and Taylor, S. G., III. (1970). *Cancer* **25**, 389.

Petersen, M. J., and Edelman, I. S. (1964). *J. Clin. Invest.* **43**, 583.

Petersen, P. (1968). *J. Clin. Endocrinol. Metab.* **28**, 1491.

Pietrek, J. (1969). *Pol. Tyg. Lek.* **24**, 373.

Pinals, R. S., and Krane, S. M. (1962). *Postgrad. Med. J.* **38**, 507.

Plimpton, C. H., and Gellhorn, A. (1956). *Am. J. Med.* **21**, 750.

Powell, D., Singer, F. R., Murray, T. M., Minkin, C., and Potts, J. T., Jr. (1972a). *Clin. Res.* **20**, 569.

Powell, D., Shimkin, P. M., Doppman, J. L., Wells, S., Aurbach, G. D., Marx, S. J., Ketcham, A. S., and Potts, J. T. (1972b). *N. Engl. J. Med.* **286**, 1169.

Powell, D., Singer, F. R., Murray, R. M., Mimkin, C., and Potts, J. T., Jr. (1973). *N. Engl. J. Med.* **289**, 176.

Raisz, L. G., and Nieman, I. (1969). *Endocrinology* **85**, 446.

Raisz, L. G., Trummel, C. L., Mundy, G. R., and Luben, R. A. (1975). *In* "Calcium Regulating Hormones" (R. V. Talmage, M. Owen, and J. A. Parsons, eds.), p. 149. Excerpta Med. Found., Amsterdam.

Randall, R. E., Jr., and Lireman, D. S. (1964). *J. Clin. Endocrinol. Metab.* **24**, 1331.

Raphael, J. C., Kleinknecht, D., and Chanard, J. (1971). *Presse Med.* **79**, 1103.

Raymond, J. P. (1968). *Presse Med.* **76**, 1465.

Ream, N. W., Perlia, C. P., Wolter, J., and Taylor, S. G., III. (1968). *J. Am. Med. Assoc.* **204**, 1030.

Rice, B. F. (1969). *Recent Prog. Horm. Res.* **25**, 283.

Rice, B. F., Ponthier, R. L., Jr., and Miller, M. C., III. (1971). *Endocrinology* **88**, 1210.

Richet, G., Ardaillon, R., Amiel, C. *et al.* (1963). *J. Urol.* **69**, 373.

Riggs, B. L., Arnaud, C. D., Reynolds, J. C., and Smith, L. H. (1971). *J. Clin. Invest.* **50**, 2079.

Robertson, R. P., Baylink, D. J., Marini, J. J., and Adkison, H. W. (1975). *J. Clin. Endocrinol. Metab.* **41**, 164.

Robertson, R. P., Baylink, D. J., Metz, S. A., and Cummings, K. B. (1976). *J. Clin. Endocrinol. Metab.* **43**, 1330.

Roof, B. S., Carpenter, B., Fink, D. J., and Gordon, G. S. (1971). *Am. J. Med.* **50**, 686.

Ross, L., and Shelley, E. (1968). *Am. J. Obstet. Gynecol.* **100**, 410.

Rothschild, E. O., Myers, W. P. L., and Lawrence, W., Jr. (1964). *Clin. Res.* **12**, 462.

Rottino, A., Hoffman, G. T., and Brondolo, B. (1952). *Proc. Soc. Exp. Biol. Med.* **80**, 339.

Rudd, F. W. (1972). *J. Urol.* **107**, 986.

Salassa, R. M., Jowsey, J., and Arnaud, C. D. (1970). *N. Engl. J. Med.* **283**, 65.

Samuelsson, S. M., and Werner, I. (1963). *Acta Med. Scand.* **173**, 539.

Sataline, L. R. (1962). *N. Engl. J. Med.* **267**, 646.

Schatten, W. E., Ship, A. G., Pieper, W. J., and Bartter, F. C. (1968). *Ann. Surg.* **148**, 890.

Schneider, A. B., and Sherwood, L. M. (1974). *Metabolism,* **23**, 975.

Scholz, D. A., Riggs, B. L., Purnell, D. C., Goldsmith, R. S., and Arnaud, D. C. (1973). *Mayo Clin. Proc.* **48**, 124.

Schussler, G. O., Verso, M. A., and Nemoto, T. (1972). *J. Clin. Endocrinol. Metab.* **35**, 497.

Seftel, L. A., and Gusberg, S. B. (1965). *Obstet. Gynecol.* **25**, 693.

Segré, G. V., Habener, J. F., Powell, D., Tregéar, G. D., and Potts, J. T., Jr. (1972). *J. Clin. Invest.* **51**, 3163.

Seifert, G., and Seeman, N. (1967). *Dsch. Med. Wochenschr.* **92**, 1104.

Seller, R. H. (1971). *Am. Heart J.* **82**, 551.

Seyberth, H. W., Segré, G. V., Morgan, J. L., Sweetnam, B. J., Potts, J. T., Jr., and Oates, J. A. (1975). *N. Engl. J. Med.* **293**, 1278.

Shackney, S., and Hasson, J. (1967). *Ann. Int. Med.* **66**, 906.

Sherwood, L. M. (1967). *N. Engl. J. Med.* **278**, 663.

Sherwood, L. M. (1971). *N. Engl. J. Med.* **284**, 839.

Sherwood, L. M., and Abe, M. (1972). *Clin. Res.* **20**, 756.

Sherwood, L. M., O'Riordan, J. L. H., Aurbach, J. D., and Potts, J. T., Jr. (1967). *J. Clin. Endocrinol. Metab.* **27**, 140.

Sherwood, L. M. (1976). *In* "The Year in Endocrinology 1975–76," (S. H. Ingbar, ed.), p. 249–76, Plenum Press, New York.

Sigurdsson, G., Woodhouse, N. J. Y., Taylor, S., and Joplin, G. F. (1973). *Br. Med. J.* **1**, 27.

Silva, O. L., Becker, K. L., Primack, A., Doppman, J. L., and Snider, R. H. (1976). *Chest* **69**, 495.

Simpsom, J. A. (1954). *Br. Med. J.* **1**, 494.

Singer, F. R., Neer, R. M., Murray, T. M., Keutman, H. T., Deftos, L. J., and Potts, J. T., Jr. (1970). *N. Engl. J. Med.* **283**, 634.

Singer, F. R., Powell, D., Minkin, C., Bethune, J. E., Brickman, A., and Coburn, J. W. (1973). *Ann. Intern. Med.* **78**, 365.

Sitrin, M. D., and Bohr, D. F. (1971). *Am. J. Physiol.* **220**, 1124.

Smith, J. P., Boronow, R. C., and Moure, J. M. (1968). *South. Med. J.* **61**, 375.

Snedecor, P. A., and Baker, W. H. (1964). *Cancer* **17**, 1492.

Soffer, A., Toribara, T., Moore-Jones, D., and Wever, D. (1960). *AMA Arch. Intern. Med.* **30**, 129.

Spaulding, S. W., and Walser, M. (1970). *J. Clin. Endocrinol. Metab.* **31**, 531.

Spencer, H., Greenberg, J., Berger, E., Perrone, M., and Laszio, D. (1956). *J. Lab. Clin. Med.* **47,** 29.

Spencer, H., Lewin, I., and Freidland, J. A. (1967). *Isr. J. Med. Sci.* **3,** 643.

Sperber, M. A. (1969). *Br. Med. J.* **3,** 176.

Spiro, H. M. (1960). *Gastroenterology* **39,** 544.

Spiro, H. M. (1970). "Clinical Gastroenterology," p. 296. Collier-Macmillan, New York.

Stanbury, S. W. (1972). *J. Clin. Endocrinol. Metab.* **1,** 239.

Steck, I. E., Deutsch, H., Reed, C. I., and Struck, H. G. (1937). *Ann. Intern. Med.* **10,** 951.

Stein, R. C. (1971). *J. Pediatr.* **78,** 861.

Steinberg, D. (1972). *Ann. Intern. Med.* **76,** 670.

Steinberg, D., Osofsky, M., and Rubin, A. D. (1971). *N. Y. State Med.* **71,** 583.

Stolbach, L. L., Krant, M. J., and Fishman, W. H. (1969). *N. Engl. J. Med.* **281,** 757.

Stone, G. E., Waterhouse, C., and Terry, R. (1961). *Ann. Intern. Med.* **54,** 977.

Streeto, J. M. (1969). *N. Engl. J. Med.* **280,** 427.

Strickland, N. J., Bold, A. M., and Medd, M. E. (1967). *Br. Med. J.* **3,** 590.

Strott, C. A., and Nugent, C. A. (1968). *Ann. Intern. Med.* **68,** 188.

Suki, W. N., Eknoyan, G., Rector, F. C., Jr., and Seldin, D. W. (1969). *Nephron* **6,** 50.

Suki, W. N., Yuim, J. J., von Minden, M., Saller-Herbert, C., Eknoyan, G., and Martinez-Maldonado, M. (1970). *N. Engl. J. Med.* **283,** 836.

Svane, S. (1964). *Acta Med. Scand.* **175,** 353.

Tambyak, J. A., and Lim, M. K. L. (1969). *Br. Med. J.* **1,** 751.

Targovnik, J. H., Rodman, H. S., and Sherwood, L. M. (1971). *Endocrinology* **88,** 1477.

Tashjian, A. H., Jr. (1969). *Biotechnol. Bioeng.* **11,** 109.

Tashjian, A. H., Jr. (1974). *N. Engl. J. Med.* **290,** 905.

Tashjian, A. H., Jr. (1975). *N. Engl. J. Med.* **293,** 1317.

Tashjian, A. H., Jr., Levine, L., and Munson, P. L. (1964). *J. Exp. Med.* **119,** 467.

Tashjian, A. H., Jr., Voelkel, E. F., Levine, L., and Goldhabed, P. (1972). *J. Exp. Med.* **136,** 1329.

Taylor, D. M., and Siemsen, A. W. (1965). *Arch. Intern. Med.* **115,** 67.

Thalassinos, N., and Joplin, G. F. (1968). *Br. Med. J.* **4,** 14.

Thomas, W. H. G., and Karat, A. B. A. (1966). *Br. Med. J.* **2,** 745.

Tremblay, R. E., and Ansell, J. S. (1964). *J. Urol.* **91,** 10.

Trudeau, W., and McGuigan, J. E. (1969). *N. Engl. J. Med.* **281,** 862.

Turchi, J. J., Flandreau, R. H., Forte, A. L., French, G. N., and Ludwig, G. D. (1962). *J. Am. Med. Assoc.* **180,** 799.

Turkington, R. W., Goldman, J. K., and Ruffner, B. W. (1966). *Cancer* **19,** 406.

Unger, R. H., and Lochner, J. (1964). *J. Clin. Endocrinol. Metab.* **24,** 823.

Voelkel, E. F., Tashjian, A. H., Jr., Franklin, R., Wasserman, E., and Levine, L. (1975). *Metab., Clin. Exp.* **24,** 973.

Vogel, S. B., Enneking, W. F., and Thomas, W. C., Jr. (1967). *Endocrinology* **80,** 404.

von Recklinghausen, F. D. (1891). As cited in Baker (1956).

Walser, M. (1958). *J. Clin. Invest.* **37,** 940.

Walser, M. (1961). *Am. J. Physiol.* **200,** 1099.

Walser, M. (1962). *J. Clin. Invest.* **41,** 1454.

Walser, M. (1970). *Mod. Treat.* **7,** 662.

Waugh, W. H. (1962). *Circ. Res.* **11,** 927.

Weidmann, P., Massry, S. G., Coburn, J. W., Maxwell, M. H., Atelson, J., and Kleeman, C. R. (1972). *Ann. Intern. Med.* **76,** 741.

West, T. E. T., Joffe, M., Sinclair, L., and O'Riordan, J. L. H. (1971). *Lancet* **1,** 675.

Wills, M. R., and McGowan, G. K. (1964). *Br. Med. J.* **1,** 1153.
Wilson, J. R., Merrich, H., and Woodward, E. R. (1961). *Ann. Surg.* **154,** 485.
Wyss, F., Studer, H., and Staub, J. J. (1971). *Internist* **12,** 215.
Zeffren, J. L., and Heinemann, H. O. (1962). *Am. J. Med.* **33,** 54.
Zidar, B. L., Shadduck, R. K., Winkelstein, A., Zelger, Z., and Hawker, C. D. (1976). *New Eng. J. Med.* **295,** 692.
Zusman, J., Brown, D. M. and Nesbit (1973). *New Eng. J. Med.* **289,** 1335.

7

Metabolic Bone Disease in Children

ROBERT STEENDIJK

I. Growth and Development of the Skeleton	634
A. Bone Structure and Development in the Fetus and Child	634
B. Chemical Determinants of Skeletal Metabolism in Infancy, Childhood, and Adolescence	638
C. Calcium Homeostasis in Pregnancy and Early Infancy	639
II. Differential Diagnosis of Hypercalcemia	643
A. Signs and Symptoms	643
B. Primary Hyperparathyroidism	644
C. Idiopathic Hypercalcemia of Infancy	648
D. Familial Benign Hypercalcemia	651
E. Vitamin D Intoxication	651
F. Immobilization	653
G. Addison's Disease	654
H. Leukemia	654
I. Sarcoidosis	654
J. Hypothyroidism	655
K. Hypophosphatasia	655
III. Differential Diagnosis of Hypocalcemia	658
A. Signs and Symptoms	658
B. Neonatal Hypocalcemia	658
C. Idiopathic Hypoparathyroidism	663
D. Surgical Hypoparathyroidism	667
E. Pseudohypoparathyroidism	667
F. Hypohyperparathyroidism	670
G. Primary Hypomagnesemia	670
H. Dwarfism and Cortical Thickening of Tubular Bones	671
IV. Normocalcemic Disorders of Mineral Metabolism	672
A. Osteoporosis	672
B. Osteogenesis Imperfecta	673

Copyright © 1978 by Academic Press, Inc.
All rights of reproduction in any form reserved
ISBN 0-12-068702-X

C. Hereditary Hyperphosphatasia 677
D. Polyostotic Fibrous Dysplasia 679
E. Vitamin C Deficiency 683
F. Osteopetrosis 683
G. Hypothyroidism 687
H. Pycnodysostosis 688
I. Hypervitaminosis A 688
J. Other Rare Diseases 688
V. Bone Disease in Disorders of Renal Function 689
A. Idiopathic Hypercalciuria 689
B. Renal Osteodystrophy 692
References 696

A variety of metabolic bone disorders that afflict adults (described in detail in other chapters in Volume I and in this volume) are also seen in children. Metabolic bone disease in growing children is a large and varied subject, since it includes all generalized skeletal disorders in which the mass, structure, growth, composition, or metabolism of bone are deranged by abnormal metabolism of any of the inorganic or organic constituents of bone tissue. The origin of these diseases may be in the bone itself or it may be a disturbance of mineral or organic metabolism not limited to bone. A number of these diseases are hereditary or congenital, others are acquired; the pathogenesis may be endocrine, nutritional, or unknown. It is difficult to classify such a large variety of disorders satisfactorily. In this chapter these disorders will be discussed with reference to the state of circulating levels of calcium and renal function. The general, nonspecific clinical disorders characterized by either hypercalcemia or hypocalcemia peculiar to the neonatal, preadolescent and adolescent years are discussed separately.

I. GROWTH AND DEVELOPMENT OF THE SKELETON

A. Bone Structure and Development in the Fetus and Child

The developing fetus does not acquire much calcium before the eighth week, when mineralization of the skeleton begins. From that time deposition of bone tissue is a rapid process, and at term the fetus contains about 28 gm of calcium or 8 gm per kg body weight (Widdowson and Spray, 1951). From a structural and dynamic point of view fetal bone differs considerably from the bone that is present during most of the life span of the individual. The primitive bone is of the woven type, characterized by irregular arrangement of the collagen fibers, a high degree of mineralization of the organic matrix, and numerous large osteocytes. This is immediately apparent from microradiographs of thin undecalcified sections of the bone (Steendijk, 1969). In the cortical areas of the long bones the layers or bands of woven bone are separated by spaces containing a vascular connective tissue. As the prenatal period progresses, these spaces gradually become filled by layers of lamellar bone, which has a lower degree of mineralization and contains smaller and less numerous osteocytes. This lamellar bone is deposited alongside the woven bone and also in cylindrical structures, the primary osteones. As a result, the cortex becomes very compact (Fig. 1) (Steendijk, 1971). During growth the bone gradually begins to assume its characteristic shape by external remodeling. Simultaneously, the marrow cavity is formed by endosteal resorption, a relatively slow process compared to periosteal deposition of new bone. Between the third and the tenth month the diameter of the femoral midshaft increases eightfold, while the diameter of the marrow cavity attains only twice its original value. This results in the very thick cortex, typical of neonatal long bones, which has been termed "physiological osteosclerosis" (Fig. 1). Internal remodeling of the cortex is completely absent until the last prenatal month, when resorption cavities begin to appear near the endosteal side of the cortex (Steendijk, 1971).

Shortly after birth endosteal resorption in the long bones is accelerated and the diameter of the marrow cavity increases so rapidly that the cortex becomes relatively thin, although bone continues to be deposited on the periosteal side (Garn, 1970). This has been observed in the tibia, femur, and metacarpals and is probably characteristic of all long bones. Simultaneously internal remodeling becomes a very active process in which primitive bone is replaced by lamellar bone in the form of secondary Haversian systems. Approximately 6 months after birth, the thin cortex and the numerous resorption cavities and growing osteones impart a histological picture termed "physiological osteoporosis" (for want of a better expression) (Fig. 1). The growth in thickness of the entire bone and of the cortex has been studied in a number of bones but mainly in the metacarpals. From measurements made on radiographs of the midshaft of the second metacarpal it has been shown that toward the end of the second year the diameter of the marrow cavity equals the diameter of the neonatal cortex (Bonnard, 1968). This means that all primitive cortical bone has been remodeled within 2 years. If the same rate of growth is assumed in the other long bones, the rate of remodeling of the skeleton is approximately 50% per year during this period. This high remodeling rate decreases rapidly until later in childhood when it approximates 10% per

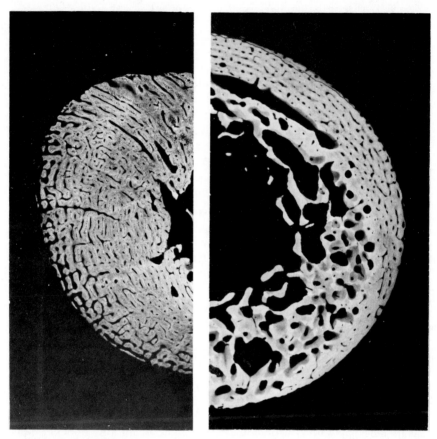

Fig. 1. Microradiographs of undecalcified cross section from the femoral midshaft of a normal newborn infant (left, physiological osteosclerosis) and of an 8-month-old infant (right, physiological osteoporosis) ($\times$ 12).

year. It rises again during the pubescence years, after which it falls to the adult value of 4–8% per annum (Steendijk, 1971). Changes in bone mass that attend early and senescent adulthood are described in detail in Chapter 6, Volume I.

The growth of the diameter of the long bones has been studied exhaustively by Garn (1970) and his associates, using the 2nd metacarpal as a reference. Changes in the cross-sectional area, total diameter, and of the marrow cavity of the metacarpal midshaft are illustrated in Fig. 2. The development shows a remarkable sex difference, beginning in early adolescence. In both sexes, between the ages of 10 and 18 years, periosteal deposition of new bone increases, but more so in males than in females. Following this increased growth rate, growth levels off and the

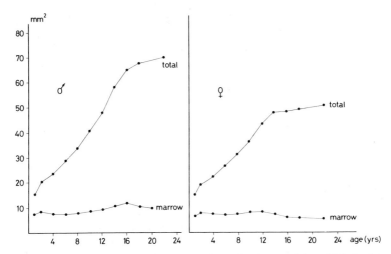

Fig. 2. Growth in boys and girls of the cross-sectional area of the midshaft of the 2nd metacarpal. Total: area surrounded by periosteum; marrow: area of marrow activity. (Drawn from data by Garn, 1970.)

rate of decrease in the diameter of the marrow cavity is greater in girls than in boys. The result is a conspicuous increase in cortical diameter much more pronounced in males than in females. Relative to the total diameter of the bone, however, the cortex of the adolescent female is thicker than in males of comparable age. This sex difference in bone dimensions results, at least in part, from the difference in the level of androgenic and estrogenic hormones in boys and girls. It is assumed that the endosteal deposition of bone in adolescence is the result of the activity of androgens and estrogens, the latter being more potent in this respect (Garn, 1970).

The amount of calcium in the body can only be measured accurately by carcass analysis and this has been done too infrequently to permit the derivation of the values that obtain throughout the growth years. From the available measurements it appears that the amount of calcium relative to body weight rises from a value of 0.8% in the neonate to 1.6% in the adult male (Widdowson, 1965). Using his metacarpal measurements and some values derived from carcass analyses, Garn (1970) has computed the annual increments in calcium content of the body. The results of these calculations show that the relative amount of calcium in the body falls in the first year of life to approximately 0.6% and then slowly rises to 1.6% in the young adult male and 1.3% in the young adult female. The initial fall (which has been documented by carcass analysis) results probably from the high rate of bone resorption in infancy. Subsequently, the rate of remodeling decreases, resulting in an increase of the average degree of bone tissue mineralization. In addition, uncalcified cartilage, mainly in the epiphyseal centers of the long bones, is replaced by bone. These characteristics of the developing skeleton contribute to the increase of the calcium content of the body. In this respect it is interesting to realize that a 5-year-old child has as much calcium per kg of body weight as a 70-year-old woman. The child, however, is less prone to sustain fractures than the aged human being, suggesting that the physical properties of bone tissue are not reflected by whole body or skeletal calcium content (see Chapter 6, Volume I).

B. Chemical Determinants of Skeletal Metabolism in Infancy, Childhood, and Adolescence

The magnitude of the changes that occur during skeletal development is reflected by the concentration of alkaline phosphatase in serum and urinary hydroxyproline content. Circulating alkaline phosphatase, which in the young and growing child is predominantly the isoenzyme produced by skeletal osteoblasts (see Chapter 3, Volume I), is approximately 4 times higher in infancy than in adulthood when the average values are 5 King-Armstrong Units in women and 7 King-Armstrong Units in men (Dent and Harper, 1962; Nordin and Smith, 1965). As noted in Chapter 3, Volume I, the skeletal alkaline phosphatase isoenzyme is also decreased in adult life when active growth has terminated. During the pubertal growth spurt the concentration of alkaline phosphatase temporarily rises, reaching values that are approximately twice those reported for adults (de Wijn, 1965; Round, 1973).

The urinary excretion of hydroxyproline (free and total) in children is also higher than in adults, both absolutely and when expressed per kg of body weight. Urinary hydroxyproline is derived primarily from bone collagen (see Chapter 1, Volume I) and is highest in infancy, although the values are very low in the early neonatal period (Morrow, et al., 1967; Klein and Teree, 1966). The normal adult level is approximately 30 mg per 24 hours, although the range is wide (Nordin and Smith, 1965). The values in 1- to 2-month-old infants may average 40–50 mg per 24 hours (Klein and Teree, 1966). Relative to body weight, these babies excrete more than 20 times as much as adults. Recently it has been shown that the excretion of hydroxyproline is highly correlated with growth rate, which is most apparent during the pubertal growth spurt (Pappas et al., 1971; Zorab et al., 1970). At this stage of development the excretion in males is higher than in females, often attaining values of 100 mg per 24 hours and more. Values of this magnitude are found in adults with hyperparathyroidism, acromegaly, or Paget's disease of bone.

The concentration of serum phosphate, which is highest before birth, declines gradually during childhood. Levels in infancy (approximately 6 mg/100 ml) are about twice as high as in adults. There is some evidence to suggest that a rise occurs in puberty, but longitudinal studies are required to confirm this (de Wijn, 1965). The serum calcium concentration averages 10.0 mg/100 ml throughout childhood and adolescence, except for the first few days of life when it is slightly lower (Bergman, 1972). Recently, Arnaud *et al.* (1973) found the concentration of immunoreactive parathyroid hormone of children to be comparable to that of adults (22 μl Eq/ml), although in young children slightly higher levels were found. It appears, therefore, that the high rate of remodeling of bone in childhood is independent of the concentration of parathyroid hormone. In the first two days of life the concentration of parathyroid hormone in serum is very low (David and Anast, 1974; Root *et al.,* 1974).

Throughout the development of the child bone growth, turnover of bone tissue and the accompanying changes in serum phosphate, serum alkaline phosphatase, and the excretion of hydroxyproline are dependent on nutritional (Park, 1964) and endocrine (Garn, 1970) factors. The most important of these are growth hormone, and somatomedin, parathyroid hormone, calcitonin, thyroxine, and the sex hormones. The many intricate interrelations between these factors have only partly been resolved and even a brief outline is beyond the scope of the present text. It should be emphasized, however, that rickets in children occurs at serum phosphorus concentrations that are at a lower end of the normal adult range. It appears, therefore, that the high levels of serum phosphorus normally seen in the growing cycles of life are essential for adequate mineralization of osteoid tissue.

It should be emphasized that metabolic bone disease in childhood is superimposed on a high rate of skeletal remodeling. Consequently certain types of metabolic bone disease are manifested by gross skeletal changes more rapidly in children than in adults. Thus, disturbances in endochondral mineralization rapidly lead to distortion in growth rate and shape of bones and are considered early signs of metabolic bone disease in young children. The differences between adults and children in this regard are exemplified by the rapid skeletal response of the latter to vitamin D deficiency, hyperparathyroidism, adrenocorticoid hormone excess, and renal failure when compared to an adult population.

C. Calcium Homeostasis in Pregnancy and Early Infancy

The developing fetus does not acquire much calcium before the eighth week, when mineralization of the fetal skeleton begins. From the third month calcium is deposited in the fetal bones at a rate that increases from approximately 10 mg per day in the third month to 250–300 mg per day in the last weeks of pregnancy. Considerable changes in the calcium metabolism of the pregnant woman occur even before the loss of calcium to the fetus becomes appreciable. The intestinal absorption of calcium increases throughout pregnancy and urinary calcium, elevated initially, decreases during the second half of pregnancy. Calcium retention increases before calcium accumulates in the body of the fetus. According to several investigators, the increased calcium retention accounts for at least 60% of the calcium delivered to the fetus. It has been concluded from measurements of cortical and medullary width of the shaft of the second metacarpal of pregnant women that bone is being deposited at the endosteal surface of the long bones (Garn, 1970). In accordance with this kinetic studies with ^{48}Ca reveal that bone accretion increases from the beginning of pregnancy until it reaches a value twice that of normal shortly before term. Bone resorption is depressed initially, but rises from the 30–34th week to values higher than in nonpregnant women of similar age. An unknown fraction of the change in calcium kinetics is the result of the increasing quantity of fetal bone, which has high rates of accretion. The fetus is not entirely responsible for these changes, since they are already apparent at an early date and persist for a short time after delivery (Heaney and Skillman, 1971).

The mechanism responsible for these changes still remains to be elucidated. Estrogenic hormones and placental lactogens, which have growth hormone-like properties, may play a role, since growth hormone increases skeletal remodeling and is known to increase endosteal deposition of bone in the adult animal. Recently, it has been found that the circulating level of immunoreactive parathyroid hormone was normal to low in the beginning of pregnancy and decreased during the 20–24th week. Subsequently, a progressive rise occurred to values of approximately twice normal in the last week. This could account for the increased bone remodeling in the latter half of pregnancy. Elevated PTH levels may also be responsible for the low urinary calcium excretion, with simultaneously elevated intestinal resorption. The stimulus for increased PTH secretion is not known. Ultrafiltrable plasma calcium is normal throughout pregnancy; however, it may be of importance in this respect that the PTH level rises concomitantly with increasing fetal bone formation (Cushard *et al.*, 1972; Root *et al.*, 1974).

Following pregnancy, the changes in calcium metabolism persist for a few weeks in nonlactating women. The influence of lactation on maternal calcium and bone metabolism is still uncertain, although a significant amount of calcium is lost to the neonate. Parathyroid hormone levels of both lactating and nonlactating women are reportedly normal 4–8 weeks after delivery. If it is assumed that a causal relationship exists between elevated circulating levels of parathyroid hormone and the growing demand of the fetus for calcium, the normal value during lactation, when the maternal loss of calcium is, in fact, greater than during pregnancy, is surprising. The increased cortical thickness of the second metacarpal gained during pregnancy is lost during lactation. Lactating women lose an average of 2.2% of the femoral calcium content during periods varying from 90 to 120 days. When pregnancy is not followed by lactation, cortical bone loss does not occur.

From animal experiments and clinical observation it appears that the fetal parathyroid glands actively regulate plasma calcium and phosphate levels in the latter half of pregnancy (Tsang *et al.*, 1976). Hypocalcemia, induced in fetal sheep by EDTA infusions, results in a rise in fetal parathyroid hormone levels without change in the calcium and parathyroid hormone in maternal blood. Injections of parathyroid extract into rat or dog fetuses result in fetal hypercalcemia, without concomitant elevations in maternal plasma calcium. Decapitation of fetal rats with removal of the parathyroid glands is, however, followed by fetal hypocalcemia. Administration of PTH to the pregnant rat results in a substantial rise of plasma calcium and only a negligible effect on fetal plasma calcium. In fetal rats, plasma phosphorus falls following administration of PTH, indicating reactivity of the fetal kidney to PTH. On the other hand, when a maternal hypercalcemia is induced by parenteral infusions, fetal plasma calcium also increases. These experimental findings collectively imply that parathyroid hormone does not cross the placenta in significant amounts (Garel and Jost, 1971). Parathyroid glands from 3- to 4-month-old fetuses can induce bone resorption *in vitro*. From clinical observations, a role of the parathyroid glands in fetal calcium homeostasis appears undeniable. Infants of pregnant women with hyperparathyroidism have severe neonatal hypocalcemia, often with tetany. These findings in an infant have occasionally led to the diagnosis of hyperparathyroidism in the mother (Van Arsdel, 1955). Hypoparathyroid women have delivered infants who developed hypercalcemia in the first few days of life. Usually, these changes in the calcium levels of the newborn infants were transient. In at least three infants of hypoparathyroid mothers bone structure was found to be abnormal radiologically and compatible with hyperparathyroidism. The symptoms of hypoparathyroidism were relieved during the second half of pregnancy but returned shortly after delivery (Landing and Kamoshita, 1970).

These clinical observations differ from the aforementioned animal experiments inasmuch as the changes in maternal calcium metabolism were chronic rather than acute. Apparently, chronic hypo- or hyper-parathyroidism in the mother may lead to the opposite condition in the fetus and newborn. This is best explained by assuming that the abnormal maternal serum calcium levels were reflected in the fetal plasma, resulting in the appropriate reaction of the parathyroid glands. Since newborn infants of hyperparathyroid mothers have never been found to show signs of the same disease, it appears that parathyroid hormone does not cross the placenta in humans to any appreciable extent.

It is not known whether the vitamin D requirements of women are higher during pregnancy and lactation than at other times (World Health Organization, 1970). Recent investigations on the metabolism of vitamin D in pregnancy suggest that the requirement for vitamin D may be increased, since plasma 25-hydroxy-vitamin D levels were often found to be low in the last months before term (Turton et al., 1977). On the basis of normal plasma-levels of 25-hydroxy-vitamin D, Fairney et al. (1977) concluded that during the first 4–6 weeks of lactation there was no indication for supplementary vitamin D. It has been well documented that newborn infants from mothers who were vitamin D-deficient during pregnancy suffer from congenital rickets (Maxwell et al., 1939; Snapper, 1965; Begum et al., 1968). Hillman and Haddad (1974) found that the vitamin D status of the newborn reflects maternal circulating levels, and that this substance (and/or its metabolites) crosses the placenta. These observations reveal that vitamin D is essential for normal fetal skeletal development. Vitamin D is present in the aequeous fraction of human milk as a water-soluble conjugate with sulfate. Its concentration was found to be 1.00 μgm/100 ml, and even higher in the first week of lactation. The quantity of vitamin D received by the infant in full lactation must be considered to meet its requirement (Lakdawala and Widdowson, 1977).

Since cow's milk is deficient in vitamin D, infant feedings should be supplemented from the first weeks of life. From the fact that supplementation with vitamin D_2 or D_3 in amounts of 100–200 IU per day prevents rickets, it can be concluded that the enzymes in liver and kidney, responsible for the biological activation of vitamin D_1 are present soon after birth (Avioli and Haddad, 1973; Hillman and Haddad, 1974).

Prematurely born infants with a very low birth weight (below 1300 gm) are likely to have an insufficient intake of vitamin D (Lewin et al., 1971). Whether they require more vitamin D than the recommended dose of 10 μgm per day has not yet been resolved. Recent studies demonstrate that unlike term infants who have the capacity to maintain normal serum 25-hydroxycholecalciferol (25-OHD) levels or to increase their levels toward the normal range, the premature infant can neither maintain normal serum 25-OHD levels in plasma nor increase their levels toward the normal range (Hillman and Haddad, 1975). Indeed, the premature infant born with a low serum 25-OHD level may experience a decrease to levels well below those seen in rachitic infants (i.e., < 6 ng/ml). The ability to maintain or to restore 25-OHD levels to normal begins somewhere between 35 to 38 weeks of gestation. Postnatally, the point at which this ability develops appears to correlate with gestation. In infants over 34 weeks gestation, this begins at 1 or 2 weeks, whereas in infants less than 34 weeks, the time before restoration is at least 3–4 weeks (Hillman and Haddad, 1974; 1975). Extremely low levels of plasma 25-OHD have been documented as long as 6–8 weeks postnatally in premature infants. The finding that premature infants cannot raise low levels of plasma 25-OHD or sustain normal levels is consistent with the hypothesis that the liver of premature infants cannot convert vitamin D to 25-OHD at rates comparable to those of term infants. Early studies in formula-fed premature infants emphasize the initiation of vitamin D prophylaxis within the first 2 weeks of life (Chisolm and Hurrican, 1962) and reveal that rickets is preventable and rates of linear growth are as rapid with vitamin D intakes of 100–200 IU per day as with intakes of 400–1200 IU per day (May and Wygent, 1939; Glaser et al., 1949), but at that time infants weighing less than 1500 gm rarely survived.

II. DIFFERENTIAL DIAGNOSIS OF HYPERCALCEMIA

A. Signs and Symptoms

The signs and symptoms of hypercalcemia are independent of the underlying cause. In older children as in adults (see Chapter 6, Volume I) the characteristic signs are thirst, polyuria, muscular weakness, fatigue, anorexia, nausea, vomiting, and constipation. In infants and very young children the syndrome is characteristically manifested by "failure to thrive." When these signs are found in a child, further examination to establish the presence of hypercalcemia is obligatory and should be done forthwith lest continued hypercalcemia lead to irreversible changes in renal function. It must be emphasized that in many cases of hypercalcemia the diagnosis has been made only after an unduly long period of time had elapsed since the appearance of the symptoms. Probably the vagueness of the syndrome and the comparative rarity of diseases with hypercalcemia lead to the delay in establishing the diagnosis. At present such delay is inexcusable considering the simplicity of the determination of serum calcium. When symptomatic hypercalcemia obtains, the serum calcium concentration is at least 12.5 mg/100 ml. When a normal concentration is found, the determination should be repeated several times since fluctuations in the concentration of serum calcium may occur. When serum calcium rises to 20 mg/100 ml and more, a hypercalcemic crisis may occur, characterized by severe dehydration, shock, hemoconcentration, and cardiac arrhythmias. The mortality is high.

B. Primary Hyperparathyroidism

The condition is very rare in infancy and childhood. At the time of writing 59 proved and 3 probable cases could be found in the literature (Bjernulf et al., 1970; Mühlethaler et al., 1967). As in adults, hyperparathyroidism may be caused by hyperplasia or adenoma of the parathyroid glands (Chapter 1). In children, these two forms differ in so many aspects that separate treatment is indicated. Primary parathyroid hyperplasia has only been seen in young children. The symptoms always start in infancy, and sometimes can be traced back to the neonatal period; the diagnosis has never been made in children over 3 years of age (Mühlethaler et al., 1967). This feature serves to distinguish the two forms of hyperparathyroidism, since adenomata are not found in children below 3 years of age. It is a serious disease, which ends fatally in a rather short time if parathyroidectomy is not performed. Of the 12 proved cases (5 boys and 7 girls), 7 patients died. Of another 3 probable cases, 1 died. The disease was familial in several instances (Bjernulf et al., 1970; Goldbloom et al., 1972; Lund, 1973; Mühlethaler et al., 1967). Consanguinity of the parents has been reported (Hillman et al., 1964) and the available evidence strongly suggests autosomal recessive inheritance of this condition. Recently a case has been reported with autosomal dominant inheritance (Spiegel et al., 1977).

The main clinical symptoms are those of hypercalcemia and failure to thrive. In addition, soft areas in the bones of the skull (craniotabes) and swelling of the osteochondral junctions of the ribs may be present. Despite a generalized hypotonia the tendon reflexes may be exaggerated. Fever and dehydration are present in the more severely ill children. Serum calcium is always markedly elevated and in the majority of the children it was over 17 mg/100 ml; in one case a value of 20 mg/100 ml was recorded. Serum phosphate is depressed, serum magnesium moderately elevated, and serum alkaline phosphatase raised. Urinary calcium may or may not be increased. Radiological examination of the long bones reveals diminished density, coarse trabecular structure, subperiosteal resorption, and pathological fractures. The picture may resemble congenital lues, since the periosteal diameter of the long bones is more uniform than in normal children. Changes resembling rickets have not been reported.

Renal function usually is normal or moderately impaired. Slight albuminuria may be present and aminoaciduria has also been found.

The only successful treatment is subtotal (or total) parathyroidectomy. This should be done as soon as possible after the diagnosis has been established (Goldbloom *et al.*, 1972). In a few cases the symptoms returned a number of months after subtotal removal of the parathyroid glands, necessitating reoperation. Postoperative maintenance has proved to be comparatively easy considering the serious preoperative condition. Although calcium usually normalizes 1–7 days after parathyroidectomy, it may be necessary to administer calcium intravenously when serum calcium falls below 8 mg/100 ml. Abnormal skeletal findings revert to normal in a matter of months, reflecting the rapid turnover of bone inherent to the age of the patient and to the disease. From the published reports it appears that the hyperplastic parathyroid glands consist predominantly of large chief cells, but occasionally hyperplasia of waterclear cells is noted. Oxyphil cells do not seem to play a role. From autopsy reports of six cases nephrocalcinosis was present in all but one. Other features were interstitial pneumonia with calcification of the alveolar walls and deposition of calcium salts in skeletal and cardiac muscle tissue, stomach, and blood vessels. In the untreated patient acute hyperparathyroidism or "parathyroid crisis" is the main cause of death. With a rapid rise of serum calcium the children become critically ill and death results from cardiac arrest. In this situation vigorous attempts may be essential to control the hypercalcemia (see Chapter 6) and parathyroidectomy should be performed as soon as possible, since this procedure may be life-saving. Children who have been successfully treated grow and develop normally; only one died 13 days after the operation. If all parathyroid tissue has been removed, they should of course be treated as hypoparathyroid patients.

It is possible that this syndrome is more frequent than would appear from the few reported cases. In view of the unspecific symptoms and the often rapidly fatal outcome, the diagnosis can easily be missed if it is not considered. It has been suggested that infantile hyperparathyroidism may be one of the causes of sudden unexpected death. In one case the diagnosis was indeed made after this event (Mühlethaler *et al.*, 1967). In establishing the diagnosis, hypercalcemia is the most important finding and no reliance should be placed on semiquantitative or quantitative estimations of urine calcium, since the excretion of calcium may be normal. If hypercalcemia is found, the disease should be differentiated from "idiopathic infantile hypercalcemia." This is not difficult, since the radiographs of the bones are completely different and serum phosphate is not low in the latter condition. Moreover, in "idiopathic infantile hypercalcemia'' serum alkaline phosphatase is normal. A special variant of parathyroid hyperplasia is constituted by the cases of supposed or proved hyperparathyroidism in infants born from mothers who were hypoparathyroid during pregnancy (Aceto *et al.*, 1966; Bronsky *et al.*, 1968). Of the four infants reported, only one had hypercalcemia. This child died at the age of 6 weeks and had hyperplastic parathyroid glands. The other three babies survived and developed normally. They were normocalcemic but had radiographic bone changes that closely resembled those seen in hyperparathyroidism. These changes disappeared spontaneously within 6 months.

Adenomata of the parathyroid glands are more frequent than hyperplasia, are equally distributed between the sexes, and occur mainly just before or during puberty. Of 48 cases reported, only 6 were diagnosed before age 10 (Bjernulf *et al.*, 1970; Mühlethaler *et al.*, 1967) (Table I). The signs and symptoms often are vague and moreover of insidious onset, which helps to explain the observed fact that in 41 cases the average time between the first clinical symptoms and the diagnosis was $2\frac{1}{2}$ years. The predominant signs, which should lead to determination of serum calcium, are those of hypercalcemia. In a number of cases neurological symptoms such as hypotonicity of the muscles, ataxic tremor, difficulty in walking, pain in the extremities, and even blindness and coma have been described. Mentally the patients become apathetic. The picture may resemble a bizarre neurological disorder (Lloyd *et al.*, 1965) (Table II). In a minority of cases deformities of the legs have been described due to changes in the metaphyses, which resembled rickets radiologically. Deformities may also result from fractures as a consequence of severe loss of

TABLE I

Age at Diagnosis of 48 Cases of Primary Hyperparathyroidism due to Adenoma[a]

Age (years)	Number of cases	Age (years)	Number of cases
0	0	9	2
1	0	10	1
2	0	11	4
3	1	12	5
4	0	13	9
5	0	14	14
6	0	15	8
7	2	16	1
8	1		

[a] From Mühlethaler *et al.* (1967) and Bjernulf *et al.* (1970).

TABLE II

Symptoms and Signs in 36 Cases of Primary Hyperparathyroidism due to Adenoma[a]

Symptoms and signs	Number	%
Physical		
Fatigue, weakness, anorexia, constipation, vomiting	21	58
Nervousness, irritability, depression, headache	4	11
Mental retardation, infantilism, blindness, dysarthria, diplopia	7	19
Alopecia	1	2.8
Gastroduodenal ulcers	2	5.6
Polyuria and polydipsia	12	33
Hypertension	6	17
Bone and joint symptoms, fractures	16	45
X ray		
Local skeletal changes	26	72
Renal lithiasis	11	31
Both	6	17

[a] From Bjernulf et al. (1970).

bone mineral. In the vast majority of the cases described, serum calcium has been elevated, although not as high as in infantile parathyroid hyperplasia (i.e., usually less than 17 mg/100 ml). Serum inorganic phosphate is low and serum alkaline phosphatase elevated. As in infants with parathyroid hyperplasia the concentration of calcium in the urine is not always increased. Polyuria is present in about one-third of the cases. Radiologically periosteal erosions are seen, mainly in the phalanges; generalized osteopenia is often present and rarely metaphyseal osteosclerosis is found, especially in the upper tibia. In a few cases the picture presented by the metaphyses resembled rickets (Lloyd et al., 1965; Lomnitz et al., 1966) and occasionally bone cysts have been seen. The lamina dura of the teeth is absent. Nephrolithiasis is relatively rare and severe impairment of renal function is exceptional, although the glomerular filtration rate is diminished in about half of the cases. Cases of hyperparathyroidism "with nephrolithiasis and without apparent bone disease" are less frequent in children than in adults. A probable explanation for this difference is the higher turnover of skeletal tissue in children, which results in an earlier manifestation of parathyroid bone disease. Cardiovascular changes include hypertension, shortened Q-T interval, and complete heart block.

Since the symptoms may be vague, serum calcium determinations in unexplained disorders, which may seem to be of psychogenic or neurological origin, are deemed essential. The finding of an elevated serum calcium level usually leads to the diagnosis. Rarely serum calcium may be normal, even in repeated determinations. In these instances, measurements of serum phosphorus, parathyroid hormone, and urine calcium should lead to the diagnosis. The elevated serum calcium should not fall following cortisol or prednisone administration but this is not always the case. Usually the symptoms abate completely after removal of the adenoma (or rarely adenomata) but if the diagnosis is made too late, residual symptoms such as EEG changes, mental impairment, and even blindness may persist. None of the children described have died. Histologically the adenomata consist of chief cells. Recurrence after complete removal of the adenomatous tissue has not been seen.

C. Idiopathic Hypercalcemia of Infancy

Although this disorder of calcium homeostasis is not as much in the forefront as it was 15 to 20 years ago, it continues to manifest itself and the pathogenesis still remains controversial. Usually two forms are distinguished: a mild and a severe one. These two forms have been separated according to degrees of clinical severity. Also, one group of patients is characterized by certain signs that are absent in the other group. This separation is still imprecise since intermediate forms have been reported. The mild and the severe form may simply represent quantitatively different expressions of the same pathological entity. As a rule the symptoms in the mild form of this disorder do not become apparent before the infant is 3–7 months old and the average birth weight of the affected child is normal (Fraser et al., 1966). The main clinical feature is failure to thrive and the main symptoms are those of hypercalcemia. On physical examination the child may be dehydrated and the tendon reflexes hyperactive; a soft precordial murmur is heard in 10% of the cases and there are no characteristic facial features. Chemical examination reveals a raised serum calcium (11–18 mg/100 ml), and a normal serum phosphate, unless elevated by severe renal failure, which is the exception rather than the rule. The serum alkaline phosphatase is normal. The α-globulins may be raised, cholesterol levels are often elevated, and acidosis may be present. Serum calcium may fluctuate spontaneously and one should not rely on a single determination to establish or rule out the diagnosis. The skeleton is usually normal radiologically, but in a number of cases the density of the metaphyseal ends of the long bones is increased; these areas appear distinct and sharply delineated. The calcium balance is strongly positive, due to increased intestinal absorption, and urinary calcium is increased.

Therapy consists of elimination of oral calcium and vitamin D and guarding the infant from direct sunlight. If the infant has been given cow's milk (which appears to be so in the majority of cases described), substitution of this for breast milk may result in immediate improvement of the physical and chemical symptoms. Administration of calcium-free milk yields even better results. At present this milk preparation is commercially available, but it may be difficult to acquire. Cow's milk with added sodium sulfate (3 gm per liter) is a very good alternative, since sulfate inhibits calcium absorption. Cortisone, in a dosage of 25–50 mg per day, results in spectacular improvement within 24 hours. It may have to be continued for a longer period, and the signs and symptoms of hyperadrenocorticism may ensue. Short-term calcitonin therapy (100 MRC units per day i.m.) is also beneficial (Job et al., 1966), although the effects of sustained therapeutic programs are unknown. Treatment in whatever form should continue until serum calcium is normalized. This may take from several months to 2 years, much longer than in ordinary straightforward cases of vitamin D intoxication. The prognosis is generally good if the disease is recognized and treated promptly. If renal damage is severe, the child may die from this complication, even after serum calcium has been corrected.

Although the essential signs and symptoms of hypercalcemia are the same as in the mild form, there are some distinctive feaures of the severe form of idiopathic hypercalcemia. The average birth weight of the affected children is below normal. The symptoms appear earlier; hypercalcemia signs present a few days after birth in approximately one-third of patients (Brunette and Gerbeaux, 1963). Most of the children have a peculiar facies, for which the term "elfin" has been introduced. The cheeks are full and pouting, the mouth is wide with full lips and receding chin; the upperlip is shaped in a cupid's bow; the bridge of the nose is flattened; the forehead is high and prominent; the eyes are rather wide apart and epicanthal folds are present; the ears are low placed and stand out prominently. Strabismus is present in some of the cases. Congenital heart disease is also present in the vast majority of the cases described. Usually this is supravalvular aortic stenosis, but pulmonary stenosis also occurs (Jue et al., 1965). All children are mentally retarded and the general condition is worse than in the mild form. Renal involvement with nephrocalcinosis usually is more severe than in the less severe form. Hypertension is often present and fever is more prominent. Physical development is delayed. Osteosclerosis of the metaphysis is a conspicuous radiological sign. Metastatic calcifications have been reported. Sex distribution is equal. Therapy is the same as in the mild form but results often are only temporary, initial success being followed by renewed elevation of serum calcium in spite of continuing treatment. Attempts at therapy with

TABLE III

Survey of Cases of the Mild and Severe Forms of Idiopathic Hypercalcemia[a]

	Mild	Severe
Number	46	37
Complete physical recovery	39	3
Fatal outcome	3	16 (15 below age 3)
Partial recovery (renal function impaired)	1	6
Physically well, but severe		
Mental deficiency	0	8
Still in active stage	3	4

[a] From Brunette and Gerbeaux (1963).

calcitonin have not yet been reported. A large proportion of the children die at an early age due to hypercalcemic crises or renal failure (Table III). If treatment is successful, the propensity to hypercalcemia eventually disappears, but mental retardation and often impairment of renal function are permanent, as is, of course, the typical facies.

Between 1953 and 1955, when in England 200 cases of idiopathic hypercalcemia were reported, the disease received much attention. It appeared that infant foods at that time often contained far more vitamin D (2000-4000 IU per day) than was needed for the prevention of rickets. Accordingly it was presumed that the disease represented vitamin D intoxication in children who were unduly sensitive to calciferol. Still the question remained why only a small part of all British children became hypercalcemic. When vitamin D intake was drastically reduced, the incidence of the disease fell, but it was not completely eradicated. In 1953–1955 the number of reported cases was 7.2 per month and it dropped to 3.0 per month in 1960–1961. According to the British Paediatric Association report on infantile hypercalcemia (1964), the marked decline in hypercalcemia did not correspond in time with the major reduction in vitamin D allowance, which took place a few years earlier. It remained speculative, therefore, whether the decrease of hypercalcemia was a consequence of the reduced intake of vitamin D. The results of this survey applied to both forms, since a distinction between the mild and the severe form was not made in these studies.

In some infants the concentration of serum vitamin D was determined. It was found to be normal in eight mildly affected children whereas it was greatly elevated in five of nine infants with the severe form; four infants had normal concentrations (Fraser et al., 1966). Results of administration of fairly large doses of vitamin D to children with the severe form were equivocal (Brunette and Gerbeaux, 1963). At present, it appears that a direct causal relation between vitamin D and infantile hypercalcemia has not been established, although there is a certain amount of evidence that implicates vitamin D in the pathogenesis of this syndrome.

It is equally difficult to define whether the two forms are separate entities or simply represent the ends of a single spectrum. The presence of "intermediate" forms argues in favor of the latter concept. It is possible that the severe form not only is at one end of a spectrum, but also begins *in utero*. This might explain the presence of supravalvular aortic stenosis and other vascular anomalies in this form, since it has been shown that early intoxication with vitamin D in animals produces strikingly similar lesions (Friedman, 1967). It might also explain the facial abnormalities, the tendency to a low birth weight, and the mental deficiency. To date both vitamin D and hypercalcemia have been incriminated in this regard. In this respect it should be emphasized that the mothers of most of the affected children were healthy and did not receive high doses of vitamin D during pregnancy. Although most of the published cases have been isolated ones, familial occurrence has been reported in at least three instances. There was no consanguinity in these cases. Recently it has been suggested that a congenital defect of the action or production of calcitonin might be responsible for the disease. This hypothesis rests on the finding that intravenous administration of calcium to older normocalcemic children with the severe form resulted in hypercalcemia, which disappeared significantly more slowly than in normal children of the same age. The implication was that bone resorption did not decline following exogenous hypercalcemia as a result of the absence of the calcitonin-mediated regulating mechanism (Forbes *et al.*, 1972).

D. Familial Benign Hypercalcemia

Recently a family has been described in which 11 members in four generations had moderately elevated serum calcium levels, low urinary calcium excretion, and normal serum parathyroid hormone levels. This benign condition was thought to be caused by an abnormal receptor mechanism for calcium ion control of parathyroid hormone secretion. Mental development was normal and the affected people were symptom free. The mode of inheritance appeared to be autosomal dominant (Foley *et al.*, 1972).

E. Vitamin D Intoxication

Intoxication with vitamin D has never been a frequent occurrence, and the incidence declined further when the potential harmful effects of large doses became known. It is not possible simply to state at which dose symptoms of intoxication may occur. This depends on the age and size of the child, on the size of the dose and the number of doses given, on the intervals between repeated dosages, on the intake of calcium, and finally, on the presence of increased bone resorption (fracture, immobilization). Most of the infants and young children with vitamin D poisoning, described by Illig and Prader (1959), had received several doses of 15 mg or more within several months before hypercalcemia was discovered. On the other hand, a 3-month dose of 7.5–10 mg has never been shown to cause poisoning in infants. Children with pneumocystis pneumonia are especially susceptible to vitamin D intoxication. At present, intoxication is mainly seen in children who are being treated for chronic hypocalcemic conditions or hypophosphatemic rickets. Once intoxication has occurred, the patient is more susceptible to repeated intoxications, even when the dose for treatment of the disease has been lowered. This may be caused by the very long half-life of vitamin D in the body (see Chapter 5, Volume I, and Chapter 2, this volume). On the other hand, symptoms of intoxication usually do not last long if the condition is quickly recognized and adequately treated.

Signs and symptoms are no different from those of other conditions with hypercalcemia. The presence of polyuria and a strongly positive Sulkowich test in the urine in children treated with high doses of vitamin D or dihydrotachysterol (DHT) constitute a warning of approaching hypercalcemia. It should be remembered that DHT is about 2 to 3 times as effective as vitamin D in raising plasma calcium and therefore is apt to cause hypercalcemia in lower doses. On the other hand, the hypercalcemia resulting from DHT therapy returns to normal at a greater rate when the drug is discontinued than that observed following cessation of vitamin D therapy. The most dangerous consequence of hypercalcemia is irreversible renal damage, resulting from hypercalciuria and peritubular deposits of calcium phosphate. When these deposits are large and numerous they are visible on plain films of the abdomen as nephrocalcinotic intrarenal deposits. Treatment should consist of prompt elimination of vitamin D and a calcium-free diet. Dehydration should be treated by ample provision of fluids. This is important, since the concentrating power of the kidney is impaired and fluid loss in the urine is increased. If promptly treated, recovery takes about 2 weeks and can be speeded up by administration of cortisone or related synthetic analogues. Rapid treatment usually results in complete recovery. Renal function returns to normal, but it is possible that small foci of calcium deposits remain and that minor functional impairment may persist. Patients treated with high doses of vitamin D should therefore be checked at regular intervals for hypercalciuria and hypercalcemia.

F. Immobilization

It is a well-known fact that following immobilization, acute paralysis of one or more limbs (poliomyelitis), and/or fracture of one or more bones, the urinary calcium rises to values that exceed the normal range (Millard et al., 1970). Severe hypercalcemia in children has only been described occasionally in such cases, but it is likely that mild to moderate elevations in serum calcium concentrations occur more frequently than previously assumed for immobilized patients. Close examination in 10 normal adults who had sustained a fracture revealed that serum calcium rose slightly above the normal range in three, whereas ionized calcium was raised in nine of these patients (Heath et al., 1972). Similar studies in children have not yet been reported. In the literature reports of six healthy pubertal children could be found who developed severe hypercalcemia following a fracture (Hyman et al., 1972). In one child an erroneous diagnosis of primary hyperparathyroidism was made and the neck was explored. All six children were severely ill and serum calciums ranged from 13.7 to 16 mg/100 ml. One had hypertensive encephalopathy (Berliner et al., 1972); otherwise, the symptoms were those of hypercalcemia.

Although the immobilization is often considered a primary causative factor, it appears most likely that immobilization per se is unlikely to result in hypercalcemia, unless accompanied by a fracture and/or paralysis. In a fractured limb, osteoporosis (mainly distal from the fracture site) develops rapidly and is visible on X-ray examination within 3 weeks from the date of the fracture. This posttraumatic osteoporosis is a more rapid process than the comparatively slowly developing bone loss of immobilization. When a fracture and subsequent immobilization is present in a child of 10–15 years, the relatively higher bone turnover attending pubescence predisposes to hypercalcemia (Lawrence et al., 1973; Levine et al., 1975). Therapy should consist primarily of mobilization and (partial) weight bearing on the fractured leg. Other measures are elimination of calcium from the diet and ample fluid therapy. Glucocorticoids may be useful therapeutic agents if the hypercalcemia is not corrected by ambulation (Lawrence et al., 1973). Since the hypercalcemia is caused by increased osteoclastic activity, calcitonin may be helpful. In immobilized children with normal serum calcium levels, calcitonin does, in fact, lower serum calcium (Illig et al., 1972).

The danger of hypercalcemia following a fracture is especially great in children with hypophosphatemic rickets, subjected to large daily doses of vitamin D and in whom osteotomy is performed to correct a deformity. In such cases the combination of osteotomy and immobilization is superimposed on the hypercalcemic response to vitamin D therapy. Severe and long-lasting hypercalcemia is likely to result and has indeed often been reported. When in such patients an osteotomy is planned, vitamin D therapy should be terminated at least 2–3 months before the operation and resumed 6–8 weeks after the operation (Steendijk *et al.*, 1968).

G. Addison's Disease

Adrenocortical failure, a rarity in childhood, may also be complicated by hypercalcemia. This is caused by the impaired secretion of cortisol; the hypercalcemia disappears in a matter of days following administration of cortisone in physiological doses (Prader *et al.,* 1959).

H. Leukemia

Hypercalcemia is an infrequent but important complication of acute lymphatic and myelogenous leukemia in childhood. The symptoms of hypercalcemia may rarely be the initial complaints of the child. Up to 1970, four cases of hypercalcemia have been reported in children under 17 years of age (Stein, 1971). The clinical symptoms are those of hypercalcemia and also those of the leukemic process itself, which may be similar (fatigue, vague pains, anorexia). Since decreased skeletal density has been noted radiologically, it has been suggested that the hypercalcemia results from rapid destruction of bone tissue by the leukemic process. On the other hand, it cannot be excluded that hypercalcemia may be caused by a substance with PTH-like activity, produced by the leukemic cells (Neiman and Li, 1972; Zidar *et al.,* 1976). The hypercalcemia of leukemic patients may be associated with demonstrable skeletal lesions, although bone disease may also be undetected radiologically. Therapy consists of the appropriate therapeutic regimen for leukemia. Hypercalcemia may also develop during therapy. In such cases symptomatic treatment is indicated with appropriate diuretics and hydration. On the other hand, hypocalcemia has repeatedly been observed in acute lymphoblastic leukemia within 24–48 hours of the initiation of therapy (Zusman *et al.,* 1973).

I. Sarcoidosis

Sarcoidosis is a rare disease in childhood and the incidence of hypercalcemia in children with this disease is not known. The pathogenesis of hypercalcemia is similar as in adult patients. Illig and Prader (1959) found that small doses of vitamin D may produce toxic effects. Therapy should include elimination of vitamin D from the diet and a diet with a low calcium content. Administration of cortisone (50–100 mg day) is followed by decreased intestinal absorption of calcium and a fall of plasma calcium to normal levels, and the condition of the patient improves rapidly.

J. Hypothyroidism

Occasionally hypothyroidism is accompanied by hypercalcemia. In a recent review calcium levels ranging from 11 to 13.5 mg/100 ml were detected in 4 of 16 cases of congenital athyrosis, in 3 of 8 cases with ectopic thyroid tissue, and in none of six cases with hypothyroidism due to enzyme defects. With one exception, these children were over 4 years of age; all were untreated (Royer *et al.,* 1968). In hypothyroid patients intestinal absorption of calcium is increased and skeletal turnover of calcium is diminished (see Chapter 4). Calcium infusion reportedly leads to higher plasma calcium levels than in normal controls (Royer *et al.,* 1968). Obviously these changes in the fate of calcium are important for the development of hypercalcemia. It is doubtful whether these patients are abnormally sensitive to vitamin D. The absence of calcitonin, however, may play a role in the propensity to hypercalcemia, since athyrotic children rendered euthyroid with thyroxine still seem to differ from normal children in the response of plasma calcium to intravenous calcium (Anast and Guthrie, 1971). Treatment consists of calcium deprivation, cortisone, and, of course, administration of thyroxine or desiccated thyroid. Rarely hypercalcemia may develop following the initiation of thyroid replacement therapy.

K. Hypophosphatasia

Hypophosphatasia is an inborn error in bone metabolism with an estimated incidence of 1:100,000 births. The severity of this inherited disease varies with the most severe cases characteristically apparent *in utero* or at birth. Within the first few weeks of life children with this disorder usually fail to thrive, manifesting gastrointestinal disturbances, interrupted febrile episodes, and convulsions. Physical examination reveals broadened epiphyses and prominent chondrocostal junctions. Radiologically the cranium is poorly mineralized and rachitic-like changes dominate the ends of the long bones (Fraser, 1957; Teree and Klein, 1968).

Serum calcium is elevated or high normal and serum phosphate is normal. The serum alkaline phosphatase is very low or even undetectable, a finding considered pathognomonic for the disease. Children and adults with this disease excrete excessive amounts of phosphoethanolamine, which is normally not detectable in plasma or urine. This substance also appears in the urine of patients with scurvy, celiac disease, hypothyroidism, hepatic disease, and erythroblastosis fetalis. Normally, phosphoethanolamine is hydrolyzed (presumably by alkaline phosphatase), liberating inorganic phosphate. It has been assumed but never substantiated that an inherited deficiency in alkaline phosphatase production leads to an accumulation of the phosphoethanolamine substrate and a defect in the calcification of bone. Attempts to define the relationship of this phosphorylated ester, alkaline phosphatase, and skeletal calcifications are still fraught with interpretive difficulties. Another alkaline phosphatase substrate, pyrophosphate, also accumulates in the plasma and urine of patients with hypophosphatasia (Russell *et al.*, 1971), and phosphatidylcholine (Eisenberg and Pimstone, 1967) is also increased in the urine of adults with this disorder.

The disease is inherited as an autosomal recessive trait, although autosomal dominant patterns have not been excluded in certain instances. Heterozygotes can be identified by plasma alkaline phosphatase values, which are subnormal for the patient's age, and the detection of either phosphoethanolamine or phosphatidylcholine in the urine (Pimstone *et al.*, 1966; Eisenberg and Pimstone, 1967). The finding of a "normal" alkaline phosphatase in patients with high urinary phosphoethanolamine content is not inconsistent, since the intestinal alkaline phosphatase isoenzyme may be the major component of the total serum alkaline phosphatase in this instance (Warshaw *et al.*, 1972).

In the severe cases the prognosis is poor. In milder cases, the symptoms may not appear before the second half of the first year or even later. Again, the picture resembles rickets, but the children are less sick and serum calcium may be normal. Deformities of the legs may draw attention to the disease. A number of patients later develop renal failure, probably as a result of the elevated plasma calcium level and progressive nephrocalcinosis. Craniostenosis may develop as in other cases of chronic rickets and craniotomy may be essential to prevent undue intracranial pressure and compression of the optic nerve (Schlesinger *et al.*, 1955). If patients survive to the age of 4 years, the disease tends to run a milder course and the prognosis becomes more favorable, although spontaneous healing of the bone lesions has rarely been reported (Pimstone *et al.*, 1966).

Histologically, an excess of osteoid tissue is found and the growth zones are broadened with irregular arrangement of the columns of cartilage cells. These changes resemble rickets (Chapters 4 and 6, Volume I). In addition, an unexplained scarcity of osteocytes has been found (Engfeldt and Zetterström, 1956). Dental lesions are prominent (Ritchie, 1964) and consist of hypoplastic deformities with crowding and early loss of deciduous and permanent teeth, probably as a result of abnormal cementogenesis. Large amounts of interglobular dentin, a dental sign of rickets, are present. Sometimes the dental changes represent the only overt manifestation of the disease (Pimstone et al., 1966).

The pathogenesis of the disease has been studied by Russell et al. (1971), who found increased levels of pyrophosphate in the plasma of these patients. They suggested that this might be the cause of the defective mineralization, since pyrophosphate is a known poison of crystal formation of apatite. The function of alkaline phosphatase might be to prevent accumulation of pyrophosphate and thereby to ensure normal mineralization. Therapeutic trials with large doses of inorganic phosphate were proposed, since this might result in elimination of pyrophosphate. This was attempted by Bongiovanni and his co-workers (1968) in two patients, with apparent favorable results. Although this seemed to confirm that pyrophosphate was the damaging substance, it was later found that feeding inorganic phosphate did not lower the plasma levels of pyrophosphate. Treatment of another patient with phosphate supplements failed to influence the course of the disease (Teree and Klein, 1968).

The patients cannot be properly treated. Vitamin D does not improve the bone lesions and may be dangerous since it may cause a (further) rise of serum calcium. Similarly, immoderate exposure of the skin to sunlight and a stimulated endogenous production of vitamin D might lead to a deterioration of the patient's condition.

In 1969 Scriver and Cameron described the case of a 3-month-old girl with the bone changes of hypophosphatasia, hypercalcemia, muscular hypotonia, and urinary excretion of phosphoethanolamine. The activity of alkaline phosphatase in serum was normal, however. It was found that the patient's plasma hydrolyzed phosphoethanolamine more slowly than normal plasma. The patient's subsequent course also closely resembled that of hypophosphatasia. Craniotomy was performed in her second year, after which her condition gradually improved. Although the authors called this disease "pseudohypophosphatasia," because of a normal "total" alkaline phosphatase level, it should be emphasized that this case most probably exemplified the need for more sophisticated isolation of alkaline phosphatase isoenzymes (Warshaw et al., 1972).

The treatment of hypercalcemia in infants and children differs only quantitatively from the therapy in adults. It must be emphasized that proper hydration of the child is of prime importance, and should be carefully guarded. Recently a new form of treatment has been used with success in children with severe hypercalcemia due to vitamin D intoxication. Najjar et al. (1972) administered frusemide intravenously in 20-mg doses in isotonic saline as often as necessary to maintain a copious diuresis. The fall of serum calcium was satisfactory and urinary calcium increased 5–10-fold. The excretion of sodium, potassium, and magnesium is also increased by frusemide and these ions must be replaced during diuretic therapy.

III. DIFFERENTIAL DIAGNOSIS OF HYPOCALCEMIA

A. Signs and Symptoms

The diagnostic signs and symptoms of hypocalcemia in older children are similar to those of adults as described in Chapter 6, Volume II. In new-born infants, however, the symptoms of hypocalcemia often are sufficiently different to merit a separate description. They may consist of fine tremors of the fingers and chin, vomiting, and rapid, shallow respirations with intercostal retractions, periods of tachypnea alternating with apnea. Laryngeal signs are uncommon. Still, generalized convulsions do appear in this age group, and the proportion of neonatal convulsions due to a primary disturbance of mineral metabolism may approximate 55% (Cockburn et al., 1973). Clearly, in new-born infants, determination of serum calcium to rule out hypocalcemia is indicated by relatively aspecific signs.

B. Neonatal Hypocalcemia

The calcium concentration of cord blood is higher than the levels observed in maternal plasma. The mean value of serum calicum in cord blood is between 11 and 12 mg/100 ml and in maternal plasma, 9.5 mg/100 ml (Saville and Kretchmer, 1960). In the first few hours after birth, serum calcium falls rapidly, reaching a nadir of approximately 9.0 mg/100 ml during the second day (Bergman, 1972). In infants fed breast milk the value rises during the remainder of the first week. If the formula contains cow's milk, serum calcium may remain low and even decrease further (Fomon, 1967). It is usually stated that the fall in serum calcium after birth is the result of the sudden interruption of the supply of calcium from the placenta, while the oral supply is still insufficient and fetal bone formation continues. It is also probable that the relative degree of parathyroid insufficiency that obtains in the immediate neonatal period and high fetal calcitonin levels play contributory roles (Hillman et al., 1977). Finally, the low serum calcium might be secondary to the rise in serum phosphate, which occurs as a consequence of the catabolic state in the first few days, and the high tubular reabsorption of phosphate, the latter resulting from parathyroid insufficiency (Tsang et al., 1976). A rise in serum phosphate from 7.0 to 9.6 mg/100 ml between the first and third days of life has been found in normal children (Connelly *et al.*, 1962). At the end of the first month of life, homeostatic control is such that various concentration ratios of calcium and phosphate in the food can be dealt with without an appreciable change in serum calcium. Serum phosphate remains partly dependent on the phosphate content of the food and is higher in children fed formulas derived from cow's milk (Fomon, 1967).

Neonatal hypocalcemia has been arbitrarily defined as a level of serum calcium below 8 mg/100 ml occurring during the first few days (Roberton and Smith, 1975; Prader and Fanconi, 1969) or weeks (Mizrahi *et al.*, 1968) of life. This early hypocalcemia may be the result of a number of widely different causes of a transient or permanent nature (Table IV), which initially closely resemble each other. In trying to establish a diagnosis, care should be taken not to overlook the possibility of permanent hypoparathyroidism. Idiopathic hypoparathyroidism may be present even when serum calcium levels are normal. Therefore, an infant with hypocalcemia should be followed continually until a nontransient form of hypocalcemia can be ruled out. Although in the majority of affected infants neonatal hypocalcemia is transient, a considerable proportion of these children appear to have enamel hypoplasia of the deciduous canines and molars, resulting in destruction of these teeth. This becomes evident at 2 to 5 years of age when the earlier hypocalcemic episodes may have been entirely forgotten. Enamel hypoplasia has been attributed to hypocalcemia, occurring during a critical period of enamel development (Stimmler *et al.*, 1973).

"First-day hypocalcemia" can be regarded as an exaggeration of the normal postpartum decrease in serum calcium. The incidence in normal full-term infants is low (i.e., 1.2%) but not negligible. In recent years, "first-day hypocalcemia" has been reported with increasing frequency in

TABLE IV

Diseases and Conditions Causing Neonatal Hypocalcemia

1. Transient neonatal hypocalcemia
   a. "First day" hypocalcemia
   b. Nutritional hypocalcemia
   c. Hypocalcemia with maternal hyperparathroidism
   d. Transient idiopathic hypoparathyroidism
2. Nontransient neonatal hypocalcemia
   a. Idiopathic hypoparathyroidism (various forms)
   b. Hypocalcemia with congenital hypomagnesemia
   c. Hypocalcemia with dwarfism and cortical
      thickening of tubular bones

children with hyaline membrane disease and fetal or neonatal distress (David and Anast, 1973; Roberton and Smith, 1975). Premature infants and infants of mothers with diabetes or toxemia of pregnancy are more prone to develop hypocalcemia. There is some evidence that prematurely born, hypocalcemic infants and their mothers may suffer from vitamin D deficiency (Rosen et al., 1974). In infants with hypocalcemia, an increased incidence of severe heart failure due to persistent ductus arteriosus has been found (Roberton and Smith, 1975). Hypocalcemia is not a feature of "small-for-dates" infants (Table V). Since classical tetany may not be the presenting sign, it is easily possible to overlook this condition and regard it as epilepsy or brain damage. Treatment is indicated when serum calcium is below 7.5 mg/100 ml and clinical symptoms occur. Several observations suggest that impaired secretion or synthesis of parathyroid hormone may be involved (David and Anast, 1973; Fairney et al., 1973; Tsang et al., 1976). In addition, the high neonatal levels of calcitonin and an increase in the secretion of growth hormone due to hypoglycemia may play a role (Bergman, 1974).

Neonatal tetany, resulting from "nutritional hypocalcemia," that is, a low Ca/P ratio and a high phosphate concentration in the formula, characteristically occurs between the fifth and tenth day of life when the feedings have reached their appropriate quantity. In the past, when diluted cow's milk was routinely administered to infants, this type of tetany was seen far more often than at present, when it has virtually disappeared. The Ca/P ratio and the phosphate concentration in breast milk are, respectively, 2.20 and 150 mg/liter. In cow's milk, diluted 50% with water, these values are 1.30 and 405 mg/liter, respectively. This hypocalcemic syndrome most probably results from a dietary-induced hyperphosphatemia, because inadequate amounts of parathyroid hormone in the infant preclude adequate phosphate excretion by the kidney. Older infants with more functionally intact parathyroid-releasing mechanisms do not become hypocalcemic on diluted cow's milk.

TABLE V

Hypocalcemia in 207 Newborns with a Birth Weight below 2500 gm[a]

Percentile	Number of infants	Ca less than 7 mg/100 ml
< 10 = small for dates	53	2 (4%)
> 10 = premature	154	33 (21%)

[a] Prader and Fanconi (1969).

Treatment of hypocalcemia when accompanied by manifest tetany should be symptomatic and directed toward the relief of tetany. Repeated intravenous administration of calcium gluconate is the treatment of choice. The amount of calcium to be given depends on the age of the child and the severity of the condition (Mizrahi *et al.*, 1968). In both infants and older children, calcium gluconate can be administered intravenously in a dosage of 10 ml of a 10% solution, at a rate of 1 ml per minute, a more rapid rate leading to bradycardia. The injection should be terminated as soon as the attack subsides. It may be repeated in a few hours if necessary. In older children, and in hypocalcemia without tetany solution of calcium chloride can be given by mouth, either with food or as a continuous intragastric drip. The total amount usually administered over a 24-hour period should approximate 100 mg Ca/kg body weight. In infants, this substance can be given with the formula, e.g., 100 mg of calcium as calcium chloride every 8 hours. The concentration of calcium chloride should not be increased, since this may cause necrosis of the gastric mucosa. Because of this danger, calcium chloride should be used cautiously. On the other hand, the calcium salt has the initial advantage of inducing a mild systemic acidosis, which raises the proportion of ionized calcium in serum. Since after 1 or 2 days the acidosis is apt to become severe, calcium chloride should not be given for more than 2 days. If therapy is still necessary after this time, the same amount of elemental calcium should be administered as the calcium gluconate or calcium carbonate salt. The acute treatment with calcium should continue until serum calcium has risen to a minimal value of over 7.5 mg/100 ml. Hypocalcemic infants should be given a formula with a low phosphate concentration containing breast milk or one of its substitutes with similar Ca/P ratios. Treatment of manifest tetany should always be prompt, since repeated convulsions may impair normal development. Recently repeated daily intravenous injections of small doses of 1,25-dihydroxycholecalciferol (0.05 μgm/Kg bodyweight) have proved to be a safe and dependable form of treatment for protracted neonatal hypocalcemia (Kooh *et al.*, 1976).

Hypocalcemia is also seen in infants born of mothers with hyperparathyroidism. In this instance hypocalcemia with clinical symptoms may occur during the first few days of life, but also much later, even when the infant is several months old (Hutchin and Kessner, 1964). Usually symptoms appear between the second and twenty-fourth day. The onset of symptoms has been observed after a change in the mode of feeding from human milk to cow's milk. This would signify that the infant's parathyroid function remains insufficient to cope with the low Ca/P ratio and high phosphate content of the formula, even at an age of several weeks to a few months, while adequate homeostasis could be maintained on breast milk. Several cases in one family have occurred before the diagnosis of hyperparathyroidism was established in the mother (Walton, 1954). The occurrence of this type of infantile hypocalcemia suggests that maternal hyperparathyroidism and the attendant hypercalcemia during pregnancy inhibits the proper development of parathyroid function in the fetus. In the affected infants, hypocalcemia may be prolonged, but eventually serum calcium levels become normal. Symptomatic treatment with calcium salts may be necessary in the most severe cases.

"Transient idiopathic hypoparathyroidism" is rare, occurs predominantly in male infants, and is at first indistinguishable from persistent congenital hypoparathyroidism. The disease is not familial and the mothers do not have hyperparathyroidism during pregnancy. The first sign of this disease (usually a generalized convulsion) occurs in the first 2 or 3 weeks of life. Serum calcium is low and serum phosphate high. These values become normal 3 to 6 days after administration of parathyroid extract (500 USP units/m²/day in three divided doses). When this treatment is discontinued a hypocalcemic, hyperphosphatemic relapse occurs within a few days (Fanconi and Prader, 1967; Balsan and Alizon, 1968). Administration of vitamin D or DHT (0.5 mg/day) is the treatment of choice. Most cases show no relapse when this medication is stopped after the third month of life. For this reason, in cases of so-called hypoparathyroidism of infancy treated with vitamin D, the medication should be discontinued at the age of 3 months to rule out the potential transient nature of the disorder (see Chapter 3).

In the majority of the children with this disorder double periosteal contours have been found on radiological analysis of the long bones. These disappear toward the age of 6 months. Double periosteal contours are also seen in 35% of full-term and premature infants before the first month of life and in 47% and 39%, respectively, when the infants are examined after the first month (Shopfner, 1966). These contours may represent rapid bone growth at the periosteum and their relation to transient hypoparathyroidism may be spurious. As to the pathogenesis of this form of hypocalcemia, it has been suggested that these children have partial hypoparathyroidism that later becomes compensated (Fanconi and Prader, 1967).

Other diseases in which hypocalcemia is of a permanent nature may also have their onset in infancy and therefore must be differentiated from the transient types of hypocalcemia (Table IV). These diseases will be dealt with separately, since they do not belong exclusively to the neonatal or infantile periods.

C. Idiopathic Hypoparathyroidism

Under the heading of "idiopathic hypoparathyroidism" are grouped cases of hypoparathyroidism of a permanent nature, occurring spontaneously during childhood. Some of the cases are apparent at birth and others do not appear until later in childhood. The incidence is rare: of 151 reported cases of idiopathic hypoparathyroidism, 100 occurred in children and only 22 had symptoms in the first 2 years of life (Table VI; Lahey *et al.*, 1963). The diagnosis is difficult and too often the children had been treated for epilepsy for some time (even years) before hypocalcemia was discovered (Moshkowitz *et al.*, 1969). The average interval between the onset of the symptoms and the diagnosis in the reported cases up to 1963 was 6.3 years (Lahey *et al.*, 1963). A finding of one normal serum calcium value does not rule out the diagnosis, since in a number of cases the hypocalcemia is intermittent. "Epileptic fits" may be produced by intercurrent illnesses and at that time serum calcium is low. However, when the child appears to be well, normal, or near-normal calcium values may be found. The diagnosis rests on the finding of hypocalcemia and hyperphosphatemia, which can be corrected by administration of parathyroid extract (200 USP units daily for 5–7 days).

The main signs and symptoms of hypoparathyroidism are similar to those occurring in adults (Chapter 3), but some features are typical for children. Enamel hypoplasia, for instance, is frequent and probably results from the susceptibility of enamel formation to the serum calcium level (Stimmler *et al.*, 1973). Mental retardation occurs and its severity may be associated with the quality of the control of the disease. It is a frequent complication, which has been found in at least 21% of affected children (Lahey *et al.*, 1963). Since mental retardation may be preventable, close scrutiny for the possible presence of hypoparathyroidism in every child with "epilepsy" and the members of its family is obligatory.

TABLE VI

Age at Onset of 151 Cases of Idiopathic Hypoparathyroidism[a]

Age group (years)	Number	Age group (years)	Number
0–2	22	21–25	3
3–5	24	26–30	6
6–10	29	31–35	8
11–15	25	36–40	6
16–20	7	over 40	21

[a] Lahey *et al.* (1963).

A classification of different forms of idiopathic hypoparathyroidism may be based on the age at onset of the symptoms, on the clinical features, or on the mode of inheritance. This is often difficult, since the inheritance pattern is not strictly known in each case and because the age at diagnosis is often years later than the age at onset of the disease. A classification of the hypoparathyroid syndromes as adapted from Barr *et al.* (1971) is noted in Table VII.

Among the cases that are diagnosed in the first year of life there is an excess of males, some of whom have male siblings with the same condition (Taitz *et al.*, 1966). The disease in these familial cases with sex-linked recessive inheritance is usually mild and the prognosis good. The remainder of the early-onset cases are sporadic with an equal sex incidence. Some children are severely ill and often die at a very young age as a result of undue susceptibility to infections, consequent upon impaired development of the immune system. These represent cases of III/IV pharyngeal pouch syndrome, first described by DiGeorge in 1965, in which the thymus and the parathyroid glands are aplastic. In these children cardiovascular anomalies, cerebral defects, and thyroid hypoplasia also occur. In addition, there are facial characteristics that may be diagnostic in typical cases: low set ears with a partly fused helix and anthelix, hypoplasia of the mandible, shortened philtrum of the upper lip, and blunted tip of the nose. Transplantation of thymus tissue has recently been performed in a number of these infants with (partial) restoration of immunocompetence and possibly an improvement of the prognosis. In a small number of children with this syndrome immunological abnormalities have not been

TABLE VII

Classification of Persistent Idiopathic Hypoparathyroidism[a]

---

1. Sporadic
   a. Most cases of isolated hypoparathyroidism (congenital, juvenile)
   b. All cases of III/IV pharyngeal pouch syndrome (congenital)
2. Sex-linked recessive (male)
   Some cases of isolated hypoparathyroidism (congenital)
3. Autosomal dominant
   Some cases of isolated hypoparathyroidism; in a few combined with moniliasis (congenital or juvenile, but also asymptomatic in adults)
4. Autosomal recessive
   a. Some cases of isolated hypoparathyroidism (congenital)
   b. Hypoparathyroidism with other diseases; mainly moniliasis, Addison's disease, and pernicious anemia (juvenile)

---

[a] Adapted from Barr *et al.* (1971).

demonstrated and the prognosis mainly depends on the cardiovascular status (Gatti *et al.*, 1972).

Idiopathic hypoparathyroidism has been reported in two generations with autosomal-dominant inheritance (Barr *et al.*, 1971). The age at diagnosis was variable; some patients presented symptoms in infancy, others at an age between 2 and 16 years, while still others were asymptomatic and were only discovered as a result of a survey of the family. These latter patients had serum calcium values below normal, but above the level at which tetany usually occurs. In one family, calcification of the basal ganglia was found in some members with normal serum calcium and phosphate values. Some of the cases in this group had monilia infections. One family member had been treated erroneously for epilepsy for 20 years!

Idiopathic hypoparathyroidism often occurs in conjunction with other diseases. As detailed quite extensively in Chapter 3, it appears that these syndromes usually are familial, with autosomal-recessive inheritance. It is not possible to discover a common denominator in these bizarre syndromes, in which moniliasis appears to occur more often than other diseases such as megaloblastic anemia, steatorrhea, Addison's disease, hepatic cirrhosis, Hashimoto's disease, diabetes mellitus, cystic fibrosis, and hypoprothrombinemia. One case of Turner's syndrome and hypoparathyroidism has been described (Tuvemo and Gustavson, 1972). The frequency of some of these syndromes is listed in Table VIII.

Moniliasis and disorders of gastrointestinal function are the most frequent complicating diseases. It has been thought that the dystrophic skin, nails, and mucous membranes in hypoparathyroidism might predispose toward infections with *Candida albicans*, but moniliasis may be present

TABLE VIII

Diseases Complicating Idiopathic Hypoparathyroidism, Based on 151 Cases[a]

Disease	Number of cases	Percent
Moniliasis	21	13.9
Addison's disease	16	10.6
Hypothyroidism	4	2.6
Cystic fibrosis	7	4.6
Steatorrhea	8	5.3
Chronic diarrhea	9	6.0
Megaloblastic anemia	6	4.8
Hypoprothrombinemia	2	2.0

[a] Lahey *et al.* (1963).

before the hypoparathyroid changes become manifest. Gastrointestinal disorders (diarrhea and steatorrhea) have been reported to persist after correction of the serum calcium and phosphate values. Steatorrhea has also been attributed to moniliasis, but the fungus has not been found in the lower intestinal tract. Of the 16 cases of Addison's disease and hypoparathyroidism, 6 had moniliasis (Stickler *et al.*, 1965). Four cases of idopathic hypoparathyroidism have been reported, two of which also had moniliasis. In the patients described the temporal sequence of these disorders is inconstant. Usually, but not always, moniliasis is first observed, and Addison's disease is preceded by hypoparathyroidism. If a patient treated for hypoparathyroidism with large doses of vitamin D develops adrenocortical insufficiency, the latter becomes apparent by repeated periods of hypercalcemia and a diminishing need for vitamin D. This is a manifestation of the little understood "antagonism" between vitamin D and cortisol (see Chapter 6, Volume I). Also, if Addison's disease and hypoparathyroidism occur simultaneously, hypocalcemia and its signs may be masked and apparent only after cortisol replacement.

The seven patients described with hypoparathyroidism and "cystic fibrosis of the pancreas" all had the sweat electrolyte disturbances common to that disorder, but only one had pulmonary disease and only two had steatorrhea. It is still doubtful whether these patients had cystic fibrosis in its classic form. Megaloblastic anemia in patients with hypoparathyroidism has also been described (Stickler *et al.*, 1965). Vitamin B_{12} deficiency could be the result of malabsorption, but in at least one case it was present with normal intestinal function. It has been fashionable to explain the coincidence of multiple endocrinopathies in the same patient with hypoparathyroidism on an autoimmune basis (Hung *et al.*, 1963). In some patients with hypoparathyroidism autoantibodies against adrenal and thyroid tissue have been detected. The idea presently is still speculative since the antibodies are not cytotoxic.

Children with hypoparathyroidism, as adults, are treated with high doses of vitamin D or dihydrotachysterol (DHT). It is not possible to give a rule of thumb according to which the doses can be calculated; this is a matter of trial and error. Therapy should be directed toward maintaining the serum calcium between 8.5 and 10.0 mg/100 ml. This can usually be achieved in infants with 10,000 IU (0.25 mg) per day. In older children 20,000 IU are administered initially with gradual increments to a maintenance dose of 0.625–1.5 mg per day. In hypoparathyroid infants, cow's milk should be avoided as much as possible, unless the calcium/phosphate ratio can be increased. In older children, the consumption of milk in moderate amounts should present no problem. In rare instances when refractoriness to large doses of vitamin D (i.e., > 50,000 IU per day) obtains, dihydrotachysterol (DHT) may prove effective. Recently, a 13-year-old girl has been described (Rosler and Rabinowitz, 1973) who was resistant to both vitamin D and DHT, but who responded to administration of magnesium (300 mg/day) in addition to moderate doses of vitamin D. As noted by Avioli (1974) and in Chapter 3, hypomagnesemia or magnesium-depleted states may, in fact, blunt the normal response to vitamin D in hypoparathyroid patients. In recent years, small daily doses (0.25–2.5 μgm) of 1,25-dihydroxycholecalciferol or 1-α hydroxycholecalciferol have been used to correct hypocalcemia and maintain normal levels of serum calcium (Russell et al., 1974; Kind et al., 1975). These observations indicate that the hypocalcemia in hypoparathyroidism is the result of impaired secretion of 1,25-dihydroxycholecalciferol, due to the absence of parathyroid hormone (Garabedian et al., 1972).

D. Surgical Hypoparathyroidism

Since surgery of the thyroid gland is performed much less frequently in children than in adults, postoperative hypoparathyroidism is a rarity. Its management is no different from that in adults and needs no special discussion (see Chapter 3).

E. Pseudohypoparathyroidism

This disease, first described by Albright et al. (1942), is usually characterized by (1) low serum calcium and high serum phosphate refractory to administration of parathyroid hormone; (2) brachymetacarpaly and brachymetatarsaly, usually of the 4th digit, but also of digits 1 and 5; and (3) metastatic calcifications in muscle and subcutaneous tissue (MacGregor and Whitehead, 1954). In addition the patients usually are small and stocky; they have a round face and brachycephalic skull (Fig. 3); mental development is retarded. The disease has rarely been described in infants, possibly because it is not recognized. Most reports concern older children and adults (see Chapter 3 for additional details). Signs of hyperparathyroidism, such as subperiosteal erosions in the phalanges on X rays of the hands, increased bone turnover (measured by microradiography), and osteitis fibrosa (found histologically and by X ray) have been described in a number of children (Kolb and Steinbach, 1962; Fanconi et al., 1964; Cohen and Vince, 1969). These findings disappeared or abated following treatment with high doses of vitamin D and normalization of the serum calcium level.

The daily dosage of vitamin D needed to keep serum calcium at or near

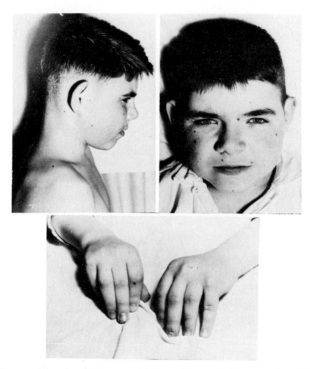

Fig. 3. Face and hands of a 6-year-old boy with pseudohypoparathyroidism. The 4th metacarpal of the left hand is short.

normal varies widely, not only between patients, but also in one patient over time. It has been observed that a dose of 75,000 units of DHT per day in a prepubertal patient had to be much reduced ater completion of growth and maturation, since the higher dosage caused hypercalcemia. In two patients (Suh *et al.*, 1970; Stögmann and Fischer, 1975) the low serum calcium did not respond to parathyroid extract, but hypercalcemia resulted from the administration of parathyroid extract once the calcium level had been normalized by vitamin D. There is presently no unified explanation for these facts, which renders this disease one of the most intriguing of the metabolic bone disorders. It has been noted that the calcitonin level in thyroid tissue of these patients is greatly increased. This appears to be a consequence rather than the cause of the low serum calcium level, since ablation of the thyroid gland has no effect on serum calcium (Suh *et al.*, 1969).

The X-ray findings of patients with pseudohypoparathyroidism were exhaustively described and reviewed by Steinbach *et al.* (1965) and by Steinbach and Young (1966). Brachymetacarpaly (Figure 3) and/or metastatic calcifications occur in all patients. However, since short metacarpals are the result of early closure of the epiphyseal disc, this sign usually is absent in infants and young children. A thickened calvarium and calcification of the basal ganglia are seen in about one-third of the patients examined. In spite of the small stature, skeletal age is accelerated in a number of patients. This leads to significant short stature in adulthood (Figure 4). Usually there are no further endocrine anomalies in pseudohypoparathyroidism, but deficiencies of thyrotropin and of prolactin have been described (Carlson *et al.*, 1977).

The disease occurs sporadically as well as in families. The mode of inheritance is uncertain (Fanconi *et al.*, 1964), although an autosomal-dominant mode of transmission is usually encountered. This does not explain the observation that the disorder occurs more often in boys than in girls. It may be that the expression of some of the features of pseudohypoparathyroidism depends on the sex of the patient. Studies of inheritance patterns are hampered by the considerable variation in the manifestations of the disease. In some patients, serum calcium rises spontaneously with age to normal values, while serum phosphate falls. They then have become similar to another group of patients, characterized by small stature, brachymetacarpaly, and round faces, a condition that

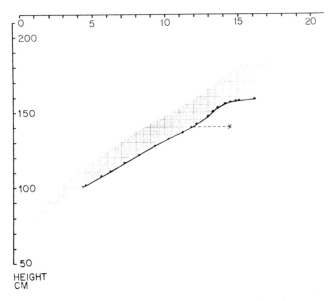

Fig. 4. Growth curve of the boy from Fig. 3. Horizontal axis represents age in years; dark area represents 10th–90th percentiles. Adult stature is relatively shorter than stature during childhood, as a result of advanced development [X = skeletal age (14.5 years) at chronological age 12.0 years].

has been termed by Albright as "pseudo-pseudohypoparathyroidism." It is better to abandon this meaningless expression and use the descriptive term "brachymetacarpal short stature" (Van der Werff ten Bosch, 1959), if only to emphasize that this disorder has no clear link with the parathyroid glands. Nevertheless, it is remarkable that both conditions occur in one family (Fanconi *et al.*, 1964). Treatment of pseudohypoparathyroidism consists of high daily doses of vitamin D or dihydrotachysterol. In 4 patients studied recently (Kooh *et al.*, 1975; Sinha and Bell, 1976) small daily doses of 1,25-dihydroxycholecalciferol (0.04–0.08 μgm/Kg bodyweight) resulted in normalization of serum calcium. In another patient treated in this manner, no effect could be obtained however (Kind *et al.*, 1975). At present there is no explanation for these conflicting results.

F. Hypohyperparathyroidism

In 1963 Costello and Dent described a 15-year-old girl who had hypocalcemia and hyperphosphatemia, while the X-ray pictures of her hands and long bones were indistinguishable from hyperparathyroidism (subperiosteal erosions and osteitis fibrosa cystica). Renal function was normal. Later, Allen *et al.* (1968) described a similar case in a 10-year-old boy. The reaction to PTH was not determined. Vitamin D or DHT was given in dosages of 0.5–1.5 mg/day, which led to healing of the bone lesions, while serum calcium and phosphate became normal. The pathogenesis of this disorder remains unexplained, but as in some cases of pseudohypoparathyroidism, there appears to be a dissociation of the effects of PTH, the action of PTH on the skeleton being notably intact while the extraskeletal effect of PTH appears blunted (Steendijk, 1971). Although the patients with hypohyperparathyroidism resemble some cases with pseudohypoparathyroidism, they clearly belong to a different group, since short stature is not apparent and metacarpals are normal. The characteristic facies is absent and their intelligence is normal.

G. Primary Hypomagnesemia

The normal plasma level of magnesium is 2.1–2.5 mg/100 ml (1.8–2.1 mEq/liter). It becomes important to consider magnesium deficiency with low plasma levels in infants with hypocalcemia and overt tetany that persists despite the restoration of serum calcium to normal. When these unexpected findings are encountered, serum magnesium levels should be ascertained. Hypomagnesemia with hypocalcemia is characterized by convulsions resistant to the usual treatment, low serum calcium, normal serum phosphate, and normal serum alkaline phosphatase values. The few cases described occurred in children who were 2–6 weeks old. Sporadic and familial cases have been reported (Strömme et al., 1969). All symptoms abate when the oral administration of magnesium is initiated in high doses (3–5 gm magnesium glycerophosphate per day, equivalent to 300–500 mg of magnesium). This treatment must be continued indefinitely (Friedman et al., 1967). The hypocalcemia is sensitive to administration of PTH but the magnesium levels remain low. This response should be contrasted with that seen in patients with hypoparathyroidism or neonatal hypocalcemia, in whom magnesium levels also may be low, but rise when the hypocalcemia is corrected (Wacker and Parisi, 1968). From investigations carried out in the few patients reported (all males, two of whom were siblings), it appears that the disease is caused by an isolated defect in intestinal absorption of magnesium or by an unknown derangement of magnesium homeostasis, which can be corrected by administration of magnesium in high doses (Paunier et al., 1968). Recent investigations into the pathogenesis of the hypocalcemia in this disease have shown that the synthesis of PTH is impaired in magnesium depletion, resulting in a "functional hypoparathyroidism" (Suh et al., 1973; Chase and Slatopolsky, 1974; Anast et al., 1976; Muldowney et al., 1970). Magnesium depletion with convulsions and with or without hypocalcemia is also a feature of protein-calorie malnutrition. It has been found that addition of magnesium to the diet results in faster recovery (Caddell and Goddard, 1967).

H. Dwarfism and Cortical Thickening of Tubular Bones

This rare familial syndrome has been described by Kenny and Linarelli in 1966, by Caffey in 1967, and by Frech and McAlister in 1968. It is characterized by extremely short stature, low birth weight, delayed closure of the large fontanel, myopia, abnormally thick cortices of the long bones, and episodic hypocalcemia with hyperphosphatemia. Mental development is normal. The only adult patient described had an uneventful puberty and measured 122 cm at 32 years of age. She had three children, one of whom had the same syndrome. He measured 40 cm at birth after a pregnancy of 37 weeks. The hypocalcemia is not continuous and may become apparent in infancy or during the adolescent years. The long bones have thick cortices with narrowing of the medullary cavity. There also is frontal bossing of the skull and the calvarium may be thin with barely distinguishable inner and outer tables. The thickening of the cortex of the long bones is exclusively on the endosteal surface (Caffey, 1967) and the periosteal diameter is normal. This serves to distinguish these bones from the type of thickening seen in Engelmann's disease (progressive diaphyseal dysplasia) in which the cortical walls are thickened internally as well as externally. Osteopetrosis can be ruled out by the shape of the bones. Superficially the face of a patient with this disease may resemble that of patients with pseudohypoparathyroidism, although brachymetacarpaly is absent and cortical thickening of long bones is prominent.

IV. NORMOCALCEMIC DISORDERS OF MINERAL METABOLISM

A. Osteoporosis

Osteoporosis in children occurs in a great many widely different diseases of which it usually is a minor feature. This symptomatic type has been ably reviewed by Royer *et al.* (1964), who found that it was the most common bone disease in children. Loss of skeletel tissue or "osteopenia" (see Chapter 6, volume I) is frequently encountered in renal disease (nephrotic syndrome, idiopathic hypercalciuria), gastrointestinal and allied disorders (celiac disease, hepatic cirrhosis, and glycogen storage disease), endocrine disorders (ovarian dysgenesis, Cushing's syndrome, in children on steroid therapy, hyperthyroidism), diseases of the musculoskeletal system (dermatomyositis, rheumatoid arthritis, fractures), and malignant diseases such as acute leukemia. Treatment of these diseases with clinical recovery often leads to conspicuous improvement of the osteopenia. Unlike the relatively slower recovery of the adult skeleton to corrective medical intervention (see Chapter 6, Volume I), childhood osteoporosis characteristically responds quite rapidly.

"Idiopathic juvenile osteoporosis" constitutes in a sense a paradoxical condition in that at a time when all tissues of the body increase in size, bone mass diminishes rapidly. About 20 cases have been described concerning children of both sexes, between the ages of 8 and 13 years, who were otherwise completely healthy (Berglund and Lindquist, 1960; Dent and Friedman, 1964b; Jowsey and Johnson, 1972). The severity of this condition appears to vary and in most cases a spontaneous remission occurs in 3–5 years (see Chapter 6, Volume I, for more details). The sign which ultimately leads to the diagnosis is usually a fracture, which occurs either spontaneously or after very slight trauma. Rarely bone pain preceeds the fractures. Serum calcium and phosphate are normal in this disorder, whereas in most instances, the alkaline phosphatase is distinctly elevated. Microradiographic analysis of undecalcified bone biopsies reveal a normal bone architecture and bone formation, although bone resorption is markedly increased. Radiologically the resorption is most evident in trabecular bone and on the endosteal surface of the cortex of the long bones. Newly formed bone, e.g. in the metaphyses of the radius and ulna, may be conspicuously radiolucent (Brenton and Dent, 1976). Rarely periosteal resorption occurs and the total diameter of the long bones decreases. The process may be very severe in the growing ends of the long bones, suggesting that, in some cases, in addition to increased resorption, bone formation may be decreased. Urinary hydroxyproline values, usually in the high normal range, are considered consistent with the increased bone resorption documented histologically (see Chapter 1, Volume I). The calcium balance is negative as a result of diminished intestinal absorption and/or small but significant elevations in urinary calcium (Jowsey and Johnson, 1972).

The pathogenesis of the disease is presently obscure. One theory holds that an imbalance in the intestinal absorption of calcium and phosphate leads to subtle but progressive increments in parathyroid hormone secretion and increased resorption of bone (Jowsey and Johnson, 1972). Administration of high doses of vitamin D and increased intake of calcium are characteristically without effect in this disease. The results of such therapy are difficult to evaluate, however, since spontaneous recovery may occur at any time during the course of the disease. Since the bone mass in these patients may never reach normal values in spite of spontaneous remissions, it has been suggested that these children therefore become symptomatic with "crush fracture osteoporosis" at a relatively early age (Dent and Friedman, 1964b; see Chapter 6, Volume I).

B. Osteogenesis Imperfecta

Osteogenesis imperfecta is a rare disorder, first described at the end of the eighteenth century and since then known by a variety of names (Freda *et al.*, 1961). Osteogenesis imperfecta may consist of several entities. In all forms the underlying metabolism and/or structure of collagen is abnormal. The clinical expression of this is "brittle bones", the severity of which varies considerably. In "osteogenesis imperfecta congenita" the child is born with multiple fractures and often does not survive since multiple rib fractures render breathing impossible. When the fractures occur beyond the infant years, the disease traditionally has been called "osteogenesis imperfecta tarda", and runs a milder course. In a study on 62 patients, Smith *et al.* (1975) recently were able to distinguish three types: A form with autosomal dominant inheritance and rather mild bone disease, blue sclerae and a reduced amount of polymeric collagen of normal stability in a skin biopsy; a severe form, which occurs spontaneously or may be recessively inherited, with congenital fractures, more normally colored sclerae, and a normal amount of polymeric skin collagen of reduced stability; finally a comparatively rare very severe form, which was lethal soon after birth and in which the skin collagen was very unstable and consisted of small non-cross-linked fibres. It was postulated that the same abnormalities would be present in bone collagen. Smith *et al.* (1975) observed that each of these subgroups might still be heterogeneous since intermediate situations can exist.

Whereas the incidence of the severe congenital forms has been estimated at 1:60,000 deliveries (Freda *et al.*, 1961), the incidence of the milder types is not well known since the diagnosis cannot be made with certainty in some children who sustain a number of fractures after apparently minor trauma but who have none of the other signs of the disease and who lose the propensity to fractures as they grow older. In the more severely effected children other conspicuous features, caused by abnormal development of mesenchymous tissues, may be present such as blue or pale blue sclerae (actually the sclerae are white but so thin that the chorioid plexus shows through), a lax cutis, and lax joint capsules. Tooth development is impaired by abnormal structure of dentine (dentinogenesis imperfecta) mainly in the severe form of the disease. The enamel is normal since it is not of mesenchymous origin. Typically the calvarium consists of multiple "Wormian bones" and is very thin and pliable at birth. Subsequently the skull may become deformed with a prominent and sunken occiput and reclining forehead. Deafness, due to otosclerosis, may occur after age 20 and is more common in the milder form of the disease. Usually the frequency of the fractures decreases with age and fractures may occur in adulthood. In a few cases, however, the diagnosis was not made before middle age, which indicates that this rule is far from universal (Table IX). Serum calcium and phosphate are characteristically normal whereas acid and alkaline phosphatases may be elevated, the latter often a result of fracture healing. The excretion of hydroxyproline is below the normal range (Riley and Jowsey, 1973).

Repeated fractures of the bones of the legs, expecially the femur, not only lead to severe and sometimes bizarre deformities, but also to shortness of stature. This is insufficient to explain the extreme shortness of stature often encountered in these children, and it must be assumed that repeated fractures near the epiphyseal discs interfere with normal growth. An inherent disorder of the growth apparatus, however, is not a feature of the disease. The fractures heal normally, sometimes by exuberant callus formation (Fig. 5a). In spite of much recent work on the biochemistry and structure of collagen in this disease, the fundamental defects are still unknown (Riley and Jowsey, 1973; Pentinnen *et al.*, 1974; Smith *et al.*, 1975). At present it seems that several distinct defects may underly the

TABLE IX

**Distribution of Age at First Fracture and
Incidence of Deafness in 174 Patients with
Osteogenesis Imperfecta**[a]

Age group (years)	Percent of patients having first fracture
Birth year	6.0
1	8.0
1–3	38.5
3–5	12.5
5–15	27.0
15	8.0

Age group (years)	Incidence of deafness
10–19	6.8%
20–29	10.3%
30–39	35.5%
40–49	32.0%
50–59	50.0%

[a] Sman (1961).

described differences in clinical expression. A change in the aminoacid sequence of the α-chain of the molecule, or a defect in the cross-linking mechanism are but two of the possibilities that have been postulated (Smith *et al.*, 1975). Recently, a failure of thin collagen fibres to aggregate extracellularly into large fibre bundles has been observed (Teitelbaum *et al.*, 1974). In the most severe congenital cases the cortex of the long bones may be entirely missing and bone tissue may consist of a sparse trabecular system of immature woven bone (see Chapter 2). In less severe cases, the width of the cortex is reduced, normal Haversian remodeling is impaired, and the primitive woven structure persists (Fig. 5b). In mild cases, bone structure may have a near-normal appearance.

A definitive therapeutic approach to this disorder is still lacking. More than a decade ago, Aeschlimann *et al.* (1966) suggested that high doses of fluoride might be of value in decreasing the frequency of the fractures. Since this report, which concerned only one child, fluoride has been tried in other patients, and with the possible exception of one patient (Kuzemko, 1970), favorable results could not be confirmed (Albright and Grunt, 1971). Short-term calcitonin treatment has been reported to increase the retention of calcium and phosphate (Castells *et al.*, 1972), but more detailed long-term studies have proved to be unrewarding. Solomons

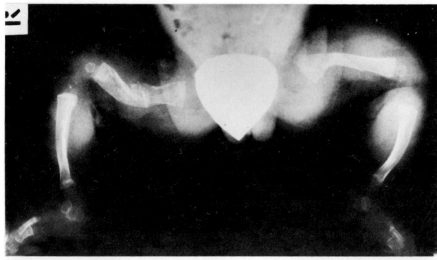

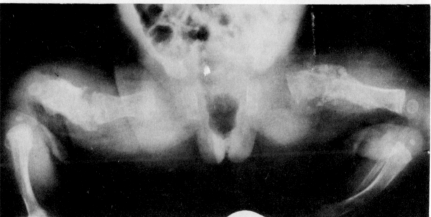

Fig. 5a. X-ray photographs of the legs of a girl with osteogenesis imperfecta (congenital type). Upper, 4 days after birth; lower, 14 days later, showing callus formation.

and Styner (1969) found that bone collagen from patients with osteogenesis imperfecta inhibited calcification in vitro. This inhibition could be reversed in vitro by pyrophosphate and magnesium ions. The therapeutic efficacy of pyrophosphate-like compounds (e.g., diphosphonates) in this disorder is unknown; the results of long-term magnesium therapy have been disappointing. Estrogens and testosterone and their derivatives have not been beneficial and should be discouraged (Cattell and Clayton, 1968), since the only effect is that of precocious puberty and/or virilization in preadolescent children. Careful orthopedic manage-

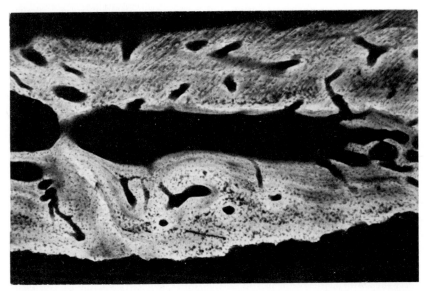

Fig. 5b. Microradiograph of undecalcified cross-section from a rib of a 5-year-old boy with osteogenesis imperfecta. The bone is mainly of the woven type. Only a few lamellae are visible. Normal Haversian remodeling is absent ($\times$ 50). (Compare with normal cortical bone in Fig. 7.)

ment, such as intramedullary rodding, may prevent the most severe deformities and facilitate early ambulation (Albright, 1973). This method is fraught with difficulties however, mainly since the results are often cancelled out by growth, which necessitates re-operation (Williams *et al.*, 1973).

The best management of these severely handicapped children who often are quite intelligent is dictated by common sense and much depends on the capacity of the parents and siblings to cope with the situation. Inventiveness, emotional stability, and a disciplined homelife are very important factors for the wellbeing of those who suffer from osteogenesis imperfecta.

C. Hereditary Hyperphosphatasia

Altogether less than 20 children have been described with this disease, the most conspicuous feature of which is a very high total serum alkaline phosphatase. In this and in other aspects, the disease resembles adult Paget's disease (Chapter 5). Although these two disorders may not be identical, the name "juvenile Paget's disease" (Woodhouse *et al.*, 1972) seems appropriate in view of this similarity.

The disease has been described under a variety of names (Woodhouse *et al.,* 1972), the best known being "congenital" or "hereditary hyper-phosphatasia." The disorder occurs in either sex with equal frequency. It has repeatedly been reported in siblings and in one instance the parents were consanguineous. The most probable mode of inheritance therefore appears to be autosomal recessive. Usually the first signs and symptoms become apparent in infancy or young childhood, but in one case the disease seems to have started *in utero*. The children refuse to walk or to use their arms and the extremities gradually become bowed and fracture easily. The skull and the bones of the face enlarge, sometimes so rapidly that the overlying skin is stretched and tightened. Pain is not always present and the skin over the affected bones may or may not be warm. In severe cases the whole skeleton may be affected. The deciduous teeth are shed early as a result of the rapidly remodeling jaws. X-ray examination of the long bones shows loss of normal cortical architecture with widening of the shafts. The trabecular pattern has been described as "cobweb" (Thompson *et al.,* 1969). The bones of the skull are irregularly thickened.

Histologically, the bone tissue shows signs of highly increased remodeling activity as in adult Paget's disease. In the long bones, this may lead to replacement of the cortex by trabecular bone. The structure of the bone remains lamellar with a few reported exceptions when woven bone was formed. In the more severely affected areas the marrow becomes fibrous. Hematopoiesis is unimpaired. Serum calcium and phosphate are normal, but alkaline phosphatase is markedly elevated to 20–40 times the normal concentration. Acid phosphatase is also increased in many instances. The level of serum uric acid is increased sometimes to twice the normal childhood value of 3.2 mg/100 ml (Eyring and Eisenberg, 1968). Renal function is unimpaired. The excretion of hydroxyproline is increased as would be expected in a disease with highly increased bone turnover. The excretion of uric acid is also elevated as a result of overproduction of this substance. Endocrine status is normal, but growth may be impaired as a result of the deformities and fractures. The prognosis for life is unknown, but may be unfavorable in the most severe cases, since the air passages may become blocked as a result of the irregular and bizarre deformation of the skull and facial bones.

As in adult Paget's disease, the pathogenesis of "juvenile Paget's disease" is unknown. Impressed by the favorable results of calcitonin in adult Paget's disease, Woodhouse and his co-workers (1972) treated a 5-year-old boy with synthetic human calcitonin. The results were remarkable: the excretion of hydroxyproline and serum alkaline phosphatase fell conspicuously and immediately after the beginning of treatment. The balance of calcium and phosphate became more positive. These favorable results continued for as long as the hormone was administered. The clinical condition improved and there were no more fractures.

D. Polyostotic Fibrous Dysplasia

Fibrous dysplasia of bone, like hereditary hyperphosphatasia, is characterized by an increase in bone turnover. There are, however, obvious differences between these two disorders, which should be viewed as separate entities. Polyostotic fibrous dysplasia, first described in 1936 by McCune and in 1937 by Albright and co-workers, is apparently more common than congenital hyperphosphatasia (Alexander, 1971). Girls are more often affected than boys and familial occurrence has not been reported. The disorder usually becomes manifest between the ages of 3 and 10 years. In about half of the girls described, the bone disorder has been accompanied by precocious puberty. Cutaneous pigmentation is a more frequent feature. Although neither early sexual maturation nor pigmentation is obligatory, the disorder has become known as a triad of three apparently unrelated conditions: bone disease, precocious puberty, and pigmentations. The "cafe-au-lait" colored areas have irregular serrated edges and have been termed by Albright "coast of Maine" type to distinguish then from similarly colored spots in neurofibromatosis, which have a smooth "coast of California" edge. The pigmentations may be present at birth and should then be regarded as a possible forerunner of bone disease. It has been said that the disease is mainly unilateral and that the pigmented areas are mainly found on the side of the bone lesions, although many exceptions to this have been noted. The extent of the pigmented areas is also unrelated to the extent of severity of the bone lesions, which vary from localized skeletal involvement to generalized bone destruction. The femur (92% of cases) and the tibia (81% of cases) are most often involved (Harris *et al.*, 1962). When the changes of fibrous dysplasia occur in the upper end of the femur, the resulting outward bowing leads to a "shepherd-crook" deformity (Albright and Reifenstein, 1948). Another feature, which is present in 50% of the cases, is a thickening of the base of the skull.

Sexual precocity is uncommon in boys with polyostotic fibrous dysplasia, but it has been reported at least in four cases (Benedict, 1962). In some patients hemihypertrophy of an entire side of the body or of a few bones, not affected by the fibrous lesions, has been described (Benedict, 1962). The precocious puberty is manifested by breast development, growth of pubic and axillary hair, and an increased rate of linear growth, unless this is compensated for by deformities of the lower extremities. Menarche occurs early but usually does not take place before the clinical signs of skeletal disease have become apparent. It may precede all osseous manifestations of the disease. Therefore, polyostotic fibrous dysplasia should be ruled out in any girl presenting with precocious puberty. From the described signs of puberty it may be deduced that this form of precocious sexual development is of cerebral or hypothalamic origin. This has been questioned by Benedict (1962) who could not find any signs of ovulation in the ovaries of three girls. Moreover, the excretion of gonadotropins has often been found to be within the normal range. Still, it is impossible to maintain that the precocious development is entirely of adrenal origin since breast development is always present. Aarskog and Tveteraas (1968) described a girl in whom polyostotic fibrous dysplasia, pigmentations, and precocious puberty developed a few years following bilateral adrenalectomy for Cushing's disease. Hyperthyroidism has been documented in this syndrome (Benedict, 1966; Zangeneh *et al.,* 1966) and enlarged parathyroid glands have been found in a small number of patients (Benedict, 1962).

Radiologically, the bone lesions resemble those of congenital hyperphosphatasia. In severe cases the cortex becomes so thin it is difficult to detect (Fig. 6). The radiographic pattern of the spongious bone resembles

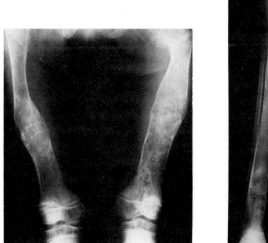
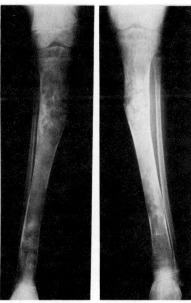

Fig. 6. X-ray photographs of upper (left) and lower (right) legs of a 6-year-old girl with severe polyostotic fibrous dysplasia. Note the very thin cortex and the "cigarette-smoke" picture of the bone tissue.

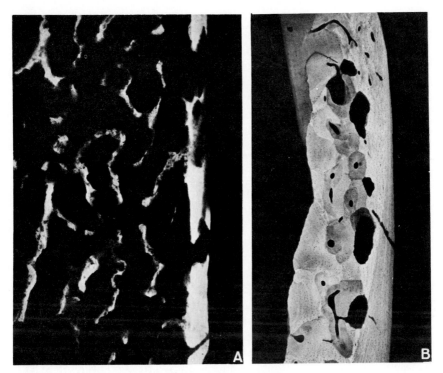

Fig. 7. A: Microradiograph of undecalcified cross-section from the fibula of a young adult male with polyostotic fibrous dysplasia. A fragmented remnant of the cortex is visible. The rest of the cortex has been replaced by irregularly shaped trabeculae of woven bone (× 30). B: Microradiograph of undecalcified cross-section from the fibula of a 7-year-old normal boy. Normal structure of cortex with Haversian remodeling (× 25).

"the wavy pattern of the smoke from the tip of a burning cigarette." Alternatively, the uniform replacement of cortex and marrow by trabecular tissue may impart a ground glass appearance of the skeleton. Microscopically the lesion consists predominantly of an abundance of woven bone and an increase in the number of osteoblasts and osteoclasts. The rate of remodeling is high. In severely affected areas the bone marrow has been completely replaced by a fibrous tissue with randomly arranged thin and coarse fibers, which virtually obliterates the hemopoietic component (Fig. 7). The bones break easily and often. Healing is rapid with abundant callus formation and gross structural deformities. Despite the fibrotic invasion of marrow tissue, signs of extramedullary hematopoiesis have never been described, even in cases with virtual complete skeletal involvement.

Serum calcium is normal; phosphate may be normal or low (below 3.0 mg/100 ml), a finding that has led some to postulate the coexistence of secondary hyperparathyroidism (Kunin, 1962). The response of a low serum phosphate to high doses of vitamin D has been variable (Ryan *et al.*, 1968). In a very severe case, recently observed by the author, serum phosphate was repeatedly below 2.5 mg/100 ml, circulating parathyroid hormone concentration was slightly elevated, and high doses of dihydrotachysterol failed to correct the low serum phosphate value. Serum alkaline phosphatase and urinary hydroxyproline may be elevated to many times the normal values and serum acid phosphatase variably increased.

The pathogenesis of polyostotic fibrous dysplasia is unknown and to date specific therapeutic regimens are wanting. Although it might be expected that administration of calcitonin would result in a decrease of the high bone turnover, several attempts with this hormone have failed to achieve this result. Unlike the results obtained with Paget's disease of bone (see Chapter 5), hypocalcemia does not occur after intravenous administration of up to 100 MRC units of porcine calcitonin, and urinary excretion of hydroxyproline has continued unabated after several weeks of treatment with intramusculary administered calcitonin (unpublished observations by the author). Administration of mithramycin (25 μg/kg/day for 5 consecutive days) has not resulted in the slightest improvement of the signs in a 7-year-old girl, although untoward elevations of SGOT, SGPT, and LDH were observed (unpublished observations by the author). This therapeutic failure of calcitonin and mithramycin, if confirmed by additional studies, suggests that the pathogenesis of the increased turnover of bone and skeletal abnormalities in this disease differ from that of Paget's disease. Recently Dent and Gertner (1976) postulated that cases of polyostotic fibrous dysplasia and osteomalacia or rickets are analogous to the syndrome of "tumor rickets," in which hypophosphatemia appears to be due to the presence of a mesenchymal tumor. In one of their patients the low serum phosphate became normal and the rickets healed when most of the bone affected by fibrous dysplasia was resected.

The prognosis in this disorder is guarded. Harris *et al.* (1962), reporting on a long-term follow-up study in 37 patients, found that the most common physical deformity (occurring in 60%) was leg length discrepancy. More than one-third of the patients had suffered three or more fractures. The course of the disease did not become stationary after the age of puberty, as had previously been claimed, and there were three deaths either from inanition after multiple fractures or from pneumonia following fracture of a number of ribs. Five patients were confined to wheelchairs. Finally, monostotic fibrous dysplasia in adults is far more common than polyostotic fibrous dysplasia. In children the monostotic form (without precocious puberty and pigmentation) is rarely encountered.

E. Vitamin C Deficiency

Presently, frank deficiency of ascorbic acid or scurvy is rare in all parts of the world, in spite of the fact that vitamin C intake is below the recommended allowance in a number of the developing nations. The reason for this discrepancy is that scurvy is detected clinically only when the deficiency is severe and of several months to a year duration. In the Western world, scurvy only occurs in neglected infants, who do not receive fruit juice or ascorbic acid for several months. In older children the disease is virtually never encountered.

The main osseous lesions of scurvy are large subperiosteal hematomas, which cause localized swelling of the legs or arms. These are so painful that the infant avoids movement, assumes a "frog-leg" position, and may appear paralyzed. The costochondral junctions are also swollen and tender. Bleeding of the gums and into the subcutaneous tissues and anemia with low serum iron concentrations are also encountered.

Apart from general osteopenia, examination of the long bones reveals a pathognomonic radiological picture. A widened zone of provisional calcification in the metaphysis appears as an opaque transverse band. On its diaphyseal side this band is bordered by an area of very irregular structure, which has been called the "Trummerfeld zone" and which represents destroyed primary spongiosa. The pathological basis of these changes is the failure of normal bone matrix to form, ascorbic acid being necessary for the maturation of the collagen fibril (Hutton *et al.,* 1967). The edges of the metaphysis may be drawn out into small spicules, which point toward the diaphysis. This spur formation results from separation of the periosteal layer by blood and subsequent mineralization of tissue remnants. In the most severe cases the periosteum becomes almost completely separated from the bone by accumulation of blood as a result of the increased hemorrhagic tendency. Epiphyseolysis may also occur. Most of the lesions heal rapidly upon administration of ascorbic acid. The subperiosteal hematomas calcify, later to be resorbed (Rang, 1969). The clinical picture of a "battered baby" may resemble scurvy very closely. It should be emphasized that vitamin C deficiency is by far the least frequent of the two syndromes.

F. Osteopetrosis

This disorder, variably listed as "marble bones disease," "Albers-Schonberg disease," and "osteosclerosis fragilis generalisata," can be separated into two forms: a severe form with autosomal-recessive inheritance and a mild form with autosomal-dominant inheritance. Approximately 150 cases of each form have been described with equal sex distribution (Johnston *et al.*, 1968). Children with the severe form commonly fall ill in the first year of life with anemia, thrombocytopenia, or a fracture. The prominent features of the disease are listed in Table X. All bones are usually involved, but the most conspicuous changes are found in the long bones. These are characterized by increased skeletal density and "flask" or "clublike" deformities, the latter resulting from absent or diminished metaphyseal cortical resorption (external remodeling) during linear growth. The abnormalities in skeletal remodeling may obtain *in utero* with newborn infants manifesting these characteristic lesions. The marrow cavity is absent (Fig. 8) and longitudinal striations in the metaphyseal regions of the long bones resemble a "celery stalk" radiographically. Despite the appearance of dense bones, fractures are also very common in this disorder. Rickets may be present in early infancy and is occasionally associated with a decrease in serum calcium and phosphate. Usually,

TABLE X

Signs and Symptoms in the Two Forms of Osteopetrosis[a]

Sign	Percent
Severe form (50 cases)	
Optic atrophy	78
Splenomegaly	62
Hepatomegaly	48
Poor growth	36
Frontal bossing	34
Fracture	28
Loss of hearing	22
Mental retardation	22
Large head	22
Lymphadenopathy	18
Osteomyelitis	18
Facial paralysis	10
Genu valgum	16
Pectus deformity	8
Mild form (133 cases)	
Symptom-free	48
Fracture	38
Osteomyelitis	10
Cranial nerve paralysis	22
Bone pain	20

[a] From Johnston *et al.* (1968).

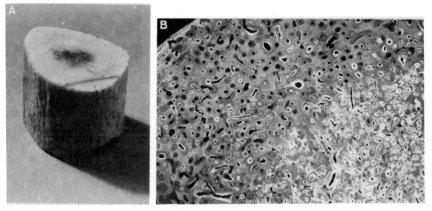

Fig. 8a. Segment of humerus from patient with osteopetrosis.

Fig. 8b. Microradiograph of undecalcified cross-section from bone of Fig. 8a. Note the absence of marrow cavity (center of bone is in lower righthand corner). Densely mineralized old bone and less densely to normally mineralized more recently deposited bone are shown (lefthand upper part of figure). (× 12).

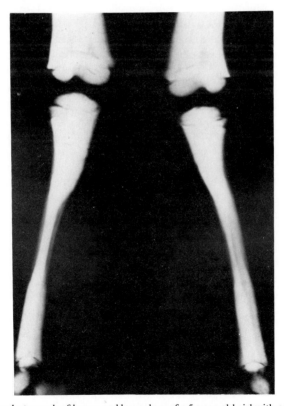

Fig. 8c. X-ray photograph of knees and lower legs of a 5-year-old girl with osteopetrosis.

685

however, these values are normal. The intestinal absorption of calcium is high and the urinary excretion is diminished.

The liver and spleen are enlarged with extramedullary hematopoiesis present in both the liver and lymph nodes. Hypersplenism is common. When the children with the severe form of osteopetrosis survive, repeated transfusions are necessary and the spleen must be removed to diminish hemolysis. It has often been stated that extramedullary hematopoiesis is a sequel of absent bone marrow, and histologically abnormal bone marrow with deficient hematopoietic tissue has indeed been observed. Extravascular hemolysis may also make a substantial contribution to the anemia (Enell and Pehrson, 1968). Cranial nerve paralysis (mainly involving the oculomotor and facialis), blindness, and deafness result from insufficient or absent growth of the foramina through which the cranial nerves pass (Johnston et al., 1968).

Microscopically bone tissue contains remnants of early fetal calcified cartilage and woven bone, indicating impairment of resorption. More specific microradiographic analysis reveals that density of the bone tissue is predominantly increased although variable. Some normally remodeled areas with secondary Haversian systems may be encountered (Fig. 8). The density of the bone radiologically is also variable. During preadolescent growth and development varying degrees of osteosclerosis are detectable in the long bones as transverse bands of increased density. These variations are related to the amount of calcium absorbed in the gut and the rate of skeletal growth and remodeling.

At present, the treatment for this severe form of osteopetrosis is less than adequate. In one instance the combination of a low calcium diet and prednisolone for 4 months resulted in improvement in the radiological appearance of the skeletal lesions (Dent et al., 1965). Subsequently the addition of cellulose phosphate (10 gm/day) decreased the intestinal absorption of calcium virtually to zero and induced hypocalcemia with tetany. The hypocalcemia responded effectively to the administration of parathyroid hormone and vitamin D. In this case, therefore, severe restriction of calcium intake and decreased calcium absorption resulted in decreased density of the bone formed at that time. The response of this patient incriminates hyperabsorption of calcium as a potential pathogenetic factor. Patients with the severe form of osteopetrosis usually die at an early age (<25 years) from anemia or infections.

Usually the benign, dominantly inherited form of the disease is not recognized before adolescence or adulthood when a fracture necessitates radiological examination. The youngest reported case was 11 months old. As noted in Chapter 4, for medullary carcinoma, investigation of family members of an affected patient may lead to an early diagnosis in an asymptomatic individual (Johnston *et al.,* 1968). The bone lesions resemble those found in the severe form, but are less extensive. The changes begin in the diaphysis, later extending to the metaphyses. The liver and spleen are of normal size; anemia and extramedullary hematopoiesis are absent. A large number of patients are completely asymptomatic. Fractures occur in 38% of reported patients and osteomyelitis, predominantly of the mandible, in 10%. Cranial involvement occurs in 22% of those affected (Johnston *et al.,* 1968). Renal tubular acidosis has also been reported in isolated cases (Vainsel *et al.,* 1971). Serum calcium, phosphate, and alkaline phosphatase are normal, but serum acid phosphatase is increased, and may prove to be a valuable genetic marker for the disease (Johnston *et al.,* 1968). The prognosis for the benign form is much better than for the severe form. Many patients approach middle age with minimal clinical discomfort.

Both forms of osteopetrosis most probably reflect the same pathogenetic process. The basic defect is still unknown. Metabolic and morphologic data accumulated in patients with the benign form are consistent with the formation of an abnormal type of bone, which fractures easily. Results of investigations with vitamin D and parathyroid hormone in one child have suggested that the bone is refractory to the calcium-mobilizing action of these substances. Hypercalcemia could only be produced by high doses of vitamin D and a high calcium diet and therefore may have been of intestinal origin (Fraser *et al.,* 1968).

Osteopetrosis has been compared to similar conditions in rabbits, grey lethal mice, bulls, and domestic fowl (Brown and Dent, 1971). In fowl, the disorder probably is of viral origin and an overproduction of calcitonin may contribute to the grey lethal mouse type (Walker, 1966). In bulls, a disease very similar to osteopetrosis may be caused by overfeeding with calcium, leading to secondary overproduction of calcitonin and decreased bone resorption (Krook *et al.,* 1969). Unlike the animal forms of osteopetrosis, calcitonin secretion is reportedly normal in patients with this disorder (Brown and Dent, 1971). It is not yet known whether the difference between the benign and malignant forms of osteopetrosis is of a quantitative or qualitative nature. The latter possibility is suggested by the different inheritance patterns.

G. Hypothyroidism

Increased bone density has occasionally been described in infants with untreated congenital hypothyroidism (Andersen, 1961). This phenomenon probably results from the increased intestinal absorption of calcium and the decreased turnover of bone, which accompany the hypothyroid state (see Chapter 4; Royer *et al.*, 1968). It is not a frequent feature of this disease and distinction from osteopetrosis is easy, since the contour of the long bones is normal. In older children with acquired hypothyroidism similar increased bone density has not been reported.

H. Pycnodysostosis

This disease recently has been distinguished from osteopetrosis (Maroteaux and Lamy, 1965) and some 40 patients have been described, many as examples of osteopetrosis (Elman, 1967; Emami-Ahari *et al.*, 1969). The condition is familial with an autosomal-recessive inheritance pattern. This disorder is characterized by increased bone density, persistently open cranial sutures, absence of normal angulation of the mandible, atrophic terminal phalanges, short stature, and a tendency to fractures. Radiologically, the bones may be indistinguishable from patients with osteopetrosis but the medullary cavity is present, although narrow. Hematopoiesis is normal and compression of the cranial nerves has not been reported. Recently, intermittently high basal levels of calcitonin have been found in a child with pycnodysostosis. The significance of this finding is not known (Baker *et al.*, 1973).

I. Hypervitaminosis A

Chronic overdosage with retinol for 6 months or more has been associated with cortical thickening of the long bones, which is only periosteal and limited to the diaphysis. Metacarpals and metatarsals are also affected. Other symptoms are hyperesthesia, hyperirritability, alopecia, and tenderness over the thickened bones. In recent years, about 20 children under 3 years of age have been described, who received between 30,000 and 150,000 μg of vitamin A per day for several months and in whom the above-mentioned symptoms developed subsequently (Davidson *et al.*, 1975). The signs disappear rapidly after interruption of the intake of vitamin A. The only permanent sequel may be diminished stature, since high doses of retinol cause premature closure of the epiphyseal discs.

J. Other Rare Diseases

A variety of extremely rare childhood disorders of bone associated with increased bone density have been reported in detail (Hinkel, 1957). Other types of metabolic disease of connective tissue and/or bone seen in children include the genetic mucopolysaccharidoses (McKusick, 1972;

Bailey, 1973), disorders of the epiphyseal plate (Rang, 1969; Bailey, 1973), and systemic bone disease of small premature infants (Griscom *et al.*, 1971).

V. BONE DISEASE IN DISORDERS OF RENAL FUNCTION

Little information is available on the urinary excretion of calcium in infants and children. The best study is that of Royer (1961), and his accumulated data are listed in Table XI. He noted that 18 of 19 normal

TABLE XI

Urinary Calcium Excretion in 74 Normal Infants and Children According to Age and Excretion[a]

Age (years)	Excretion of calcium in urine in mg/kg/24 hours						
	0–1	1–2	2–3	3–4	4–5	5–6	6–7
0–1	1	4	2	1			
1–3	5	4	2				
3–6	4	2	3	3	2		
6–9	4	5	7	1	2	1	1
9–12	2	3					
12–18	5	4	2	1	1	2	
Total: 74	21	22	16	6	5	3	1

[a] From Royer (1961).

children under 3 years of age excreted less than 3 mg/kg/24 hours. Of all 74 children examined, 88% excreted less than 3 mg/kg/24 hours and 25% less than 1 mg/kg/24 hours. Calcium excretion was found to be largely independent of calcium intake, but a low phosphate diet caused urinary calcium to increase. In view of these findings, urinary calcium greater than 6 mg/kg/24 hours in children can be considered abnormal; excretion rates of 4–6 mg/kg/24 hours should be suspect and calcium levels less than 0.5 mg/kg/24 hours considered low.

A. Idiopathic Hypercalciuria

Increased excretion of calcium in infants and children can be caused by the conditions listed in Table XII. The nonrenal causes have been dealt with earlier in this chapter. In this section, attention will be focused on the hypercalciuria of renal origin. As with a number of other conditions

TABLE XII

Differential Diagnosis of Childhood Hypercalciuria

A. Nonrenal causes
   1. Excessive intestinal absorption of calcium
      a. Excess vitamin D and calcium
      b. Sarcoidosis
   2. Hypercalcemia
   3. Increased resorption of bone
      a. Immobilization
      b. Idiopathic and symptomatic osteoporosis
B. Renal causes
   1. Idiopathic hypercalciuria
   2. Hypercalciuria in other disorders of renal function
      a. Renal tubular acidosis
      b. Bartter's syndrome
      c. Wilson's disease

involving calcium metabolism, idiopathic hypercalciuria may be more frequent than would appear from the small number of cases described in the literature. If urinary calcium determinations are not performed as a matter of routine in children with suspected metabolic disease, the diagnosis, and the appropriate therapy, may be missed to the detriment of the patients. The syndrome is not uniform. If hypercalciuria is regarded as the predominant sign, two types can be distinguished: one with, and one without rickets.

Idiopathic hypercalciuria without rachitic skeletal changes has been well described in the past (Royer, 1967; Fanconi, 1963; Beilin and Clayton, 1964). The children, mainly boys, were found to have the disease between the ages of 1 and 18 years. In a number of the older children, the signs had been present, unrecognized, for a number of years (Chapter 2, Volume I). The hypercalciuria is severe (6–20 mg/kg/24 hours) and the patients are small (4–5 standard deviations below the mean for age) but well-proportioned and weight is about normal for height. Skeletal age is retarded. Routine radiological surveys reveal generalized osteopenia. Apart from the hypercalciuria, the concentrating ability to the kidney is reduced and the resulting polyuria is resistant to Pitressin. Most children have proteinuria (0.4–3 gm per day), with predominant excretion of globulin, indicating renal tubular origin of the protein. Glomerular filtration rate, hydrogen ion excretion, and excretion of amino acids are all within normal limits. Both nephrocalcinosis and nephrolithiasis may occur and renal biopsy may reveal focal interstitial nephritis. Serum values for calcium, phosphate and alkaline phosphatase, creatinine, sodium, and potassium are normal in this childhood form of idiopathic hypercalciuria.

It is necessary to distinguish this disease from other forms of short stature, cystinosis, or the Fanconi syndrome, nephrogenic diabetes insipidus, and other causes of hypercalciuria. The cause of the short stature is unclear. Although it has been assumed that calcium deficiency might explain the impairment of growth, more detailed studies of growth hormone and somatomedin secretion and activity are lacking. The hypercalciuria can be decreased by the institution of low sodium or low calcium diets and the oral administration of sodium phytate or hydrochlorothiazide. The treatment of choice is a low sodium diet (less than 10 mEq/day), the latter resulting in a striking decrease of urinary calcium excretion (Royer, 1967). This regime results in improvement of the calcium balance (which is usually negative or insufficiently positive) and increase in linear growth rates. The polyuria may or may not improve. Vitamin D improves the calcium balance, but does not cause a reduction in urinary calcium loss; it may in fact produce nephrocalcinosis. Although a low calcium diet reduces renal calcium excretion it also reduces calcium retention and therefore should not be prescribed for prolonged periods of time. Sodium phytate in a dosage of 1.8–9 gm per day (sodium phytate theoretically binds 100 mg of calcium per gram) has been used with encouraging results. This mode of therapy however, has the same disadvantage as a low calcium diet (Beilin and Clayton, 1964). Although hydrochlorothiazide (1–5 mg/kg/day) reduces calcium excretion, it may lead to a variety of systemic complaints, which have been ascribed to the induction of hyponatremia (Fanconi, 1963). Improvement of the diabetes insipidus is not always achieved with this drug.

Idiopathic hypercalciuria with rickets has only been described in boys and is rare. Hypercalciuria is accompanied by a low serum phosphate (Dent and Friedman, 1964a); nephrocalcinosis and nephrolithiasis have not been described. Amino aciduria and proteinuria of the tubular type do occur, but acidosis is absent. The rachitic bone lesions and the low serum phosphate respond favorably to vitamin D in doses of 0.25 mg/day. Although this medication leads to a further increase of urinary calcium excretion, the calcium balance becomes more positive. Children with this form of idiopathic hypercalciuria are small before therapy, and catch-up growth is rare during treatment. As in the adult type of idiopathic hypercalciuria (see Chapter 2, Volume I) it is assumed that the childhood variant of this disorder is the result of an intrinsic impairment of the reabsorption of calcium in the proximal tubule, which may be either congenital or acquired. The accompanying polyuria and proteinuria also point to a renal origin of the disease. It is not known whether the rachitic form is pathologically similar to the nonrachitic form, except for the presence of complicating secondary hyperparathyroidism, leading to hypophosphatemia and rickets. To date, studies of serum parathyroid hormone levels as reported by Coe *et al.* (1973) for adults have not been reported for children.

Recently hypercalciuria has also been described in two children with chronic hypocalcemia, hyperaldosteronism, and increased plasma renin activity (Fanconi *et al.*, 1971). Although treatment with potassium and spironolactone led to improvement of the condition, the hypercalciuria persisted. The cause of the syndrome was thought to be congential dysfunction of the proximal renal tubule.

Another disease in which hypercalciuria, sometimes with rachitic changes and nephrocalcinosis, has been described is hepatolenticular degeneration or Wilson's disease (Litin *et al.*, 1959). An accumulation of copper in the kidney results in tubular destruction with glycosuria, amino aciduria, phosphaturia, and sometimes hypercalciuria. The syndrome of renal tubular acidosis also presents with hypercalciuria and rickets and is described in detail in Chapter 5, Volume I.

B. Renal Osteodystrophy

The pathogenesis of renal osteodystrophy is the same in children as in adults, and is discussed in detail in Chapter 2. Important childhood manifestations of the disorder which deserve emphasis are the bone lesions that lead to malformations, epiphyseolysis, and crippling, and the growth failure.

As in adults, osseous manifestations of chronic renal failure usually do not become clinically apparent in children before the glomerular filtration rate has dropped to at least 20–25% of its normal value. If severe renal failure is present from birth, severe bone lesions always occur in the course of several years. But if renal function has been adequate until the mid-childhood years, bone lesions may not be visible radiographically for a considerable period of time. Perhaps this is due to an accompanying decrease in the rate of remodeling, which is also responsible for the stunting of growth. Histologically the bone lesions consist of rickets, osteitis fibrosa, osteoporosis, and osteosclerosis either singly or in combination. It apppears that osteosclerosis is remarkably frequent and may occur in as many as 50% of the cases in which the bone is involved. It is predominantly found in the spine (Haust *et al.*, 1964). Rachitic changes may predominate in some children whereas hyperparathyroidism is the dominant skeletal lesion in others. If moderate to severe rachitic changes are present, signs of osteitis fibrosa such as subperiosteal erosions can be found in virtually all cases. Microscopically bone tissue shows abundant resorption and rachitic changes (Fig. 9). Osteitis fibrosa without rachitic

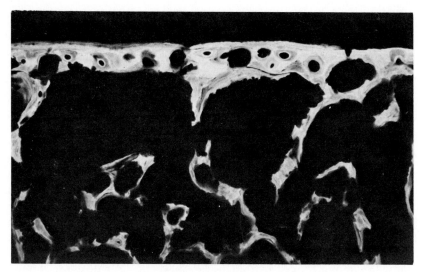

Fig. 9. Microradiograph of undecalcified cross-section of a rib from a 13-year-old boy who died after several years of severe chronic renal failure ($\times$ 75). Signs of rickets (irregular mineralization of bone, radiolucent cement lines) and of osteitis fibrosa (greatly increased resorption of bone) are abundantly present.

changes is only encountered in the most severe cases of renal osteodystrophy. Such cases usually have a long history of renal functional impairment.

In severe renal osteodystrophy epiphyseolysis frequently occurs. When this involves the femoral heads, it causes coxa vara with loss of height. Occasionally the femoral neck is no longer discernible radiologically in these cases. Destruction of the epimetaphyseal areas at other sites leads to bizarre changes in the shape of the limbs with varying, but usually high, degrees of invalidity. Ritz *et al.* (1973), who studied microscopically the metaphyseal region in severe renal disease, found that the primary spongiosa had been replaced by irregularly shaped trabeculae of woven bone, surrounded by fibrous marrow tissue. These trabeculae were rarely and irregularly connected with the cartilage plate, an observation that is consistent with the occurrence of epiphyseolysis. In children with epiphyseolysis osteitis fibrosa is more advanced than in those without (Mehls *et al.*, 1975).

Stunting of growth in children with chronic renal failure may be very severe and has been found to persist in spite of conspicuous improvement of the bone lesions by treatment with high doses of vitamin D. Serum somatomedin is low (Saenger *et al.*, 1974). Regular dialysis does not appear to improve the growth rate (Broyer *et al.*, 1972), whereas successful homotransplantation has a variable effect on growth (Grushkin and Fine, 1973), although somatomedin rises to normal values (Saenger *et al.*, 1974). Some catch-up growth may occur after transplantation, but normal height is rarely achieved. This is due in part to the necessity of administering large doses of adrenocortical steroids and to the fact that severe coxa vara with displacement of the femoral head is not corrected spontaneously, despite improvement of the diffuse skeletal osteodystrophy.

The aims of all forms of treatment should be to keep serum calcium as close to normal as possible, to bring serum phosphate down to *but not below* normal range, and to prevent the development of (or more commonly, alleviate) secondary hyperparathyroidism. In these respects there is little difference between therapy in adults and children (see Chapter 2). Lowering of serum phosphate by a low phosphate diet and aluminum hydroxide should be approached with caution in children since this form of therapy may lead to hypophosphatemic lesions (Dodge and Travis, 1965). In the presence of rachitic bone lesions, the indication for treatment with vitamin D or dihydrotachysterol is clear. The dose for children usually ranges between 0.1 and 1 mg per day. Initially, a low dose should be administered and great care must be taken to increase the dose slowly and to avoid hypercalcemia. If administration of vitamin D (or dihydrotachysterol) is carefully controlled, significant improvement may occur within the course of 1 or 2 years as is shown in Fig. 10. Although it is not always possible to achieve such spectacular results, significant improvement usually obtains (Dent *et al.*, 1961). Once the rachitic lesions have disappeared radiologically the daily dose of vitamin D should be drastically reduced or omitted altogether, until the lesions reappear. Unduly long administration of high doses of vitamin D inevitably leads to hypercalcemia.

In patients with a normal serum calcium concentration and minimal or no radiological signs of bone disease, the indication for vitamin D is uncertain. Again, the risk of hypercalcemia is comparatively high. On the other hand, as noted in Chapter 2, the activity of the parathyroid glands may be significantly increased despite the apparent absence of bone lesions on routine radiographs. At present, the best approach is to administer vitamin D or 25-hydroxycholecalciferol (25-OHD) when the circulating parathyroid hormone levels are elevated in order to prevent the development and progression of disabling bone disease. The dosage of vitamin D or 25-OHD should depend on the serum levels of parathyroid hormone and calcium. The ideal doses of either medication is that which lowers the serum concentration of parathyroid hormone to normal, without the occurrence of hypercalcemia. Experience with the administration of 1α-hydroxy-cholecalciferol in children is still limited (Postlethwaite *et*

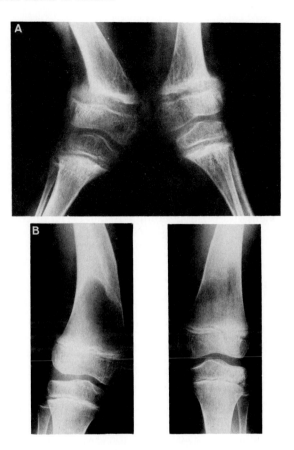

Fig. 10. X-ray photograph of the knees of a 12-year-old boy with severe renal osteodystrophy (GFR 7%). A, before treatment; B, after 3 years of treatment with 0.2–0.6 mg of
dihydrotachysterol per day. In both femora the site of the metaphysis at the beginning of
treatment is still visible. The boy did not use his legs during the first year of treatment.

al., 1976). Administration of sodium bicarbonate by mouth is sometimes
indicated to combat the acidosis (Dent *et al.,* 1961). As noted for adults
with renal disease, parathyroidectomy in childhood and adolescence may
also prove therapeutic for the osteodystrophy (Fine *et al.,* 1972).

Experience with the results of renal hemodialysis in children is still
limited (Fine *et al.,* 1972; Broyer *et al.,* 1972). It appears that rachitic bone
lesions tend to respond favorably to dialysis in patients on vitamin D in
doses of 0.1–0.75 mg per day. On the other hand, osteitis fibrosa may
improve, remain stationary, become worse, or in fact develop during
dialysis. This remarkable difference in reaction of the bone to what must

be regarded as an identical therapeutic regimen is unexplained, but the development of hyperparathyroid bone disease during dialysis appears to be related to the duration of the azotemia (Potter *et al.*, 1974). As noted in Chapter 2, parathyroidectomy may be indicated during dialysis if the bone lesions progress despite administration of vitamin D or 25-OHD, aluminum hydroxide and oral calcium supplements. Renal homotransplantation in children now has been performed in a fairly large number of patients and the results appear to confirm the original observations of Fine *et al.* (1970). Radiological signs of osteodystrophy disappear within the first 4–12 months following successful grafting of a kidney in the majority of cases. It is of great interest that this improvement occurs despite the large dosages of prednisone that are commonly administered. Coxa vara, genu valgum, and other orthopedic conditions, which tend to complicate renal osteodystrophy, are characteristically unaffected by transplantation. Slipping of the upper femoral epiphysis may become a real hazard in children with viable transplants. Weight gain secondary to better eating habits as well as increased activity are obviously predisposing factors in this regard.

REFERENCES

Aarskog, D., and Tveteraas, E. (1968). *J. Pediatr.* **73,** 89.
Aceto, T., Jr., Batt, R. E., Bruck, E., Schultz, R. B., and Perez, Y. R. (1966). *J. Clin. Endocrinol. Metab.* **26,** 487.
Aeschlimann, M. I., Grunt, J. A., and Crigler, J. A. (1966). *Metab. Clin. Exp.* **15,** 905.
Albright, F., and Reifenstein, E. C. (1948). ''The Parathyroid Glands and Metabolic Bone Disease,'' p. 263. Williams & Wilkins, Baltimore, Maryland.
Albright, F., Butler, A. M., Hampton, A. D., and Smith, P. (1937). *N. Engl. J. Med.* **216,** 727.
Albright, F., Burnett, C. H., Smith, P. H., and Parsons, W. (1942). *Endocrinology* **30,** 992.
Albright, J. A. (1973). *In* ''Disproportionate Short Stature'' (J. A. Bailey, II, ed.), p. 230. Saunders, Philadelphia, Pennsylvania.
Albright, J. A., and Grunt, J. A. (1971). *J. Bone Joint Surg., Am. Vol.* **53,** 1415.
Alexander, F. W. (1971). *Arch. Dis. Child.* **46,** 91.
Allen, E. H., Millard, F. J. C., and Nassim, J. R. (1968). *Arch. Dis. Child.* **43,** 295.
Anast, C. S., and Guthrie, R. A. (1971). *Pediatr. Res.* **5,** 668.
Anast, C. S., Winnacker, J. L., Forte, L. R., and Burns, T. W. (1976). *J. Clin. Endocrinol. Metab.* **42,** 707.
Andersen, J. J. (1961). *Acta Paediatr. Scand., Suppl.* **125,** 100.
Arnaud, S. B., Goldsmith, R. S., Stickler, G. B., McCall, J. T., and Arnaud, C. D. (1973). *Pediatr. Res.* **7,** 485.
Avioli, L. V. (1974). *Am. J. Med.* **57,** 34.
Avioli, L. V., and Haddad, J. G. (1973). *Metab., Clin. Exp.* **22,** 507.
Bailey, J. A., II, ed. (1973). ''Disproportionate Short Stature.'' Saunders, Philadelphia, Pennsylvania.

THE BRITISH SCHOOL OF OSTEOPATHY
1-4 SUFFOLK STREET, LONDON SW1Y 4HG
TEL: 01-930 9254-8

Baker, R. K., Wallach, S., and Tashjian, A. H., Jr. (1973). *J. Clin. Endocrinol. Metab.* **37,** 46.

Balsan, S., and Alizon, M. (1968). *Arch. Fr. Pediatr.* **25,** 1151.

Barr, D. G. D., Prader, A., Esper, U., Rampini, S., Marrian, V. J., and Forfar, J. O. (1971). *Helv. Paediatr. Acta* **26,** 507.

Begum, R., Dal Coutinho, R., Darmaday, T. L., and Yudkin, S. (1968). *Lancet* **1,** 1048.

Beilin, L. J., and Clayton, B. E. (1964). *Arch. Dis. Child.* **39,** 409.

Benedict, P. H. (1962). *Metab., Clin. Exp.* **11,** 30.

Benedict, P. H. (1966). *Am. J. Dis. Child.* **111,** 426.

Berglund, G., and Lindquist, B. (1960). *Clin. Orthop. Relat. Res.* **17,** 259.

Bergman, L. (1972). *Biol. Neonate* **20,** 346.

Bergman, L. (1974). *Acta Paediatr. Scand., Suppl.* **248,** 1.

Berliner, B. C., Shenker, I. R., and Weinstock, M. S. (1972). *Pediatrics* **49,** 92.

Bjernulf, A., Hall, K., Sjögren, I., and Werner, I. (1970). *Acta Paediatr. Scand.* **59,** 249.

Bongiovanni, A. M., Album, M. M., Root, A. W., Hope, J. W., Marino, J., and Spencer, D. M. (1968). *Am. J. Med. Sci.* **255,** 163.

Bonnard, G. D. (1968). *Helv. Paediatr. Acta* **23,** 445.

Brenton, D. P., and Dent, C. E. (1976). *In* "Inborn Errors of Calcium and Bone Metabolism" (H. Bickel and J. Stern, eds.), p. 222. MTP Press, Lancaster.

British Paediatric Association. (1964). *Br. Med. J.* **1,** 1659.

Bronsky, P., Kiamko, R. T., Moncada, R., and Rosenthal, I. A. (1968). *Pediatrics* **42,** 606.

Brown, D. M., and Dent, P. B. (1971). *Pediatr. Res.* **5,** 181.

Broyer, M., Loirat, C., and Kleinknecht, G. R. (1972). *Acta Paediatr. Scand.* **61,** 677.

Brunette, M., and Gerbeaux, S. (1963). *Can. Med. Assoc. J.* **89,** 1074.

Caddell, J. L., and Goddard, D. R. (1967). *N. Engl. J. Med.* **276,** 533 and 535.

Caffey, J. (1967). *Am. J. Roentgenol., Radium Ther. Nucl. Med.* (N.S.) **100,** 1.

Carlson, H. E., Brickman, A. S., and Bottazzo, G. F. (1977). *N. Engl. J. Med.* **294,** 612.

Castells, S., Inamdar, S., Baker, R. K., and Wallach, S. (1972). *J. Pediatr.* **80,** 757.

Cattell, H. S., and Clayton, B. (1968). *J. Bone Joint Surg., Am. Vol.* **50,** 123

Chase, L. R., and Slatopolsky, E. (1974). *J. Clin. Endocrinol. Metab.* **38,** 363.

Chisholm, J. J., and Hurrican, H. E. (1962). *J. Pediatr.* **60,** 206.

Cockburn, F., Brown, J. K., Belton, N. R., and Forfar, J. O. (1973). *Arch. Dis. Child.* **48,** 99.

Coe, F. L., Canterbury, J. M., Firpo, J. J., and Reiss, E. (1973). *J. Clin. Invest.* **52,** 134.

Cohen, R. D., and Vince, F. P. (1969). *Arch. Dis. Child.* **44,** 96.

Connelly, J. P., Crawford, J. D., and Watson, J. (1962). *Pediatrics* **30,** 425.

Costello, J. M., and Dent, C. E. (1963). *Arch. Dis. Child.* **38,** 397.

Cushard, W. G., Jr., Creditor, M. A., Canterbury, J. M., and Reiss, E. (1972). *J. Clin. Endocrinol. Metab.* **34,** 767.

David, L., and Anast, C. S. (1973). *In* "Clinical Aspects of Metabolic Bone Disease" (B. Frame, A. M. Parfitt, and H. Duncan, eds.), Int. Congr. Ser. No. 270, p. 661. Excerpta Med. Found., Amsterdam.

David, L., and Anast, C. S. (1974). *J. Clin. Invest.* **54,** 287.

Davidson, S., Passmore, R., Brock, J. F., and Truswell, A. S. (1975). "Human Nutrition and Dietetics," 6th ed., p. 148. Churchill, London.

Dent, C. E., and Friedman, M. (1964a). *Arch. Dis. Child.* **39,** 240.

Dent, C. E., and Friedman, M. (1964b). *Q. J. Med.* **34,** 177.

Dent, C. E., and Gertner, J. M. (1976). *Q. J. Med.* **45,** 411.

Dent, C. E., and Harper, C. M. (1962). *Lancet* **1,** 559.

Dent, C. E., Harper, C. M., and Philpot, G. R. (1961). *Q. J. Med.* **30,** 1.

Dent, C. E., Smellie, J. M., and Watson, L. (1965). *Arch. Dis. Child.* **40,** 7.
de Wijn, J. F. (1965). *Helv. Paediatr. Acta* **20,** 497.
DiGeorge, A. M. (1965). *J. Pediatr.* **67,** 907.
Dodge, W. F., and Travis, L. B. (1965). *Pediatrics* **35,** 792.
Elsenberg, E., and Pimstone, B., (1967). *Clin. Orthop. Relat. Res.* **52,** 199.
Elman, S. M. (1967). *J. Bone Joint Surg., Am. Vol.* **49,** 153.
Emami-Ahari, Z., Zarabi, M., and Javid, B. (1969). *J. Bone Joint Surg., Br. Vol.* **51,** 307.
Enell, H., and Pehrson, M. (1968). *Acta Paediatr. Scand.* **47,** 279 and 529.
Engfeldt, B., and Zetterström, R. (1956). *Bone Struct. Metab., Ciba Found. Symp., 1955* p. 258.
Eyring, E. J., and Eisenberg, E. (1968). *J. Bone Joint Surg., Am. Vol.* **50,** 1099.
Fairney, A., Jackson, D., and Clayton, B. E. (1973). *Arch. Dis. Child.* **48,** 419.
Fairney, A., Naughten, E., and Oppé, T. E. (1977). *Lancet* **2,** 739.
Fanconi, A. (1963). *Helv. Paediatr. Acta* **18,** 306.
Fanconi, A., and Prader, A. (1967). *Helv. Paediatr. Acta* **22,** 342.
Fanconi, A., Heinrich, H. G., and Prader, A. (1964). *Helv. Paediatr. Acta* **19,** 181.
Fanconi, A., Schachenmann, G., Nussli, R., and Prader, A. (1971). *Helv. Paediatr. Acta* **26,** 144.
Fine, R. N., Rosoff, L., Grushkin, C. M., Donnell, G. N., and Lieberman, E. (1970). *J. Pediatr.* **76,** 32.
Fine, R. N., Isaacson, A. S., Payne, V., and Grushkin, C. M. (1972). *J. Pediatr.* **80,** 243.
Foley, T. P., Jr., Harrison, H. C., Arnaud, C. D., and Harrison, H. E. (1972). *J. Pediatr.* **81,** 1060.
Fomon, S. J. (1967). "Infant Nutrition," p. 146. Saunders, Philadelphia, Pennsylvania.
Forbes, G. V., Bryson, M. F., Manning, J., Amirhakim, G. H., and Reina, J. C. (1972). *Acta Paediatr. Scand.* **61,** 305.
Fraser, D. (1957). *Am. J. Med.* **22,** 730.
Fraser, D., Kidd, B. S. L., Kooh, S. W., and Paunier, L. (1966). *Pediatr. Clin. North. Am.* **13,** 503.
Fraser, D., Kooh, S. W., Chan, A. M., and Cherian, A. G. (1968). *Calcif. Tissue Res.* **2,** Suppl., 52.
Frech, R. S., and McAlister, W. H. (1968). *Radiology* **91,** 457.
Freda, V. J., Vosburgh, G. J., and DiLiberti, C. (1961). *Obstet. Gynecol.* **18,** 535.
Friedman, M., Hatcher, G., and Watson, L. (1967). *Lancet* **1,** 703.
Friedman, W. F. (1967). *Am. Heart J.* **73,** 718.
Garabedian, M., Holick, M. F., DeLuca, H. F., and Brogle, I. T. (1972). *Proc. Natl. Acad. Sci. U.S.A.* **69,** 1673.
Garel, J. M., and Jost, A. (1971). *Ann. Endocrinol.* **32,** 253.
Garn, S. M. (1970). "The Earlier Gain and Later Loss of Cortical Bone." Thomas, Springfield, Illinois.
Gatti, R. A., Gershanik, J. J., Levkoff, A. H., Wertelecki, W., and Good, R. A. (1972). *J. Pediatr.* **81,** 920.
Glaser, K., Parmalee, A. H., and Hoffman, W. S. (1949). *Am. J. Dis. Child.* **77,** 1.
Goldbloom, R. B., Gillis, D. A., and Prasad, M. (1972). *Pediatrics* **49,** 514.
Griscom, N. T., Craig, J. N., and Neuhauser, E. B. D. (1971). *Pediatrics* **48,** 883.
Grushkin, C. M., and Fine, R. N. (1973). *Am. J. Dis. Child.* **125,** 514.
Harris, W. H., Didley, H. R., and Barry, R. J. (1962). *J. Bone Joint Surg., Am. Vol.* **44,** 207.

Haust, M. D., Landing, B. H., Holmstrand, K., Currarino, G., and Smith, B. S. (1964). *Am. J. Pathol.* **44,** 141.

Heaney, R. P., and Skillman, T. G. (1971). *J. Clin. Endocrinol. Metab.* **33,** 661.

Heath, H., Earll, J. M., Schaff, M., Piechocki, J. T., and Li, T. K. (1972). *Metab. Clin. Exp.* **21,** 663.

Hillman, D. A., Scriver, C. R., Pedvis, S., and Shragovitch, L. (1964). *N. Engl. J. Med.* **270,** 483.

Hillman, L. S., and Haddad, J. G. (1974). *J. Pediatr.* **84,** 742.

Hillman, L. S., and Haddad, J. G. (1975). *J. Pediatr.* **86,** 928.

Hillman, L. S., Rojanasathit, S., Slatopolsky, E., and Haddad, J. G. (1977). *Pediatr. Res.* **11,** 739.

Hinkel, C. L. (1957). *Clin. Orthop. Relat. Res.* **9,** 85.

Hung, W., Migeon, C. J., and Parrott, R. H. (1963). *N. Engl. J. Med.* **269,** 658.

Hutchin, P., and Kessner, D. M. (1964). *Ann. Intern. Med.* **61,** 1109.

Hutton, J. J., Tappel, A. L., and Udenfriend, S. (1967). *Arch. Biochem. Biophys.* **118,** 231.

Hyman, L. R., Boner, G., Thomas, J. C., and Segar, W. E. (1972). *Am. J. Dis. Child.* **124,** 723.

Illig, R., and Prader, A. (1959). *Helv. Paediatr. Acta* **14,** 618.

Illig, R., Budliger, H., Kind, H. P., and Prader, A. (1972). *Helv. Paediatr. Acta* **27,** 225.

Job, J. C., Milhaud, G., Gorce, F., Boigne, J. M., and Rossier, A. (1966). *Arch. Fr. Pediatr.* **23,** 643.

Johnston, C. C., Lavy, N., Lord, T., Vellios, F., Merritt, A. D., and Deiss, W. P., Jr. (1968). *Medicine (Baltimore)* **47,** 149.

Jowsey, J., and Johnson, K. A. (1972). *J. Pediatr.* **81,** 511.

Jue, K. L., Noren, G. R., and Anderson, R. C. (1965). *J. Pediatr.* **67,** 1130.

Kenny, F. M., and Linarelli, L. (1966). *Am. J. Dis. Child.* **111,** 201.

Kind, H. P., Prader, A., DeLuca, H. F., and Gugler, E. (1975). *Lancet* **1,** 1145.

Klein, L., and Teree, J. M. (1966). *J. Pediatr.* **69,** 266.

Kolb, F. O., and Steinbach, H. L. (1962). *J. Clin. Endocrinol. Metab.* **22,** 59.

Kooh, S. W., Fraser, D., DeLuca, H. F., Holick, M. F., Belsey, R. E., Clark, M. B., and Murray, T. M. (1975). *N. Engl. J. Med.* **293,** 840.

Kooh, S. W., Fraser, D., Toon, R., and DeLuca, H. F. (1976). *Lancet* **2,** 1105.

Krook, L. V., Lutwak, L., and McEntee, K. (1969). *Am. J. Clin. Nutr.* **22,** 115.

Kunin, A. S. (1962). *Metab., Clin. Exp.* **11,** 978.

Kuzemko, K. A. (1970). *Arch. Dis. Child.* **45,** 581.

Lahey, M. E., McMordaunt, R., and Robins, M. M. (1963). *Clin. Pediatr.* **2,** 43.

Lakdawala, D. R., and Widdowson, E. M. (1977). *Lancet* **1,** 167.

Landing, B. H., and Kamoshita, S. (1970). *J. Pediatr.* **77,** 842.

Lawrence, G. D., Loeffler, R. G., Martin, L. G., and Connor, T. B. (1973). *J. Bone Joint Surg., Am. Vol.* **55,** 87.

Levine, C., Greer, R. B., and Gordon, S. L. (1975). *J. Trauma* **15,** 70.

Lewin, P. K., Reid, M., Reilly, B. J., Swyer, P. R., and Fraser, D. (1971). *J. Pediatr.* **78,** 207.

Litin, R. B., Randall, R. V., Goldstein, N. P., Power, M. N., and Diessner, G. R. (1959). *Am. J. Med. Sci.* **238,** 615.

Lloyd, H. M., Aitken, R. E., and Ferrier, T. M. (1965). *Br. Med. J.* **2,** 853.

Lomnitz, E., Sepulveda, L., Stevenson, C., and Barzelatto, J. (1966). *J. Clin. Endocrinol. Metab.* **26,** 309.

Lund, H. T. (1973). *Acta Paediatr. Scand.* **62,** 317.

McCune, D. J. (1936). *Am. J. Dis. Child.* **52,** 743.

MacGregor, M. E., and Whitehead, T. P. (1954). *Arch. Dis. Child.* **29,** 398.

McKusick, V. A. (1972). "Hereditable Disorders of Connective Tissue," 4th ed. Mosby, St. Louis, Missouri.

Maroteaux, P., and Lamy, M. (1965). *J. Am. Med. Assoc.* **191,** 715.

Maxwell, J. P., Pi, H. T., Lin, H. A. C., and Kuo, C. C. (1939). *Proc. R. Soc. Med.* **32,** 287.

May, E. W., and Wygent, T. M. (1939). *Arch. Pediatr.* **56,** 426.

Mehls, O., Ritz, E., Krempien, B., Gilli, G., Willich, E., and Schäfer, K. (1975). *Arch. Dis. Child.* **50,** 545.

Millard, F. J. C., Nassim, J. R., and Woolen, J. W. (1970). *Arch. Dis. Child.* **45,** 399.

Mizrahi, A., London, R. D., and Gribetz, D. (1968). *N. Engl. J. Med.* **278,** 1163.

Morrow, G., Kivirikko, K. I., and Prockop, D. J. (1967). *J. Clin. Endocrinol. Metab.* **27,** 365.

Moshkowitz, A., Abrahamov, A., and Pisanti, S. (1969). *Pediatrics* **44,** 401.

Mühlethaler, J. P., Schärer, K., and Antener, I. (1967). *Helv. Paediatr. Acta* **22,** 529.

Muldowney, F. P., McKenna, T. J., Kyle, L. H., Freaney, R., and Swan, M. (1970). *N. Engl. J. Med.* **282,** 61.

Najjar, S. S., Aftimos, S. E., and Kurani, R. F. (1972), *J. Pediatr.* **81,** 1171.

Neiman, R. S., and Li, H. C. (1972). *Cancer* **30,** 942.

Nordin, B. E. C., and Smith, D. A. (1965). "Diagnostic Procedures in Disorders of Calcium Metabolism," p. 68. Churchill, London.

Pappas, A. M., Miller, M. E., Anderson, M., and Green, W. T. (1971). *Clin. Orthop. Relat. Res.* **74,** 241.

Park, E. A. (1964). *Pediatrics* **33,** 815.

Paunier, L., Radde, I. C., Kooh, S. W., Cohen, P. E., and Fraser, D. (1968). *Pediatrics* **41,** 385.

Pentinnen, R. P., Lichtenstein, J. R., Martin, G. R., and McKusick, V. A. (1974). *Proc. Natl. Acad. Sci. U.S.A.* **72,** 586.

Pimstone, B., Eisenberg, E., and Silverman, S. (1966). *Ann. Intern. Med.* **65,** 722.

Postlethwaite, R. S., Hill, L. F., and Houston, I. B. (1976). *Arch. Dis. Child.* **51,** 236.

Potter, D. E., Wilson, C. J., and Ozonoff, M. B. (1974). *J. Pediatr.* **85,** 60.

Prader, A., and Fanconi, A. (1969). *In* "Mineral Metabolism in Paediatrics" (D. Barltrop and W. L. Burland, eds.), p. 3. Blackwell, Oxford.

Prader, A., Uehlinger, E., and Illig, R. (1959). *Helv. Paediatr. Acta* **14,** 607.

Rang, M. (1969). "The Growth Plate and its Disorders," p. 44. Livingstone, Edinburgh.

Riley, F. C., and Jowsey, J. (1973). *Pediatr. Res.* **9,** 757.

Ritchie, G. MacL. (1964). *Arch. Dis. Child.* **39,** 584.

Ritz, E., Krempien, B., Mehls, O., Malluche, H., Strobel, Z., and Zimmerman, H. (1973). *Nephron* **10,** 195.

Robertson, N. R. C., and Smith, M. A. (1975). *Arch. Dis. Child.* **50,** 604.

Root, A., Grushkin, A, Reber, R. M., Stopa, A., and Duckett, G. (1974). *J. Pediatr.* **85,** 329.

Rosen, J. F., Roginsky, M., Nathenson, G., and Finberg, L. (1974). *Am. J. Dis. Child.* **127,** 220.

Rosler, A., and Rabinowitz, D. (1973). *Lancet* **1,** 803.

Round, J. M. (1973). *Br. Med. J.* **3,** 137.

Royer, P. (1961). *Helv. Paediatr. Acta* **16,** 320.

Royer, P. (1967). *Acta Paediatr. Scand., Suppl.* **172,** 186.

Royer, P., Gerbeaux-Balsan, S., and Mathieu, M. (1964). *In* "l'Ostéoporose" (D. J. Hioco, ed.), p. 95. Masson, Paris.

Royer, P., Mathieu, M., and Balsan, S. (1968). *Ann Endocrinol.* **29,** 610.

Russell, R. G. G., Bisaz, S., Donath, A., Morgan, D. B., and Fleisch, H. (1971). *J. Clin. Invest.* **50,** 961

Russell, R. G. G., Smith, R., Walton, R. J., Preston, C., Basson, R., Henderson, R. G., and Norman, A. W. (1974). *Lancet* **2,** 14.

Ryan, W. G., Nibbe, A. F., Schwartz, T. B., and Ray, R. D. (1968). *Metab., Clin. Exp.* **17,** 988.

Saenger, P., Wiedemann, E., Schwartz, E., Korth-Schutz, S., Lewy, J. E., Riggio, R. R., Rubin, A. L., Stenzel, K. H., and New, M. I. (1974). *Pediatr. Res.* **8,** 163.

Saville, P., and Kretchmer, N. (1960). *Biol. Neonate* **2,** 1.

Schlesinger, B., Luder, J., and Bodian, M. (1955). *Arch. Dis. Child,* **30,** 265.

Scriver, C. S., and Cameron, D. (1969). *N. Engl. J. Med.* **281,** 604.

Shopfner, C. E. (1966). *Am. J. Roentgenol., Radium Ther. Nucl. Med.* [N.S.] **97,** 154.

Sinha, T. H., and Bell, N. H. (1976). *N. Engl. J. Med.* **294,** 612.

Sman, G. (1961). "Osteogenesis Imperfecta in Sweden." Svenska Bok Forlaget, Stockholm.

Smith, R., Francis, R. J. O., and Bauze, R. J. (1975). *Q. J. Med.* **44,** 555.

Snapper, I. (1965). "Chinese Lessons to Western Medicine," p. 21. Grune & Stratton, New York.

Solomons, C. C., and Styner, J. (1969). *Calcif. Tissue Res.* **3,** 318.

Spiegel, A. M., Harrison, H. E., Marx, S. J., Brown, E. M., and Aurbach, G. D. (1977). *J. Pediatr.* **90,** 269.

Steendijk, R. (1969). *In* "Mineral Metabolism in Paediatrics" (D. Barltrop and W. L. Burland, eds.), p. 51. Blackwell, Oxford.

Steendijk, R. (1971). *Clin. Orthop. Relat. Res.* **77,** 247.

Steendijk, R., Nielsen, H. K. L., and Kraai, A. (1968). *Helv. Paediatr. Acta* **23,** 627.

Stein, R. C. (1971). *J. Pediatr.* **78,** 861.

Steinbach, H. L., and Young, D. A. (1966). *Am. J. Roentgenol., Radium Ther. Nucl. Med.* [N.S.] **97,** 49.

Steinbach, H. L., Ruhde, U., Honsson, M., and Young, D. A. (1965). *Radiology* **85,** 670.

Stickler, G. B., Peyla, T. L., Dower, J. C., and Logan, G. B. (1965). *Clin, Pediatr.* **4,** 276.

Stimmler, L., Snodgrass, G. J. A. I., and Jaffe, A. (1973). *Arch. Dis. Child.* **48,** 217.

Stögmann, W., and Fischer, J. (1975). *Am. J. Med.* **59,** 140.

Strömme, J. H., Nesbakken, R., Normann, T., Skjörten, F., Skyberg, D., and Johannesen, B. (1969). *Acta Paediatr. Scand.* **58,** 433.

Suh, S. M., Kooh, S. W., Chan, A. W., Fraser, D., and Tashjian, A. H., Jr. (1969). *J. Clin. Endocrinol. Metab.* **29,** 429.

Suh, S. M., Fraser, D., and Kooh, S. W. (1970). *J. Clin. Endocrinol. Metab.* **30,** 609.

Suh, S. M., Tashjian, A. H., Jr., Matsuc, N., Parkinson, D. K., and Fraser, D. (1973). *J. Clin. Invest.* **52,** 153.

Taitz, L. S., Salvador, C. Z., and Schwartz, E. (1966). *Pediatrics* **38,** 412.

Teitelbaum, S. L., Kraft, W. J., Lang, R., and Avioli, L. V. (1974). *Calcif. Tissue Res.* **17,** 75.

Teree, T. M., and Klein, L. (1968). *J. Pediatr.* **72,** 41.

Thompson, R. C., Gaull, G. E., Horwitz, S. J., and Schenk, R. K. (1969). *Am. J. Med.* **47,** 209.

Tsang, R. C., Donovan, E. F., and Steichen, J. J. (1976). *Pediatr. Clin. North Am.* **23,** 611.

Turton, C. W. G., Stanley, P., Stamp, T. C. B., and Maxwell, J. D. (1977). *Lancet* **1,** 222.

Tuvemo, T., and Gustavson, K. H. (1972). *Acta Paediatr. Scand.* **61,** 724.

Vainsel, M., Fondu, P., Cadranel, S., Rocmans, C., and Gepts, W. (1971). *J. Clin. Invest.* **50.** 2137.

Van Arsdel, P. P. (1955). *J. Clin. Endocrinol. Metab.* **15,** 680.

Van der Werff ten Bosch, J. J. (1959). *Lancet* **I,** 69.

Wacker, W. E. C., and Parisi, A. F. (1968). *N. Engl. J. Med.* **278,** 712.

Walker, D. G. (1966). *Z. Zellforsch. Mikrosk. Anat.* **72,** 100.

Walton, R. L. (1954). *Pediatrics* **13,** 227.

Warshaw, J. B., Littlefield, J. W., Fishman, W. H., Ingus, M. R., and Stolbach, L. L. (1972). *Acta Paediatr. Scand.* **61,** 429.

Widdowson, E. M. (1965). *In* "Human Body Composition" (J. Brozek, ed.), p. 31. Pergamon, Oxford.

Widdowson, E. M., and Spray, C. M. (1951). *Arch. Dis. Child.* **26,** 205.

Williams, P. F., Cole, W. H. J., Bailey, R. W., Dubow, H. I., Solomons, C. C., and Millar, E. A. (1973). *Clin. Orthop. Relat. Res.* **96,** 288.

Woodhouse, N. J. Y., Fisher, M. T., Sigurdsson, G., Joplin, G. F., and MacIntyre, I. (1972). *Br. Med. J.* **4,** 267.

World Health Organization. (1970). *W.H.O., Tech. Rep. Ser.* **452,** 34.

Zangeneh, F., Lulejian, G. A., and Steiner, M. M. (1966). *Am. J. Dis. Child.* **111,** 644.

Zidar, B. L., Shadduck, R. K., Winkelstein, A., Zeigler, Z., and Hawker, C. D. (1976). *N. Engl. J. Med.* **295,** 692.

Zorab, P. A., Clark, S., Harrison, A., and Seel, J. R. (1970). *Arch. Dis. Child.* **45,** 763.

Zusman, J., Brown, D. M., and Nesbit, M. E. (1973). *N. Engl. J. Med.* **289,** 1335.

THE BRITISH SCHOOL OF OSTEOPATHY
1-4 SUFFOLK STREET, LONDON SW1Y 4HG
TEL: 01-930 9254-8

Index

A

Abnormalities, multiple congenital,
  idiopathic hypoparathyroidism and,
  272–273
Acid, secretion, hyperparathyroidism and,
  85
Acid-base balance, hypercalcemia and, 607
Acidosis
  hyperchloremic, 68
    differential diagnosis and, 108
  parathyroid hormone and, 161
  renal, improvement of, 69
  renal osteodystrophy and, 165–166
  renal tubular, 68
Acid phosphatase
  hereditary hyperphosphatasia and, 678
  Paget's disease and, 545
Acromegaly
  parathyroid tumors and, 62
  pseudohypoparathyroidism and, 381
Acute parathyroid intoxication, pancreatitis
  and, 86
Addison's disease
  hypercalcemia and, 654
  idiopathic hypoparathyroidism and, 276
Adenoma
  benign, primary hyperparathyroidism
    and, 51–58
  double, occurrence of, 123
  ectopic, 52
  hyperplasia and, 58
  parathyroid, spontaneous infarction, 93

retroesophageal, 52
unusual location of, 123
Adenyl cyclase-cyclic and adenosine
  monophosphate, response to parathyroid hormone and, 325, 329
Adolescence, chemical determinants of
  skeletal metabolism in, 638–639
Adrenal insufficiency
  hyperparathyroidism and, 114
  transient neonatal, 258
β-Adrenergic receptors, parathyroid hormone release and, 45
Adrenocorticotropic hormone, medullary
  thyroid carcinoma and, 472
Alcoholism, chronic, hypocalcemia and, 260
Alkaline phosphatase
  differential diagnosis and, 108
  hypercalcemia and, 606
  hyperparathyroidism and, 95
  hypoparathyroidism and, 301–303
  serum
    Paget's disease and, 527, 543–545
    postoperative, 124
    uremia and, 172, 174
Alkalosis
  metabolic, treatment of, 414
  tetany and, 291
Alopecia totalis, idiopathic hypoparathyroidism and, 277–278
Aluminum intoxication, symptoms of, 196
Amyloidosis, systemic, 250
Anephric subjects
  25-hydroxycholecalciferol and, 190

serum calcium in, 159
vitamin D metabolism in, 155
Angioid streaks, Paget's disease and, 505, 550, 565
Ankylosing spondylitis
  genetics and, 493
  hyperparathyroidism and, 90–91
  Paget's disease and, 513
Antibodies
  adrenal, idiopathic hypoparathyroidism and, 282
  calcitonin and, 561–563
  prolactin-cell, idiopathic hypoparathyroidism and, 282
Anticonvulsants, osteomalacia and, 363
Anti-rachitic activity, assayable, uremia and, 153, 160
Antisera, parathyroid hormone, 101
Antitetanisches Präparat 10, therapy with, 406–407
Arteriography, selective, location of parathyroid tissue by, 104–107
Arthralgia, uremia and, 166
Arthritis
  dialysis and, 180
  gouty, 180
Articular system, hyperparathyroidism and, 88–91
L-Asparaginase, hypoparathyroidism and, 247
Assays, standardization, 102–103
Autoimmunity, idiopathic hypoparathyroidism and, 279, 281

B

Band keratopathy, hyperparathyroidism and, 92
Barium swallow, location of parathyroid gland by, 104
Basal ganglia, calcification of, 371, 381–382
Battered baby, scurvy and, 683
Bicarbonate, reabsorption of, 12
Blood flow, parathyroid hormone and, 15
Bone
  biochemical defects, renal disease and, 194–195
  calcium influx into, 6
  changes in ectopic and primary hyperparathyroidism, 603–604

collagen
  degradation of, 192
  Paget's disease and, 533
  synthesis, 193
  crystal maturation, 191
  density, hyperparathyroidism and, 72
  development in fetus and child, 634–638
  formation, modulation of, 8
  healing, Paget's disease and, 520
  histology of, 494
  hungry, 221, 226, 410
  metabolism, lactation and, 640–641
  pagetic, composition of, 534
  parathyroid hormone and, 5
  periosteal, formation of, 168
  remodeling of, 8–9
  resorption of, 5
    acidosis and, 165
    1,25-dihydroxycholecalciferol and, 157
    thiazide diuretics and, 117–118
  turnover
    hyperparathyroidism and, 71–72
    thyroid hormone deficiency and, 450–451
    uremic, tetracycline and, 188
    vasculature, Paget's disease and, 565
Bone cysts, hyperparathyroidism and, 80
Bone disease
  in disorders of renal function
    idiopathic hypercalciuria, 689–692
    renal osteodystrophy, 692–696
  hemodialysis and, 183–187
Bone pain, uremia and, 166
Bone-stimulating factor, dialysis and, 185–186
Brachydactyly
  familial, 297
  pseudohypoparathyroidism and, 296, 381
Brachymetapodia,
  pseudohypoparathyroidism and, 391
Brachyphalangia,
  pseudohypoparathyroidism and, 387
Brachytelephalangia,
  pseudohypoparathyroidism and, 389–390
Breast cancer, hypercalcemia and, 587–589
Bronchial carcinoma, endocrine disturbances and, 601–602
Brown tumors
  hyperparathyroidism and, 77, 80
  uremia and, 167

C

Cafe-au-lait pigmentation, polyostotic
  fibrous dysplasia and, 679
Calcification
  cardiac, detection of, 182
  ectopic, hyperparathyroidism and, 91
  endochondrial, renal rickets and, 176
  intracranial, 292
  metastatic, 120
    idiopathic hypercalcemia and, 649
  periosteal, hypervitaminosis A and, 115
  progressive vascular, 201–202
  pulmonary, nonuremic patients and,
    181–182
  soft tissue
    hemodialysis and, 187
    pseudohypoparathyroidism and, 391, 393
  tetracycline and, 188
  vascular, uremia and, 167
Calcific periarthritis, Paget's disease and,
  547–548
Calcific tenosynovitis, dialysis and, 180
Calcinosis cutis, dialysis and, 180–181
Calcitonin
  acute effects, Paget's disease and, 540–
    542
  bioassay, 473–479
  chemistry, 458
  ectopic production, 476–479
  hypercalcemia and, 618
  idiopathic hypercalcemia and, 649
  medullary thyroid carcinoma, 461, 475
    clinical features, 466–468
    diagnosis, 468–472
    embryology, 462
    histopathology, 462–466
    treatment, 472–473
  in newborn, 252
  Paget's disease and, 558–564
  parathyroid hormone secretion and, 44, 45
  physiology, 458–459
    bone and bone minerals, 459–460
    gastrointestinal tract, 460–461
    kidney, 460
  plateau response to, 560–561
  pseudohypoparathyroidism and, 366
  recent developments, 479–481
  renal failure and, 152
  resistance to, 561–563

  vitamin D metabolism and, 154
Calcium
  absorption
    control of, 163
    1,25-dihydroxycholecalciferol and, 157,
      158
    uremia and, 161–162
  adenylyl cyclase and, 45
  blood, parathyroid hormone secretion
    and, 34, 35, 36, 44
  calculated T_m, 9
  clearance of, 9
  dialysate concentrations, 185
  homeostasis in pregnancy and early in-
    fancy, 639–643
  influx into bone, 6
  infusion, 95
  intake
    monitoring of, 196
    supplementation of, 196–197
  intestinal transport, 13
    regulation of, 152
  ionized, 252
  kinetics, hypoparathyroid and
    pseudohypoparathyroid patients, 341
  malabsorption, renal osteodystrophy,
    151–153
  reabsorption of, 12
  serum
    hypertension and, 582
    postoperative nadir, 124
    pseudohypoparathyroidism and,
      298–299
  supplementation
    postoperative, 129–130
    therapy and, 412–413
  total-body, osteomalacia and, 171
  transport, sites of, 151–152
  vitamin D metabolism and, 154
Calcium balance, tumor-associated hypercalcemia and, 590–591
Calcium metabolism
  thyroid hormone deficiency and, 451
  thyroid hormone excess and, 455–457
Calcium oxalate, soft tissues and, 177
Calcium phospahate
  amorphous, maturation of, 188
  soft tissues and, 177
Calcium X phosphorus product
  osteitis fibrosa and, 171

soft tissue calcification and, 178
Calcium pyrophosphate dihydrate, deposi-
    tion of, 88
Calcium tolerance, hypothyroidism and,
    451
Candida albicans
    hypoparathyroidism and, 665–666
    infections, 274–276
Capital epiphysis, slipped, 376
Carbonic anhydrase, parathyroid hormone
    and, 11
Carcinoma
    medullary, parathyroid hormone secre-
        tion and, 44–45
    parathyroid, surgery and, 123
    primary hyperparathyroidism and, 51, 54,
        59–64
Cardiac disease, hypocalcemia and, 401
Cardiovascular complications, Paget's dis-
    ease and, 548–549
Cardiovascular lesions, idiopathic hypercal-
    cemia of infancy and, 119
Cardiovascular system
    hypercalcemia and, 582–584
    primary hyperparathyroidism and, 91
Cartilage, TCA cycle, uremia and, 194
Cataracts
    bilateral, 372
    renal failure and, 178–179
Chamberlain's line, Paget's disease and, 508
Children
    bone development in, 634–638
    chemical determinants of skeletal
        metabolism in, 638–639
    hyperparathyroidism in, 92–93, 644–648
    treatment of hypercalcemia in, 657–658
    uremic bone disease in, 175–177
Chloride-to-phosphate ratio
    hyperparathyroidism and, 69
    sarcoidosis and, 112
Cholecalciferol, therapy and, 406, 409
Chondrocalcinosis
    hyperparathyroidism and, 88–89
    Paget's disease and, 547–548
Chvostek's sign, hypocalcemia and, 130
Citrate
    metabolism, 9
    Paget's disease and, 542–543
Colchicine, hypocalcemia and, 17
Collagen metabolism
    Paget's disease

bone collagen, 533
    collagenolysis, 533–534
    hydroxyproline and hydroxylysine
        excretion, 535–536
    nondialyzable urinary hydroxyproline,
        536–540
    other collagen peptides, 536
    renal insufficiency and, 191–192
Congestive heart failure, calcification and,
    182
Convulsions
    metabolic, 255
    postoperative, 221
Corticosteroids, hypercalcemia and, 617–
    618
Cortisone suppression test
    sarcoidosis and, 112
    vitamin D intoxication and, 115
Cottonwool pattern, Paget's disease and,
    508
Craniotabes, hyperparathyroidism and, 644
Creatine phosphokinase, hypoparathy-
    roidism and, 404–405
Cretins, calcium metabolism in, 451
Crib deaths, parathyroid glands and, 273
Cyclic adenosine 3′:5′-monophosphate
    calcium mobilization and, 7
    excretion of, 322, 324
    ion reabsorption and, 12
    parathyroid hormone and, 17, 45
    pseudohypoparathyroidism and, 321
    urinary, 15
Cyclic adenosine monophosphate/creatinine
    ratio, parathyroid hormone and, 253
Cytomegalic inclusion disease,
    hypoparathyroidism and, 251

D

Deafness, osteogenesis imperfecta and, 675
Deformities
    flask or clublike, osteopetrosis and, 684
    varus or valgus, uremic children and, 177
Dental abnormalities, hypocalcemia and,
    399–400
Deoxyribonucleic acid, synthesis, vitamin
    D_3 and, 157
Diagnosis
    differential
        adrenal insufficiency, 114
        general, 107–108

hypercalcemia, 605, 607–608, 643–658
  alkaline phosphatase and, 606
  degree of hypercalcemia, 606
  electrolyte and acid-base balance, 607
  elevated parathyroid hormone, 607
  general state of debilitation, 606–607
  hypophosphatemia and, 606
  radiographic and biopsy evidence, 606
hypervitaminosis A, 115–116
idiopathic hypercalcemia of infancy,
      119
malignancy, 108–109
mild alkali syndrome, 118–119
Paget's disease, 504–505
prolonged immobilization, 118
sarcoidosis, 109–113
thiazide drug administration, 116–118
thyrotoxicosis, 113–114
vitamin D intoxication, 114–115
primary hyperparathyroidism
  general considerations, 93–95
  radioimmunoassay for parathyroid
      hormone, 97–107
  special tests, 95–97
Dialysis, peritoneal, calcification and, 185–
      186
Diet
  hypercalcemia and, 615–616
  renal osteodystrophy and, 195–197
Di George syndrome, characterization of,
      272
Digitalis, hypercalcemia and, 583–584
Dihydrotachysterol
  hydroxylation of, 159
  hypoparathyroidism and, 666–667
  resistance to, 410
  therapy and, 406, 407, 408
1,25-Dihydroxycholecalciferol
  biological half-life of, 156
  bone resorption and, 157
  defective production of, 152
  formation of, 154, 158
  hypocalcemia and, 667
      postoperative, 130
  levels, hypoparathyroidisms and, 362
  production of, 14
  sarcoidosis and, 111
  therapy with, 410–411, 412
  uremia and, 199–200
24,25-Dihydroxycholecalciferol, formation
      of, 154–155

Diphosphonates, Paget's disease and, 555–
      558
Distal tubules
  calcification, hypercalcemia and, 585
  phosphate clearance and, 11
  phosphate reabsorption and, 11, 13
Diuretics, hypercalcemia and, 615
Dwarfism, hypocalcemia and, 671–672
Dyschondroplasia,
      pseudohypoparathyroidism and, 304

E

Ectodermal changes, *see also* Skin
  dystrophic, idiopathic hypoparathy-
      roidism and, 275
  hypocalcemia and, 399
Ectopic bone formation,
      pseudohypoparathyroidism and, 304
EDTA, *see* Ethylenediaminetetraacetate
Electroencephalogram, hypercalcemia and,
      579–580
Electrolytes, hypercalcemia and, 607, 611–
      615
Electromyographic findings, spasmophilia
      and, 293–294
Electrophoresis, serum proteins, differential
      diagnosis and, 108
Elfin facies, idiopathic hypercalcemia and,
      649
Ellsworth-Howard test
  conditions for, 310
  hypoparathyroidism and, 309
  usefulness of, 314
Endocrine cataract, 292
Endocrinological disorders
  medullary thyroid carcinoma and, 468
Endocrinopathies
  hereditary, hyperparathyroidism man-
      agement issues and, 121–123
  idiopathic hypoparathyroidism and, 279
Enemas, phosphate-containing, 196
Epilepsy, idiopathic hypoparathyroidism
      and, 663
Epinephrine, parathyroid hormone secre-
      tion and, 44, 45
Epiphyseal dysgenesis, thyroid hormone
      deficiency and, 448, 450
Epiphyseal slipping, renal rickets and, 176
Epiphyseolysis
  renal osteodystrophy and, 693
  renal rickets and, 176

Ergocalciferol
   pseudohypoparathyroidism and, 360–361
   therapy and, 406–407, 409
Ethylenediaminetetraacetate
   calcitonin secretion and, 469
   hypercalcemia and, 617
   hypocalcemia and, 238–242
   parathyroid reserve and, 243–244
   resistance to parathyroid hormone and,
      319
   spasmophilia and, 295–296
Etiology, primary hyperparathyroidism,
      50–64
Extremities, Paget's disease and, 513–518

                         F

Facies, idiopathic hypercalcemia and, 649
Familial benign hypercalcemia, differential
      diagnosis, 651
Feces, calcium excretion, hyperthyroidism
      and, 455
Feedback loop, vitamin D metabolism and,
      154
Fetus, bone development in, 634–638
Fibrous dysplasia, Paget's disease and, 505
Fractures, Paget's disease and, 518–522
Fructose intolerance, hereditary, 69
Furosemide, hyperparathyroidism and,
      120–121

                         G

Gangrene, soft tissue calcification and, 178
Gastrin
   levels, hyperparathyroidism and, 85–86
   calcitonin secretion and, 470
Gastrointestinal motility, idiopathic hypo-
      parathyroidism and, 285
Gastrointestinal tract
   calcitonin and, 460–461
Gastrointestinal system
   hypercalcemia and, 580–582
   hyperparathyroidism and, 84–88
Gels, aluminum-containing, prescription of,
      196
Genetics
   idiopathic hypoparathyroidism
      familial cases, 278–283
      moniliasis and endocrinopathies, 274–
         278

   sporadic cases, 271–274
   Paget's disease and, 492–493
Giant-cell granuloma, hyperparathyroidism
      and, 77
Giant cell tumor, Paget's disease and, 527–
      530
Glucagon
   calcitonin secretion and, 470
   Paget's disease and, 558
   parathyroid hormone secretion and, 44
   secretion, hyperparathyroidism and,
      87–88
Glucocorticoids
   diagnosis of hyperparathyroidism and,
      96–97
   hypoparathyroidism and 259–260
   sarcoidosis and, 110–111
   vitamin D intoxication and, 115
Glucose, intolerance, 161
Glucose reabsorption,
      pseudohypoparathyroidism and, 320–
      321
Gonadal dysgenesis,
      pseudohypoparathyroidism and, 381
Gout, Paget's disease and, 546–547
Ground substance, bone matrix and, 8
Growth
   thyroid hormone deficiency and, 448–450
   thyroid hormone excess and, 452–454
Growth hormone, skeleton and, 640
Gustatory abnormalities,
      pseudohypoparathyroidism and, 394–
      395

                         H

Heartblock, calcification and, 182
Hematomas, subperiosteal, scurvy and, 683
Hemochromatosis, hypoparathyroidism
      and, 247–248
Hemodialysis
   bone disease and, 183–187
   hypercalcemia and, 621
Heparin, dialysis osteopenia and, 185
Hepatitis, idiopathic hypoparathyroidism
      and, 280
Hereditary hyperphosphatasia, polyostotic
      fibrous dysplasia and, 680–681
Histomorphometric data, idiopathic and
      pseudohypoparathyroidism, 364
Honeycomb skull, Paget's disease and, 508

Hungry bone disease, 221, 226, 416
Hydration, hypercalcemia and, 611
1-α-Hydroxycholecalciferol
  hypoparathyroidism and, 667
  postoperative hypocalcemia and, 130
  renal osteodystrophy and, 200–201
25-Hydroxy cholecalciferol
  advanced renal failure and, 160
  hepatic formation, 154
  hydroxylation of, 14
  levels, uremia and, 159
  pregnancy and, 642
  renal osteodystropy and, 694
  sarcoidosis and, 111
  uremia and, 190, 199
25-Hydroxydihydrotachysterol
  activity of, 408
  therapeutic efficacy, 198
1α-Hydroxylase, activation of, 14
Hydroxylysine, excretion, Paget's disease
  and, 535–536
Hydroxyproline
  collagen turnover and, 192
  excretion of, 17
    calcitonin and, 459–460
    in children, 638, 639
    hyperthyroidism and, 456
    Paget's disease and, 535
  matrix dissolution and, 8
  urinary, 95
    nondialyzable, 536–540
    total, 225, 404
Hyperaldosteronism, secondary, uremia
  and, 153
Hyperaluminemia, symptoms of, 196
Hypercalcemia
  adrenal insufficiency and, 114
  clinical occurrence, 585–587
    breast cancer, 587–589
    lung tumors and others associated with
      hypercalcemia, 590
    myeloma, leukemia and lymphoma, 589
  corticoids and, 112
  cretinism and, 451
  differential diagnosis, 107–108
    Addison's disease, 654
    familial benign, 651
    hypophosphatasia, 655–658
    hypothyroidism, 655
    idiopathic hypercalcemia of infancy,
      648–651

    immobilization, 653–654
    leukemia, 654
    primary hyperparathyroidism, 644–648
    sarcoidosis, 654–655
    signs and symptoms, 643–644
    vitamin D intoxication, 651–652
  ectopic, 604–605
  effects of
    cardiovascular, 582–584
    gastrointestinal, 580–582
    kidney, 584–585
    nervous system, 578–580
  hyperthyroidism and, 456–457
  hypervitaminosis A and, 115–116
  malignant disease and, 108–109, 578
  mild-alkali syndrome and, 118–119
  Paget's disease and, 545–546
  parathyroid hormone and, 7
    biosynthesis, 43
    secretion, 34
  pathogenesis of tumor-associated
    calcium balance and, 590–591
    differential diagnosis, 605–608
    ectopic parathyroid hormone produc-
      tion, 595–604
    mechanisms, 591–595
    new hypercalcemic syndromes, 604–
      605
    other calcium disorders associated with
      tumors, 608–610
  posttransplantation, 203
  primary hyperparathyroidism and, 48
  prolonged immobilization and, 118
  radioimmunoassay for parathyroid hor-
    mone and, 103–104
  regulation of mineral flow and, 8
  sarcoidosis and, 110
  thiazide diuretics and, 96, 116, 118
  thyroid carcinoma and, 219
  thyrotoxicosis and, 113–114
  treatment, 610–611
    comparison of available modalities,
      621–622
    dietary control, 615–616
    evaluation of methods, 612–613
    hydration and electrolyte replacement,
      611–615
    in infants and children, 657–658
    mobilization, 615
    nonspecific therapy, 617–621
    specific therapy, 616–617

vitamin D intoxication and, 114–115
Hypercalcemic crisis
  pancreatitis and, 86
  treatment of, 621
Hypercalciuria, 95
  hyperthyroidism and, 10
  idiopathic, 94
    thiazide diuretics and, 116–117
  immobilization and, 118
  mild-alkali syndrome and, 118
  Paget's disease and, 545–546
  sarcoidosis and, 110
Hypercementosis, Paget's disease and, 510
Hyperchloremia, sarcoidosis and, 112
Hypermagnesemia, secondary hypopara-
    thyroidism and, 258–259
Hypernatremia, as complication, 614
Hypernephroma, ectopic parathyroid hor-
    mone production and, 601
Hyperosteoidosis, renal disease and, 188
Hyperparathyroidism
  articular system and, 88–91
  asymptomatic, 49–50
  bone density and, 72
  cardiovascular system and, 91
  complications of, 49
  cortisone suppression test and, 112
  cure of, 54
  ectopic, 41
  failure to correct surgically, 128
  gastrointestinal symptoms, 84–88
  heriditary aspects, 61
  magnesium clearance and, 131–132
  hypercalcemia and, 644–648
  maternal, 257–258
  mental disturbances and, 83–84
  neuromuscular system and, 81–83
  normocalcemic, 93–94
  operations, parathyroid function and,
    220–224
  osteocytic osteolysis and, 73
  other manifestations and complications,
    92–93
  pancreatitis and, 581–582
  persistent, reoperation and, 129
  plasma standard, 101–102
  postoperative management, 123–132
  primary, 48–49
    adenoma and, 646–647
    clinical manifestations, 65–93

diagnosis, 93–107
  differential diagnosis, 107–119
  etiology and pathology, 50–64
  incidence, 49–50
  treatment, 119–132
  pruritis and, 181
  renal symptoms, 65–70
  sarcoidosis and, 109–113
  secondary
    dialysis and, 185
    mineralization and, 188–189
    parturition and, 35
    renal osteodystrophy and, 160–164
    reversal of, 200
    soft tissue calcification and, 179
    suppression of, 187
    treatment of, 201
  skeletal disease and, 70–81
  subclinical, 89
  surgical approach, 222–223
  tertiary, 161
Hyperphosphatasia
  congenital, Paget's disease and, 505
  hereditary, 677–679
Hyperphosphatemia
  neonatal, 254
  posttransplantation, 203
  pseudohypoparathyroidism and, 298–301
  renal failure and, 163–164
Hyperplasia, primary hyperparathyroidism
    and, 52, 58
Hypertension
  hypercalcemia and, 582
  hyperparathyroidism and, 91
  thiazide diuretics and, 118
Hyperthyroidism, hypercalcemia and, 113
Hypertrophic osteoarthropathy, hyper-
    thyroidism and, 454
Hyperuricemia
  Paget's disease and, 546–547
  primary hyperparathyroidism and, 89–90
Hyperventilation, tetany and, 291
Hypervitaminosis A
  hyperparathyroidism and, 115–116
  mineral metabolism and, 688
Hypocalcemia
  chronic alcoholism and, 260
  differential diagnosis
    dwarfism and cortical thickening of
      tubular bones, 671–672

hypo-hyperparathyroidism, 670
idiopathic hypoparathyroidism, 663–667
neonatal, 658–662
primary hypomagnesemia, 670–671
pseudohypoparathyroidism, 667–670
signs and symptoms, 658
surgical hypoparathyroidism, 667
hypomagnesemia and, 261, 290
hypoparathyroidism and, 402–403
incidence of, 227
induction of, 238–239
intestinal motility and, 285–286
neonatal, 641
dieases and conditions causing, 659
early, 251–253
late, 254–255
nutritional, 660
pancreas and, 286–287
parathyroid hormone and, 6, 34
persistent, 221
postoperative, 124, 128–130, 228–229
pseudohypoparathyroidism and, 298–299
signs and symptoms
cardiac disease, 401
dental abnormalities, 399–400
ectodermal changes, 399
neurologic features, 395–398
ocular findings, 400–401
tumors and, 609–610
Hypo-hyperparathyroidism
hypocalcemia and, 670
osteitis fibrosa and, 371, 373
vitamin D and, 360
Hypomagnesemia
correction of, 290, 410
idiopathic hypoparathyroidism and, 278
neonatal, 254
parathyroid extract and, 263
patient data, 265
postoperative, 130–132, 221
primary, 255–257
hypocalcemia and, 670–671
resistance to PTH and, 261–268
Hypoparathyroidism
L-asparaginase and, 247
biological findings, 402–405
congenital idiopathic, 255
cytomegalic inclusion disease and, 251
experimental, 283

functional, 252, 253, 262–263, 671
hemochromatosis and, 248
infarction of parathyroid adenoma and, 249
latent, tests for, 236–245
masked, 235
metabolic defect in, 14
in newborn
early hypocalcemia, 251–253
late hypocalcemia, 254–255
primary hypomagnesemia, 255–257
parathyroidectomy and, 58
parathyroid hormone and, 239
parathyroid trauma and, 250
permanent, 222, 231–232, 233
postoperative, 129, 130, 218–245, 665
causes and determining factors, 229–234
natural history, 234–236
pseudoidiopathic, 268–269
radiation damage and, 245–247
responses to parathyroid extract, 350
secondary
hypermagnesemia and, 258–259
maternal hyperparathyroidism and, 257–258
serum phosphate and, 227
symptoms of, 235
tetany and, 237
thyroid surgery and, 224–245
transient, 223–224
treatment of, 405–415
vitamin D intoxication and, 114
Hypoparathyroidism-Addison's disease-moniliasis, 283
other endocrinopathies and, 277
Hypophosphatasia, hypercalcemia and, 655–658
Hypophosphatemia
hypercalcemia and, 606
primary hyperparathyroidism and, 48
Hypophosphatemic osteomalacia, tumors and, 608–609
Hyposthenuria, hypercalcemia and, 584
Hypothyroidism
bone turnover and, 450–451
hypercalcemia and, 655
mineral metabolism and, 687–688
TSH levels and, 383–384

Hyproprotein, uremia and, 192
Hytakerol, principal component of, 467

I

Idiopathic hypercalcemia of infancy
  differential diagnosis and, 648–651
  hyperparathyroidism and, 119
Idiopathic hypercalciuria, causes for, 689–690
Idiopathic hypoparathyroidism, 250, 269–270
  complicating diseases, 665
  differential diagnosis, 309–310, 663–667
  genetic classification and physiopatholog-ical considerations, 271–283
  incidence, 270–271
  persistent, classification of, 664
  spasmophilia and, 290–296
  steatorrhea and, 283–290
  transient, 662
Idiopathic infantile hypercalcemia, hyper-parathyroidism and, 645–646
Idiopathic juvenile osteoporosis, 672–673
Immobilization
  hypercalcemia and, 653–654
  hyperparathyroidism and, 118
Immunity, cell-mediated, idiopathic hypo-parathyroidism and, 276
Infancy
  calcium homeostasis in, 639–643
  chemical determinants of skeletal metabo-lism in, 638–639
Infants
  hyperparathyroid mothers and, 661–662
  idiopathic hypoparathyroidism in, 272
  premature, vitamin D and, 642–643
  treatment of hypercalcemia in, 657–658
Intestinal malabsorption
  hypocalcemia and, 290
  pseudohypoparathyroidism and, 287
Intestine
  mucosal growth, vitamin D_3 and, 157
  parathyroid hormone and, 13–14
Ion transport, kidney and, 9
Isoproterenol, parathyroid hormone release and, 45

J

Jaws, Paget's disease and, 509

K

Kidney
  calcitonin and, 460
  hypercalcemia and, 584–585
  hyperparathyroidism and, 65–70
  ion transport and, 9
  parathyroid hormone metabolism and, 33
  resistance to parathyroid hormone and, 319
  thiazide diuretics and, 117

L

Lactase deficiency,
  pseudohypoparathyroidism and, 287
Lactation
  bone metabolism and, 640–641
  calcitonin and, 481
  parathyroidectomy and, 15
  vitamin D requirement and, 642
Lamina dura, hyperparathyroidism and, 77
Leukemia
  hypercalcemia and, 589, 654
  hypocalcemia and, 609–610
Lipase, hypocalcemia and, 286
Liver
  microsomal cytochrome P-450 enzyme, 160
  parathyroid hormone metabolism and, 33
Liver disease, idiopathic hypoparathy-roidism and, 281
Lung tumors, hypercalcemia and, 590
Lymphoma, hypercalcemia and, 589

M

Magnesium
  deficiency of, 262
  dialysate concentrations, 185
  parathyroid hormone release and, 44
  reabsorption of, 12
  serum, hypocalcemia and, 610
Magnesium clearance, hyperparathyroidism and, 131
Main d'accoucheur, appearance of, 293
Malabsorption syndrome, Paget's disease and, 550–551
Malignancy
  differential diagnosis and, 108–109
  hypercalcemia and, 586

Paget's disease and, 522–530
Medullary carcinoma, familial, 122
Medullary thyroid carcinoma
  clinical features, 466–468
  diagnosis, 468–472
  embryology, 462
  histopathology, 462–466
  treatment, 472–473
Mental disturbances
  hyperparathyroidism and, 83–84
  hypocalcemia and, 398
Mental retardation,
    pseudohypoparathyroidism and, 296,
    394
Metacarpal shortening,
    pseudohypoparathyroidism and, 389
Metaphyses, celery stalk, osteopetrosis and,
    684
Metastases, parathyroid glands and, 248–
    249
Methionine, selenium-labeled, parathyroid
    tissue and, 104
Microradiography, bone turnover and, 71
Microtubules, bone cells and, 17
Mild-alkali syndrome, hyperparathyroidism
    and, 118–119
Mineralization, defect in, 188
Mineral metabolism
  normocalcemic disorders
    hereditary hyperphosphatasia, 677–679
    hypervitaminosis A, 688
    hypothyroidism, 687–688
    osteogenesis imperfecta, 673–677
    osteopetrosis, 683–687
    osteoporosis, 672–673
    other rare diseases, 688–689
    polyostotic fibrous dysplasia, 679–683
    pycnodysostosis, 688
    vitamin C deficiency, 683
  Paget's disease and, 530–533
Mithramycin
  hypercalcemia and, 618–619
  Paget's disease and, 553–555
Mitochondria, renal, hydroxylation by, 158
Mixed phase, Paget's disease, 494, 497–498
Mobilization, hypercalcemia and, 615
Moniliasis
  idiopathic hypoparathyroidism and, 274–
    276
  steatorrhea and, 289
Mucopolysaccharidoses, genetic, 688

Multiple endocrine syndrome, genetic as-
    pects of, 62
Multiple-endocrine-neoplasia
  neuroectoderm dysplasia and, 64
  type I, 61–62, 63
  type II, 61, 62–63
Multiple neoplasia syndromes, hereditary,
    61–64
Muscle
  weakness and atrophy, hyper-
    parathyroidism and, 81–82
  weakness, uremia and, 182–183
Musculoskeletal system, renal failure and,
    166
Myeloma, hypercalcemia and, 589
Myocardial contractility, hypercalcemia
    and, 583
Myopathy, hyperparathyroidism and, 82–83

N

Nephrocalcinosis
  cretinism and, 451
  hyperparathyroidism and, 65–67
  uremia and, 181
Nephrolithiasis, hyperparathyroidism and,
    65–68, 94
Nervous system, hypercalcemia and, 578–
    580
Neurofibromatosis, pigmentation and, 679
Neuromuscular system, hyper-
    parathyroidism and, 81–83
Neuropsychiatric functions, hyper-
    parathyroidism and, 83–84
Neutron activation
  dialysis and, 186
  total-body calcium and, 171
Newborn
  hypoparathyroidism
    early hypocalcemia, 251–253
    late hypocalcemia, 254–255
    primary hypomagnesemia, 255–257
    secondary hypoparathyroidism in, 257–
      258
Norepinephrine, parathyroid hormone and,
    45
5′-Nucleotidase, Paget's disease and, 545

O

Ocular findings, hypocalcemia and, 400–401
Ossifications, ectopic, 373–374, 393–394

Osteitis fibrosa
  alkaline phosphatase and, 124
  epiphyseolysis and, 693
  maintenance hemodialysis and, 191
  osteosclerosis and, 171
  pseudohypoparathyroidism and, 372–373
  secondary hyperparathyroidism and, 167
  soft tissue calcification and, 178
Osteitis fibrosa cystica, hyper-
    parathyroidism and, 67, 70, 71, 73, 75,
    76
Osteoarthritis, hyperparathyroidism and, 90
Osteoarthropathy, hypertropic, bronchial
    carcinoma and, 601–602
Osteoblast(s)
  function of, 8
  parathyroid hormone and, 74
Osteoblastic metastases, hypocalcemia and,
    609
Osteoblastic phase, Paget's disease, 494,
    499–504
Osteoblastomas, hyperparathyroidism and,
    80
Osteochondrodystrophy,
    pseudohypoparathyroidism and, 393–
    394
Osteoclast(s), parathyroid hormone and, 74
Osteoclast-activating factor, leucocytes
    and, 595
Osteoclastic activity, parathyroid hormone
    and, 188
Osteoclastic responses, bone resorption
    and, 7
Osteoclastomas, hyperparathyroidism and,
    80
Osteocytic osteolysis
  Paget's disease and, 501–504
  parathyroid hormone and, 188
Osteodystrophy
  1, 25-dihydroxy D₃ and, 199–200
  healing of, 203
Osteogenesis imperfecta, in children, 673–
    677
Osteolysis, osteocytic, 7, 9, 73, 75
Osteolytic phase, Paget's disease, 494–497
Osteomalacia
  Ca X P product and, 171
  hallmark of, 188
  hyperparathyroidism and, 75
  pseudohypoparathyroidism and, 362–363
  renal failure and, 185

symptomatic bone disease and, 166–167
Osteomalacic osteodystrophy, frequency of,
    166
Osteopenia, hyperparathyroidism and, 70,
    71, 73, 80
Osteopetrosis, signs and symptoms, 683–
    687
Osteoporosis
  in children, 672–673
  dialysis and, 186
  hyperparathyroidism and, 70
  Paget's disease and, 510
Osteoporosis circumscripta, Paget's disease
    and, 506–507
Osteosarcoma, serum alkaline phosphatase
    and, 544–545
Osteosclerosis
  dialysis and, 186
  idiopathic hypercalcemia and, 649
  renal disease and, 168–171, 192
  secondary hyperparathyroidism and, 77
Ovarian failure, idiopathic hypoparathy-
    roidism and, 279, 281

                         P

Paget's disease
  complications
    associated neoplasias, 522–530
    fractures, 518–522
  drug treatment
    calcitonin, 558–564
    diphosphonates, 555–558
    glucagon, 558
    indications, 551
    miscellaneous drugs, 552
    mithramycin, 553–555
    phosphate, 553
    sodium fluoride, 552–553
  etiology of, 564–567
  focal manifestations, 505–506
    jaws, 509
    pain, 506
    pelvis and extremities, 513–518
    skull, 506–509
    spine, 509–513
  histopathology, 494–504
    differential diagnosis, 504–505
  historical, 490
  incidence and epidemiology, 490–493
  juvenile, 678–679

metabolic aspects
  acute effects of calcitonin, 540–542
  citrate, 542–543
  collagen, 533–540
  mineral, 530–533
  other phosphatases, 545
  serum alkaline phosphatase, 543–545
mild, indications for treatment, 552
mixed phase, 494, 497–498
nature of, 490
osteoblastic phase, 494, 499–504
osteoclastic phase, 494–497
serum procollagen in, 539
systemic complications and associated
    diseases
  calcific periarthritis and chondro cal-
    cinosis, 547–548
  cardiovascular complications, 548–549
  hypercalciuria, renal calculi and hyper-
    calcemia, 545–546
  hyperuricemia and gout, 546–547
  malabsorption syndrome, 550–551
  pseudoxanthoma elasticum, angioid
    streaks and skin changes, 549–550
Pain, Paget's disease and, 506
Pancreas, calcifications of, 87
Pancreatic disease, idiopathic hypoparathy-
    roidism and, 287
Pancreatic juice, hypocalcemia and, 286
Pancreatitis, hyperparathyroidism and,
    86–88, 581–582
Papilledema, hypoparathyroidism and, 398
Parathyroid adenoma, infarction of, 249
Parathyroid crisis, 249
Parathyroidectomy
  subtotal, hypoparathyroidism and, 58
  total, transplantation and, 204
  uremic osteodystrophy and, 201–203
Parathyroid extract, patient responses to,
    350
Parathyroid gland
  activity of, 45
  cellular atrophy in, 125
  function, provocative tests of, 236–242
  hepatitis and, 280
  metastatic involvement, 248–249
  nonsurgical damage, 250–251
  primary hyperplasia, surgical treatment,
    123
  secretory reserves, 37–38
  trauma to, 249–250

tumors, acromegaly and, 62
Parathyroid hormone
  abnormal, 268–269
  action of, 188
    on bone, kidney and intestine, 4
  adenylcyclase-cyclic AMP and, 329–330
  amino- and carboxy-terminal determi-
    nants, 101
  biosynthesis of, 3, 38–42
  calcium-conserving action, 10
  cAMP/creatinine ratio and, 253
  cellular effects, 74
  chemical composition, 18
  degradation or inactivation, 30, 46
  disappearance from circulation
    half-time, 32
    chronic renal failure and, 32
  ectopic production, 595–604, 607–608
  feedback regulation, 4–5
  fragments of, 3
    biological activity, 21, 22–23, 28
    circulating, 28–32
    immunoreactivity, 24, 25
    secretion, 31, 32
  heterogeneity of recognition sites, 101
  homogeneous preparations, 18
  hypomagnesemia and, 263
  hypoparathyroidism and, 239
  immunoassay, nonparallel slope of re-
    sponse, 24–25
  immunoreactive, 101
    in circulation, 32
    heterogeneity of, 24, 31, 32
    hypomagnesemia and, 265
    newborns and, 252–253
    pregnancy and, 253
    species of, 327–328
  injected, volume of distribution, 33
  inorganic phosphate and, 163
  maintenance hemodialysis and, 191
  metabolic clearance, 161
  metabolic fate, 3
  peripheral clearance and metabolism,
    26–32
  precursors of, 40
  purification of, 18
  radioimmunoassay, 97–107
  resistance to, 259–261, 296, 308–325
    hypomagnesemia and, 261–268
  secretion
    calcium and, 34, 35

hypomagnesemia and, 131
phosphate and, 45
rate, 36, 37
suppression of, 99–100
sequence analysis, 18–20
structure-activity relationships, 22
synthetic peptide, bioassay of, 21–22
therapy and, 414–415
thiazide diuretics and, 117
vitamin D metabolism and, 154
Parathyroid insufficiency, demonstration of,
241–242
Parathyroiditis
atrophic, 250
experimental, 283
Parathyroid reserve, estimation of, 243–244
Parathyroid tissue, abnormal, localization
of, 104–107
Pathology
primary hyperparathyroidism, 50–64
renal osteodystrophy, 187–191
Pelvis, Paget's disease and, 513–518
Peptic ulcer
hypercalcemia and, 580–581
hyperparathyroidism and, 84–86
Peptides, collagen, Paget's disease and, 536
Periarthritis, prevention of, 180
Periarticular disorders, hyperparathyroidism and, 88
Peritoneal dialysis, hypercalcemia and, 621
Pernicious anemia, idiopathic hyperparathyroidism and, 277
Personality disturbances, postoperative, 221
Pheochromocytoma, familial, 122
Phlyctenular kerato-conjunctivitis,
idiopathic hypoparathyroidism and, 277
Phosphate
deficiency, reversal of, 204
depletion of, 69
excretion of, 9
homeostasis, renal failure and, 164
hypercalcemia and, 619–621
inorganic, renal cortical, 154
intake, monitoring of, 196
intravenous, hyperparathyroidism and,
121
parathyroid hormone secretion and, 45
reabsorption of, 11, 95, 96, 156–157
restriction, dermal calcification and, 181
serum
in childhood, 639

EDTA and, 241
functional hypoparathyroidism and, 252
hypoparathyroidism and, 227
thyroid surgery and, 235
supplementation, Paget's disease and, 553
Phosphate clearance
delay of, 241
diagnosis of hyperparathyroidism and,
95–96
distal tubule and, 11
hypoparathyroidism and, 403
parathyroid hormone and, 9
Phosphaturia, parathyroid hormone and, 11
Phosphaturic response, parathyroid hormone and, 9
Phosphorus
dietary, absorption of, 162–163, 164
inorganic, serum levels, 94–95
plasma, hyperthyroidism and, 457
serum
pseudohypoparathyroidism and, 298–
299
sarcoidosis and, 110
Photon absorptiometry
bone mineral loss and, 167
dialysis and, 186
Phytate
latent hypoparathyroidism and, 242–243
mineralization and, 237–238
Pigmentation
coast of California, 679
coast of Maine type, 679
Plateau response, calcitonin and, 560–561
Platybasia, Paget's disease and, 508–509
Pneumocystis pneumonia, vitamin D intoxication and, 652
Polyendocrine disorders, 283
Polyostosis, Paget's disease and, 505
Polyostotic fibrous dysplasia
pathogenesis, 682
symptoms of, 679–681
Pregnancy
calcitonin and, 479
calcium homeostasis in, 639–643
hyperparathyroidism and, 92
hypocalcemia and, 35
immunoreactive parathyroid hormone
and, 253
vitamin D requirement and, 642
Prematurity, hypocalcemia and, 251
Pre-proparathyroid hormone

biosynthesis of, 38, 40, 42
sequences, 20
Primary hyperparathyroidism, *see* Hyperparathyroidism
Procollagen, in sera, Paget's disease and,
539
Proparathyroid hormone
biological activity, 23
biosynthesis, 38–42
calcium and, 43, 44
control of, 42–46
sequences, 20
Proparathyroid hormone-cleaving enzyme,
hypercalcemia and, 43
Propranolol, parathyroid hormone release
and, 45
Prostaglandins
medullary thyroid carcinoma and, 472
production, tumors and, 595
pseudohyperparathyroidism and, 109
Protein
restriction, vitamin deficiency and, 196
synthesis
parathyroid hormone and, 8
regulation of, 153
vitamin D and, 157
Protein kinase, activation of, 17
Proteinuria, hypercalcemia and, 585
Protrusio acetabuli, Paget's disease and,
515, 516
Proximal tubule
parathyroid hormone and, 13
phosphate and, 11
Pruritis
dermal calcification and, 180–181
severe, parathyroidectomy and, 202
Pseudoencapsulation, parathyroid
hyperplasia and, 58
Pseudogout, hyperparathyroidism and,
88–89
Pseudohypoparathyroidism, 376
acquired secondary, 284
adenyl cyclase-cyclic adenosine
monophosphate system and, 325–330
associated endocrinopathies, 382–385
blood chemistries, 298–303
borderline, 299
EDTA infusion and, 319
as an entity, 374
end-organ resistance to parathyroid hormone and, 308–325

general, 296–298
genetics of, 304–308
hypocalcemia and, 667–670
incidence, 303–304
familial, 305–308
intestinal malabsorption and, 287
malignant disease and, 108–109
metabolic defect in, 14
normocalcemic, 297, 367
parathyroid extract and, 309–311
pathogenesis of, 355–367
responses to parathyroid extract, 350
special forms and related conditions,
intermittently normal serum calcium
values, 367–372
related conditions, 380–382
roentgenologic osteitis fibrosa, 372–377
type II, 377–380
special studies
normalization of serum calcium with
vitamin D, 338–351
total parathyroidectomy, 351–354
twin sisters, 331–338
type II, 322, 374
typical signs of, 385–395
Pseudo-pseudohypoparathyroidism
definition of, 371
occurrence of, 297
Puberty, adenomata of parathyroid glands
and, 646–647
Pycnodysostosis, signs and symptoms, 688
Pyridoxine, collagen formation and, 195–
196
Pseudoxanthoma elasticum, Paget's disease
and, 549

R

Radiation damage, hypoparathyroidism and,
245–247
Radioimmunoassay, 42
calcitonin, 473
hyperparathyroidism and, 24
parathyroid hormone, 97–100
general diagnostic use, 100–104
location of abnormal tissue, 104–107
plasma hormonal species and, 31
Radiological changes
thyroid hormone deficiency and, 450
thyroid hormone excess, 454–455
Receptor(s), parathyroid hormone and, 22,
34

Receptor binding,
  pseudohypoparathyroidism and, 358–
  359
Red eye syndrome, renal failure and, 179
Reexploration, persistent hyperparathyroidism and, 129
Rehydration, hyperparathyroidism and,
  120–121
Renal calculi, Paget's disease and, 545–546
Renal cell carcinoma, hypercalcemia and,
  598
Renal disease, calcitonin and, 164
Renal failure
  advanced, 25-hydroxy D₃ and, 160
  chronic, 158
  chronic
    characterization of, 151
    in children, 693
Renal function
  disorders, bone disease and, 689–696
  hyperparathyroidism and, 69
Renal insufficiency
  calcium transport and, 152
  chronic, secondary hyperparathyroidism,
    and 159
Renal osteodystrophy
  in children, 692–696
  clinical correlates, 166–177
  nature of bone lesions
    biochemical defects, 191–195
    histological manifestations, 187–191
  pathogenesis
    acidosis, 165–166
    altered vitamin D metabolism, 153–160
    malabsorption of calcium, 151–153
    secondary hyperparathyroidism, 160–
      164
  soft tissue calcification and, 177–183
  therapeutic management
    dietary factors, 195–197
    parathyroidectomy, 201–203
    transplantation, 203–205
    vitamin D, 197–198
    vitamin D metabolites and synthetic
      analogues, 198–201
    vitamin D resistant, theatment of, 200–
      201
Renal phosphate threshold, theoretical, 309
Renal rickets, characterization, 175–177
Resorption
  subperiosteal, 76–77
  dialysis and, 186

Rickets, hypophosphatemic, hypercalcemia
  and, 653–654
Roentgenograms
  routine, hyperparathyroidism and, 76
  uremia and, 167
Rugger jersey sign, uremia and, 169

S

Salmon calcitonin, resistance to, 562
Sarcoidosis
  differential diagnosis and, 109–113
  hypercalcemia and, 615, 654–655
Sarcoma, Paget's disease and, 524–527
Scurvy, occurrence of, 683
Seabright-Bantam syndrome, parathyroid
  hormone resistance and, 308
Second messengers, parathyroid hormone
  and, 17
Sedimentation rate, differential diagnosis
  and, 108
Sensorineural loss, Paget's disease and, 509
Serotonin, medullary thyroid carcinoma
  and, 472
Set-point error, radioimmunoassay and, 99
Sex, postoperative complications and, 233
Sexual precocity, polyostotic fibrous
  dysplasia and, 679–680
Skeletal disease, hyperparathyroidism and,
  70–81
Skeletal fractures, uremia and, 166
Skeletal metabolism
  chemical determinants in infancy, child-
    hood and adolescence, 638–639
  thyroid hormone deficiency
    histopathology, 450
    metabolic studies, 450–451
    radiological changes, 450
  thyroid hormone excess
    histopathology, 454
    metabolic studies, 455
    radiological changes, 454–455
Skeleton
  calcitonin and, 459
  demineralization, 153
  growth and development
    calcium homeostasis in pregnancy and
      early infancy, 639–643
    chemical determinants in infancy,
      childhood and adolescence, 638–
      639
    in fetus and child, 634–638

resistance to parathyroid hormone and, 319
Skin, necrosis, hyperparathyroidism and, 92
Skin changes, Paget's disease and, 549–550
Skull, Paget's disease and, 506–509
Sodium, reabsorption of, 12
Sodium fluoride, Paget's disease and, 552–553
Sodium infusion, hypercalcemia and, 611, 614
Sodium sulfate, calciuresis and, 614
Sodium transport, calcium and, 11
Somatomedin
  childhood renal insufficiency and, 175
  renal osteodystrophy and, 693–694
Spasmophilia
  diagnostic criteria, 295
  hypoparathyroidism and, 290–296
Spine, Paget's disease and, 509–513
Squamous cell tumors, hypercalcemia and, 602
Stature
  hypothyroidism and, 451
  pseudohypoparathyroidism and, 385, 387
Steatorrhea
  hyperparathyroidism and, 87
  hypomagnesemia and, 264
  idiopathic hypoparathyroidism and, 283–290
  moniliasis and, 289
  treatment of, 290
Strontium, parathyroid hormone secretion and, 44
Subperiosteal resorption, uremia and, 167
Sudden infant death syndrome, parathyroid glands and, 273
Surgery
  hyperparathyroidism and, 123
  primary hyperparathyroidism and, 222–223
Sweat, calcium excretion, hyperthyroidism and, 455

T

Tetany
  chronic constitutional, 292–293, 296
  hypocalcemia and, 395–398
  hypoparathyroidism and, 237
  latent, 293
  neonatal, 252, 258, 660–661
  normocalcemic, 291, 292

postoperative, 220
recalcification and, 226
Tetracycline
  osteomalacia and, 188
  uptake, deficiency of, 189
Therapy, medical, hyperparathyroidism and, 120–121
Thiazide diuretics, hyperparathyroidism and, 96, 116–118
Thyroid
  carcinoma, hypercalcemia and, 219
  medullary carcinoma, 61
    parathyroid hormone secretion and, 44–45
  surgery, hypoparathyroidism and, 224–245
Thyroidectomy, total, hypoparathyroidism and, 232–233
Thyroid hormone
  deficiency
    calcium metabolism, 451
    clinical sequelae, 451–452
    growth and maturation, 448–450
    skeletal metabolism, 450–451
  excess
    calcium metabolism, 455–457
    clinical sequelae, 457
    growth and maturation, 452–454
    skeletal metabolism, 454–455
Thyroiditis, idiopathic hypoparathyroidism and, 279
Thyroid stimulating hormone, pseudohypoparathyroidism and, 383–384
Thyroid surgery, hypocalcemia and, 235
Thyrotoxicosis
  hyperparathyroidism and, 113–114
  hypocalcemia and, 225
Thyrotropin releasing hormone, pseudohypoparathyroidism and, 384
Tooth, development, parathyroid hormone and, 15
Toxic goiter, hypoparathyroidism and, 229
Toxins, uremic, 153
Trace metals, renal hydroxylation and, 160
Trade off hypothesis, secondary hyperparathyroidism and, 162–164
Transplantation, renal osteodystrophy and, 203–205
Treatment
  primary hyperparathyroidism
    general, 119–121

management issues in hereditary endo-
    crinopathies, 121–123
postoperative management, 123–132
surgery, 123
Tricarboxylic acid cycle, alteration, uremia
    and, 194
1,24,25-Trihydroxycholecalciferol, forma-
    tion of, 155–156
Trummerfeld zone, scurvy and, 683
Tumors
    other associated calcium disorders
        hypocalcemia, 609–610
        hypophosphatemic osteomalacia, 608–
            609
Tumoral calcinosis, renal failure and, 179–
    180

                        U

Uremia
    biochemical findings, 172, 174
    bone pain and, 166
    chronic
        acidosis and, 165
        parathyroidectomy and, 202
        serum vitamin D and, 153
        skeletal defects and, 194
    phosphate absorption and, 163–164
    serum magnesium in, 197
    roentgenographic changes and, 167
    soft tissue calcification and, 178
    transplantation and, 204
    vitamin D intoxication and, 198
Uric acid, gouty arthritis and, 180
Urine
    calcium excretion, hyperthyroidism and,
        455, 456
    total hydroxyproline in, 225

                        V

Venous sampling, location of parathyroid
    tissue and, 104

Vertebrae, framed, Paget's disease and, 511
Vertebral crush fractures, hyperpara-
    thyroidism and, 70–71
Viral infection, Paget's disease and, 566–567
Viscera, calcification of, 177–178
Vitamin A, levels, chronic renal disease
    and, 161
Vitamin C
    collagen formation and, 195–196
    deficiency, mineral metabolism and, 683
Vitamin D
    abnormal metabolites, 158
    deficiency, 8
        steatorrhea and, 284
    hydroxylation, 254, 361
    hypoparathyroidism and, 666–667
    intermediary metabolism, 260
    intoxication, differential diagnosis, 651–
        652
    metabolism, alterations in, 153–160
    renal osteodystrophy and, 694
    requirement in pregnancy or lactation, 642
    resistance to, 153, 198, 410
        uremia and, 190, 199
    sensitivity, sarcoidosis and, 110, 111
    therapy, renal disease and, 197–198
5,6-trans-Vitamin D_3, biological effects, 200
Vitamin D intoxication
    glucocorticoids and, 110–111
    hyperparathyroidism and, 114–115

                        W

Woven bone, osteosclerosis and, 170, 192

                        Z

Zollinger-Ellison syndrome
    hereditary aspects, 63
    management of, 122–123

A
B
C 8
D 9
E 0
F 1
G 2
H 3
I 4
J 5